NEUROLOGY SECRETS

Third Edition

NEUROLOGY SECRETS

Third Edition

LOREN A. ROLAK, MD

Director
The Marshfield Clinic Multiple Sclerosis Center
Marshfield, Wisconsin
Clinical Associate Professor of Neurology
University of Wisconsin
Madison, Wisconsin
Adjunct Associate Professor of Neurology
Baylor College of Medicine
Houston, Texas

HANLEY & BELFUS, INC./Philadelphia

Publisher: HANLEY & BELFUS, INC.
                    Medical Publishers
                    210 South 13th Street
                    Philadelphia, PA 19107
                    (215) 546-7293; 800-962-1892
                    FAX (215) 790-9330
                    Web site: http://www.hanleyandbelfus.com

Note to the reader: Although the information in this book has been carefully reviewed for correctness of dosage and indications, neither the authors nor the editor nor the publisher can accept any legal responsibility for any errors or omissions that may be made. Neither the publisher nor the editor makes any warranty, expressed or implied, with respect to the material contained herein. Before prescribing any drug, the reader must review the manufacturer's current product information (package inserts) for accepted indications, absolute dosage recommendations, and other information pertinent to the safe and effective use of the product described.

Library of Congress Cataloging-in-Publication Data

Neurology secrets / |edited by| Loren A. Rolak.—3rd ed.
      p. ; cm.—(The Secrets Series®)
   Includes bibliographical references and index.
   ISBN 1-56053-465-6 (alk. paper)
    1. Nervous system—Diseases—Examinations, questions, etc.. I. Rolak, Loren A. II.
Series.
   |DNLM: 1. Nervous System Diseases—Examination Questions. WL 18.2 N493 2001|
RC356.N48 2001
616.8'076—dc21

                                                                    2001024688

NEUROLOGY SECRETS, 3rd edition   ISBN 1-56053-465-6

Last digit is the print number: 9   8   7   6   5   4   3   2

CONTENTS

1. Clinical Neuroscience. 1
   Dennis R. Mosier, M.D., Ph.D.

2. Clinical Neuroanatomy. 15
   Sudhir S. Athni, M.D., Igor M. Cherches, M.D., and Brian Loftus, M.D.

3. Approach to the Patient with Neurologic Disease 53
   Loren A. Rolak, M.D.

4. Myopathies. 59
   Yadollah Harati, M.D., FACP, and Kathryn Copeland, M.D.

5. Neuromuscular Junction Diseases 71
   Clifton L. Gooch, M.D., and Tetsuo Ashizawa, M.D.

6. Peripheral Neuropathies. 83
   Yadollah Harati, M.D., FACP, and Robert J. Kolimas, M.D.

7. Radiculopathy and Degenerative Spine Disease 99
   Steven B. Inbody, M.D.

8. Myelopathies 111
   Richard M. Armstrong, M.D., FRCPC

9. Brainstem Disease 121
   Eugene C. Lai, M.D., Ph.D.

10. Cerebellar Disease 137
    Eugene C. Lai, M.D., Ph.D.

11. Basal Ganglia and Movement Disorders 147
    Philip A. Hanna, M.D., Francisco Cardoso, M.D., and Joseph Jankovic, M.D.

12. Autonomic Nervous System. 181
    Yadollah Harati, M.D., FACP, and Hazem Machkhas, M.D.

13. Demyelinating Disease. 201
    Loren A. Rolak, M.D.

14. Dementia. 209
    Rachelle S. Doody, M.D., Ph.D.

15. Aphasia and Behavioral Neurology 219
    David B. Rosenfield, M.D.

16. Dysarthria, Dysfluency, and Dysphagia. 229
    David B. Rosenfield, M.D.

17. Vascular Disease. 237
    David Chiu, M.D., and John P. Winikates, M.D.

18. Neuro-Oncology. 249
    Everton A. Edmondson, M.D.

19. Pain Syndromes 261
    Steven B. Inbody, M.D.

20. Headaches.. 273
    Howard S. Derman, M.D.

21. Seizures and Epilepsy.. 283
    Paul A. Rutecki, M.D.

22. Sleep Disorders... 301
    James D. Frost, Jr., M.D.

23. Neurologic Complications of Systemic Disease 309
    R. Glenn Smith, M.D., Ph.D., and Loren A. Rolak, M.D.

24. Infectious Diseases, Including AIDS 329
    Maria E. Carlini, M.D., and Richard L. Harris, M.D.

25. Pediatric Neurology 343
    Angus A. Wilfong, M.D., FRCPC

26. Electroencephalography... 367
    Richard A. Hrachovy, M.D.

27. Electromyography 389
    James M. Killian, M.D.

28. Neuroradiology... 397
    Loren A. Rolak, M.D.

29. Neurologic Emergencies... 399
    Loren A. Rolak, M.D.

30. Neurology Trivia... 401
    Loren A. Rolak, M.D.

INDEX 417

CONTRIBUTORS

Richard M. Armstrong, M.D., FRCPC
Associate Professor, Department of Neurology, Baylor College of Medicine, Houston, Texas

Tetsuo Ashizawa, M.D.
Professor, Department of Neurology, Baylor College of Medicine, Houston, Texas

Sudhir S. Athni, M.D., M.B.A.
Department of Neurology, Neurology of Central Georgia; Macon Northside Hospital, Macon, Georgia

Francisco Cardoso, M.D.
Associate Professor, Department of Psychiatry and Neurology, The Federal University of Minas Gerais; Chief, Neurology Service, Hospital des Clinicas-UFMG, Minas Gerais, Brazil

Maria E. Carlini, M.D.
Assistant Professor, Department of Internal Medicine, Section of Infectious Diseases, University of Texas–Houston Medical School, Houston, Texas

Igor M. Cherches, M.D.
Department of Neurology, Baylor College of Medicine; Texas Medical Center, Houston, Texas

David Chiu, M.D.
Assistant Professor, Department of Neurology, Baylor College of Medicine; The Methodist Hospital, Houston, Texas

Kathryn J. Copeland, M.D.
Assistant Professor, Department of Neurology, University of Louisville School of Medicine; Staff Physician, University of Louisville Hospital, Louisville, Kentucky

Howard S. Derman, M.D.
Associate Professor, Department of Neurology, Baylor College of Medicine; The Methodist Hospital, Houston, Texas

Rachelle Smith Doody, M.D., Ph.D.
Effie Marie Cain Professor in Alzheimer's Disease Research, Department of Neurology, Baylor College of Medicine; Active Staff, The Methodist Hospital, Houston, Texas

Everton A. Edmondson, M.D.
Neurologist in Private Practice, Houston, Texas

James D. Frost, Jr., M.D.
Professor, Department of Neurology, Section of Neurophysiology, Baylor College of Medicine; The Methodist Hospital, Houston, Texas

Clifton L. Gooch, M.D.
Department of Neurology, Columbia University College of Physicians and Surgeons; Director, EMG Laboratory, Columbia Presbyterian Medical Center, New York-Presbyterian Hospital, New York, New York

Philip A. Hanna, M.D.
Assistant Professor, New Jersey Neuroscience Institute, Seton Hall University; JFK Medical Center, Edison, New Jersey

Yadollah Harati, M.D., FACP
Professor, Department of Neurology, Section of Neuromuscular Diseases, Baylor College of Medicine; Executive Director, Neurology Care, Houston Veterans Affairs Medical Center, Houston, Texas

Richard L. Harris, M.D.
Professor of Medicine, Associate Dean of Graduate Medical Education, Baylor College of Medicine; Director, Infection Control, The Methodist Hospital, Houston, Texas

Richard A. Hrachovy, M.D.
Professor, Department of Neurology, Baylor College of Medicine; Director, EEG Laboratory, Houston Veterans Affairs Medical Center, Houston, Texas

Steven B. Inbody, M.D.
Director, Consultative Neurology, Texas Medical Center, Houston, Texas

Joseph Jankovic, M.D.
Professor, Department of Neurology, and Director, Parkinson's Disease Center and Movement Disorders Clinic, Department of Neurology, Baylor College of Medicine; The Methodist Hospital, Houston, Texas

James M. Killian, M.D.
Professor and Vice Chairman, Department of Neurology, Baylor College of Medicine; Deputy Chief and Senior Attending, The Methodist Hospital, Houston, Texas

Robert J. Kolimas, M.D.
Assistant Professor, Department of Neurology, Baylor College of Medicine; Director, Neurology Outpatient Service, Houston Veterans Affairs Medical Center, Houston, Texas

Eugene C. Lai, M.D., Ph.D.
Associate Professor, Department of Neurology, Baylor College of Medicine, Houston, Texas

Brian Loftus, M.D.
Neurologist, Diagnostic Clinic of Houston, Houston, Texas

Hazem Machkhas, M.D.
Assistant Professor, Department of Neurology, Baylor College of Medicine; Houston Veterans Affairs Medical Center, Houston, Texas

Dennis R. Mosier, M.D., Ph.D.
Assistant Professor, Department of Neurology; MDA Neuromuscular Clinic, Baylor College of Medicine; Neurology Service, Houston Veterans Affairs Medical Center, Houston, Texas

Loren A. Rolak, M.D.
Clinical Associate Professor, Department of Neurology, University of Wisconsin Medical School, Madison, Wisconsin; Adjunct Associate Professor, Department of Neurology, Baylor College of Medicine, Houston, Texas; Director, The Marshfield Clinic Multiple Sclerosis Center, Marshfield, Wisconsin

David B. Rosenfield, M.D.
Professor, Departments of Neurology and Otolaryngology and Communications Sciences; Director, Stuttering Center, Speech Motor Control Laboratory, Baylor College of Medicine, Houston, Texas

Paul A. Rutecki, M.D.
Associate Professor, Departments of Neurology and Neurosurgery, University of Wisconsin Medical School; William S. Middleton Veterans Affairs Hospital, Madison, Wisconsin

Robert Glenn Smith, M.D., Ph.D.
Assistant Professor, Department of Neurology, Baylor College of Medicine; Interim Chief of Neurology Service, Ben Taub General Hospital; Director, Outpatient Neurology Clinics, Harris County Hospital District, Houston, Texas

Angus A. Wilfong, M.D., FRCPC
Assistant Professor, Departments of Neurology and Pediatrics, Medical College of Wisconsin; Children's Hospital of Wisconsin, Milwaukee, Wisconsin

John P. Winikates, M.D.
Assistant Professor, Department of Neurology, Baylor College of Medicine, Houston, Texas

FOREWORD

The excitement of neurology is related not only to new information developing from the tremendous advances in basic neurosciences, but also to the elegance of the nervous system itself and to the increasingly sophisticated methods that we use to learn how it functions and how it can be disturbed in disease. There are a large number of textbooks in the field, as well as a large number of computerized learning systems in medicine. But none of them has yet replaced the effectiveness of the Socratic approach to education, both in an academic and in a clinical setting. In neurology, as well as in other areas of medicine, one of the most difficult tasks is knowing how to ask the right questions. For the medical student just starting out, pertinent questions relate to where the lesion may be and to the tempo of the process, which may suggest the etiology. For the house officer, the questions may relate more to the patterns of symptoms and signs characteristic of certain diseases, whereas for the practitioner the prognosis of untreated disease and the efficacy of various therapies may be the focus of inquiry. For all individuals concerned with problem solving in neurologic disease, asking the right question the right way is of greatest importance.

In preparing this third edition, Dr. Loren Rolak and members of the Department of Neurology at Baylor College of Medicine have employed the question and answer approach, which is the hallmark of The Secrets Series®. Every question in every chapter has been reviewed, with some deletions and many additions. A new chapter on clinical neuroscience has been added to make the book as current as possible. The book is intended to cover the kinds of questions commonly encountered in an academic institution on teaching rounds for medical students and residents, and also in clinical problem solving in the office. *Neurology Secrets* is not intended to be an in-depth approach to disease etiology and pathogenesis. Instead, it is intended to phrase questions in a way that provides "the big picture." From that point on, the student—and all of us continue to be students for our entire careers—must use original source material as well as the patients themselves to continue the educational process.

The authors have been extremely successful in accomplishing their goals, and all of us will benefit. No field will change more than the field of neurology in the future, and *Neurology Secrets* lets you in on the ground floor of what promises to be one of the most exciting voyages ever taken—one that results in an understanding of our humanity through an understanding of the brain.

Stanley H. Appel, M.D.
Professor and Chairman
Department of Neurology
Baylor College of Medicine
Houston, Texas

PREFACE TO THE THIRD EDITION

During the process of revising this edition, it became obvious how much the practice of neurology has advanced in just the last few years. The management of almost every neurologic disease required changes, and in many cases our understanding of basic sciences and of disease processes has been fundamentally altered. Even the way doctors and patients learn and communicate has changed now that use of the Internet is prevalent. Therefore, in this new edition, many answers were rewritten, new questions added, and old ones deleted. The bibliographies now contain appropriate Web sites for further reference. Neurology is one of the most dynamic medical specialties, but this revised edition should enable the reader to continue asking the right questions and finding the right answers.

Loren A. Rolak, M.D.

1. CLINICAL NEUROSCIENCE

Dennis R. Mosier, M.D., Ph.D.

1. Why is it important to understand the molecular and cellular mechanisms underlying normal and abnormal nervous system function?

The answer to this question could easily require a book. Listed below are several advantages to the practicing clinician:

1. Enhancement of diagnostic possibilities and treatment options
2. More appropriate selection of diagnostic tests and interpretation of test results
3. Prediction of drug side effects and interactions
4. Selection of optimal drug regimens
5. Aid to critical review of novel concepts and therapies
6. Understanding of the rationale for current clinical trials
7. Provision of a background for communicating information to patients and families

2. Name several types of cellular alterations that can lead directly to neurologic disease.

The following is only a partial list:

1. Altered volume regulation (e.g., cytotoxic edema)
2. Anatomic alterations
   - Loss of neurons
   - Loss of axons
   - Loss of synaptic connections
   - Inappropriate synaptic connections
3. Deafferentation (e.g., loss of receptors in sensory end organs)
4. Altered membrane excitability
5. Failure of axonal conduction
6. Disordered synaptic function
7. Altered excitation-contraction coupling in muscle

CELLULAR ANATOMY

3. Describe the major types of glial cells in the CNS and their influence on neurologic disease.

1. **Astrocytes**—large glial cells that stabilize extracellular potassium concentrations and limit the accumulation of extracellular glutamate by specific uptake mechanisms. Astrocytes proliferate in response to many CNS insults and may release neuronal growth factors and form barriers to the spread of infection.

2. **Oligodendroglia**—myelin-forming glial cells. Myelin antigens may form targets for autoimmune attack in multiple sclerosis.

3. **Ependymal cells**—neuroepithelial cells lining the ventricular system, choroid plexus, and central canal of the spinal cord.

4. **Microglia**—resident mononuclear phagocytic cells that become reactive in degenerative diseases and demyelinating disorders as well as in more acute CNS insults. They produce numerous cytokines (which regulate inflammatory processes), present antigens to T-cells, and secrete a number of cytotoxic factors (e.g., free radicals, low–molecular-weight neurotoxins). Thus, activated microglia have the potential to amplify neuronal injury in a number of CNS disorders and may represent a target for therapeutic intervention.

4. What are the components of the blood-brain barrier?

The blood-brain barrier is not a single barrier but a composite of many systems that act to control the entry of substances from the blood to the brain:

1. Capillary **endothelial cells** linked by tight junctions and expressing specialized uptake systems for particular metabolic substrates (e.g., glucose, amino acids)

2. A prominent **basement membrane** between endothelia and adjacent cells

3. Pericapillary **astrocytes** with end-feet adjacent to capillaries

A similar system exists for the choroidal epithelium (blood-cerebrospinal fluid [CSF] barrier).

5. Which regions of the brain lack a significant blood-brain barrier?

Brain regions that lack a significant blood-brain barrier tend to be midline structures located near ventricular spaces. They include the area postrema, organum vasculosum of the lamina terminalis (OVLT), subfornical and subcommissural organs, median eminence of the hypothalamus, and neurohypophysis.

6. Under what conditions is the integrity of the blood-brain barrier compromised?

• Inflammation or infection
• Osmotic injury
• Malignant hypertension
• Neovascularization (particularly around tumors)
• Cerebral ischemia and reperfusion
• Seizure activity

Compromise of the blood-brain barrier often can be demonstrated by contrast enhancement in radiographic studies or suspected when acute elevations of CSF protein are observed. Consequences of blood-brain barrier (or blood-CSF barrier) compromise include vasogenic edema, enhanced penetration of antibiotics or other drugs, and increased entry of potentially toxic substances from the systemic circulation.

NERVE CONDUCTION

7. What is the Nernst equation?

The Nernst equation describes the membrane potential (E) needed to balance an ionic concentration gradient across the membrane so that the net flux of the ion across the membrane is zero (e.g., the ion is in equilibrium):

$$E = (RT/zF) \ln (C_o/C_i)$$

C_o is the concentration of a given ion outside a cell membrane; C_i is the concentration of the same ion within the cell; and RT/zF is approximately $+25$ mV at room temperature for monovalent cations such as potassium (K^+). The resting membrane potential in neurons depends most strongly on the K^+ concentration gradient, although other ions such as sodium (Na^+) and chloride (Cl^-) contribute to a lesser extent. Thus, even small changes in the extracellular K^+ concentration can result in significant changes in the membrane potential.

8. What is an action potential?

The action potential, as classically defined, is an all-or-nothing, regenerative, directionally propagated, depolarizing nerve impulse. In axons, the rising (depolarizing) phase of the action potential is mediated by activation of voltage-dependent Na^+ currents, which depolarizes the membrane toward the Nernst potential for sodium. Repolarization of the membrane potential is influenced by two processes: (1) voltage-dependent inactivation of Na^+ currents and (2) voltage-dependent activation of K^+ currents, which hyperpolarizes the membrane potential toward the Nernst potential for potassium. In many axons, a hyperpolarization potential, mediated by one or more K^+ currents, follows the action potential. When Na^+ currents are largely inactivated, a new action potential cannot be initiated (absolute refractory period). When Na^+ currents are recovering from inactivation and K^+ currents are maximally activated, action potentials can sometimes be generated, but only by very strong stimulation (relative refractory period).

9. What is saltatory conduction?

In myelinated axons, currents underlying the action potential flow from one node of Ranvier to another, propagating the action potential by depolarizing distant sites rather than adjacent membrane. This "jumping" of the impulse from node to node, which greatly increases the conduction velocity, is termed saltatory conduction (from Latin *saltare*, to leap).

SYNAPSES

10. How are signals transmitted across chemical synapses?

At a commonly studied excitatory chemical synapse, the neuromuscular junction, the following events occur:

1. Depolarization of the presynaptic motoneuron terminal by an arriving action potential

2. Activation of voltage-dependent calcium (Ca^{2+}) channels

3. Entry of Ca^{2+}, which locally increases intraterminal calcium concentrations

4. Synchronized, quantal release of neurotransmitter from the presynaptic terminal (According to the vesicle hypothesis of release, neurotransmitter packaged in synaptic vesicles is released into the synaptic cleft by exocytosis.)

5. Diffusion of neurotransmitter across the synaptic cleft

6. Binding of neurotransmitter to specific receptors on the postsynaptic membrane

7. Receptor-mediated opening of ion channels that mediate an excitatory postsynaptic potential (an endplate potential at the neuromuscular junction)

8. Initiation of an action potential in the postsynaptic cell if the postsynaptic potential reaches the threshold of activation of postsynaptic Na^+ channels

At the neuromuscular junction, the transmitter (acetylcholine) is rapidly hydrolyzed by the enzyme acetylcholinesterase. At most inhibitory synapses, the postsynaptic potential is hyperpolarizing, making it more difficult for excitatory potentials in the postsynaptic cell to reach threshold for action potential generation. Binding of neurotransmitter to receptors may induce second-messenger activation at some synapses, in addition to changes in ionic conductances.

11. Name several synaptic vesicle-associated proteins. Describe their relevance to neurologic disease.

Vesicle-associated protein	Significance
Synaptophysin	Used as a marker of neuronal differentiation in tumors
	Used to identify synapses (e.g., when counting synapse numbers in studies of dementing illnesses)
Synaptobrevin	Cleaved by tetanus toxin, botulinum toxins B, D, F, and G
SNAP-25	Cleaved by botulinum toxins A and E
Syntaxin	Cleaved by botulinum toxin C1
Synaptotagmin	Putative Ca^{2+} sensor for evoked transmitter release
Vesicular monoamine transporters (VMAT1,2)	Uptake of monoamines into synaptic vesicles; inhibited by reserpine

Many vesicle-associated proteins are now known to be specific for certain cell types or organelles, suggesting the potential for selective manipulation of their functions to achieve experimental and therapeutic goals.

Lin RC, Scheller RH: Mechanisms of synaptic vesicle exocytosis. Annu Rev Cell Dev Biol 16:19–49, 2000.

12. Can synapses undergo modification?

Synapses are not static structures. They are constantly modified in the nervous system through alterations of connectivity (e.g., sprouting and new synapse formation or retraction of synaptic connections) and alterations in the efficacy of synaptic transmission (e.g., use-dependent facilitation, potentiation, or depression of the function of individual synapses). Induction of both types of synaptic modifications, often referred to as synaptic plasticity, may occur at central and peripheral synapses.

13. Briefly describe the cellular processes thought to subserve learning and memory.

In most models, the major biologic basis for learning and memory is thought to derive from changes in synaptic function:

Long-term potentiation (LTP) is a long-lasting increase in the amplitude of a synaptic response following stimulation. LTP can be induced by weak but temporally contiguous stimulation of separate input pathways to the same postsynaptic neuron (associative LTP), mimicking the behavioral phenomenon of classical conditioning. Induction of LTP appears to require postsynaptic elevations of Ca^{2+}, probably via Ca^{2+}-permeable glutamate receptors, but the mechanism by which LTP is expressed (i.e., whether it is a pre- or postsynaptic alteration) is an area of considerable debate.

Long-term depression (LTD) can produce long-term reductions in synaptic strength. Long-term changes in synaptic function may underlie not only normal processes, such as learning and memory, but also the establishment of chronic pain states and recovery from CNS insults.

Martin SJ, Grimwood PD, Morris RG: Synaptic plasticity and memory: An evaluation of the hypothesis. Annu Rev Neurosci 23:649–711, 2000.

Sweatt JD: The neuronal MAP kinase cascade: A biochemical signal integration system subserving synaptic plasticity and memory. J Neurochem 76:1–10, 2001.

NEUROTRANSMITTERS

14. How is a chemical substance established as a neurotransmitter?

As classically proposed, the following features should be demonstrated to establish that a given substance is acting as a neurotransmitter:

1. Presence of the substance within neuron terminals.
2. Release of the substance with neuronal stimulation.
3. Application of the exogenous substance to the postsynaptic membrane (at physiologic concentrations) reproduces the effects of stimulation of the presynaptic neuron.
4. The concentration-response curve of the substance applied to the postsynaptic membrane is affected by drugs in the same way as normal postsynaptic responses are affected.
5. A local mechanism exists for inactivation of the substance (e.g., enzymatic degradation, uptake into nerve terminals or glia).

15. What is Dale's principle? List exceptions to this maxim.

Dale's principle, as modified by J.C. Eccles, states that a given neuron contains and releases only one neurotransmitter and exerts the same functional effects at all of its termination sites. For example, a spinal motoneuron contains and releases the same neurotransmitter (acetylcholine), which generates the same effect (excitation) at both of its termination sites (neuromuscular junction and recurrent collateral synapse to the Renshaw cell). This useful generalization allows us to describe neurons in terms of their principal transmitters and functions (e.g., a glutamatergic excitatory neuron or a cholinergic inhibitory neuron). However, the assertions of Dale's principle are not universally true:

1. Some neurons may contain and release more than one transmitter or release neuromodulatory peptides and nonpeptide substances from the same terminal.
2. The same nerve terminal can release different proportions of neurotransmitter or modulatory substances at different times, depending on the history of prior stimulation.
3. A transmitter released from a single neuron may have differing effects at different synapses.
4. Separate clusters of postsynaptic receptors with opposing functions may coexist under a single synaptic terminal.

These exceptions to Dale's principle expand the range of possible mechanisms for modulating synaptic efficacy in vivo and challenge the tendency to oversimplify explanations of neuronal function.

Tsen G, et al: Receptors with opposing functions are in postsynaptic microdomains under one presynaptic terminal. Nat Neurosci 3:126–132, 2000.

16. **Name several important loci and functions of the neurotransmitter acetylcholine.**
    At **peripheral synapses**, acetylcholine acts as the principal neurotransmitter of:
    • Motoneurons innervating striated muscle
    • Preganglionic autonomic neurons innervating ganglia
    • Postganglionic parasympathetic neurons
    • Sympathetic sudomotor fibers
    The functions of **central cholinergic synapses** and the receptor subtypes mediating their effects are generally less well defined than at peripheral synapses. Central cholinergic pathways or nuclei include:
    • Olivocochlear bundle (efferent regulation of auditory inputs)
    • Pedunculopontine nuclei (modulation of sleep states)
    • Septohippocampal projections (regulation of the hippocampal theta rhythm, which can influence processes subserving learning and memory)
    • Projections to the neocortex from basal forebrain nuclei (particularly the nucleus basalis of Meynert, which is thought to be involved early in Alzheimer's disease)
    • Local interneurons in the striatum (regulation of motor activity)

17. **Name and describe the two major types of acetylcholine (ACh) receptors.**
    1. **Nicotinic ACh receptors** (nAChRs) are located at the skeletal neuromuscular junction, in autonomic ganglia, and in the brain. The nicotonic AChR at the neuromuscular junction, when activated by ACh, acts as a nonselective cation channel. It is the major antigenic target in most cases of myasthenia gravis. Mutations in genes encoding subunits of neuronal nicotinic receptors have been linked to some inherited frontal lobe epilepsies.
    2. **Muscarinic ACh receptors** (mAChRs) are located in parasympathetic effector sites and in the brain. Activation of mAChRs may open or close ionophores, activate guanylate cyclase, or initiate other signal transduction mechanisms. Modulation of brain muscarinic AChRs can affect sleep-wake states and modify seizure thresholds; it is under investigation as an intervention to improve cognitive function in patients with dementing illnesses.
    Both types of ACh receptors can be located at presynaptic or postsynaptic sites.

18. **What is the most abundant excitatory neurotransmitter in the CNS? By what mechanisms does it induce its effects?**
    Glutamate, an excitatory amino acid neurotransmitter, is synthesized from α-ketoglutarate by transamination and from glutamine by the enzyme glutaminase. After release from the presynaptic terminal, glutamate may interact with several types of receptors, including:
    1. NMDA (*N*-methyl-*D*-aspartate) receptors
    2. AMPA (α-amino-3-hydroxy-5-methyl-4-isoxazole) receptors
    3. Kainate receptors
    4. Metabotropic glutamate receptors
    The NMDA and some types of AMPA receptors are permeable to calcium as well as to monovalent cations. These receptors are thought to be critically involved in Ca^{2+}-dependent processes underlying learning and memory and (if excessively stimulated) may contribute to Ca^{2+}-dependent processes that mediate neuronal injury.

19. **What is GABA? How does it exert its action(s)?**
    Gamma-aminobutyric acid (GABA) is a neurotransmitter synthesized from glutamate via the enzyme glutamic acid decarboxylase (GAD). After secretion into a synapse, its action is terminated by uptake via a specific GABA transporter. GABA is metabolized via GABA transaminase to succinic semialdehyde. GABA receptors include $GABA_A$ and $GABA_B$ receptors. Receptors of the $GABA_A$ type (the majority of GABA receptors) act as chloride channels, exercising largely inhibitory effects. Many drugs act on GABA pathways. $GABA_A$ receptors are modulated by barbiturates and benzodiazepines; baclofen is an agonist for $GABA_B$ receptors. Vigabatrin (γ-vinyl GABA), a potent anticonvulsant, inhibits GABA transaminase. Of interest,

anti-GAD antibodies have been reported in most patients with stiff-person syndrome, which presents with continuous, involuntary muscular activity.

20. Discuss the synthesis, secretion, actions, and termination of action of the neurotransmitter dopamine.

Synthesis of catecholamines

1. Tyrosine → L-hydroxyphenylalanine (L-DOPA) via tyrosine hydroxylase (TH)
2. L-DOPA → dopamine via DOPA decarboxylase
3. Dopamine → norepinephrine via dopamine β-hydroxylase (DBH)
4. Norepinephrine → epinephrine via phenylethanolamine N-methyltransferase (PNMT)

Secretion. Dopamine is transported from the cytoplasm into synaptic vesicles by vesicular monoamine transporters (VMATs) prior to release from the nerve terminal. Under certain circumstances, cytoplasmic dopamine may be released nonexocytotically by reversal of amino acid transporters located in the plasma membrane.

Actions. Five types of dopamine receptors (D1 through D5) have been identified, each exhibiting a distinct pharmacologic profile as well as a unique neuroanatomic distribution. D1-like receptors (D1 and D5) have historically been recognized as the dopamine receptors that stimulate adenylate cyclase via stimulatory G proteins. In contrast, D2-like receptors (D2A, D2B, D3, and D4) generally inhibit adenylate cyclase via pertussis toxin-sensitive G proteins. More recent studies have identified multiple second-messenger systems that can be activated by dopamine receptors.

Termination of action. The action of dopamine is terminated primarily by reuptake via specific transporters. Dopamine is also inactivated by catabolism. Intracellular dopamine is oxidatively deaminated by monoamine oxidase to homovanillic acid (HVA), and extracellular dopamine is methylated by catechol-O-methyltransferase (COMT) to produce dihydroxyphenylacetic acid (DOPAC).

Fon EA, et al: Vesicular transport regulates monoamine storage and release but is not essential for amphetamine action. Neuron 19:1271–1283, 1997.

21. List the major functions of dopamine in the nervous system.

1. Motor control (via nigrostriatal projections)
2. Modulation of short-term or working memory (via projections from ventral tegmental area to prefrontal cortex)
3. Behavioral reinforcement (via mesolimbic projections)
4. Hypothalamic regulation of pituitary function (e.g., by inhibiting prolactin secretion)
5. Modulation of brain regions controlling emesis (e.g., area postrema of the medulla)
6. Dopaminergic neurons are also present in the olfactory bulb and the retina as well as in enteric neurons; in these systems the exact role of dopamine is less well defined.

22. What is serotonin? Where does it act in the nervous system?

Serotonin, or 5-hydroxytryptamine (5-HT), is an indoleamine neurotransmitter originally described in **enterochromaffin cells** of the gut. It is produced from the amino acid tryptophan by the actions of tryptophan hydroxylase (yielding 5-hydroxytryptophan as an intermediate) and an aromatic amino acid decarboxylase. The action of released 5-HT is terminated by reuptake into nerve terminals; its major metabolite is 5-hydroxyindoleacetic acid (5-HIAA), which is formed following oxidative deamination by monoamine oxidase. Serotonergic neurons are found in the **raphe nuclei** of the brainstem. More rostral neurons project to diencephalic and telencephalic structures, whereas more caudal neurons project to the inferior olive and spinal cord. N-acetylation of serotonin by cells of the **pineal gland** (via 5-HT N-acetyltransferase) is followed by O-methylation (via hydroxyindole O-methyltransferase, or HIOMT) to produce the hormone melatonin. Multiple receptor subtypes for 5-HT have been described. The 5-HT_{1B} and 5-HT_{1D} receptors, which are found on **trigeminal nerve terminals supplying cranial blood vessels** and meninges, modulate the vasodilatation associated with migraine headaches. 5-HT_3 receptor antagonists such as ondansetron, which have both peripheral and central actions, are effective in suppressing nausea and vomiting.

23. What is denervation supersensitivity?

Two to three weeks after the loss of an innervating neuron, the postsynaptic membrane of an innervated cell develops increased sensitivity to the neurotransmitter that was released by the presynaptic terminal of the innervating neuron. Denervation of skeletal muscle results in increased expression and extrajunctional spread of postsynaptic nicotinic acetylcholine receptors. This response may underlie the potentially life-threatening reaction observed when patients with neuromuscular disorders are given the nicotinic cholinergic agonist, succinylcholine, which acts as a depolarizing muscle relaxant.

ION CHANNELS

24. What is an ion channel? How does it work?

Ion channels, formed from one or more membrane-spanning protein subunits that form an aqueous pore, allow the selective and rapid flux of ions across cell membranes. Channels respond to (are gated by) specific stimuli, such as changes in the transmembrane voltage gradient (voltage-gated channels), chemical agonists (ligand-gated channels), or mechanical stretch or pressure. Channel gating is believed to induce a molecular conformational change, termed **activation**, which opens an aqueous pore through which ions may pass. **Inactivation** is typically a slower process that acts to close the channel even in the presence of an activating stimulus; the channel must recover before it is again susceptible to activation. Single ion channels are also characterized by a specific **conductance**, which is a measure of permeability of the cell membrane to a given ion. **Selective permeability** for particular ions is a feature of many ion channels. Ion channels also may be regulated by local ion concentrations (e.g., Ca^{2+}, H^+), phosphorylation, association with other channels or regulatory proteins, changes in synthesis or internalization, and other factors. Alterations in any of these molecular properties (kinetics, conductance, selective permeability, or regulation) may cause ion channel dysfunction at the molecular level, which may lead to disease.

25. What are ion channelopathies? How do they present clinically?

Ion channelopathies, or disorders in which the clinical presentation results primarily from ion channel dysfunction, frequently present with brief exacerbations or episodes of clinical symptoms. In such disorders (e.g., periodic paralysis), interictal function is typically normal, and attacks are often triggered by specific factors (e.g., exercise, temperature changes, startle responses, drugs). Therapies, in addition to symptom management and treatment of underlying causes of the ion-channel abnormality (e.g., autoimmunity), have been directed at identification and avoidance of triggering factors as well as use of drugs that ameliorate the specific ion-channel dysfunction observed at the molecular level.

Ackerman MJ, Clapham DE: Ion channels—basic science and clinical disease. N Engl J Med 336:1575–1586, 1997.

26. Name the major physiologic effects of potassium channels in neurons. Discuss the mechanism of action of therapeutic potassium channel blockers.

Potassium channels in neurons (1) contribute to the resting membrane potential; (2) shorten action potential duration; (3) contribute to afterhyperpolarization following an action potential (thus prolonging the relative refractory period for action potential generation); (4) terminate burst firing by neurons; (5) mediate oscillatory activity in some spontaneously firing neurons; and (6) mediate some types of inhibitory postsynaptic potentials (IPSPs).

Currently available K^+ channel blockers (4-aminopyridine and 3,4-diaminopyridine), which are rather nonselective among different channel subtypes, prolong action potential duration. In the Lambert-Eaton myasthenic syndrome, action potential prolongation can extend the voltage-dependent opening of Ca^{2+} channels in nerve terminals, increasing Ca^{2+} entry and promoting transmitter release. In some patients with multiple sclerosis, prolongation of the action potential, by extending the duration of current flow, is thought to reduce the likelihood of conduction block in demyelinated axons. At higher doses, K^+ channel blockers can induce seizure activity, possibly by promoting spontaneous firing and burst firing in neurons.

27. In which disorders affecting the nervous system have abnormalities of potassium channel function been suggested to play a critical role?

1. **Ataxia-myokymia syndrome** (EA-1), presenting as dominantly inherited myokymia and episodic ataxia, has been associated with mutations in the gene *KCNA1* (located on chromosome 12p), which encodes a delayed rectifier K^+ channel expressed in brain and peripheral nerve.

2. Two of the **dominantly inherited long Q-T syndromes** (LQT1 and LQT2), which may present as syncopal seizures as well as syncope and sudden cardiac death, are associated with mutations in genes encoding delayed rectifier K^+ channels expressed in the heart (*KvLQT1* on chromosome 11p15 and *HERG* on chromosome 7q35-36).

3. A **recessive long Q-T syndrome** (Jerve-Lange-Nielsen syndrome), which exhibits sensorineural hearing loss, also may result from mutations in *KvLQT1*, which is expressed in the stria vascularis of the inner ear as well as in the heart.

4. Recently, syndromes of dominantly inherited **benign familial neonatal convulsions**, which may be associated with an increased risk of adult epilepsy, have been linked to mutations in *KCNQ2* (on chromosome 20q13) and *KCNQ3* (on chromosome 8q24), which encode delayed rectifier K^+ channels expressed in the brain.

5. Some cases of **Isaac's syndrome**, which presents as acquired neuromyotonia, have been suggested to result from an antibody-mediated autoimmune attack on K^+ channels in motor nerves.

6. **Acquired long Q-T syndrome associated with nonsedating antihistamines** such as terfenadine may predispose to sudden death in susceptible people or when serum concentrations are elevated by coadministration of erythromycin. Terfenadine has been shown to block HERG K^+ channels, which may contribute to its toxicity.

7. Some **snake toxins** (e.g., dendrotoxin from the African green mamba) exhibit potent K^+ channel blocking activity.

Curran ME, et al: A molecular basis for cardiac arrhythmia: HERG mutations cause long QT syndrome. Cell 80:795–803, 1995.

Hart IK, et al: Autoantibodies detected to expressed K^+ channels are implicated in neuromyotonia. Ann Neurol 41:238–246, 1997.

Biervert C, et al: A potassium channel mutation in neonatal human epilepsy. Science 279:403–406, 1998.

28. Name the major functions of calcium in excitable cells.

The following is only a partial list:
1. Regulation of membrane excitability (by extracellular Ca^{2+} concentration)
2. Action potential mediation
3. Stimulus-secretion coupling (e.g., neurotransmitter release)
4. Mediation of some stimulation-induced changes in synaptic efficacy
5. Regulation of ion channel function
6. Regulation of many enzymes
7. Regulation of axoplasmic transport
8. Modulation of axonal outgrowth during development
9. Excitation-contraction coupling in skeletal and cardiac muscle
10. Regulation of gene expression

Ghosh A, Greenberg ME: Calcium signaling in neurons: Molecular mechanisms and cellular consequences. Science 268:239–247, 1995.

29. What are the different types of calcium channels? What do they do?

• **Voltage-gated calcium channel** (VGCC) types located on plasma membranes

T	Transient; activated at low voltages
L	Long-acting (slowly inactivating); activated at high voltages; found in skeletal and cardiac muscle and some central neurons
N	Activated at intermediate voltages; present in many central neurons; mediate transmitter release in autonomic neurons

P/Q Activated at high voltages; present in many central neurons; mediate transmitter release at skeletal neuromuscular junctions

R Resistant to other VGCC blockers

- **Ligand-gated calcium channels** located on plasma membranes, such as NMDA-sensitive glutamate receptors
- **Intracellularly located calcium channels**, including a ryanodine-sensitive channel in endoplasmic reticulum.

30. In which neurologic disorders is alteration or dysfunction of calcium channels believed to play a critical role?

Disorder	Alteration
Lambert-Eaton myasthenic syndrome	Autoimmune attack on P/Q-type voltage-gated Ca channel at motoneuron terminals
Hypokalemic periodic paralysis	Mutation in *CACNL1A3* gene (1q31-32): coding for the skeletal muscle dihydropyridine-sensitive voltage-gated Ca^{2+} channel
Malignant hyperthermia	Mutation in *RYR1* gene (19q13): coding for the skeletal muscle ryanodine receptor
Familial hemiplegic migraine and episodic ataxia type 2	Mutation in *CACNL1A4* gene (19p13): coding for P/Q type Ca^{2+} channel in brain

Ophoff RA, et al: Familial hemiplegic migraine and episodic ataxia type 2 are caused by mutations in the Ca^{2+} channel gene *CACNL1A4*. Cell 87:543–552, 1996.

NEURONAL INJURY AND DEATH

31. What is the excitotoxicity hypothesis? Why is it important?

The excitotoxicity concept seeks to correlate overstimulation of neurons (by chemical or electrical means) with cell injury or death. In the CNS, excitotoxicity is hypothesized to occur in the context of processes (e.g., ischemia, seizure activity, some neurodegenerative diseases) that lead to elevated extracellular concentrations of excitatory amino acids such as glutamate.

According to the glutamate hypothesis of excitotoxicity, interaction of high levels of glutamate with calcium-permeable glutamate receptors (NMDA receptors and some forms of the AMPA receptor) results in increased calcium entry, which may injure susceptible cells. Much of the damage induced by short-term ischemia in animal models of stroke can be blocked by antagonists of glutamate receptors, and a number of clinical trials are under way to test these agents in patients with acute stroke. Riluzole, a drug with effects on glutamate receptor function, has shown limited efficacy in patients with amyotrophic lateral sclerosis.

Excitotoxic damage is also thought to occur in the slow-channel syndrome, a congenital myasthenic syndrome associated with progressive endplate myopathy.

Choi DW: Excitotoxic cell death. J Neurobiol 23:1261–1276, 1992.

Gomez CM, et al: Slow-channel transgenic mice: A model of postsynaptic organellar degeneration at the neuromuscular junction. J Neurosci 17:4170–4179, 1997.

32. What are free radicals? What is their relationship to neuronal injury?

Free radicals are molecules with one or more unpaired electrons. Many of the free radical species produced in living cells, such as superoxide anion (O_2^-) and hydroxyl radical (OH), arise from oxygen in the electron-transport chain. Free radical-induced biochemical alterations have been documented in ischemic stroke as well as many neurodegenerative diseases. The challenge has been to establish whether these changes initiate cell injury, amplify other pathologic processes, or occur simply as late markers of cell injury. Mutations in *SOD1*, the gene coding for Cu/Zn superoxide dismutase, a key enzyme involved in oxygen free-radical metabolism, have been associated with one form of familial amyotrophic lateral sclerosis. Two basic strategies are being tested to modify free radical-induced damage in neurologic illness: antioxidants, which reduce free-radical production, and free-radical scavengers, which react with free radicals to trap unpaired electrons in relatively unreactive species.

33. Discuss the differences between necrotic and apoptotic neuronal death.

Necrotic cell death is generally triggered by an insult that overwhelms cellular homeostatic mechanisms and proceeds by cell swelling, disruption of organelles, and eventual lysis of dying cells. Spillage of necrotic cell contents, including proteolytic enzymes and toxic by-products of metabolism, into the extracellular environment is thought to be deleterious to adjacent cells.

In contrast, the characteristic features of **apoptotic cell death** are chromatin condensation, DNA fragmentation, cell membrane blebbing, loss of the nuclear membrane, and eventual fragmentation of the cell into easily phagocytosed "apoptotic bodies."

In apoptosis, damage to adjacent cells resulting from products of a dying cell is thought to be minimized. Apoptotic cell death is believed to be a major means of cell death induced by irradiation (tumor cells), glucocorticoids (lymphocytes), cell death mediated by cytotoxic T-lymphocytes, and growth-factor withdrawal. A phase of apoptotic cell death occurs during normal development in many cell groups of the CNS, most notably in bulbar and spinal motoneurons. Early-onset forms of spinal muscular atrophy have been linked to mutations in neuronal apoptosis inhibitory protein (NAIP) as well as in survival motor neuron (*smn*) genes. Enhanced susceptibility to apoptosis induced by normally sublethal insults has been documented in animal models of adult-onset neurodegenerative illnesses; the contribution of this form of cell death to the corresponding human disorders remains to be defined.

34. What are adhesion molecules? How may they play a role in neurologic disease?

Cell adhesion to other cells and to the extracellular matrix regulates many cellular functions, including neurite outgrowth during development, cell growth, cell recognition, immune responses, and responses to mechanical stress. Examples of specialized molecules involved in cell adhesion include:

1. ICAM-1 (an intercellular adhesion molecule), which is upregulated in endothelial cells after cerebral ischemia and may potentiate injury by binding to and facilitating invasion of neutrophils into ischemic brain tissue.

2. Merosin (a muscle isoform of laminin), an extracellular matrix component that binds α-dystroglycan (a member of the muscle dystrophin-glycoprotein complex). It is deficient in one form of congenital muscular dystrophy.

3. Mutations in the gene for L1CAM (L1-neural cell adhesion molecule) are associated with an X-linked syndrome of mental retardation, hydrocephalus, and agenesis of the corpus callosum.

4. Cell adhesion molecules with known signaling functions also may serve as receptors for pathogenic organisms or regulate their entry. For instance, entry of the retrovirus HTLV-1 (a cause of tropical spastic paraparesis) into susceptible cells is inhibited by CD82 adhesion molecules (tetraspanins).

Finckh U, et al: Spectrum and detection rate of L1CAM mutations in isolated and familial cases with clinically suspected L1-disease. Am J Med Genet 92:40–46, 2000.

Pique C, et al: Interaction of CD82 tetraspanin with HTLV-1 envelope glycoproteins inihibits cell-to-cell fusion and virus transmission. Virology 276:455–465, 2000.

35. What is a neurotrophic factor?

During development, the survival of many types of neurons requires one or more factors derived from the targets that the neurons innervate. The most famous of the neurotrophic factors, or factors that promote the survival and growth of neurons, is nerve growth factor (NGF), which influences sympathetic ganglia and dorsal root ganglia. Other factors, such as BDNF (brain-derived neurotrophic factor), CNTF (ciliary neurotrophic factor), GDNF (glial cell-derived neurotrophic factor), and CT-1 (cardiotrophin-1), have been shown to influence other subsets of neurons, including motoneurons. Although primary deficiency of neurotrophic factors has not been shown to cause any of the major human neurodegenerative diseases, growing evidence indicates that these factors can regulate neuronal properties even in the adult nervous system and may have survival-promoting effects on neurons injured by a variety of causes. Recently, a trial of insulinlike growth factor 1 (IGF-1) reported beneficial effects on disease progression in patients with amyotrophic lateral sclerosis.

Lai EC, et al: Effect of recombinant human insulin-like growth factor-1 on progression of ALS. A placebo-controlled study. Neurology 49:1621–1630, 1997.

36. What is a molecular chaperone?

It is becoming increasingly clear that most proteins are not assembled into functioning structures or organelles by simple self-aggregation or self-assembly. Chaperones are proteins that enhance the folding of amino acid sequences into appropriate conformations that increase the speed and/or accuracy of assembly. Chaperones also may recognize aberrantly folded proteins and target them for rapid disassembly. Molecules with chaperone-like activity are implicated in cellular responses to heat shock and other forms of stress, aggregation of amyloid proteins, and the tagging of abnormal proteins for degradation by proteasomal pathways. Abnormal chaperone function has been documented in a number of neurodegenerative disorders, including the expanded triplet repeat diseases. Mutations in the gene for a small heat-shock chaperone protein, alpha B-crystallin, are linked to myopathies marked by the pathologic accretion of desmin, an intermediate filament expressed in muscle.

Gregersen N, et al: Defective folding and rapid degradation of mutant proteins is a common disease mechanism in genetic disorders. J Inherit Metab Dis 23:441–447, 2000.

Vicart P, et al: A missense mutation in the alpha B-crystallin chaperone gene causes a desmin-related myopathy. Nat Genet 20:92–95, 1998.

MOLECULAR BIOLOGY

37. What is the fundamental principle of molecular biology?

The fundamental principle of molecular biology states that the flow of genetic information in cells is from DNA to RNA to protein. Synthesis of RNA from a DNA template is called transcription, whereas synthesis of protein from an RNA template is called translation. A notable exception to this principle is the replication of certain RNA viruses (retroviruses), in which DNA can be synthesized from an RNA template by reverse transcriptase.

38. Distinguish among gene, allele, polymorphism, and mutation.

A **gene** is the nucleic acid sequence carrying the information representing a particular polypeptide. **Alleles** are any of the alternative forms (sequence variants) of a gene or genetic locus. Any locus at which multiple alleles exist as stable components in a population is termed **polymorphic**. In common usage, a non–disease-causing genetic variant is termed a benign polymorphism. A **mutation** is a change in DNA sequence (which may or may not result in detectable effects). Obviously, alleles, including those which are now considered benign polymorphisms, resulted from mutations in the past.

39. Name several types of genomic alterations that can lead to disease.

1. Single base-pair substitutions—may alter a single amino acid or stop the DNA from being read.

2. Insertion or deletion of one or more base pairs—alter the reading frame (frameshift).

3. Repetition of sequences of base pairs (e.g., triplet repeat mutations).

4. Duplication of a gene or chromosome (e.g., *PMP22* gene duplication in Charcot-Marie-Tooth disease 1A).

5. Chromosomal deletion or translocation.

6. Imprinting—due to differential activity of paternal and maternal copies of a gene.

7. Alterations of a regulatory protein (e.g., a promoter region) that controls expression of one or more downstream genes.

8. Alteration in a gene with widespread effects on DNA transcription (e.g., the methyl-CpG binding protein 2 or MeCP-2 gene in Rett syndrome) may cause misregulation of a large number of distant genes.

Matsuura T, et al: Large expansion of the ATTCT pentanucleotide repeat in spinocerebellar ataxia type 10. Nat Genet 26:191–194, 2000.

40. What is the polymerase chain reaction (PCR)?

PCR is a process used to amplify a region of DNA, allowing it to be detected with high sensitivity. It requires knowledge of the DNA sequence on either side of a target region ("flanking sequence"). DNA primers matching the flanking sequence are used to initiate copying of the target region DNA by a heat-stable DNA polymerase. The resulting DNA strands undergo denaturation with heat to separate the strands; then the primers are allowed to bind again, with synthesis of new complementary strands. This cycle is repeated until the desired amplification of the target region DNA is achieved.

41. What are functional cloning and positional cloning?

Two principal strategies have been used to isolate genes underlying human genetic disorders:

1. **Functional cloning** is based on identification of the protein that is altered in a disorder, with subsequent sequencing of the protein and design of cDNA probes to try to find the gene coding for the protein. This approach requires prior knowledge of the defective protein, which is not available for most inherited diseases.

2. The more recent approach is **positional cloning** (reverse genetics), in which the gene responsible for a disease phenotype is mapped to a chromosomal location, usually by analysis of markers linked to it or by identifying an associated genetic defect (chromosomal translocation or deletion). This candidate region is then physically mapped, cloned, and ultimately sequenced to identify genetic mutations associated with the disease phenotype. The task of identifying the function(s) of the altered protein product and the mechanism(s) by which it produces disease then begins. In many cases, the second task may prove more difficult than the task of isolating the disease gene.

42. What are trinucleotide or triplet repeats? How have they been linked to neurologic diseases?

In many genes, short blocks of repeated sequences (e.g., CAGCAG… or CTGCTG…) normally occur. Expansions of these trinucleotide or triplet repeat sequences beyond their normal size have recently been associated with a number of neurodegenerative disorders, including:

- Fragile X syndromes
- Myotonic dystrophy (DMPK or myotonic dystrophy protein kinase gene)
- Huntington's disease (huntingtin gene)
- X-linked spinobulbar muscular atrophy (androgen receptor gene)
- Dentatorubral-pallido-luysian atrophy
- Spinocerebellar atrophies (notably SCA1 [ataxin-1 gene] and SCA6 [*CACNL1A4*, coding for a P/Q-type voltage-gated Ca^{2+} channel])
- Friedreich's ataxia (frataxin gene)

For most of these disorders, longer repeat size is associated with an earlier age of onset and/or more severe phenotype. The length of expanded repeats is characteristically unstable, and often lengthens further with successive generations, producing the clinical phenomenon of **anticipation** (earlier onset and more severe phenotype with successive generations).

Ashizawa T, Zoghbi HY: Diseases with trinucleotide repeat expansions. In Appel SH (ed): Current Neurology, vol. 17. Amsterdam, IOS Press, 1997.

43. How can a disease exhibiting autosomal dominant inheritance result from loss of function of the gene product?

Most biologic systems operate with significant reserve capacity so that approximately 50% loss of function (as may occur with loss of expression of a single gene copy) does not result in disease. Hence, autosomal dominant disorders have often been thought to result from **gain-of-function mutations**, in which the altered gene product acts in a novel manner (e.g., expression in the wrong cell type, altered regulation, or acquisition of toxic properties). However, it is becoming increasingly clear that many dominantly inherited disorders could also result from **loss of function** of the gene product. If the altered gene product not only loses its function but also prevents the product from the normal gene copy from acting normally, the mutation is said to be a **dominant negative mutation**. This mutation may occur when the protein product functions in dimers or multimers or in complexes with other proteins. **Haploinsufficiency** is said to occur when establishment of a normal phenotype requires more of the gene product than a single gene copy can produce. A state of haploinsufficiency may involve not only reduction of gene dosage but also factors preventing compensatory upregulation of product from the remaining gene.

44. Discuss the prion hypothesis and its relevance to neurologic disease.

The transmissible spongiform encephalopathies are caused by proteinaceous agents that resist inactivation by procedures that modify nucleic acids. The prion hypothesis states that infectivity is transmitted solely by an altered protein and does not require DNA or RNA. Production of altered protein in infected cells would result from a conformational change in a normal host protein (PrP or prion protein) that is catalyzed by interactions with an abnormal form of the same protein. This hypothesis requires that the information necessary for replication be contained within the conformation of the protein itself, representing a challenge to the fundamental principle of molecular biology (see question 37). Human prion diseases include kuru, Creutzfeldt-Jakob disease, Gerstmann-Straussler-Scheinker disease, fatal familial insomnia, and variant CJD or "mad cow" disease.

Telling GC, et al: Evidence for the conformation of the pathologic isoform of the prion protein enciphering and propagating prion diversity. Science 274:2079, 1996.

45. Do axotomized CNS neurons have the potential for significant regeneration?

CNS axons can regenerate when exposed to a peripheral nerve environment but fail to regrow when exposed to the CNS environment, presumably because the CNS expresses factors that actively inhibit axon growth. Glia at injury sites express proteoglycans that inhibit regeneration. Certain axon guidance factors in the CNS, such as the semaphorins, may repel or inhibit outgrowing axons. CNS myelin itself expresses a number of inhibitors of axon growth, including the protein Nogo. Interactions between these proteins and their receptors provide targets for potential therapeutic intervention to increase axonal regeneration in the damaged CNS.

David S, Aguayo AJ: Axonal elongation into peripheral nervous system "bridges" after central nervous system injury in adult rats. Science 214:931–933, 1981.

Fournier AE, GrandPre T, Strittmatter SM: Identification of a receptor mediating Nogo-66 inhibition of axonal regeneration. Nature 409:341–346, 2001.

46. What is a stem cell?

Stem cells are cells with the potential to give rise to precursors of different cell types and exhibit capacity for self-renewal. Stem cells may be pluripotent (able to give rise to precursors of many different cell types) or unipotent (apparently committed to a particular liineage). They have the capacity, at least theoretically, to regenerate injured tissues. Increasing evidence has shown that neural stem cells exist not only during CNS development but also in the adult CNS. Moreover, bone marrow-derived hematopoietic stem cells (mesodermal origin) recently were induced to differentiate along neuronal lines (ectodermal lineage), thus providing another potential source of neuronal cells for transplantation.

Gage FH: Mammalian neural stem cells. Science 287:1433, 2000.

Mezey E, Chandross KJ: Bone marrow: A possible alternative source of cells in the adult nervous system. Eur J Pharmacol 405:297–302, 2000.

47. Name several potential obstacles to successful neuronal transplantation in humans.

The following is only a partial list:
1. Appropriate differentiation of neurons (e.g., from stem cells)

2. Maintaining stability of neuronal phenotype over time
3. Regulating neurotransmitter production and cell proliferation
4. Making connections with both upstream and downstream targets
5. Reintegration into functioning neural networks (i.e., "relearning")
6. Protection from ongoing disease processes
7. Ethical issues with cells derived from human embryos

At present it is unknown which of these obstacles will pose serious challenges to the success of neuronal transplants. The dyskinesias encountered recently in a trial of implanted embryonic dopaminergic neurons in Parkinson's disease suggest that unregulated cellular outputs may be a significant problem for some approaches. However, the potential for improvement using cell transplants may be quite large, and a number of clinical trials are under way to evaluate the safety and efficacy of neuronal transplantation in a variety of CNS disorders.

Freed CR, et al: Transplantation of embryonic dopamine neurons for severe Parkinson disease. N Engl J Med 344:710–719, 2001.

48. Describe some of the challenges encountered in producing successful "gene therapy" for CNS neuromuscular disorders.

1. Loss of function, which can be corrected with replacement of nonfunctioning genes, accounts for only a percentage of genetic disorders. Disorders resulting from a toxic gain of function may require suppression of abnormal gene product or actual correction of the defective DNA sequences, a more formidable task.

2. Most vectors for introducing DNA into cells are inefficient (i.e., only a minority of cells successfully express the introduced gene).

3. Expression of proteins from viral vectors on cell surfaces may trigger host immune responses.

4. Introduction of the normal protein itself may trigger host immune responses.

5. Expression of introduced DNA may be transient.

6. Vectors may introduce genes into nontarget cells.

7. Integrated DNA sequences may be regulated abnormally.

This is only a partial list. Despite these challenges, the promise of correcting genetic disorders at a fundamental level has spurred a high level of research aimed at bringing gene therapies to clinical trial. The recent results from replacement of the gene encoding for adenosine deaminase in T cells of patients with one form of severe immunodeficiency have further stimulated interest in extending gene therapeutic approaches to brain and neuromuscular disorders.

BIBLIOGRAPHY

1. Bloom F, Zigmond MJ, Landis SC, Squire LR: Fundamental Neuroscience. New York, AP Professional, 1999.
2. Bostock H, Kirkwood PA, Pullen AH (eds): The Neurobiology of Disease: Contributions from Neuroscience to Clinical Neurology. Cambridge, Cambridge University Press, 1996.
3. Hille B: Ionic Channels of Excitable Membranes, 2nd ed. Sunderland, MA, Sinauer, 1992.
4. Schwartz LM, Osborne BA (eds): Cell Death (Methods in Cell Biology, vol 46). San Diego, Academic Press, 1995.
Website
http://thalamus.wustl.edu/course

2. CLINICAL NEUROANATOMY

Sudhir S. Athni, M.D., Igor M. Cherches, M.D., and Brian Loftus, M.D.

EMBRYOLOGY

1. How is the neural tube formed?

Beginning around the 18th gestational day, a midline notochordal thickening anterior to the blastopore forms the neural plate. A midsagittal groove appears in the plate—the neural groove—and the sides elevate to form the neural folds. As the folds fuse, the neural tube is formed. Some cells at the edges of the fold do not fuse into the tube and become neural crest cells.

2. What types of cells are derived from the neural crest cells?

Neural crest cells give rise to (1) unipolar sensory cells, (2) postganglionic cells of sympathetic and parasympathetic ganglia, (3) chromaffin cells of the adrenal medulla, (4) some microglial cells, (5) pia mater, (6) some arachnoid cells, (7) melanocytes, and (8) Schwann cells.

3. What are the alar plate and the basal plate?

As the neural tube is formed, a longitudinal groove appears on each side and divides the neural tube into a dorsal half, or alar plate, and a ventral half, or basal plate. The **alar plate** gives rise to the prosencephalon, the sensory and coordinating nuclei of the thalamus, the sensory neurons of the cranial nerves, the coordinating nuclei including cerebellum, inferior olives, red nucleus, quadrigeminal plate, and the posterior horn area (sensory) of the spinal cord. The **basal plate** stops at the level of the diencephalon and gives rise to the motor neurons of the cranial nerves and anterior horn (motor) area of the spinal cord.

4. What is the process of formation of the ventricles, prosencephalon, mesencephalon, and rhombencephalon?

Around the end of the first gestational month, a series of bulges anterior to the first cervical somites appears. The first bulge is the prosencephalon, or forebrain. The cavity of this bulge forms the lateral ventricles and third ventricle. Secondary outpouchings from the forebrain are called optic vesicles and eventually form the retina, pigment epithelium, and optic nerve. The second bulge is the mesencephalon, or midbrain. The cavity of this bulge forms the cerebral aqueduct. The third bulge is the rhombencephalon, or hindbrain. This cavity gives rise to the fourth ventricle.

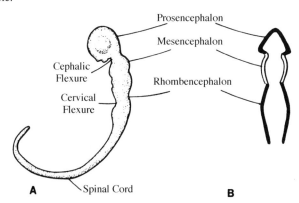

Development of the nervous system in the fourth week (*A* and *B*) of gestation.

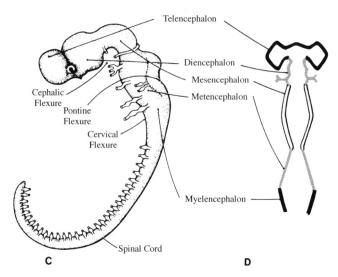

Development of the nervous system in the sixth week (*C* and *D*) of gestation. (From Gilman S, Newman SW: Manter and Gatz's Essentials of Clinical Neuroanatomy and Neurophysiology, 8th ed. Philadelphia, F.A. Davis, 1992, with permission.)

5. Which structures arise from the prosencephalon, mesencephalon, and rhomben-cephalon?

The **prosencephalon** develops into the telencephalon, which includes the cerebral cortex and basal ganglia, and the diencephalon, which includes the thalamus and the hypothalamus. The **mesencephalon** gives rise to the midbrain. The **rhombencephalon** gives rise to the meten-cephalon (pons + cerebellum) and myelencephalon (medulla).

Embryonic Divisions of the Central Nervous System

EMBRYONIC DIVISIONS		ADULT DERIVATIVES	VENTRICULAR CAVITIES
Forebrain (prosencephalon)	Telencephalon	Cerebral cortex Basal ganglia	Lateral ventricles
	Diencephalon	Thalamus Hypothalamus Subthalamus Epithalamus	Third ventricle
Midbrain (mesencephalon	—	Tectum Cerebral peduncles	Aqueduct
Hindbrain (rhombencephalon)	Metencephalon	Cerebellum Pons	Fourth ventricle
	Myelencephalon	Medulla	
Spinal cord	—	Spinal cord	No cavity

MUSCLE

6. What is the histologic organization of skeletal muscle?

Skeletal muscle is composed of long, thin, cylindrical, multinucleated cells called muscle fibers (or myofibrils). Each fiber has a motor endplate at its neuromuscular junction and is surrounded by connective tissue called endomysium. Groups of fibers, or a fascicle, are surrounded by a connective tissue layer called the perimysium. Fascicles are grouped together and surrounded by epimysium.

7. What is found at the A band, H band, I band, and Z line?
   The **A band** contains the thin filaments (actin) and the thick filaments (myosin). The **H band** is the portion of the A band that contains only myosin, and the **I band** is the portion that contains only actin.The actin is anchored at the **Z line**.

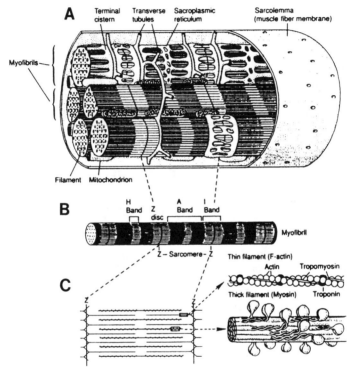

The histologic anatomy of the human skeletal muscle. (From Kandel E, Schwartz JH, Jessell TM (eds): Principles of Neuroscience, 3rd ed. New York, Elsevier, 1991, p 549, with permission.)

8. How does the muscle contract?
   When the sarcoplastic reticulum is depolarized, calcium ions enter the cell and bind to troponin. This causes a conformational change that allows exposure of the actin binding site to myosin. The myosin attaches to the actin binding site and flexes, causing the actin filament to slide by the myosin filament. Adenosine triphosphate (ATP) is required to allow the myosin-actin crossbridge to release and the muscle to relax.

9. What is meant by the term "motor unit"?
   The motor unit is one motor nerve (lower motor neuron) and all muscle fibers that it innervates.

The Muscle Stretch Reflex

10. What type of nerve fiber innervates the muscle?
   An anterior horn motor neuron, called an alpha motor neuron, innervates the muscle. It is the final common pathway for muscle contraction.

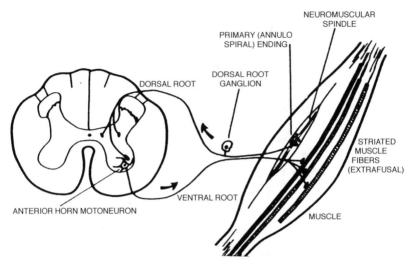

Diagram of the muscle stretch reflex. (From Garoutte B: Survey of Functional Neuroanatomy, 2nd ed. Greenbrae, CA, Jones Medical Publications, 1992, p 60, with permission.)

11. What are Renshaw cells?

Renshaw cells are interneurons that are stimulated by the alpha motor neuron and then, by a feedback mechanism, inhibit the alpha motor neuron, causing autoinhibition.

12. In the spinal cord, which nerve fibers synapse on the alpha motor neuron?

Both the corticospinal tract and afferent Ia sensory nerves regulate the alpha motor neuron by synapsing on it in the anterior horn of the spinal cord.

13. What is the function of the Ia nerve fiber?

When the muscle spindle is stretched, the Ia sensory nerve, through the dorsal root, monosynaptically stimulates the alpha motor neuron, which fires and contracts (shortens) the muscle. Thus, the muscle stretch reflex maintains tone and tension in the muscle.

14. Is the Ia reflex monosynaptic or polysynaptic?

It is monosynaptic, but it initiates a polysynaptic inhibition of the antagonist muscle group.

15. What is the role of the gamma efferent nerve?

The gamma efferent nerve fibers keep the muscle spindles "tight" by innervating and contracting the intrafusal fibers in the muscle spindle. This process ensures that the spindle remains sensitive to any stretch.

16. Where does the Ib fiber originate?

The Ib fiber originates from the Golgi tendon organ, another structure that monitors muscle stretch and acts to inhibit muscle contraction.

17. Where does the Ib neuron synapse?

At the spinal cord level, the Ib sensory nerve polysynaptically inhibits the alpha motor neuron to prevent muscle contraction and stimulates the gamma efferent fiber to reset the muscle tone.

LUMBOSACRAL PLEXUS AND LEG INNERVATION

18. Which roots make up the lumbar plexus?

Roots of L1,2,3,4 and sometimes T12 make up the lumbar plexus.

19. What are the two largest branches of the lumbar plexus?

1. **Obturator nerve (L2,3,4).** It leaves the pelvis through the obturator foramen and supplies the adductors of the thigh.

2. **Femoral nerve (L2,3,4).** It exits the pelvis with the femoral artery and supplies the hip flexors and knee extensors. Distally it continues as the saphenous nerve to supply sensation to the medial anterior knee and medial distal leg, including the medial malleolus.

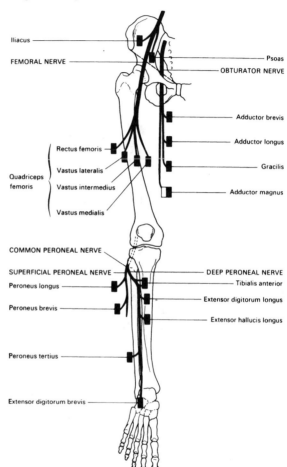

Diagram of the nerves and muscles on the anterior aspect of the lower limb. (From Medical Research Council: Aids to the Examination of the Peripheral Nervous System, London, 1976, with permission.)

20. What are the other branches of the lumbar plexus?

1. **Iliohypogastric nerve (L1)**—sensation to skin over hypogastric and gluteal areas; to abdominal muscles

2. **Ilioinguinal nerve (L1)**—sensation to skin over groin and scrotum (labia)

3. **Genitofemoral nerve (L1,2)**—enters the internal inguinal ring and runs in the inguinal canal

4. **Lateral femoral cutaneous nerve (L2,3)**—sensation to skin over anterior and lateral parts of the thigh

21. Which nerve is at risk during appendectomy (McBurney's incision)?

The iliohypogastric nerve may be cut as it passes between the external and internal oblique muscles. This results in weakness in the area of inguinal canal, putting the patient at risk for direct inguinal hernia.

22. What is meralgia paresthetica?

Meralgia paresthetica is numbness and tingling in the lateral thigh secondary to compression of the lateral femoral cutaneous nerve as it runs over the inguinal ligament. It commonly occurs in obese or pregnant patients.

23. Which nerve supplies the gluteus maximus?

The inferior gluteal nerve (L5, S1,2) supplies the gluteus maximus muscle.

24. What is the largest nerve in the body?

The sciatic nerve (L4,5, S1,2,3), the largest nerve in the body, is composed of the common peroneal nerve (L4,5, S1,2) in its dorsal division and the tibial nerve (L4,5, S1,2,3) in its ventral division.

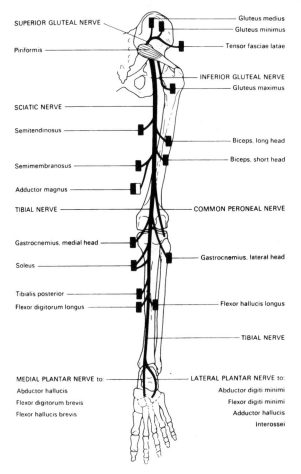

SUPERIOR GLUTEAL NERVE

Piriformis

SCIATIC NERVE

Semitendinosus

Semimembranosus

Adductor magnus

TIBIAL NERVE

Gastrocnemius, medial head

Soleus

Tibialis posterior

Flexor digitorum longus

MEDIAL PLANTAR NERVE to:
Abductor hallucis
Flexor digitorum brevis
Flexor hallucis brevis

Gluteus medius
Gluteus minimus
Tensor fasciae latae
INFERIOR GLUTEAL NERVE
Gluteus maximus

Biceps, long head
Biceps, short head

COMMON PERONEAL NERVE

Gastrocnemius, lateral head

Flexor hallucis longus

TIBIAL NERVE

LATERAL PLANTAR NERVE to:
Abductor digiti minimi
Flexor digiti minimi
Adductor hallucis
Interossei

Diagram of the nerves and muscles on the posterior aspect of the lower limb. (From Medical Research Council: Aids to the Examination of the Peripheral Nervous System, London, 1976, with permission.)

25. What is the only nerve in the sacral plexus that emerges through the greater sciatic foramen, superior to the piriformis muscle?

The superior gluteal nerve (L4,5 and S1) supplies the gluteus medius and minimus and tensor fascia lata (abduction and medial rotation of the thigh).

26. Which nerve supplies the inferior buttock and posterior thigh?

The posterior femoral cutaneous nerve (S1,2,3), which runs with the inferior gluteal nerve, supplies the inferior buttock and posterior thigh.

27. Which nerve supplies the structures in the perineum?

The pudendal nerve (S2,3,4) supplies the perineum.

28. What is the only muscle supplied by the sciatic nerve that receives innervation exclusively from the dorsal division (i.e., peroneal component) of the sciatic nerve?

The biceps femoris has only dorsal innervation. This point is important clinically in trying to differentiate lesions caused by damage to the common peroneal nerve vs. the sciatic nerve itself.

29. Which muscles are supplied by the tibial nerve?

The tibial nerve supplies plantarflexors and invertors of the foot.

30. What are the two divisions of the common peroneal nerve?

1. **Deep peroneal nerve**—dorsiflexion of the foot and toes and sensation to a small area of skin between the first and second toes.

2. **Superficial peroneal nerve**—evertors of the foot and sensation to the skin of the dorsal and lateral foot.

BRACHIAL PLEXUS AND ARM INNERVATION

31. The brachial plexus comprises which roots?

The brachial plexus comprises the ventral rami of C5,6,7,8 and T1.

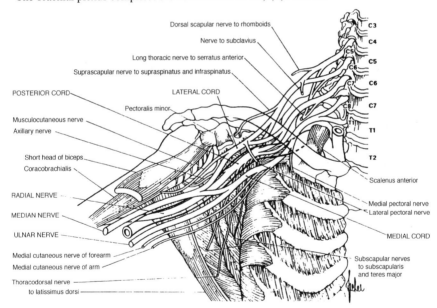

The brachial plexus. (From Tindall B: Aids to the Examination of the Peripheral Nervous System. London, W.B. Saunders, 1990, with permission.)

32. Which nerves arise from the ventral rami of the roots before formation of the brachial plexus?

1. **Dorsal scapular nerve**, from C5 to rhomboid and levator scapula muscles; responsible for elevation and stabilization of the scapula.

2. **Long thoracic nerve**, from C5,6,7 to serratus anterior responsible for abduction of the scapula.

Testing these nerves is useful in trying to differentiate between root and plexus lesions. If there is a deficit in one of these nerves (clinically or electrically), the lesion is proximal to the plexus.

33. Which roots form the three trunks of the brachial plexus?
(1) Superior trunk, formed by C5 and C6; (2) middle trunk, formed by C7; and (3) lower trunk, formed by C8 and T1.

34. Which nerves originate from the cervical roots before formation of the brachial plexus?
Dorsal scapular nerve (C5) and long thoracic nerve (C5, C6, C7).

35. What is the only nerve from the trunks of the brachial plexus?
The suprascapular nerve (C5) comes off the upper trunk and supplies the supraspinatus (abduction) and infraspinatus (external rotation) of the shoulder.

36. Which vascular structure is associated with the three cords of the brachial plexus?
The lateral cord (C5,6,7), medial cord (C8, T1), and posterior cord (C5,6,7,8) are named in relationship to the axillary artery.

37. What are the nerves off the cords of the brachial plexus?
Lateral cord
1. Lateral pectoral nerve (C5,6,7)—to pectoralis minor
2. Musculocutaneous nerve (C5,6)—to brachialis and coracobrachialis (elbow flexion)
3. Median nerve (partial; C6,7)—to pronator teres, flexor carpi radialis, part of flexor digitorum superficialis, part of palmaris longus

Medial cord
4. Medial pectoral nerve (C8, T1)—to pectoralis major (shoulder adduction)
5. Ulnar nerve (C8, T1)—ulnar wrist and long finger flexors
6. Median nerve (partial; C8, T1)—long finger flexors and small hand muscles
7. Medial brachial cutaneous nerve—skin over medial surface of arm and proximal forearm
8. Medial antebrachial cutaneous nerve—skin over medial surface of forearm

Posterior cord
9. Upper subscapular nerve (C5,6)—to subscapularis (medial rotation of the humerus)
10. Thoracodorsal nerve (C6,7,8)—to latissimus dorsi (shoulder adduction)
11. Lower subscapular nerve (C5,6)—to teres major (adducts the humerus)
12. Axillary nerve (C5, C6)—to deltoid (abduction of the humerus) and teres minor (lateral rotation of humerus)
13. Radial nerve (C5,6,7,8 and T1)—to extensor muscles of upper limb.
(See figures, next page.)

38. What is Erb's palsy?
Erb's palsy is an injury to the upper brachial plexus (C5, C6) resulting from excessive separation or stretch of the neck and shoulder (such as from a sliding injury or from pulling on an infant's neck during delivery). The result is decreased sensation in the C5 and C6 dermatomes and paralysis of scapular muscles. The arm may be held in adduction, with the fingers pointing backward, so-called waiter's tip position. Distal strength in the upper extremity remains intact.

39. What is Klumpke's palsy?
Klumpke's palsy results from maximal abduction of the shoulder, causing injury to the lower brachial plexus (C8 and T1) and leading to weakness and anesthesia in a primarily ulnar distribution.

40. What is Parsonage-Turner syndrome?
Parsonage-Turner syndrome is an acute brachial plexus neuritis, commonly also affecting the long thoracic, musculocutaneous, and axillary nerves. It causes patchy upper extremity weakness and numbness, usually accompanied by pain. Symptoms are bilateral in 20% of patients. This condition is associated with diabetes, systemic lupus erythematosus, and polyarteritis nodosa and may follow immunizations or viral infections. One-third of patients recover within 1 year and 90% within 3 years.

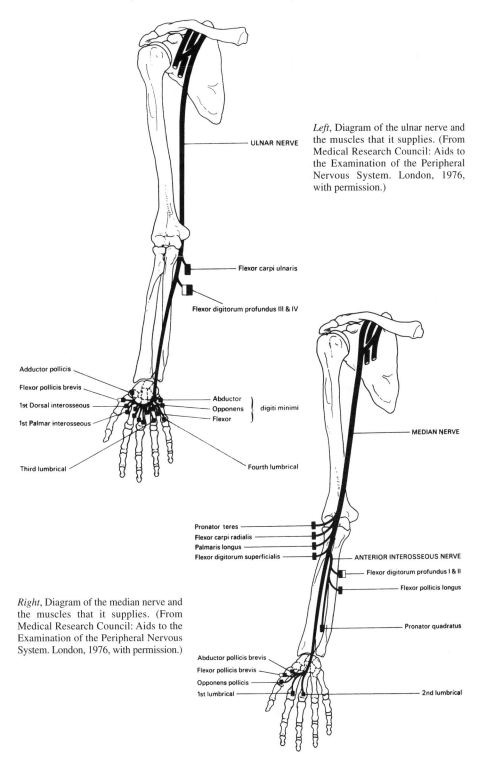

Left, Diagram of the ulnar nerve and the muscles that it supplies. (From Medical Research Council: Aids to the Examination of the Peripheral Nervous System. London, 1976, with permission.)

ULNAR NERVE

Flexor carpi ulnaris

Flexor digitorum profundus III & IV

Adductor pollicis

Flexor pollicis brevis

1st Dorsal interosseous

1st Palmar interosseous

Third lumbrical

Abductor

Opponens } digiti minimi

Flexor

Fourth lumbrical

MEDIAN NERVE

Pronator teres

Flexor carpi radialis

Palmaris longus

Flexor digitorum superficialis

ANTERIOR INTEROSSEOUS NERVE

Flexor digitorum profundus I & II

Flexor pollicis longus

Pronator quadratus

Right, Diagram of the median nerve and the muscles that it supplies. (From Medical Research Council: Aids to the Examination of the Peripheral Nervous System. London, 1976, with permission.)

Abductor pollicis brevis

Flexor pollicis brevis

Opponens pollicis

1st lumbrical

2nd lumbrical

41. What deficit results from poorly fitting crutches?

Pressure from crutches results in a lesion of the posterior cord or the radial nerve, leading to weakness of the elbow, wrist, and digits.

42. Which nerve is commonly affected in shoulder dislocation or fracture of the humerus?

The axillary nerve is affected, resulting in a lesion that causes decreased abduction of the shoulder and anesthesia over the lateral part of the proximal arm.

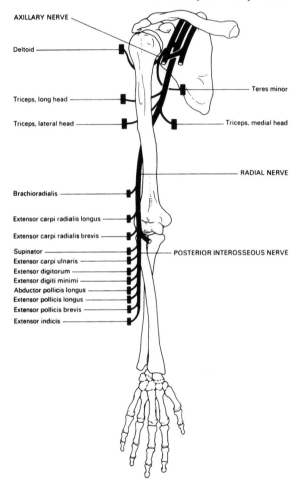

Diagram of the axillary and radial nerves and the muscles that they supply. (From Medical Research Council: Aids to the Examination of the Peripheral Nervous System. London, 1976, with permission.)

43. What is thoracic outlet syndrome (TOS)?

Classically, TOS consists of decreased upper extremity pulses, with tingling and numbness in the medial aspect of the arm secondary to compression of the medial cord of the brachial plexus and the axillary artery by a cervical rib or other structures.

ROOTS AND DERMATOMES

44. What is found in the ventral nerve root?

The ventral nerve root contains principally motor axons.

45. What is found in the dorsal nerve root?

The dorsal nerve root contains principally sensory axons.

46. What synapse is found in the dorsal root ganglia?

There is no synapse in the dorsal root ganglia. The dorsal root ganglia is made up of unipolar cell bodies for the sensory system.

47. What are the dermatomes of the following landmarks: thumb, middle finger, little finger, breast nipple, umbilicus, medial knee, big toe, and little toe?

Thumb	C6		Umbilicus	T10
Middle finger	C7		Medial knee	L3
Little finger	C8		Big toe	L4
Breast nipple	T4		Little toe	S1

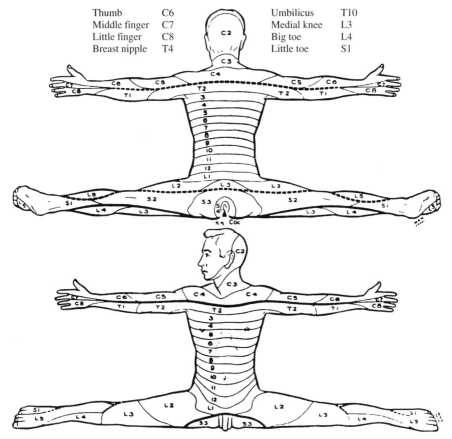

The dermatomes corresponding to each spinal root. (From Garoutte B: Survey of Functional Neuroanatomy, 2nd ed. Greenbrae, CA, Jones Medical Publications, 1991, p 76, modified with permission.)

48. What are the common signs and symptoms of lumbar radiculopathies?

Lumbar radiculopathies cause back pain with radiation below the knee. The pain increases with a Valsalva maneuver or leg stretch (such as the straight leg raising test). Weakness or numbness may develop in the distribution of the involved root. An S1 radiculopathy diminishes ankle reflexes, whereas an L4 radiculopathy decreases knee reflexes. Statistically, an L5 radiculopathy is more common than S1, followed by L4. This is because the intervertebral discs at these levels are under greatest pressure from the curvature of normal lumbar lordosis and thus are most vulnerable to herniation and compression of the spinal roots.

49. What are the common signs and symptoms of cervical radiculopathies?

Cervical radiculopathies usually involve the lower cervical roots (C6, C7, and C8). Patients typically complain of pain in the back of the neck, frequently with radiation to the arm in a dermatomal distribution. Paresthesias are often present in one or two digits. Absent biceps, brachioradialis, or triceps reflexes suggest lesions of C5, C6, and C7, respectively, and these muscles also may lose strength.

SPINAL CORD: Gross Anatomy

50. How is the spinal cord organized?

Sections of the spinal cord cut perpendicular to the length of the cord reveal a butterfly-shaped area of gray matter with surrounding white matter. The white matter consists mainly of longitudinal nerve fibers, carrying the ascending and descending tracts up and down the cord. Midline grooves are present on the dorsal and ventral surfaces (the dorsal median sulcus and ventral median fissure). The gray matter of the cord contains dorsal and ventral enlargements known as dorsal horns and ventral horns.

51. In a given transverse section of the spinal cord, how is the gray matter subdivided?

The gray matter can be subdivided into groups of nuclei. When the spinal cord is cut along its length, these nuclei appear to be arranged in cell columns or laminae. Rexed divided the cord into 10 laminae. Each lamina extends the length of the cord, with lamina I at the most dorsal aspect of the dorsal horn, lamina IX at the most ventral aspect of the ventral horn, and lamina X surrounding the central canal. Lamina II is also called the substantia gelatinosa and is the area of synapse for the spinothalamic tract. Lamina IX is the site of the cell bodies for the anterior horn motor cells.

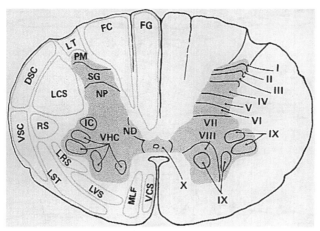

Diagram of the cross-section of the spinal cord in the lower cervical region, showing the major ascending and descending tracts, spinal nuclei, and Rexed's laminae. DSC = dorsal spinocerebellar tract; FC = fasciculus cuneatus; FG = fasciculus gracilis; IC = intermedial lateral cell column; LCS = lateral cortical spinal tract; LRS = lateral reticular spinal tract; LST = lateral spinothalamic tract; LT = Lissauer's tract; LVS = lateral vestibular spinal tract; MLF = medial longitudinal fasciculus; ND = nucleus dorsalis; NP = nucleus proprius; PM = posteromarginal nucleus; RS = rubrospinal tract; SG = substantia gelatinosa; VCS = ventral cortical spinal tract; VHC = ventral horn cell columns; VSC = ventral spinocerebellar tract. (From Gilman S, Newman SW: Manter and Gatz's Essentials of Clinical Neuroanatomy and Neurophysiology, 8th ed. Philadelphia, F.A. Davis, 1992, with permission.)

52. What are the major ascending tracts in the spinal cord?

The major ascending tracts are (1) dorsal columns, (2) spinothalamic tract, (3) dorsal spinocerebellar tract, and (4) ventral spinocerebellar tract.

53. What are the major descending tracts in the spinal cord?

The major descending tracts are (1) intermediolateral columns, (2) lateral corticospinal tract, (3) lateral reticulospinal tract, (4) lateral vestibulospinal tract, (5) medial longitudinal fasciculus, and (6) ventral corticospinal tract.

54. Going from rostral to caudal, what are the five divisions of the spinal cord?

The five divisions of the spinal cord are cervical, thoracic, lumbar, sacral, and coccygeal.

55. At what vertebral level does the spinal cord end?

The spinal cord ends at vertebral level L1–L2.

56. How many spinal nerves exit from each region of the spinal cord?

Spinal nerves exit the spinal cord in pairs: 8 cervical, 12 thoracic, 5 lumbar, 5 sacral, and 1 coccygeal. Each spinal nerve is composed of the union of the dorsal sensory root and the ventral motor root.

57. What is the filum terminale?

Although the spinal cord ends at the lower border of vertebral level L1, the pia mater continues caudally as a connective tissue filament, the filum terminale, which passes through the subarachnoid space to the end of the dural sac, where it receives a covering of dura and continues to its attachment to the coccyx.

58. What is the cauda equina?

The lumbar and sacral spinal nerves have very long roots, descending from their respective points in the spinal cord to their exit points in the intervertebral foramina. These roots descend in a bundle from the conus, termed the cauda equina for its resemblance to a horse's tail.

59. Describe the blood supply of the spinal cord.

The one anterior spinal artery and the two posterior spinal arteries travel along the length of the cord to supply blood to the cord. These arteries originate from the vertebral arteries. Other arteries replenish the anterior and posterior spinal arteries and enter the spinal canal through the intervertebral foramina in association with the spinal nerves. They are called radicular arteries if they supply only the nerve roots, and radiculospinal arteries if they supply blood to both the roots and the cord. Each radiculospinal artery supplies blood to approximately six spinal cord segments, with the exception of the great radicular artery of Adamkiewicz, which usually enters with the left second lumbar ventral root (range T10–L4) and supplies most of the caudal third of the cord. (See diagram, p. 105.)

Sensory: Dorsal Columns and Proprioception

60. What type of information is carried in the dorsal columns?

The dorsal columns convey tactile discrimination, vibration, and joint position sense.

61. What type of receptors are stimulated to sense this information?

Muscle spindles and Golgi tendon organs perceive position sense, pacinian corpuscles perceive vibration, and Meissner corpuscles perceive superficial touch sensation needed for tactile discrimination. Pacinian and Meissner corpuscles are examples of mechanoreceptors.

62. What type of peripheral nerve fiber is involved with transmission of dorsal column information?

Large, myelinated, fast-conducting nerve fibers carry dorsal column–type information.

63. What is the pathway by which this information reaches the cerebral cortex?

Sensation on skin → afferent sensory nerve → dorsal column on ipsilateral side (fasciculus gracilis and cuneatus) → lower medulla → synapse in nucleus gracilis and cuneatus → arcuate fibers → cross to the contralateral side into the medial lemniscus → ascend to the ventralis posterolateralis (VPL) nucleus of the thalamus → synapse → through the posterior limb of the internal capsule → postcentral gyrus of the cortex.

64. Where do dorsal column fibers decussate? At what locations do they synapse?
The dorsal columns decussate in the lower medulla, after synapsing in the nucleus gracilis and cuneatus. They also synapse in the VPL of the thalamus before going to the cortex.

Sensory: Spinothalamic

65. What type of information is carried in the spinothalamic tract?
The spinothalamic tract conveys pain, temperature, and crude touch.

66. What type of peripheral nerve fiber is involved with transmission of spinothalamic information?
Small, myelinated, and unmyelinated fibers carry spinothalamic-type information.

67. What is the pathway by which this information reaches the cerebral cortex?
Sensation on skin → afferent sensory nerve → substantia gelatinosa of the ipsilateral dorsal horn → synapse → cross via the anterior white commissure → contralateral spinothalamic tract → ascend to the VPL nucleus of the thalamus → synapse → through the posterior limb of the internal capsule → postcentral gyrus of the cortex.

68. Where do the spinothalamic fibers decussate? At what locations do they synapse?
These fibers decussate at the level they enter the spinal cord, after synapsing in Rexed's lamina II (substantia gelatinosa). They also synapse in the VPL of the thalamus before going to the cortex.

69. What type of receptors are stimulated to sense this information?
Pain and temperature are perceived by naked terminals of A-delta and C fibers and by many specialized chemoreceptors that are excited by tissue substances released in response to noxious and inflammatory stimuli. Substance P is thought to be the neurotransmitter released by A-delta and C fibers at their connections with the interneurons in the spinal cord.

70. Where in the internal capsule do the afferents travel from the VPL thalamic nucleus?
The sensory tracts from the VPL travel in the posterior aspect of the posterior limb of the internal capsule.

71. To which anatomic locations do the afferents from the VPL project?
They project to the postcentral gyrus (Brodmann's area 3,1,2; also called somatosensory I), and to somatosensory II (the posterior aspect of the superior lip of the lateral fissure).

Sensory: Spinocerebellar

72. Which pathway carries proprioception from the lower limbs to the cerebellum?
Proprioception travels from the legs to the cerebellum in the dorsal columns.

73. Where does cerebellar proprioception for the lower limb synapse?
These fibers synapse in the midthoracic level of the spinal cord in the nucleus dorsalis of Clark.

74. Where is the spinocerebellar tract located?
The spinocerebellar tract lies lateral to corticospinal in the cord.

Motor: Corticospinal

75. Where do the motor fibers originate?
The motor fibers originate from the precentral gyrus (Brodmann's area 4). Initiation of movement arises from the premotor cortex (Brodmann's area 6), which lies anterior to the precentral gyrus.

76. Where do the motor fibers travel in the internal capsule?

The corticospinal fibers travel in the anterior portion of the posterior limb of the internal capsule. The motor fibers to the face (corticobulbar fibers) travel in the genu of the internal capsule.

77. Which cranial nerve exits the midbrain in close proximity to the corticospinal fibers?

Cranial nerve III exits the midbrain in close proximity to the corticospinal fibers, which explains the symptoms of a common vascular syndrome. In Weber's syndrome, a stroke in this location causes an ipsilateral third nerve palsy with contralateral hemiparesis.

78. Where do the motor fibers decussate?

The corticospinal tract decussates in the lower ventral medulla, and most fibers continue in the cord as the lateral corticospinal tract, with a small percentage descending in the ventral corticospinal tract.

79. On what type of neurons in the spinal cord do the corticospinal fibers synapse?

In the spinal cord, the corticospinal fibers synapse on the alpha and gamma motor neurons in Rexed's lamina IX.

Motor: Other Tracts

80. What is the reticulospinal tract?

The reticulospinal tract also originates in the precentral gyrus, but instead of descending uninterrupted to the spinal cord, these fibers synapse in the reticular formation of the brainstem as they descend to the spinal cord. They mainly have an inhibitory effect on the alpha and gamma motor neurons.

81. What is the vestibulospinal tract?

The vestibulospinal tract is the efferent from the lateral vestibular nucleus. This tract descends the spinal cord, residing lateral to the spinothalamic tract, and coordinates motor and vestibular performance.

82. What is the medial longitudinal fasciculus (MLF)?

The medial longitudinal fasciculus is primarily an efferent of the lateral vestibular nucleus. This tract ascends to the sixth, fourth, and third cranial nuclei. Other major components of the MLF are interneurons originating from the PPRF (see question 155).

BRAINSTEM

Cranial Nerves

83. What are the three parts of the brainstem?

The brainstem consists of the midbrain, pons, and medulla.

84. What is the reticular formation?

The reticular formation is a loosely organized longitudinal collection of interneurons that fill the central core of the brainstem, which is concerned with modulating awareness and behavioral performance.

85. Name the 12 cranial nerves.

I	Olfactory	IV	Trochlear	VII	Facial	X	Vagus
II	Optic	V	Trigeminal	VIII	Auditory	XI	Spinal accessory
III	Oculomotor	VI	Abducens	IX	Glossopharyngeal	XI	Hypoglossal

86. What are general somatic afferent nerves? Which cranial nerves carry them?

General somatic afferent fibers carry extroceptive (pain, temperature, touch) and propriocep-tive impulses. Cranial nerves for proprioception: III, IV, V, VI, XII; for pain, temperature, and touch: V, VII, IX, X.

87. What are general visceral afferent nerves? Which cranial nerves carry them?

General visceral afferent fibers carry impulses from the visceral structures, and cranial nerves IX and X contain these fibers.

88. What are special somatic afferent nerves? Which cranial nerves carry them?

Special somatic afferent fibers carry sensory impulses from the special senses (vision, hear-ing, equilibrium), and cranial nerves II and VIII contain these fibers.

89. What are special visceral afferent nerves? Which cranial nerves carry them?

Special visceral afferent fibers carry impulses from the olfactory and gustatory senses, and cranial nerves I (olfactory) and VII, IX, and X (gustatory) contain these fibers.

90. What are general somatic efferent nerves? Which cranial nerves carry them?

General somatic efferent fibers carry motor impulses to somatic skeletal muscles. In the head, the tongue and extraocular muscles are of this type. Cranial nerves III, IV, VI, and XII carry these fibers.

91. What are general visceral efferent nerves? Which cranial nerves carry them?

General visceral efferent fibers carry parasympathetic autonomic axons. The following cra-nial nerves carry general visceral efferent fibers:

1. **Cranial nerve III** (Edinger-Westphal nucleus): the preganglionic fibers from the Edinger-Westphal nucleus terminates in the ciliary ganglion, and the postganglionic fibers innervate the pupil.

2. **Cranial nerve VII** (superior salivatory nucleus): the preganglionic fibers from the supe-rior salivatory nucleus terminate in the pterygopalatine and submandibular ganglion. The post-ganglionic fibers innervate the lacrimal gland (from the pterygopalatine ganglion) and the submandibular and sublingual gland (from the submandibular ganglion).

3. **Cranial nerve IX** (inferior salivatory nucleus): the preganglionic fibers from the inferior salivatory nucleus terminate in the otic ganglion, and the postganglionic fibers innervate the parotid gland.

4. **Cranial nerve X** (dorsal motor nucleus): the dorsal motor nucleus innervates the abdomi-nal viscera.

92. What are special visceral efferent nerves? Which cranial nerves carry them?

Special visceral efferent fibers innervate skeletal muscle derived from the branchial arches. Cranial nerves V (muscles of mastication, first branchial arch), VII (muscles of facial expression, second branchial arch), IX (stylopharyngeus muscle, third branchial arch), X (muscles of the soft palate and pharynx, fourth branchial arch), and XI (muscles of the larynx/sternocleido-mastoid/trapezius, sixth branchial arch) carry them.

Midbrain

93. What are the three anatomic subdivisions of the midbrain?

The midbrain can be divided into the tectum, regmentum, and cerebral crus. (See figure, next page.)

94. What is the quadrigeminal plate?

The quadrigeminal plate is formed by the tectum and the superior and inferior colliculi.

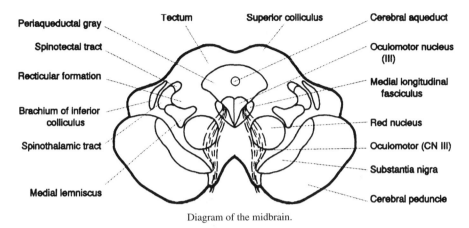

Diagram of the midbrain.

95. What is the substantia nigra?

The substantia nigra, a motor nucleus in the basal ganglia system, lies anterior to the tegmentum but posterior to the crus (pyramidal tract) in the midgrain.

96. Which disease affects the substantia nigra? What is the pathology?

The primary efferent neurotransmitter from the substantia nigra is dopamine. Parkinson's disease damages the substantia nigra. Pathologically, the neurons lose their melanin and the nucleus becomes depigmented. Many neurons also contain inclusion bodies called Lewy bodies.

97. What is the red nucleus?

The red nucleus is a globular mass located in the ventral portion of the tegmentum of the midbrain. It is a relay center for many of the efferent cerebellar tracts. The crossed fibers of the superior cerebellar peduncle pass through and around its edges.

98. What is the Edinger-Westphal nucleus?

The Edinger-Westphal nucleus, in the posterior midbrain, supplies parasympathetic fibers that terminate in the ciliary ganglion via cranial nerve III. It is mainly involved in pupillary constriction and the light accommodation reflex.

99. What is the function of cranial nerve III?

Cranial nerve III innervates all the extraocular muscles except for the lateral rectus and superior oblique. In innervates the medial rectus, superior rectus, inferior rectus, and inferior oblique muscles.

100. Where does cranial nerve III originate and exit the brainstem?

Cranial nerve III, the oculomotor nerve, exits the brainstem medially from the midbrain, between the posterior cerebral artery and the superior cerebellar artery.

101. What is the function of cranial nerve IV?

Cranial nerve IV, the trochlear nerve, innervates the superior oblique muscle.

102. What is the route of cranial nerve IV?

Cranial nerve IV travels posteriorly and medially, crosses the midline, wraps around the midbrain, and exits the brainstem laterally between the posterior cerebral artery and superior cerebellar artery. It has the longest intracranial route (approximately 7.5 cm) of any cranial nerve. It then travels through the cavernous sinus and enters the orbit through the superior orbital fissure. Because it crosses the midline, the right trochlear nerve innervates the left superior oblique muscle.

103. In a superior oblique palsy, which way would the patient tilt his or her head?

If the left superior oblique muscle is weak, then tilting the head to the right would reduce the diplopia, and tilting the head to the left would worsen the diplopia. So patients tilt their head away from the affected eye.

Pons

104. Which cranial nerves exit at the pontomedullary junction?

Cranial nerve VI exits medially and cranial nerves VII and VIII exit laterally.

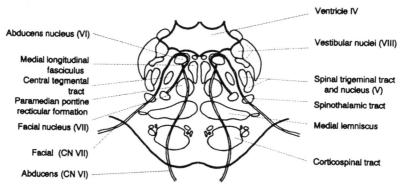

Anatomy of the pons.

105. Where does cranial nerve V exit the brainstem?

Cranial nerve V, the trigeminal nerve, exits the brainstem laterally at the mid-pons level. It divides into three main branches: V1 = ophthalmic; V2 = maxillary; and V3 = mandibular.

106. What are the four subdivisions of the trigeminal nucleus?

Mesencephalic nucleus (which is a nucleus
   of unipolar cell bodies similar to the
   dorsal root ganglion, with no synapse)

Chief sensory nucleus
Descending spinal nucleus
Motor nucleus

107. What type of information does cranial nerve V carry?

The trigeminal nerve carries sensation (general somatic afferent) from the anterior two-thirds of the face, and motor innervation (special visceral efferent) to the muscles of mastication (medial/lateral pterygoid, masseter, temporalis), the mylohyoid, anterior belly of the digastric, tensor tympani, and tensor palati.

108. What is the pathway by which sensation from the face reaches the cortex?

After cranial nerve V enters the brainstem, the afferent nerves split into two parts: those carrying dorsal column–type information and those carrying spinothalamic-type information. The former goes to the ipsilateral chief sensory nucleus of V (mid-pons) → synapse → enters the contralateral trigeminal lemniscus (which lies medial to the medial lemniscus) → VPM nucleus of the thalamus → synapse → through the posterior limb of the internal capsule to the postcentral gyrus. The pain-carrying fibers become the spinal tract of V → descend from mid-pons to lower medulla → synapse in the spinal nucleus of V → cross diffusely to form the contralateral trigeminal lemniscus (at mid-pons) → VPM nucleus of the thalamus → synapse → through the posterior limb of the internal capsule to the postcentral gyrus.

109. What is the function of cranial nerve VI?

Cranial nerve VI, the abducens nerve, abducts the eye.

110. What is the function of cranial nerve VII?

Cranial nerve VII, the facial nerve, innervates the muscles of facial expression (special visceral efferent), innervates the lacrimal, submandibular, sublingual, and parotid glands (general visceral efferent), supplies taste sensation to the anterior two-thirds of the tongue (special visceral afferent), and supplies sensation to the external ear (general somatic afferent).

111. How does the nucleus for cranial nerve VII receive higher cortical input?

The innervation to the muscles of facial expression can be separated into the muscles of the upper part of the face and the muscles of the lower part of the face. The supranuclear input responsible for the movement of the upper facial musculature is a bilateral input from the cortex to the nucleus. The supranuclear input responsible for the movement of the lower facial musculature is only a contralateral input from the cortex to the facial nucleus.

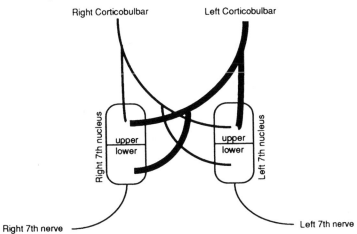

112. What is the difference between an upper motor neuron (central) and lower motor neuron (peripheral) facial weakness?

If the patient with a facial droop can move the upper facial muscles (i.e., wrinkle the forehead), the lesion is supranuclear on the contralateral side. The lesion is somewhere in the contralateral corticobulbar tracts above the facial nerve nucleus (e.g., in the crus or in the genu of the internal capsule). If the patient cannot voluntarily move any muscle involved in facial expression, either upper or lower facial musculature, the lesion is localized to the facial nucleus or the peripheral facial nerve on the ipsilateral side.

113. What is Möbius syndrome?

Möbius syndrome is congenital absence of both facial nerve nuclei, resulting in a facial diplegia. Patients also may have associated absence of the abducens nuclei.

114. What is the function of cranial nerve VIII?

Cranial nerve VIII, the vestibulocochlear nerve, has two functionally distinct sensory divisions: the vestibular nerve and the cochlear (or auditory) nerve. The vestibular nerve responds to position and movement of the head, serving functions often identified as equilibrium. The cochlear nerve mediates auditory functions.

Medulla

115. Which nerves exit in the postolivary fissure?

The glossopharyngeal nerve (cranial nerve IX), vagus nerve (cranial nerve X), and the spinal accessory nerve (cranial nerve XI) exit the brainstem in the postolivary fissure.

116. What is the nucleus ambiguus?

It is a cigar-shaped nucleus that lies in the depths of the medulla. It innervates the volitional muscles of the pharynx by way of both cranial nerves IX and X and the larynx (for phonation) via cranial nerve X. The larynx and pharynx have bilateral cortical input.

117. What is the nucleus solitarius?

It is the nucleus in the medulla that receives afferent information from the larynx (via cranial nerve X) and posterior pharynx and mediates the gag and cough reflexes (cranial nerves IX and X). Pain sensation from these areas enters the brainstem through cranial nerves IX and X but terminates in the descending spinal tract of the trigeminal nerve.

118. What is the salivatory nucleus?

The superior salivatory nucleus sends efferent autonomic fibers (general visceral efferent) through cranial nerve VII to innervate the lacrimal, submandibular, and sublingual glands as well as the mucous membranes of the nose and hard and soft palate. The inferior salivatory nucleus sends efferent autonomic fibers via cranial nerve IX to innervate the parotid gland.

119. What is the gustatory nucleus?

The gustatory nucleus is the nucleus in the medula that receives afferent sensory information for the sensation of taste. Taste from the anterior two-thirds of the tongue is innervated by the chorda tympani (cranial nerve VII), the posterior one-third of the tongue is innervated by cranial nerve IX, and the epiglottis is innervated by cranial nerve X.

120. Describe the function of cranial nerves IX and X (glossopharyngeal-vagal complex).

Cranial nerve IX (the glossopharyngeal nerve) and cranial nerve X (the vagus nerve) are usually considered together because of their overlapping functions. Both cranial nerves travel together intracranially, and both exit the cranial vault through the jugular foramen. The nucleus ambiguus innervates the volitional muscles of the pharynx through both cranial nerves IX and X, and the larynx via cranial nerve X. Sensation from the larynx enters the medulla via cranial nerve X to terminate in the nucleus solitarius. Taste fibers from the posterior one-third of the tongue travel via cranial nerve IX, and taste from the epiglottis via cranial nerve X. They terminate in the gustatory nucleus. Cranial nerve IX also supplies parasympathetic innervation to the parotid, originating in the inferior salivatory nucleus. Branches of cranial nerve X, the vagus nerve, continue beyond the larynx to innervate the heart, lungs, and abdominal viscera, providing primarily parasympathetic input.

121. What is the function of cranial nerve XI?

Cranial nerve XI, the spinal accessory nerve, is a small nerve of about 3500 motor fibers that arises from the upper cervical and lower medullary anterior horn cells and supplies the sternocleidomastoid and trapezius muscles. It exits the cranial vault via the jugular foramen.

122. What is the jugular foramen syndrome?

Because cranial nerves IX, X, and XI exit the cranial vault through the jugular foramen, the jugular foramen syndrome is a constellation of symptoms arising from a lesion (typically a tumor) at the level of the jugular foramen that compromises the function of these cranial nerves. Symptoms include loss of taste to the posterior two-thirds of the tongue; paralysis of the vocal cords, palate, and pharynx; and paralysis of the trapezius and sternocleidomastoid (SCM) muscles.

123. If the left spinal accessory nerve is cut, which functions are lost?

Because cranial nerve XI supplies the SCM and the trapezius, these muscles are weakened. Because the left SCM is involved in turning the head to the right, a lesion of the left cranial nerve XI results in an inability to turn the head to the right. The left trapezius also loses function, and the patient would not be able to shrug the left shoulder.

124. Which nerves exit in the preolivary fissure?

Cranial nerve XII, the hypoglossal nerve, exits the brainstem from the preolivary fissure.

125. If the left hypoglossal nucleus is injured, which way does the tongue deviate?

Lesioning the nucleus is similar to lesioning the peripheral nerve. The left hypoglossal nerve innervates the left tongue muscles, which, if acting alone, pushes the tongue to the right. The right hypoglossal nerve innervates the right tongue muscles, which, if acting alone, pushes the tongue to the left. Normally these muscles work together to push the tongue forward without deviation. If the left hypoglossal nucleus is lesioned, the right hypoglossal muscles act unopposed. The tongue thus deviates to the left, or, in other words, the tongue deviates toward the affected side.

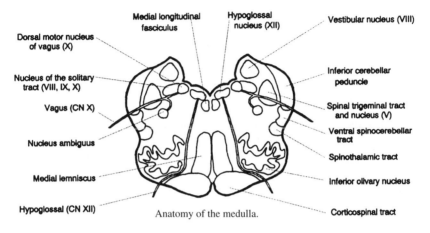

Anatomy of the medulla.

Breathing

126. Identify the disorders of respiration in a–d below. (Answers in caption)

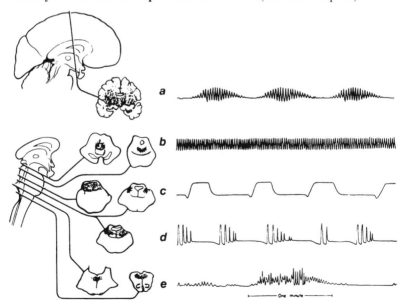

Diagram showing the location of lesions causing various characteristic patterns of respiration: a = Cheyne-Stokes; b = central neurogenic hyperventilation; c = apneustic; d = cluster; e = ataxis. (From Plum F, Posner J: The Diagnosis of Stupor and Coma, 3rd ed. Philadelphia, F.A. Davis, 1986, p 65, with permission.)

127. What is Cheyne-Stokes breathing? Where is the lesion that causes it?

Cheyne-Stokes breathing is a crescendo-decrescendo pattern of periodic breathing in which phases of hyperpnea regularly alternate with apnea. Cheyne-Stokes respirations are seen most often with lesions affecting both cerebral hemispheres.

128. What is central neurogenic hyperventilation? What causes it?

Central hyperventilation is a sustained, rapid, deep hyperpnea. It is produced by lesions in the low midbrain to upper one-third of the pons.

129. What is apneustic breathing? What causes it?

Apneusis is a prolonged respiratory cramp, a pause at full inspiration. Apneustic breathing may occur after damage to the mid or caudal pons.

130. What is cluster breathing? When does it occur?

Cluster breathing, a disorderly sequence of breaths with irregular pauses between the breaths, may result from damage to the lower pons or upper medulla.

131. What is ataxic breathing? Where is the lesion that causes it?

It is a completely irregular pattern of breathing in which both deep and shallow breaths occur randomly. The respiratory rate tends to be slow. The lesion that causes it is in the central medulla.

Posturing

132. What is decorticate posturing? What causes it?

Decorticate posturing is a stereotyped response to noxious stimuli. In the upper extremity, it consists of flexion of the arm, wrist, and fingers; in the lower extremity, of extension, internal rotation, and plantar flexion. Decorticate posturing most often occurs in comatose patients with lesions below the thalamus but above the red nucleus.

133. What is decerebrate posturing? In whom does it occur?

Decerebrate posturing is a stereotyped response to noxious stimuli. It consists of extension, adduction, and hyperpronation in the upper extremity and extension with plantar flexion in the lower extremity. Comatose patients with lesions below the red nucleus but above the vestibular nucleus may have decerebrate posturing.

Vestibular Apparatus

134. What are the five receptors of the vestibular apparatus, and what do they sense?

Three semicircular canals that are oriented 90° to each other sense rotational acceleration in all three planes. One horizontally oriented utricle and one vertically oriented saccule sense linear acceleration.

135. Where does the vestibular information synapse?

The vestibular nerve, carrying sensory data from the receptors, divides and synapses in four vestibular nuclei grouped together in the medulla: the superior, inferior, medial, and lateral vestibular nuclei.

136. What is the output from these nuclei?

The vestibulospinal tracts and the MLF are the two efferent tracts from the vestibular nuclei.

137. Where do the vestibulospinal tracts travel in the spinal cord?

The lateral vestibulospinal tract travels ventrolateral to the spinothalamic tract in the cord, whereas the medial vestibulospinal tract runs in the descending MLF.

138. Where do the vestibular nuclei project?

Vestibular nuclei project to (1) the oculomotor nuclei (cranial nerves III, IV, and VI), (2) cranial nerve XI, (3) cervical nuclei for head and neck position, (4) fastigial nuclei of the cerebellum, and (5) reticular formations of the brainstem.

139. What is the response of a normal person to cold water injected in the left ear?

Injecting cold water in to the left ear causes slow eye movements toward the left, followed by a fast phase of nystagmus back to the right.

140. What is the expected response of a comatose patient with an intact brainstem to cold water in the left ear?

The patient will have slow eye deviation toward the left ear. The fast phase nystagmus is absent.

Hearing

141. Which structures constitute the external ear? Middle ear? Inner ear?

The **external ear** is composed of the pinna, the external auditory canal, and the tympanic membrane. The **middle ear** is composed of the tympanic membrane, ossicles (malleus, incus, stapes), and oval window. The ossicles function as an impedance matching device between air and fluid during the travel of the sound wave. The **inner ear** is composed of part of the oval window, the cochlea, and the round window.

142. Which compartments of the cochlea are filled with perilymph?

- **Scala vestibuli.** It is separated from the scala tympani by Reissner's membrane.
- **Scala tympani.** It is separated from the scala media by the basilar membrane.
- **Scala media.** The third compartment is filled with endolymph and is located between Reissner's and the basilar membranes.

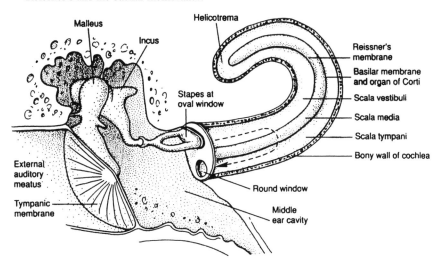

Anatomy of the hearing apparatus. (From Kandel E., Schwartz JH, Jessell TM (eds): Principles of Neuroscience, 3rd ed. New York, Elsevier, 1991, p 369, with permission.)

143. What is the pathway traveled by the cochlear fluid pressure wave initiated by a sound wave?

The stapes transmits the pressure to the round window and from it to the perilymph of the scala vestibuli, which, in turn, sets up vibrations of Reissner's membrane, resulting in a wave in the scala media. The basilar membranes move next and transmit the pressure to the scala tympani and from there to the oval window.

144. What is the arrangement of the neuroepithelial cells of the organ of Corti?

1. The outer hair cells (arranged in 3 rows) rest on the basilar membrane, with their stereocilia inserted into the tectorial membrane; these cells are able to contract and initiate the flow of endolymph toward the inner hair cells.

2. The inner hair cells (1 row) sit on the bone; they do not contract. These cells respond to the movement of endolymph and provide most of the afferent input to the spiral ganglion.

145. How does the organ of Corti serve as an audiofrequency analyzer?

The anatomic arrangement allows frequency analysis of sounds:

1. The basilar membrane responds to high frequencies at its base and to low frequencies at its apex.

2. The hair cells in the base of the cochlear duct have short and fat stereocilia, which are stimulated by high frequencies.

3. The hair cells in the apex of the cochlea have long and thin stereocilia, which respond best to low frequencies.

146. What is the anatomy of the auditory pathway?

Spiral ganglion → auditory nerve (cranial nerve VIII) → dorsal and ventral cochlear nuclei at the junction of the medulla and pons → trapezoid body (at this point 50% of the axons cross over to the other side) → superior olivary nucleus → lateral lemniscus → inferior colliculus → medial geniculate body → transverse gyrus of Heschl (area 41, partly buried in the sylvian fissure).

147. Apart from the main auditory pathway, where else does acoustic information travel?

The alternate pathways, which mediate acoustic reflexes, travel (1) to cranial nerves V and VII, (2) from the inferior colliculus to the motor centers, and (3) to the reticular activating system.

148. At what level is there crossing of information between the left and right ascending tracts?

The crossing of axons occurs on every level from the trapezoid body to the medial geniculate body.

149. To produce unilateral deafness, where could the lesion be?

The lesion must be at the cochlear nucleus or more peripheral, because of multiple crossovers above the cochlear nucleus.

150. What is Weber's test?

A vibrating tuning fork is placed in the middle of the forehead. In patients with conduction deafness, the sound is localized to the affected ear (bone > air conduction). In patients with sensorineural deafness, the signal is localized to the healthy ear.

151. What is Rinne's test?

A vibrating tuning fork is placed on the mastoid bone; when the patient can no longer hear it, it is removed and placed next to the ear. Thus, bone conduction is compared with air conduction. In conduction deafness, bone > air conduction. In sensorineural deafness, air > bone conduction.

152. What is the innervation of the external ear canal?

The external ear canal is supplied by cranial nerves V3, VII, IX, and X.

153. Damage to which structures results in hyperacusis?

1. **Facial nerve** (VII)—innervates the stapedius muscle, which retracts the stapes from the round window.

2. **Trigeminal nerve** (V)—supplies the tensor tympani, which inserts into the malleus and tenses the tympanic membrane, thus preventing it from vibrating.

154. What is the pathway for the feedback loop?

When auditory input reaches the superior olive, it sends signals to the olivocochlear bundle through the VIII nerve; the signals then terminate on the outer hair cells or afferent fibers in the spiral ganglia.

Eye Movements

155. What is the paramedian pontine reticular formation (PPRF)?

The PPRF is a collection of cells lying in the pons adjacent to the nucleus of cranial nerve VI, and is an important center for horizontal gaze. Efferent fibers from the PPRF project to the ipsilateral abducens (VI) nucleus, and to the contralateral oculomotor (III) nucleus through the MLF, stimulating both eyes to move horizontally.

156. What is the difference between saccades and smooth pursuit movements?

Saccades are fast conjugate eye movements that are under voluntary control. Saccades are generated in the contralateral frontal lobe (Brodmann's area 8). Smooth pursuits are slow involuntary movements of eyes fixed on a moving target. Pursuit movements to one side are generated in the ipsilateral occipital lobe (Brodmann's areas 18 and 19).

157. What is the pathway for saccades?

Fibers from the frontal eye field (Brodmann's area 8) pass through the genu of the internal capsule, decussate at the level of the upper pons, and synapse in the PPRF.

158. What is the pathway for smooth pursuit?

The pathway for smooth pursuit is not clearly defined but appears to arise in the anterior occipital lobe (Brodmann's areas 18 and 19) and travel to the ipsilateral PPRF.

159. What is the brainstem area for vertical gaze?

Near the superior colliculus, there are subtectal and pretectal centers that control vertical eye movements and project to cranial nuclei III, IV, and VI.

160. What are the pathways for voluntary vertical eye movements?

Vertical movements are driven symmetrically from both frontal lobes. When activated bilaterally, fibers from Brodmann's area 8 project via the frontopontine tract to act upon bilateral cranial nuclei III, IV, and VI, which then innervate their respective muscles.

CEREBELLUM

161. Describe the anatomic divisions of the cerebellum.

The cerebellum is anatomically divided into the two hemispheres, the midline vermis, and the flocculonodulus. (See diagram, p. 127.)

162. What are the functions of each cerebellar "lobe"?

The hemispheres are involved in appendicular control, the vermis is involved in axial control, and the flocculonodular lobe is involved in vestibular balance.

163. What are the three layers of the cerebellar cortex?

Outermost molecular cell layer
Middle Purkinje cell layer
Innermost granular cell layer.

164. What types of cells are located in each of these layers?

The **molecular layer** contains (1) stellate cells, (2) basket cells, (3) dendrites of Purkinje cells, (4) dendrites of Golgi type II cells, and (5) axons of granule cells. The **Purkinje layer** contains the cell bodies of Purkinje cells. The **granular layer** contains (6) granule cells, (7) Golgi type II cells, and (8) glomeruli (synaptic complexes that contain mossy fibers, axons and dendrites of Golgi type II cells, and dendrites of granule cells.)

165. What is the afferent fiber from the inferior olives? Through which peduncle does it reach the cerebellum?
The afferent fiber from the inferior olives is the climbing fiber. It enters the cerebellum through the inferior cerebellar peduncle.

166. What is Mollaret's triangle?
Mollaret's triangle is a physiologic connection between the red nucleus, inferior olives, and dentate nucleus of the cerebellum. A lesion in this pathway can cause palatal myoclonus.

167. What are the deep nuclei of the cerebellum (medial to lateral)?
Medial to lateral, the cerebellar deep nuclei are fastigial, globus, emboliform, and dentate.

168. What are the primary inputs and outputs of the cerebellum?
Cerebellar function can be conceptualized as a feedback loop, with input arriving from an origin, synapsing in a cerebellar nucleus, and then projecting back, often to the same origin.

Cerebellar Connections

CEREBELLAR PEDUNCLE	CONNECTED TO:	TRACTS THAT RUN IN THE PEDUNCLE
Superior (SCP)	Midbrain	Dentatorubrothalamic (DRT) and ventral spinocerebellar (VSC)
Middle (MCP)	Pons	Corticopontocerebellar
Inferior (ICP)	Medulla	All other tracts to/from the cerebellum

ORIGIN	INFLOW TRACT	INFLOW PEDUNCLE	CEREBELLAR NUCLEUS	OUTFLOW PEDUNCLE	OUTFLOW TRACT	DESTINATION
Precentral gyrus	CPC	MCP	Dentate	SCP	DRT	Precentral gyrus
Spinal cord	SC	ICP	Fastigial	ICP	—	Vestibular nucleus
Vestibular nucleus	VC	ICP	Vestibular	ICP	LVS (MLF)	Spinal cord

Superior cerebellar peduncle = SCP; middle cerebellar peduncle = MCP; inferior cerebellar peduncle = ICP; corticopontocerebellar = CPC; spinocerebellar = SC; vestibulocerebellar = VC; lateral vestibulospinal = LVS; and medial longitudinal fasciculus = MLF.

169. Where do the frontopontocerebellar fibers travel in the internal capsule?
They travel in the anterior limb of the internal capsule.

170. Where do the frontopontocerebellar fibers synapse?
The fibers synapse in the mid-pons prior to decussating.

171. What type of fiber originating in the cerebellar cortex is inhibitory on the deep cerebellar nuclei?
Purkinje fibers originate in the cerebellar cortex and synapse on the deep nuclei as an inhibitory neuron.

172. Where does the dentatorubrothalamic tract synapse?
These fibers synapse in the ventrolateral (VL) nucleus of the thalamus before ascending to the cortex.

BASAL GANGLIA

173. What are the basal ganglia?
   The basal ganglia are a collection of nuclei, largely concerned with motor control, composed primarily of the corpus striatum, and the lenticular complex. (See diagram, p. 137.)

174. What are the parts of the corpus striatum?
   The corpus striatum is composed of the putamen and caudate.

175. What is the lenticular complex?
   The lenticular complex, or lentiform nucleus, is composed of the globus pallidus and putamen.

176. Which structure is the lateral border of the caudate?
   The anterior limb of the internal capsule is the lateral border of the caudate.

177. What is the major outflow of the basal ganglia?
   The major outflow of the basal ganglia projects from the medial globus pallidus as a fiber bundle known as the lenticular fasciculus (Forel's field H2). Another bundle from the medial globus pallidus loops around the internal capsule as the ansa lenticularis. It then merges in Forel's field H with the lenticular fasciculus and with fibers from the dentatorubrothalamic tract. These fibers then continue as the thalamic fasciculus (Forel's field H1) and synapse in the thalamic nuclei: centromedian, ventral lateral, and ventral anterior. These thalamic nuclei then relay information up to the motor cortex.

178. Is there any other output from the medial globus pallidus?
   Yes. Apart from the lenticular fasciculus and the ansa lenticularis, a third fiber tract leaves the medial globus pallidus as the pallidotegmental tract and descends onto the pedunculopontine nucleus in the midbrain, where neurons help to regulate posture. This is the only descending tract from the basal ganglia.

179. Is there any output from the basal ganglia that does not originate in the medial globus pallidus?
   The only other output is a small tract (pallidosubthalamic fibers) that leaves the lateral globus pallidus to synapse in the subthalamic nucleus.

180. What is the major input to the basal ganglia?
   The major input is from the motor cortex and the thalamic nuclei. The basal ganglia function, simplistically, as a feedback loop: cerebral cortex → basal ganglia → thalamus → cerebral cortex.

THALAMUS

181. What structure lies lateral to the thalamus? Medial to the thalamus?
   The posterior limb of the internal capsule is the lateral border of the thalamus. The third ventricle lies medial to the thalamus.

182. What are the anatomic structures encountered by going medial to the lateral starting from the massa intermedia?
   Massa intermedia → thalamus → posterior limb of the internal capsule → globus pallidus → putamen → external capsule → extreme capsule

183. What is the anatomy of the thalamus?
   The intermedullary lamina divides the thalamus into an anterior, medial, and lateral group. The lateral group is further divided into a ventral and dorsal tier. Each group contains specific nuclei:

Anterior group: Anterior nucleus
Medial group: Dorsomedial nucleus (DM)
Lateral group: Dorsal tier
                  Lateral dorsal nucleus (LD)
                  Lateral posterior nucleus (LP)
                  Pulvinar
             Ventral tier
                  Ventral anterior nucleus (VA)
                  Ventral lateral nucleus (VL)
                  Ventral posterolateral nucleus (VPL)
                  Ventral posteromedial nucleus (VPM)
                  Lateral geniculate (LG)
                  Medial geniculate (MG)

    Other nuclei that are often considered part of the thalamus include (1) **reticular nucleus**—a small group of neurons that projects to other thalamic nuclei and may help regulate cortical activity; (2) **midline nuclei**—diffuse neurons connected to the hypothalamus; and (3) **centromedian (CM)**—an intralaminar nucleus that is part of the reticular formation which activates the cortex.

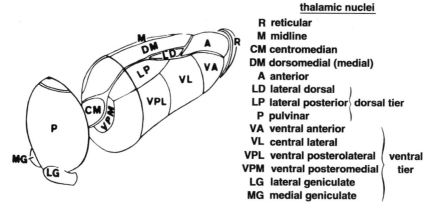

thalamic nuclei

R reticular
M midline
CM centromedian
DM dorsomedial (medial)
A anterior
LD lateral dorsal ⎫
LP lateral posterior⎬ dorsal tier
P pulvinar ⎭
VA ventral anterior ⎫
VL central lateral ⎪
VPL ventral posterolateral ⎬ ventral
VPM ventral posteromedial ⎪ tier
LG lateral geniculate ⎪
MG medial geniculate ⎭

Diagram of the major nuclei of the thalamus. (From Dunkerley GB: A Basic Atlas of the Human Nervous System. Philadelphia, F.A. Davis, 1975, p 89, with permission.)

184. What are the inputs to and from the main thalamic nuclei?

Connections of the Thalamic Nuclei

THALAMIC NUCLEUS	PRINCIPAL INPUT	PRINCIPAL OUTPUT	FUNCTION
LP	Parietal lobe	Parietal lobe	Sensory integration
LD	Cingulate gyrus	Cingulate gyrus	Emotional expression
Pulvinar	Association areas of cortex	Association areas of cortex	Sensory integration
DM	Amygdala, olfactory, and hypothalamus	Prefrontal cortex	Limbic
MG	Auditory relay nuclei (from inf. colliculus)	Auditory cortex-area 41,42	Hearing
LG	Optic tract	Visual cortex-area 17	Vision
Anterior	Mammillary body	Cingulate gyrus	Limbic
VA	Globus pallidus	Premotor cortex	Motor

(Table continued on following page.)

Connections of the Thalamic Nuclei (Continued)

THALAMIC NUCLEUS	PRINCIPAL INPUT	PRINCIPAL OUTPUT	FUNCTION
VL	Cerebellum	Premotor and motor cortices	Motor
VPM	Trigeminal lemniscus	Post central gyrus	Somatic sensation (face)
VPL	Medial lemniscus and spinothalamic	Post central gyrus	Somatic integration (body)
CM	Reticular formation, globus pallidus, hypothalamus	Basal ganglia (striatum)	Sensory integration, smell, limbic

185. What is the limbic lobe?

The limbic lobe is not a true lobe of the brain but rather a functional collection of structures that regulate higher activities such as memory and emotion. It is commonly said to include (1) cingulate gyrus, (2) parahippocampal gyrus, (3) hippocampal gyrus, and (4) uncus.

186. What is Papez's circuit?

This is a route by which the limbic system communicates between the hippocampus, thalamus, hypothalamus, and cortex. It forms a circuit from the hippocampal formation → fornix → mammillary body → mammillothalamic tract → anterior group of thalamus → cingulate gyrus → cingulate bundle → hippocampus (**Note:** the amygdala is not part of the classic Papez circuit).

OLFACTION

187. What are the olfactory receptor cells?

The receptor cells are bipolar neurons that pass from the olfactory mucosa through the cribiform plate to the olfactory bulb. Collectively, the central processes of the olfactory receptor cells constitute cranial nerve I.

188. What is the anatomy of the olfactory pathway?

1. In the olfactory bulb, the axons of receptor cells synapse on dendrites of mitral and tufted cells (forming a glomerulus).

2. The axons of mitral and tufted cells compose the olfactory tract, which soon divides into medial and lateral stria. Medial stria fibers cross to the contralateral side via the anterior commissure, while the lateral stria fibers terminate in the anterior perforated substance, amygdaloid complex and lateral olfactory gyrus (which is the primary olfactory cortex).

3. From the lateral olfactory gyrus (prepiriform area), fibers project to the entorhinal cortex, the medial dorsal nucleus of the thalamus, and the hypothalamus.

189. What is unique about the projection of olfactory information to the cerebral cortex?

Unlike other sensory modalities, olfaction reaches the cortex without relay through the thalamus.

190. What are the most common causes of anosmia?

1. Rhinitis/nasal congestion
2. Smoking
3. Head injury
4. Craniotomy
5. Subarachnoid hemorrhage
6. Meningiomas of the olfactor groove
7. Zinc and vitamin A deficiency
8. Hypothyroidism
9. Congenital (Kallmann's syndrome)
10. Dementing diseases (Alzheimer's, Parkinson's)
11. Multiple sclerosis

VISION

191. What is the arrangement of cones and rods in the retina?
The six million cones are concentrated toward the center and the 120 million rods are in the periphery of the retina. In the fovea, located centrally within the macula, each cone is served by a single ganglion cell, resulting in very high resolution. In the periphery, many rods project to a single ganglion cell, giving high sensitivity but lower resolution.

192. What are the primary functions of rods?
Rods are concerned with night vision and are most sensitive between the blue and green wavelengths.

193. What are the primary functions of cones?
Cones are concerned with color vision and daytime vision. The three types of cones are tuned, via visual pigments, to different frequencies in the blue, green, and red wavelength ranges.

194. What is the afferent pathway for the pupillary light reflex?
Retinal ganglion cells concerned with the light reflex travel with the optic nerve and tract and then break away to project down to the midbrain pretectal nucleus. From the pretectal nucleus, fibers project bilaterally, decussating via the posterior commissure to each Edinger-Westphal nucleus.

195. Which nucleus mediates pupil constriction?
The Edinger-Westphal nucleus, or preganglionic parasympathetic nucleus of cranial nerve III, mediates pupillary constriction.

196. What is the pathway for pupillary dilatation?
This pathway has three neurons. First-order fibers descend from the ipsilateral hypothalamus through the brainstem and cervical cord to T1–T2. They synapse on ipsilateral preganglionic sympathetic fibers, exit the cord, travel up the sympathetic chain as second-order neurons to the superior cervical ganglion, and then synapse on postganglionic sympathetic fibers. The third-order neurons travel via the internal carotid artery to the orbit and innervate the radial smooth muscle of the iris.

197. What is Horner's syndrome?
Horner's syndrome is an interruption of the sympathetic supply to the eye, resulting in the classic triad of ptosis, miosis, and anhydrosis.

198. Describe the pharmacologic tests to diagnose Horner's syndrome.
Instill 2% cocaine solution in both eyes, which dilates the pupils by preventing the reuptake of the sympathetic neurotransmitter norepinephrine. If one eye fails to dilate, a diagnosis of Horner's syndrome can be made, because failure to dilate indicates an interruption of the sympathetic supply (norepinephrine) to that eye. To further localize the lesion, one can use amphetamine in the affected eye, which displaces norepinephrine from the nerve terminal and dilates the pupil. If the pupil dilates in response to this test, the lesion affects the third-order neuron, causing denervation hypersensitivity. Otherwise, the lesion is in the first- or second-order neurons.

199. What is the anatomy of the lesion that causes an afferent pupillary defect?
An afferent pupillary defect means the pupil will not react to light. The lesion must be prechiasmal and almost always involves the optic nerve.

200. What is the test for an afferent pupillary defect (Marcus Gunn pupil)?
The swinging flashlight test determines an afferent pupillary defect. Shine a light into the normal eye and the pupil constricts (the affected eye also constricts consensually). Quickly move the light onto the opposite affected eye, and the pupil dilates. Removing the light from the normal

pupil causes it and the affected pupil, responding consensually, to dilate. The affected pupil thus seems to dilate when the swinging light hits it.

201. What is the value of the pupillary reflex for diagnosing third-nerve palsies?

Because the parasympathetic fibers travel along the outside of the third nerve, they are usually damaged by nerve compression, resulting in pupillary dilatation. Third-nerve palsies that cause pupillary dilatation are usually masses (e.g., tumors, aneurysms), whereas palsies that do not involve the pupil are usually medical (e.g., ischemia, vasculitis).

202. What is the pathway for pupillary constriction that occurs with convergence?

The pathway begins in the occipital lobe (Brodmann's area 18) and projects to the Edinger-Westphal nucleus bilaterally. The details of how pupils constrict during convergence are poorly understood.

203. What is an Argyll Robertson pupil?

An Argyll Robertson pupil, one form of light-near dissociation, is an irregular pupil that does not constrict to light but does constrict to accommodation. This finding is quite specific for CNS syphilis. Light-near dissociation with a regular pupil can be found in many diseases and is not specific for CNS syphilis.

204. What is the pathway of the optic nerve?

The ganglion cells from the nasal half of the retina travel in the optic nerve, where they decussate in the optic chiasm and join the contralateral optic tract to the lateral geniculate body. The ganglion cells from the temporal half of the retina travel in the optic nerve, stay in the ipsilateral optic tract, and project to the lateral geniculate body. Thus, the contralateral visual field is projected from each eye to the lateral geniculate body.

205. What thalamic nucleus is concerned with vision?

The lateral genicular body is the thalamic nucleus that handles vision.

206. What is the pathway of the optic radiation?

Second-order neurons from the lateral geniculate body project to the calcarine cortex (Brodmann's area 17). The superior visual field fibers wrap around the temporal horn on their way to the inferior lip of the calcarine fissure. The macular area is served by the most medial area of the calcarine cortex.

Visual Fields

207. Where is the lesion that causes a field defect in only one eye?

If only one eye is affected, the lesion must be prechiasmal.

208. Where is the lesion that causes left homonymous hemianopsia? Bitemporal hemianopsia? Binasal hemianopsia?

Left homonymous hemianopsia can arise from the right optic tract, right lateral geniculate body, right optic radiations, or the right occipital cortex. **Bitemporal hemianopsia** is caused by midline chiasmal lesions such as pituitary lesions (from below) or craniopharyngeal tumors (from above). **Binasal hemianopsia** can be caused only by simultaneous lesions on the lateral optic nerves or chiasm, such as bilateral internal carotid artery aneurysms.

209. What is a junctional scotoma?

A junctional scotoma results from a lesion at the junction of the optic nerve and chiasm. It causes an ipsilateral central scotoma and a superior temporal defect in the other eye. It occurs because some optic nerve fibers from the inferior temporal retina, when they decussate in the chiasm, travel forward for a few millimeters in the contralateral nerve; they are thus affected by a lesion in that nerve.

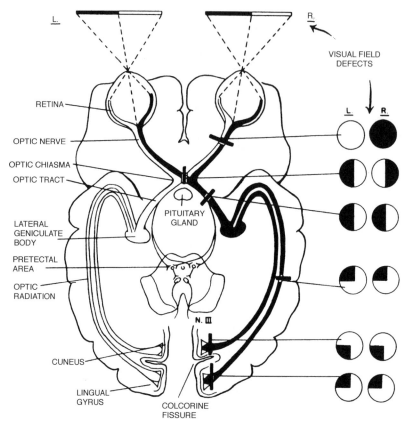

Diagram of the visual system showing the location of lesions responsible for the most common visual field defects. (From Gilman S, Newman SW: Manter and Gatz's Essentials of Clinical Neuroanatomy and Neurophysiology, 5th ed. Philadelphia, F.A. Davis, 1978, p 113, with permission.)

210. Where is the lesion that causes superior quadrantanopsia?

Superior quadrantanopsia usually results from damage to the inferior optic radiations. This may occur in Meyer's loop, which is the bundle of inferior optic radiations that swings forward into the temporal lobe.

211. What visual field results from a right occipital lobe infarction?

A right occipital lobe infarction causes a left homonymous hemianopsia with macular sparing.

CORTEX

212. What are the layers of the cerebral cortex?

The layers of the cerebral cortex are

      I. Molecular layer   IV. Inner granular layer
      II. Outer granular layer   V. Inner pyramidal or ganglion layer
     III. Outer pyramidal layer   VI. Multiform layer

Afferent fibers activated by various sensory stimuli terminate in layers IV, III, and II. These signals are then transmitted to adjacent superficial and deep layers through multiple interconnections. All the efferent fibers originate in layer V.

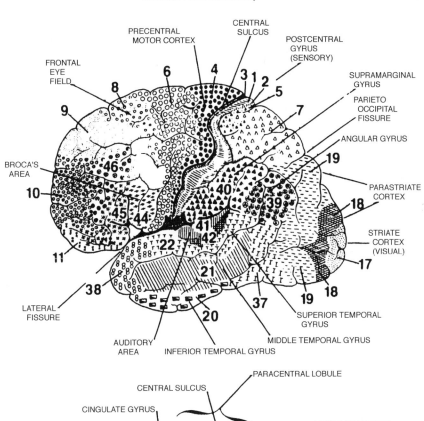

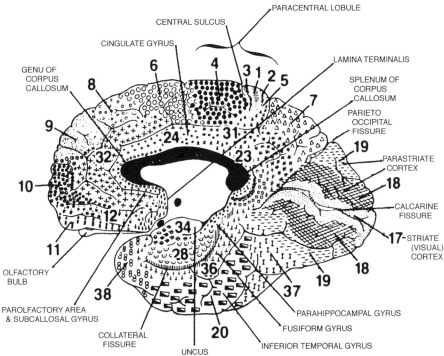

The superficial anatomy of the cerebral cortex showing Brodmann's areas. (From Garoutte B: Survey of Functional Neuroanatomy, 2nd ed. Greenbrae, CA, Jones Medical Publications, 1992, p 144, with permission.)

213. What is the columnar organization of the cortex?

Cortical neurons are arranged in cylindrical columns, each containing 100–300 neurons, which are heavily interconnected up and down through the cortical layers. Throughout the somatosensory system, cells responding to one modality are grouped together in the columns. All neurons in the column receive input from the same area and therefore comprise an elementary functional module of cortex.

214. What is the line of Gennari?

The fourth layer of the occipital cortex in area 17 is divided by a greatly thickened band of myelinated fibers, which is grossly visible and is called the line of Gennari. This stripe also gives the name of striate cortex to that area of the brain. Brodmann's areas 18 and 19 lack the line of Gennari.

215. In what cortical cell layer are the Betz cells located?

Betz cells give rise to efferent motor tracts (corticospinal fibers) and lie in cortical layer V.

216. What is the function of the frontal lobe?

The frontal lobes (both right and left) are involved in voluntary eye movements, somatic motor control, planning and sequencing of movements, and emotional affect. The left frontal lobe is crucial for motor control of speech (Broca's area).

217. What is the function of the temporal lobe?

The temporal lobes (both right and left) handle auditory and visual perception, learning and memory, emotional affect, and olfaction. The dominant temporal lobe influences comprehension of speech (Wernicke's area). The nondominant temporal lobe mediates prosody and spatial relationships.

218. What is the function of the parietal lobe?

The parietal lobes (both right and left) handle cortical sensation, motor control, and visual perception. The dominant parietal lobe also handles ideomotor praxis. The nondominant parietal lobe controls spatial orientation.

219. What is the function of the occipital lobe?

The occipital lobes (both right and left) mainly handle visual perception and involuntary smooth pursuit eye movements.

220. In which lobe is visual-spatial information processed?

It is mainly processed in the nondominant parietal lobe.

221. Where is language processed?

Language is primarily processed in Broca's area (posterior inferior frontal gyrus, Brodmann's area 44) and Wernicke's area (posterior part of the superior temporal gyrus, posterior part of Brodmann's area 22), in the dominant hemisphere.

222. Where is the lesion that causes achromatopsia (inability to match colors and hues)?

Achromatopsia results from a lesion of the dominant occipital lobe (Brodmann's area 18) and is a feature of the syndrome of alexia without agraphia.

223. What is Exner's area?

Exner's area lies superior to Broca's area, in Brodmann's area 8; if damaged, agraphia without aphasia results.

CIRCULATION

224. What is meant by the terms anterior and posterior circulation?

The anterior circulation refers to the common carotid and its distal ramifications, including the internal carotid, middle cerebral, and anterior cerebral arteries. The posterior circulation refers to the vertebral and basilar arteries and their branches, including the posterior cerebral artery.

225. Which vessels make up the circle of Willis?

1. The **anterior circulation**, composed of the middle cerebral arteries, anterior cerebral arteries, and the anterior communicating artery which connects the two anterior cerebral arteries.

2. The **posterior circulation**, composed of the posterior cerebral arteries.

3. The **posterior communicating artery**, which connects the middle cerebral with the posterior cerebral arteries, thus forming a true circle.

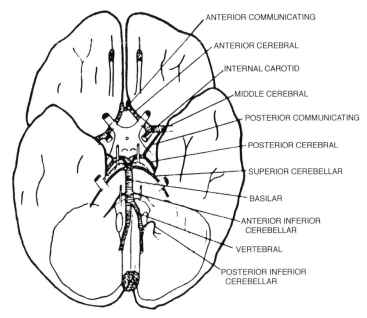

Diagram of the blood vessels that form the circle of Willis at the base of the brain. (From Garoutte B: Survey of Functional Neuroanatomy, 2nd ed. Greenbrae, CA, Jones Medical Publications, 1992, p 15, with permission.)

226. If the right anterior cerebral artery is occluded proximally, how does the circle of Willis protect the patient from becoming symptomatic?

If the occlusion is slow enough for the blood flow to accommodate, the right anterior cerebral artery receives blood from the contralateral internal carotid, via the left anterior cerebral and anterior communicating arteries.

227. What region is supplied by the anterior cerebral artery? Middle cerebral artery? Posterior cerebral artery?

The **anterior cerebral artery** supplies the medial (midline) cerebral hemispheres, superior frontal lobes, and superior parietal lobes. The **middle cerebral artery** supplies the inferior frontal, inferolateral parietal, and lateral temporal lobes. The **posterior cerebral artery** supplies the occipital lobes and medial temporal lobes.

228. What is the first intracranial branch off of the internal carotid artery?
The ophthalmic artery.

229. What is the blood supply to the deep brain nuclei?
The basal ganglia are supplied by small lenticulostriate arteries arising from the middle cerebral artery, whereas the thalamus is supplied by perforating thalamogeniculate arteries from the posterior cerebral artery. The blood supply of the thalamus comes from the posterior circulation.

230. What is the name of the artery that supplies the genu of the internal capsule?
The recurrent artery of Heubner, which is one of the named anteromedial lenticulostriate arteries, supplies the genu of the internal capsule.

231. Which artery is the first branch off of the basilar artery?
The anterior inferior cerebral artery (AICA).

232. What is the blood supply to the brainstem?
The brainstem receives its blood supply exclusively from the posterior circulation, including the vertebrals and basilar artery. The medulla receives its blood supply from the vertebrals via medial and lateral perforating arteries. The pons and midbrain receive their blood from the basilar via the medial and lateral perforating arteries.

233. What is the blood supply to the cerebellum?
The cerebellum receives its blood supply from the three cerebellar vessels:
1. Posterior inferior cerebellar artery (PICA), off of the vertebrals.
2. Anterior inferior cerebellar artery (AICA), the first branch off of the basilar.
3. Superior cerebellar artery (SCA), the last branch off of the basilar.

234. Which nerves exit the brainstem area between the posterior cerebral artery and superior cerebellar artery?
Cranial nerve III exits between the vessels medially, whereas cranial nerve IV exits between them laterally. Aneurysms of these blood vessels may thus damage these cranial nerves.

CEREBROSPINAL FLUID (CSF)

235. What anatomic structure or structures produce CSF?
The majority of CSF is produced by the choroid plexus. A small amount of CSF is also produced by the blood vessels in the subependymal region and pia.

236. Where is the choroid plexus located?
The choroid plexus is located within the ventricular system, mainly in the lateral and fourth ventricles.

237. What is the rate of CSF production?
The rate is approximately 25 cc/hr (approximately 500 cc/day).

238. How much CSF does an average adult normally have?
The average male adult has approximately 100–150 cc of CSF.

239. What is communicating hydrocephalus? Noncommunicating hydrocephalus?
Communicating hydrocephalus occurs when there is dilatation of the ventricles due to obstruction of CSF flow outside the ventricular system (i.e., distal to the foramen of Magendie), so the CSF communicates with the subarachnoid space. Noncommunicating hydrocephalus occurs when there is dilatation of the ventricles due to an obstruction of CSF flow within the ventricular system at or above the foramen of Magendie.

240. What is the route of CSF from production to clearance?

Choroid plexus → lateral ventricle → interventricular foramen of Monro → third ventricle → cerebral aqueduct of Sylvius → fourth ventricle → two lateral foramina of Luschka and one medial foramen of Magendie → subarachnoid space → arachnoid granulations → dural sinus → venous drainage.

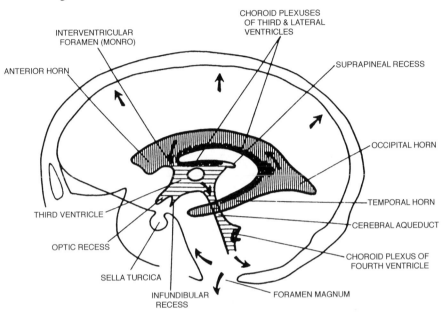

Diagram of cerebrospinal fluid. (From Garoutte B: Survey of Functional Neuroanatomy, 2nd ed. Greenbrae, CA, Jones Medical Publications, 1992, p 27, with permission.)

241. What space is invaded by a lumbar puncture?

During a lumbar puncture, the needle enters the subarachnoid space.

242. What is the ideal spinal level to do a lumbar puncture?

The ideal level for a lumbar puncture is below the conus medullaris at approximately vertebral level L4–L5.

BIBLIOGRAPHY

1. Carpenter D: Human Neuroanatomy, 8th ed. New York, Macmillan, 1990.
2. Garoutte B: Survey of Functional Neuroanatomy, 2nd ed. Greenbrae, CA, Jones Medical Publications, 1992.
3. Gilman S, Newman SW: Manter and Gatz's Essentials of Clinical Neuroanatomy and Neurophysiology, 9th ed. Philadelphia, F.A. Davis, 1996.
4. Kandel E, Schwartz JH, Jessell TM (eds): Principles of Neuroscience, 3rd ed. New York, Elsevier, 1991.
5. Patten JP: Neurological Differential Diagnosis, 2nd ed. London, Springer, 1996.
6. Plum F, Posner J: The Diagnosis of Stupor and Coma, 3rd ed. Philadelphia, F.A. Davis, 1986.
7. Tindall B: Aids to the Examination of the Peripheral Nervous System. London, W.B. Saunders, 1990.
Websites
www.anatomy.wisc.edu
www.bethisraelny.org/inn/anatomy/anatomy.html
www.lib.uchicago.edu/hw/neuroanatomy

3. APPROACH TO THE PATIENT WITH NEUROLOGIC DISEASE

Loren A. Rolak, M.D.

1. What is the first question to be answered in any patient with neurologic disease?

Where is the lesion? The neurologist, unlike most other physicians, approaches patients from an anatomic perspective, leaving issues of physiology and etiology to be addressed later. The first step in evaluating patients with neurologic symptoms is to localize the lesion to a specific part of the nervous system.

2. What is the best way to localize a lesion?

The history and physical examination accurately localize most lesions of the nervous system. The brain is unique among organs for its high degree of specialization. Because each part of the peripheral nerves, spinal cord, and brain have such specialized functions, damage to each region produces unique clinical effects. Identification of specific signs and symptoms, therefore, permits localization, sometimes within a millimeter, to discrete parts of the nervous system. Pioneer neurologists of the past century referred to the brain as "eloquent"—it speaks directly to the clinician.

3. What are the most important regions for anatomic localization?

For clinical purposes, the great complexity of neuroanatomy can be simplified to a few major regions. Lesions should be localized to one of the following regions:

1. Muscle	4. Root	7. Cerebellum
2. Neuromuscular junction	5. Spinal cord	8. Subcortical brain
3. Peripheral nerve	6. Brainstem	9. Cortical brain

4. How are symptoms localized to these neuroanatomic regions?

The history is the most important part of the neurologic evaluation of a patient. Although precise localizing information can be gleaned from the neurologic physical examination, asking the proper questions during the history accurately localizes most neurologic lesions.

A helpful system for diagnosis is to begin distally and ask patients questions about each part of the neurologic anatomy, working proximally through the muscle, neuromuscular junction, peripheral nerve, root, spinal cord, cerebellum, brainstem, and subcortex and ending with the cortex of the brain. By sequentially asking about each of these areas, the patient can be "examined" thoroughly. If localization of the lesion is still not clear after a careful history directed at each anatomic region, do not begin the physical examination yet—go back and take a better history.

5. Which clinical features of muscle disease can be elicited by history?

Muscle disease (myopathy) causes proximal symmetric weakness without sensory loss. Questions, therefore, should elicit these symptoms.

1. **Proximal leg weakness:** Can the patient get out of a car, off the toilet, or up from a chair without using the hands?

2. **Proximal arm weakness:** Can the patient lift or carry objects such as grocery bags, garbage bags, young children, school books, or briefcases?

3. **Symmetric weakness:** Does the weakness affect both arms or both legs? (Although generalized processes such as myopathies are often slightly asymmetric, weakness confined to one limb or one side of the body is seldom caused by a myopathy.)

4. **Normal sensation:** Is there numbness or other sensory loss? (Although pain and cramping may occur in some myopathies, actual sensory changes should not occur with any disease that is confined to the muscle.)

6. After a history of muscle disease is elicited, what findings can be expected on physical examination?

The examination should show proximal symmetric weakness without sensory loss. The muscles are usually normal in size, without atrophy or fasciculations, and muscle tone is usually normal or mildly decreased. Reflexes are also normal or mildly decreased.

7. Which clinical features of neuromuscular junction disease can be elicited by history?

Fatigability is the hallmark of diseases affecting the neuromuscular junction. Although these disorders resemble myopathies, causing proximal symmetric weakness without sensory loss, the weakness worsens with use and recovers with rest. Because strength improves with rest, fatigability does not usually manifest as a steadily progressive decline in function; rather, it presents as waxing and waning weakness. When the muscles fatigue, the patient must rest, leading to recovery of strength, which permits further use of the muscles, causing fatigue, which necessitates rest and recovery again. This cycle of worsening with use and recovery with rest produces a variability or fluctuation in strength that is highly characteristic of neuromuscular junction diseases.

8. After a history of neuromuscular junction problems is elicited, what findings can be expected on physical examination?

Examination should show fatigable proximal symmetric weakness without sensory loss. Repetitive testing weakens the muscles, which regain their strength after a brief period of rest. Sustained muscular activity also may lead to fatigability, such as the development of ptosis with persistent upward gaze. The weakness is often extremely proximal, involving muscles of the face, eyes, and jaw. The muscles are normal in size, without atrophy or fasciculations, with normal tone and reflexes. There is no sensory loss.

9. Which clinical features of peripheral neuropathies can be elicited by history?

Unlike myopathies and neuromuscular junction disease, weakness caused by peripheral neuropathies is often distal rather than proximal. It is also often asymmetric and accompanied by atrophy and fasciculations. Sensory changes almost always accompany neuropathies. The history should elicit these symptoms:

1. **Distal leg weakness:** Does the patient trip, drag the feet, or wear out the toes of shoes?
2. **Distal arm weakness:** Does the patient frequently drop things or have trouble with the grip?
3. **Asymmetric weakness:** Are the symptoms confined to one localized area? (Some neuropathies cause a symmetric stocking-and-glove weakness and numbness, especially those due to metabolic conditions such as diabetes. However, most neuropathies are asymmetric.)
4. **Denervation changes:** Is there a wasting or shrinkage of the muscle (atrophy) or quivering and twitching within the muscle (fasciculations)?
5. **Sensory changes:** Has the patient felt numbness, tingling, or paresthesias?

10. After a history of peripheral neuropathy is elicited, what findings can be expected on physical examination?

Examination should reveal distal, often asymmetric weakness with atrophy, fasciculations, and sensory loss. Muscle tone may be normal but is often decreased. Reflexes are usually diminished. Because involvement of autonomic fibers is common in peripheral neuropathies, trophic changes, such as smooth, shiny skin, vasomotor changes (e.g., swelling or temperature dysregulation), and loss of hair or nails, may occur.

11. Which clinical features of root diseases (radiculopathies) can be elicited by history?

Pain is the hallmark of root disease. Otherwise, radiculopathies often resemble peripheral neuropathies because of their asymmetric weakness with evidence of denervation (atrophy and fasciculations) and sensory loss. The weakness, while asymmetric, may be either proximal or distal, depending on which roots are involved. (The most common radiculopathies in the legs affect the L5 and S1 roots, causing distal weakness, whereas the most common radiculopathies in the arms affect the C5 and C6 roots, which innervate proximal regions.) The history, therefore, should elicit symptoms similar to a neuropathy with the added component of pain. The pain is usually described as sharp, stabbing, hot, and electric, and it typically shoots or radiates down the limb.

12. After a history of a radiculopathy is elicited, what findings can be expected on physical examination?

As is the case with a peripheral neuropathy, the physical examination shows asymmetric muscle weakness with atrophy and fasciculations. Tone is normal or decreased, and the reflexes in the involved muscles are diminished or absent. Weakness is confined to one myotomal group of muscles, such as those innervated by the C6 root in the arm or the L5 root in the leg. Similarly, sensory loss occurs in a dermatomal distribution. Maneuvers that stretch the root often aggravate the pain, such as straight leg raising or neck rotation.

13. Which clinical features of spinal cord disease can be elicited by history?

Spinal cord lesions usually cause a triad of symptoms:

1. **A sensory level is the hallmark of spinal cord disease.** Patients usually describe a sharp line or band around their abdomen or trunk, below which there is a decrease in sensation. The symptom of a sensory level is essentially pathognomonic for spinal cord disease.

2. **Distal, symmetric, spastic weakness.** The muscle, neuromuscular junction, nerves, and roots make up the peripheral nervous system, but the spinal cord is in the central nervous system and so has special motor properties. Damage to the spinal cord produces upper motor neuron lesions, affecting the pyramidal (or corticospinal) tract. However, the weakness mimics that of a peripheral neuropathy, because it is distal more than proximal. In actual clinical practice, almost all processes affecting the cord are symmetric. Upper motor neuron lesions cause spasticity, but this increase in tone may cause few noticeable symptoms—it is best extracted from the history by asking about stiffness in the legs.

3. **Bowel and bladder problems.** Sphincter dysfunction commonly accompanies cord lesions because of involvement of the autonomic fibers within the cord.

14. Which questions should be asked during the history to elicit the symptoms of spinal cord disease?

1. **Distal leg weakness:** Does the patient drag toes or trip?
2. **Distal arm weakness:** Does the patient drop things or have trouble with the grip?
3. **Symmetric symptoms:** Does the process involve the arms and/or legs approximately equally?
4. **Sensory level:** Is a sensory level present? Patients often describe it as a band, belt, girdle, or tightness around the trunk or abdomen.
5. **Sphincter dysfunction:** Is there retention or incontinence of bowel or bladder? (The bladder is usually involved earlier, more often, and more severely than the bowel in spinal cord lesions.)

15. After a history of spinal cord disease is elicited, what findings can be expected on physical examination?

The physical examination in a patient with spinal cord disease usually shows a sensory level below which all sensory modalities are diminished. The sensory (and motor) tracts in the spinal cord are somatotopically organized; distinctive anatomic layering and lamination to the pathways result in greatest damage to fibers from the legs and lower part of the body in the majority of spinal cord lesions. Because most leg fibers lie laterally and are easily compressed, spinal disease usually affects the legs more than the arms. In addition, the level of the symptoms detected clinically does not always correspond to the true anatomic site of the damage. For example, a mass pressing on the spinal cord may cause a sensory level and weakness any place at or below the actual anatomic level of the lesion.

The patient also may have urinary retention or incontinence and may lose superficial reflexes, including the anal wink, bulbocavernosus, and cremasteric reflexes. The examination shows evidence of upper motor neuron damage:

1. Distal weakness greater than proximal weakness
2. Greater weakness of the extensors and antigravity muscles than of the flexors
3. Increased tone (spasticity)
4. Increased reflexes
5. Clonus
6. Extensor plantar response (positive Babinski signs)
7. Absent superficial reflexes
8. No significant atrophy or fasciculations

16. Which clinical features of brainstem disease can be elicited by history?

Cranial nerve symptoms characterize brainstem disease. The brainstem is essentially the spinal cord with embedded cranial nerves. Thus, brainstem lesions cause many of the symptoms of spinal cord disease accompanied by symptoms of cranial nerve impairment.

Like the spinal cord, the brainstem contains "long tracts," or pathways that extend from the brain down through the spinal cord. The major long tracts are the pyramidal (corticospinal) tract for motor function, the spinothalamic tract carrying pain and temperature sensations up to the thalamus, and the dorsal columns carrying position and vibration sense up to the thalamus. Because of the decussation of these tracts, lesions in the brainstem do not produce a horizontal motor or sensory level as they do in the spinal cord but rather produce a vertical motor or sensory level—that is, hemiparesis or hemianesthesia affecting one side of the body.

Lesions affecting the cranial nerves in the brainstem often produce symptoms referred to as the "Ds":

Symptoms of Cranial Nerve Damage

CRANIAL NERVE	SYMPTOMS
III	Diplopia
IV	Diplopia
V	Decreased facial sensation
VI	Diplopia
VII	Decreased strength and drooping of the face
VIII	Deafness and dizziness
IX	Dysarthria and dysphagia
X	Dysarthria and dysphagia
XI	Decreased strength in neck and shoulders
XII	Dysarthria and dysphagia

17. Which questions elicit symptoms of combined cranial nerve and long tract dysfunction?

1. **Long tract signs:** Does the patient have hemiparesis or hemisensory loss?

2. **Cranial nerve signs:** Does the patient have diplopia, dysarthria, dysphagia, dizziness, deafness, or decreased strength or sensation over the face?

3. **Crossed signs:** Because the long tracts cross but the cranial nerves generally do not, brainstem lesions often produce symptoms on one side of the face and the opposite side of the body. For example, a lesion in the pons that affects the pyramidal tracts and the facial (VII) nerve will cause weakness of that side of the face and the opposite, crossed side of the body. Brainstem disease often produces bilateral or crossed findings.

18. After a history of brainstem disease is elicited, what findings can be expected on physical examination?

The physical examination in brainstem disease is almost like a mathematical equation:

$$\text{cranial nerves} + \text{long tracts} = \text{brainstem disease.}$$

Examination of the cranial nerves may reveal ptosis, pupillary abnormalities, extraocular muscle paralysis, diplopia, nystagmus, decreased corneal and blink reflexes, facial weakness or numbness, deafness, vertigo, dysarthria, dysphagia, weakness or deviation of the palate, decreased gag reflex, or weakness of the neck, shoulders, or tongue.

Long tract abnormalities may include hemiparesis, which shows an upper motor neuron pattern of distal extensor weakness with hyperreflexia, spasticity, and a positive Babinski sign. Hemisensory loss may occur to all modalities.

19. Which clinical features of cerebellar disease can be elicited by history?

Cerebellar disease causes incoordination, clumsiness, and tremor, because the cerebellum is responsible for smoothing out and refining voluntary movements. Questions, therefore, should focus on these symptoms:

1. **Clumsiness in the legs:** Does the patient have a staggering, drunken walk? (Most laymen describe cerebellar symptoms in terms of alcohol and drunkenness, probably because drinking alcohol impairs the cerebellum. The characteristic ataxic, wide-based, staggering gait of the person intoxicated by alcohol is a reflection of cerebellar dysfunction.)

2. **Clumsiness in the arms:** Does the patient have difficulty with targeted movements, such as lighting a cigarette or placing a key in a lock? (Cerebellar tremor is worse with voluntary, intentional movements that require accurate placement.)

3. **Brainstem symptoms:** Are brainstem symptoms present? (Because the cerebellar inflow and outflow must pass through the brainstem and the blood supply to the cerebellum arises from the same vessels that supply the brainstem, cerebellar disease is almost always accompanied by some brainstem abnormalities as well, and vice versa.)

20. After a history of cerebellar disease is elicited, what findings can be expected on physical examination?

The patient's gait is staggering, wide-based, and ataxic, causing difficulties especially with tandem walking. Patients may require support to avoid falling. Fine coordinated movements of the legs are impossible, such as sliding a heel down a shin or tracing patterns on the floor with the foot. The cerebellar tremor is most visible in the upper extremities, which waver and wobble with attempts to touch a specific target, such as the examiner's finger or the patient's own nose. Rapid alternating movements are irregular in rate and rhythm.

21. How can the history determine whether disease of the brain is subcortical or cortical?

The history can differentiate subcortical from cortical disease by focusing on four major areas:

1. The presence of specific cortical deficits
2. The pattern of motor and sensory deficits
3. The type of sensory deficits
4. The presence of visual field deficits

22. What specific deficits are seen with cortical lesions?

The most useful symptom of cortical disease in the dominant (usually left) hemisphere is aphasia. The history, therefore, should focus on any difficulties with language functions, including not only speech but also writing, reading, and comprehension. A lesion affecting the left side of the brain that does not affect language function is unlikely to be cortical.

In the nondominant (usually right) hemisphere, cortical dysfunction is more subtle but usually causes visual-spatial problems. Patients with nondominant cortical lesions often have neglect and denial, including inattention to their own physical signs and symptoms. This finding can be difficult to elicit on history, however, and sometimes depends on the physical examination. Note also that seizures are almost always cortical in origin.

23. How does the pattern of motor and sensory deficits differentiate cortical from subcortical involvement?

The motor homunculus in the primary and supplemental motor strips is spread upside-down over a vast expanse of gray matter. Neurons controlling the lower extremities reside between the two hemispheres, in the interhemispheric fissure, whereas neurons moving the trunk, arms, and face are draped upside-down over the superficial cortex. Cortical lesions, therefore, often involve the face, arm, and trunk but spare the legs, which are protected in the interhemispheric fissure. Cortical lesions thus cause an incomplete hemiparesis, affecting the face and arm but not the leg.

Of course, fibers to the leg descend and merge with those to the face and arm as the pyramidal tract forms deep within the brain, subcortically, to run in the internal capsule, cerebral peduncles, and the pyramids themselves. Therefore, even a small subcortical lesion can affect all of these conjoined fibers. Subcortical lesions thus cause a complete hemiparesis, affecting face, arm, and leg.

The sensory homunculus has a similar somatotropic arrangement that results in an analogous pattern of localization.

24. How does the type of sensory deficit differentiate cortical from subcortical lesions by history?

Most of the primary sensory modalities reach "consciousness" in the thalamus and do not require the cortex for their perception. A patient with severe cortical damage can still feel pain, touch, vibration, and position. A history of significant numbness or sensory loss, therefore, suggests a subcortical lesion.

Cortical sensory loss is more refined and usually involves complicated sensory processing such as two-point discrimination, accurate localization of perceptions, stereognosis, and graphesthesia. These symptoms can be difficult to elicit by history alone.

25. How do visual symptoms differentiate cortical from subcortical disease by history?

Visual pathways run subcortically for most of their length. Visual impulses in the optic nerves may cross in the chiasm and run through the optic tracts, lateral geniculate bodies, and optic radiations before synapsing in the occipital cortex. Cortical lesions, such as those affecting the motor strip, sensory strip, or language areas, are too superficial to affect these visual fibers and thus do not cause visual field deficits. Subcortical lesions often affect the visual fibers, producing visual field cuts. Therefore, a history of visual field loss suggests a subcortical lesion. (Of course, a strictly cortical lesion in the occipital lobes produces visual symptoms, but it does not affect motor, sensory, or other functions and so does not cause confusion with the typical picture of a subcortical lesion.)

26. After a history of cortical or subcortical disease is elicited, what findings can be expected on physical examination?

Physical examination findings parallel the historical deficits.

1. **Cortical dysfunction:** The patient may show aphasia, visual-spatial dysfunction, or seizures.

2. **Motor involvement:** Physical examination shows upper motor neuron weakness affecting the face and arm in a cortical lesion and the face, arm, and leg in a subcortical lesion.

3. **Sensory dysfunction:** In subcortical disease, the examination shows problems with primary sensory modalities, such as decreased pinprick and vibration, but in cortical disease it shows relatively normal sensation with impaired higher sensory processing, such as graphesthesia and stereognosis.

4. **Visual dysfunction:** Patients with subcortical disease may have visual field cuts, but patients with cortical disease do not.

27. How accurate are the history and physical examination for diagnosing neurologic disease?

The clinical examination is highly accurate in localizing neurologic disease. Once a lesion has been localized to one of the broad anatomic regions, an etiology usually suggests itself. For example, if a lesion can be localized to the peripheral nerve, it is usually easy to develop a differential diagnosis for peripheral neuropathies (such as diabetes, alcoholism) and a diagnostic plan (e.g., blood testing, nerve conduction studies). The anatomy usually implies an etiology.

Organized questioning and examination of the nervous system in this fashion are an excellent way to approach the neurologic patient.

BIBLIOGRAPHY

1. Caplan L: The Effective Clinical Neurologist. Cambridge, Blackwell Scientific Publications, 1990.
2. Haerer A: Dejong's The Neurologic Examination, 5th ed. Philadelphia, J.B. Lippincott, 1992.

4. MYOPATHIES

Yadollah Harati, M.D., F.A.C.P., and Kathryn Copeland, M.D.

1. What is a myopathy?

The term *myopathy* implies a disorder involving predominantly the muscle rather than the anterior horn cell, peripheral nerve, or neuromuscular junction.

2. What signs and symptoms are suggestive of a myopathy?

Proximal symmetric weakness, which may be acute, subacute, or chronic
Reduced, preserved, or enlarged muscle bulk
Muscle pain or discomfort with palpation (myalgia)
Muscle stiffness or cramps
Asthenia and fatigue
Myoglobinuria

3. Define myoblast, myotube, myofiber, and myofibril.

A **myoblast** is a postmitotic, mononucleated cell capable of fusion and contractile protein synthesis. **Myotubes** are long, cylindrical, multinucleated (syncytial) cells formed from the fusion of myoblasts. When their central nuclei are shifted to a subsarcolemmal position in the later stages of development, they are called **myofibers**. The appearance of central nuclei within an otherwise normal adult muscle is a useful sign of muscle regeneration. Each adult myofiber is packed with numerous **myofibrils**, largely composed of hexagonal arrangements of thick and thin contractile filaments. Myosin is the major constituent of the thick filaments, whereas actin is the contractile protein of the thin filaments.

4. Describe the embryonic origin of skeletal muscle.

Muscles develop from mesodermal cell populations arising in the somite. The connective tissues around the muscles have a different embryologic origin and are derived from the somatopleural mesoderm.

5. What is a motor unit?

A motor unit consists of a motor neuron, its single axon, the associated neuromuscular junctions and terminal axon branches, and the many muscle fibers that they supply. All muscle fibers belonging to a single motor unit are of the same histochemical and physiologic type.

6. What are the most common causes of muscle pain?

The most common complaints of muscle pain have a nonmuscular etiology such as vascular insufficiency, joint disease, or neuropathy. The vast majority of myopathies are painless. Myopathies associated with pain include inflammatory myopathies, metabolic myopathies, mitochondrial myopathies, and some muscular dystrophies (limb-girdle, Becker's muscular dystrophy). In general, in patients with a normal exam and a normal serum creatine kinase (CK) level, muscle pain is usually not myopathic in origin.

7. How do we grade functional weakness?

The most widely used system was developed by the Medical Research Council (MRC) of Great Britain. The MRC system grades strength from 0 to 5. The addition of plus (+) or minus (–) further quantifies strength:

  0 No movement
  1 Trace movement
  2 Able to move, but not against gravity

3 Able to move full range against gravity
4 Able to move against some resistance
5 Normal strength

In addition, the clinician may observe the patient performing the following maneuvers to look for subtle weakness:

1. Arise from a chair with arms folded
2. Walk the length of the examining room on toes, on heels, and tandem
3. Hop on either foot
4. Perform deep knee bends
5. Climb a step
6. Horizontally abduct arms and reach the vertex of the head
7. Lift up head from table
8. Arise from supine position with hands overhead
9. Lift head and shoulders, and extend the neck while in a prone position

8. What is Gower's sign?

This term describes the maneuver of rising from a supine position in the presence of marked proximal weakness. The patient must roll to a prone position, push off the floor, lock the knees, and push the upper body upward by "climbing up" the legs with the hands. Although Gower's sign is associated with children with myopathies, it is present in any patient with marked proximal weakness.

9. What are the most valuable tests for evaluating patients with suspected muscle disease?

A diagnosis often can be established by supporting the clinical findings with results from three key tests: (1) serum CK levels, (2) electromyography (EMG), and (3) muscle biopsy.

10. Which myopathies are associated with elevated serum CK levels in adults?

CK catalyzes the reversible reaction of adenosine triphosphate (ATP) and creatine to form adenosine diphosphate (ADP) and phosphocreatine. It is elevated in many myopathies due to myofiber disruption or degeneration. Examples include:

• Inflammatory myopathies (e.g., polymyositis-dermatomyositis)
• Alcoholic myopathy
• Drug-induced myopathies (clofibrate, aminocaproic acid, lovastatin and similar drugs)
• Infectious myopathies (AIDS, trichinosis, toxoplasmosis)
• Hypothyroid myopathy
• Metabolic myopathies (acid-maltase deficiency, late-onset myophosphorylase or phospho-fructokinase deficiency)
• Genetic myopathies (e.g., Becker muscular dystrophy, limb-girdle muscular dystrophy)

The CK level may be normal in patients with an ongoing myopathy normally associated with an elevated CK. Examples include profound muscle wasting and selected conditions such as hyperthyroidism. The actual value is often helpful in differentiating myopathies. For example, in an older patient with subacute weakness, a CK value ≤ 600 is more suggestive of inclusion body myopathy (IBM) than polymyositis (PM), in which CK is typically much higher (up to 50 times normal in severe cases).

11. What conditions other than myopathies are associated with an elevated CK level?

• Exercise
• Increased muscle bulk
• Muscle trauma (needle injection, EMG, surgery, edema, vigorous exercise, or contusion)
• Viral illnesses
• African American race
• Drug use (including alcohol and cholesterol-lowering agents)
• Eating licorice

- Hypothyroidism
- Hypoparathyroidism
- Malignant hyperthermia
- Neurogenic disease (e.g., amyotrophic lateral sclerosis)
- Benign hereditary hypercreatininemia

Typically CK levels are increased less than threefold in these conditions, whereas CK levels greater than fivefold often prove to have an underlying myopathic etiology.

12. After unaccustomed exercise, normal people often have pain and soreness of muscles. Does the type of exercise play any role in the extent of muscle pain and damage?

Yes. In the face of a markedly elevated CK level in a healthy person engaged in exercises, it is important to ask about the type of exercise. Activities that involve **concentric** contractions of muscles (shortening of muscles) produce less muscle pain and damage than activities involving **eccentric** contraction (lengthening of muscles). An example of concentric contraction is the shortening of the muscle that occurs in the flexed leg during climbing stairs. Eccentric contraction is the lengthening of the muscle in the extended leg that supports the body during walking downstairs. Elevation of CK level by 10- to 100-fold after even 30 minutes of vigorous eccentric leg exercises has been observed. Because such exercises may be especially damaging to an already diseased muscle, physical therapists should be made aware of any disease state.

13. What is the approach to evaluating a persistent but incidental elevation of serum CK?

Perform an EMG if symptoms of weakness, myalgia, cramps, or tenderness are present. If the EMG findings are suggestive of a myopathy, a muscle biopsy may be considered If both the exam and EMG are normal, follow the patient clinically. A muscle biopsy in this setting rarely yields any useful information.

14. When is a muscle biopsy indicated? How is the muscle site chosen?

Muscle weakness with associated laboratory or electrophysiologic evidence of a myopathy are indications to pursue a muscle biopsy. Selection of the most appropriate muscle for biopsy is important, and several factors need to be considered, including availability of normative data for the site. Although affected muscles are ideal to biopsy, moderately affected muscles are better than severely affected muscles because fibrosis and fatty replacement of the muscle, which are characteristic of end-stage muscle disease, may not provide adequate information. In addition, muscles affected by other conditions (e.g., radiculopathy or trauma) should be avoided if possible. In general, the biceps or deltoid muscles in the upper extremity or the vastus lateralis muscle in the lower extremity are selected. Because upper extremity muscles are more vascular, they may have a higher diagnostic yield when a vasculitic process is suspected.

15. What basic stains are typically used to evaluate a myopathy? What morphologic features of a myopathy may be seen on biopsy?

Both the hematoxylin and eosin (H&E) and the modified Gomori trichrome stains provide useful general information about the muscle structures and cellular details. In addition, the modified Gomori trichrome stain allows visualization of the mitochondrial activity and collection by staining red (ragged red fibers). The ATPase stain defines the fibers by their histochemical type. Reduced nicotinamide adenine dinucleotide trazolium reductase (NADH-TR) also differentiates type 1 and type 2 fibers and provides information about the oxidative activity of muscle fibers.

Morphologic features of a myopathy include muscle fiber necrosis, phagocytosis and regeneration, increased central nuclei, fiber hypertrophy and rounding, variation in fiber size and shape, and increased endomysial connective tissue.

16. How many fiber types are recognized by muscle histochemistry?

Type 1 fibers are slow-twitch, red fibers; type 2 fibers are fast-twitch, white fibers. The two major subtypes of type 2 fibers are types 2A and 2B. The histochemical and physiologic properties of each fiber type are determined by the anterior horn cell that innervates it.

17. What are ragged red fibers?

A ragged red fiber is a muscle fiber with an accumulation of subsarcolemmal and intermy-ofibrillar material that stains red with modified Gomori trichrome stain. This red-stained material is actually mitochondria that are abnormal in size and structure when viewed by electron microscopy. Although ragged red fibers are typically seen in mitochondrial myopathies, they may occur in other conditions are a nonspecific finding in an otherwise normal biopsy from an elderly patient.

18. What are tubular aggregates?

Tubular aggregates are clusters of tubular proliferation arising from the sarcoplasmic reticulum affecting type 2 fibers. They have a red appearance with modified Gomori trichrome stain, stain dark with NADH-TR, and do not react to serine dehydratase (SDH). They may be seen in periodic paralysis and occasionally in other conditions.

19. What are the general categories of myopathies?
- Inflammatory myopathies (e.g., polymyositis, dermatomyositis)
- Muscular dystrophies (e.g., Duchenne, myotonic)
- Congenital myopathies (e.g., central-core, centronuclear myopathy)
- Metabolic myopathies (e.g., myophosphate deficiency, phosphofructokinase deficiency)
- Mitochondrial myopathies (e.g., Kearns-Sayre syndrome)
- Toxic myopathies (e.g., alcohol, zidovudine)
- Endocrine myopathies (e.g., hypothyroidism, hypoadrenalism)
- Infectious myopathies (e.g., trichinosis, AIDS)

20. How are the polymyositis (PM) and dermatomyositis (DM) syndromes classified?
1. Adult polymyositis and dermatomyositis
2. Childhood and juvenile dermatomyositis
3. Dermatomyositis associated with other diseases (connective tissue disorders, malignancy)
4. Polymyositis associated with other diseases (connective tissue diseases, malignancy)
5. Inclusion body myositis (myopathy)

21. What are the clinical features of PM and DM?

The history and pattern of weakness (subacute weakness greatest in the upper extremities and neck flexors) are similar in DM and PM, and both are responsive to immunosuppression. Pharyngeal weakness is also common in both (about 30% of cases). Approximately 5% of patients develop symptomatic systemic involvement, including fever, weight loss, cardiac arrhythmias and conduction abnormalities, and pulmonary involvement. The presence of anti-Jo-1 antibody is a marker for interstitial lung disease. Both PM and DM also have been associated with malignancies, in particular lung, GI, breast, and ovarian cancers. Most experts agree that patients should be screened with routine blood work, chest radiograph, mammography, and pelvic and rectal exams. Patients over the age of 50 with DM are at higher risk of developing cancer and should be watched closely. Although EMG findings vary according to the stage of the disease, fibrillation and sharp wave potentials are present in most patients (including the paraspinous muscles).

Unique to DM are cutaneous manifestations that typically present at the same time as the weakness. The characteristic heliotrope rash involves the eyelids, cheeks, nose, neck, elbows, and knees. Gottron's papules are often seen on the knuckles. Skin may become scaly and atrophic, and the nail beds may appear shiny and red. Although PM is an adult disease, DM occurs in both children and adults. The skin manifestations are much more common in children.

22. What is inclusion body myositis (IBM)?

IBM is now considered the most common cause of chronic myopathy in patients 50 years of age or older. Characteristically, the painless weakness and atrophy are gradual in onset and more commonly involve the quadriceps, finger flexors, and foot dorsiflexors. Dysphagia is common. There is early loss of patellar reflexes, and a mild neuropathy may be present. CK levels are either normal or only mildly elevated. Electrodiagnostic evaluation reveals mixed myopathic and neurogenic changes. Muscle biopsy shows varying degrees of inflammation, cytoplasmic "rimmed" vacuoles and eosinophilic inclusion bodies, and small angular atrophic and denervated fibers. The vacuoles contain strong ubiquitin immunoreactivity, localized to cytoplasmic tubulofilaments and beta-amyloid proteins.

23. What are the major pathologic changes on light microscopy in the muscle biopsies of patients with PM, DM, and IBM?

Both PM and DM have:

1. Inflammatory infiltrate
   • Perivascular (more in DM)
   • Endomysial or perimysial (more in DM)
2. Fiber necrosis, phagocytosis
3. Perifascicular atrophy (especially in DM of childhood)
4. Variation and rounding of muscle fibers; occasional angular and atrophic fibers
5. Capillary loss or necrosis (more in DM)
6. Eosinophilic cytoplasmic inclusions and rimmed vacuoles, denervation changes, and interstitial infiltration (also in IBM)

24. What does the muscle biopsy photograph below signify?

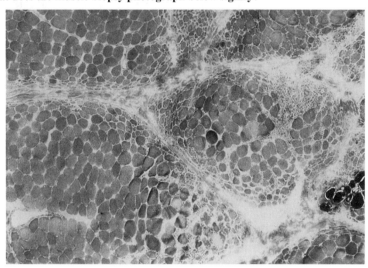

This is the typical finding of perifascicular atrophy. The muscle fibers at the periphery of the muscle fascicles are smaller, whereas the fibers in the deepest part of the fascicle are of normal size. This type of atrophy is generally recognized to be a conspicuous feature of childhood dermatomyositis and, to a lesser extent, adult dermatomyositis. Even in the absence of inflammation, this biopsy is characteristic. The pattern of atrophy is probably due to capillary changes and involves mainly muscle fibers near the perimysial connective tissue, because these fibers are less likely to have collateral circulation.

25. What is the classic facial appearance of a patient with adult-onset myotonic dystrophy?

The characteristic appearance of a patient with myotonic dystrophy (MyD) is important to recognize. Facial weakness and temporalis muscle atrophy give rise to a narrow, hatchet-faced appearance. In addition, patients develop frontal baldness, ptosis, and neck muscle atrophy early in the disease.

26. What is the most common muscular dystrophy in adults? How does it present?

MyD, which has an estimated prevalence of about 1/20,000 of the population. MyD is a multisystem disorder with an autosomal dominant pattern of inheritance, but severity and degree of systemic involvement vary considerably. The most common form of the disease presents in the second decade of life, but there is also a congenital form. The first symptom is usually myotonia, which presents as difficulty in relaxing the grip; hand weakness and gait difficulties are also common presenting complaints.

27. What systems are involved in MyD?

Cardiac. Conduction problems are a major cause of morbidity and mortality. About 90% of patients have EKG abnormalities, and complete heart block and sudden death are well recognized. Prophylactic pacemaker implantation is needed in patients with conduction block.

Respiratory. Excessive daytime sleepiness is common because of a combination of weakness of the diaphragm and intercostal muscles, decreased response to hypoxia, alveolar hypoventilation, hypercapnia, and abnormalities of brainstem neuroregulatory mechanisms.

Gastrointestinal. Smooth muscle involvement results in many symptoms, including abdominal pain, dysphagia, emesis, diarrhea, and bowel incontinence.

Central nervous system symptoms include impaired intelligence, apathy, reluctance to seek or follow medical advice, and personality disorders.

Skeletal muscle symptoms include atrophy, weakness, and myotonia.

Endocrine. Testicular atrophy and insulin resistance are common; overt diabetes is uncommon.

Other symptoms include frontal balding, cranial hyperostosis, air sinus enlargement, and minor sensory neuropathy.

28. What are the characteristics of the MyD gene?

The mutation in MyD is an expansion of a trinucleotide (CTG) repeat in the protein kinase gene on the long arm of chromosome 19. In normal people, the number of repeats is less than 37, whereas in MyD it ranges from 50 to a few thousand. The size of the expanded repeat closely correlates with the severity and age of onset of MyD and generally increases in successive generations within a family, providing a molecular basis for the clinical observed phenomenon known as anticipation (progressively earlier onset of the disease in successive generations). The exact consequences of the mutation at the molecular level are currently under investigation. The MyD gene codes for a protein kinase termed myotonia-protein kinase, which is thought to modulate ion channel function. Of note, in a number of cases with clinical features of MyD, an expansion of CTG repeats is not found.

29. Describe the salient features of the Duchenne muscular dystrophy gene.

The gene is large (2.5×10^6 base pairs), located in the short arm of the X chromosome, and codes for a structural protein called dystrophin. It is by far the largest gene characterized to date, consisting of 2.3 million base pairs and occupying approximately 1% of the human X chromosome. Dystrophin is a protein located in the subsarcolemmal region of the muscle fiber. It is expressed predominantly in skeletal, cardiac, and smooth muscle. Mutations within the gene cause Duchenne muscular dystrophy (DMD), Becker muscular dystrophy (BMD), X-linked myoglobinuria, and quadriceps myopathy. In about 30% of cases of DMD, the mutation has not been identified. Approximately 65% of cases have mutations in which one or more exons are missing, and the remaining cases are due to exon duplication.

30. What organs other than skeletal muscle are involved in DMD?

About 90% of patients have EKG abnormalities, but symptomatic involvement occurs in less than 1% of patients. Although the heart may be enlarged with minimal fibrosis, the myocardial muscle fibers do not undergo necrosis or other myopathic changes. There is also an increased incidence of gastrointestinal hypomotility that may lead to intestinal pseudo-obstruction and gastric dilatation. Finally, pachygyria and smaller than normal brains have been noted in some patients with DMD. In addition, an association between mental retardation and mutations causing central exon deletions has been observed.

31. What are the most important congenital myopathies?
1. Central-core disease
2. Nemaline myopathy
3. Centronuclear myopathy
4. Congenital fiber type disproportion
5. Reducing-body myopathy
6. Myopathy associated with tubular aggregates
7. Fingerprint-body myopathy
8. Sarcotubular myopathy
9. Multicore myopathy
10. Trilaminar myopathy
11. Cytoplasmic body myopathy
12. Familial myopathy with lysis of myofibril in type 1 fibers

32. Is there a relationship between malignant hyperthermia and central-core disease?
Central-core disease is a congenital myopathy. Malignant hyperthermia is a reaction to general anesthetics. Both conditions are transmitted by an autosomal dominant pattern of inheritance, and the genes for both diseases are located next to each other on chromosome 19 (19 q12–q13.2). Some patients with central-core disease are susceptible to malignant hyperthermia. They and their family members must be cautioned about the possibility of malignant hyperthermia reactions to anesthetics.

33. What features are suggestive of a metabolic myopathy?
Clinical features suggestive of a metabolic myopathy include exercise-related muscular pain, stiffness, or cramps and myoglobinuria. Some disorders are associated with fixed or progressive weakness.

34. How are metabolic myopathies classified?
According to the metabolic pathway that is impaired:

Glycogen is metabolized to either lactic acid or pyruvate, providing energy during both high-intensity activity and anaerobic states. During aerobic conditions, pyruvate enters the TCA cycle to generate more energy through oxidative metabolism.

Lipid metabolism is a source of energy at rest and with sustained submaximal exercise. Long-chain fatty acids and transported into the mitochondria, where carnitine palmitoyl transferase (CPT) catalyzes the reaction, forming acylcarnitine esters that are oxidized to acetyl-CoA and ATP. Acetyl-CoA then enters the TCA cycle.

Phosphocreatine and the **purine** nucleotide cycle are utilized during brief high-intensity exercise. Phosphocreatine restores the level of ATP from ADP, and CK is the enzyme that catalyzes the transfer of the phosphoryl group in these reactions.

The **mitochondria** produce enzymes that mediate the oxidation of pyruvate, glucose, and fatty acids under aerobic conditions by producing a hydrogen ion gradient.

35. What is acid-maltase deficiency? Give the differential diagnosis.
Acid-maltase deficiency (type II glycogenosis) is an autosomal recessive disorder caused by a deficiency of the lysosomal enzyme alphaglycoside (acid maltase). It can present at any age and has three different forms: infantile (Pompe's disease), childhood, and adult onset. The adult form, presenting in the third or fourth decade of life with insidious painless limb-girdle weakness, is frequently misdiagnosed as polymyositis, motor neuron disease, myotonic dystrophy, or limb-girdle muscular dystrophy. The respiratory muscles are disproportionately affected. The CK level is usually mildly elevated (2–10 times normal), and lactate production is normal. The EMG shows abundant complex repetitive discharges in addition to myopathic changes and spontaneous activity. If the discharges are not overt, the EMG findings resemble polymyositis. Therefore, a muscle biopsy may be necessary to make the diagnosis. Characteristic findings are those of a vacuolar myopathy. The vacuoles themselves contain PAS-positive material with a prominent acid phosphatase activity. Similar vacuoles also occur in chloroquine myopathy. There is no effective treatment, although a high-protein, low-carbohydrate diet has resulted in slight benefit.

36. What is the McArdle's disease? How is it treated?

Myophosphorylase deficiency (McArdle's disease) is characterized by muscle cramps and stiffness with exercise and intermittent myoglobinuria. A "second-wind" phenomenon in which the symptoms disappear after a brief rest and do not recur with resumed mild exercise has been described. Absence of myophosphorylase blocks carbohydrate metabolism, and lipids must be used for energy metabolism at rest and during exercise. Because this source of energy is insufficient for intense exercise, symptoms develop.

Treatment begins with counseling about the risks of exercise-induced rhabdomyolysis. Patients should be instructed to adjust their lifestyle to avoid strenuous exercise and to seek prompt medical attention and treatment if myoglobinuria develops. Treatments aimed at bypassing the biochemical block by supplying the muscle with a glycolytic intermediate (i.e., glucose, fructose) appear to increase work capacity in some patients, but their long-term use results in undesirable weight gain and usually proves disappointing. Injection of glucagon to promote hepatic glycogenolysis and to increase blood glucose concentration has inconsistent results, and repeated injections are objectionable for prolonged treatment. High-fat and low-carbohydrate diets have no demonstrable effect. However, diets high in amino acids (especially alanine) may be beneficial. In vivo P31-NMR spectroscopy and exercise performance are partially normalized by a high-protein diet but unaffected by intravenous amino acid infusion. This finding suggests that intramuscular protein stores provide an alternative energy substrate and are capable of partially correcting the metabolic deficits.

37. A 19-year-old man with a history of exercise-induced severe muscle cramps and exercise intolerance was forced by his trainer in a military camp to run up 50 flights of stairs. A few hours later, he noted dark (Coca-Cola–colored) urine and had fever, chills, and severe muscle soreness. CBC showed a normal WBC count, mild anemia, and an increased reticulocyte count. What is the differential diagnosis?

The patient most likely has muscle phosphofructokinase (PFK) deficiency (type VII glycogenosis, or Tarui's disease). He could have McArdle's disease, but hemolytic anemia with an elevated reticulocyte count strongly favors PFK deficiency. Normally, erythrocyte PFK is composed of both muscle (M) type and RBC (R) type subunits. Patients with PFK deficiency lack the M subunit. The inheritance pattern in most cases of PFK deficiency is autosomal recessive, and reduced erythrocyte PFK activity may be demonstrated in otherwise asymptomatic patients. Muscle PFK deficiency results in blockage of glycolysis. Clinical manifestations of PFK deficiency closely resemble those of McArdle's disease and include exercise intolerance that develops soon after vigorous activity and causes muscle fatigue, stiffness, and pain; it resolves within a few minutes to several hours.

38. What are the clinical features of myopathic carnitine deficiency?

Carnitine plays an essential role in the metabolism of fatty acids by muscle fiber. Carnitine deficiency causes slowly progressive weakness of limb, neck, and trunk muscles beginning in early childhood or mid-adult life. Cardiomyopathy (sometimes fatal) and peripheral neuropathy also may be seen, but myalgias and muscle cramps are rare. CK level is normal or mildly elevated. The carnitine level (free and acyl) is usually reduced in muscle, but not in serum or liver, and there is an excess of lipid globules in muscle fibers. Treatment with regular oral intake of L-carnitine (50–100 mg/kg/day in divided doses) usually results in improvement of muscle strength. Some patients also may improve with riboflavin or prednisone.

39. What symptoms are classic for a mitochondrial myopathy?

Although the degree of impairment varies, most mitochondrial myopathies are associated with nonfluctuating, insidiously progressive ptosis and ophthalmoplegia. Actual diplopia is rare. Other involved organ systems include:

- Cardiac (conduction abnormalities and cardiomyopathy)
- Gastrointestinal (pseudo-obstruction)
- Endocrine (diabetes, goiter, short stature)
- Central nervous system (ataxia, deafness, seizures, cerebrovascular ischemia, neuropathy)

• Skin (lipomas)
• Eye (retinitis pigmentosa, cataracts)

40. What are the most important myopathies due to point mutations in mitochondrial DNA?
1. Myoclonic epilepsy with ragged red fibers (MERRF)
2. Mitochondrial encephalomyopathy with lactic acidosis (MELAS)
3. Some myopathies with cardiomyopathy

41. What are the three major symptoms of periodic paralysis?
Periodic paralysis refers to rare diseases characterized by episodic spells (lasting minutes to days) of flaccid weakness involving a few or almost all skeletal muscles. Cranial and respiratory muscles are usually spared, and strength recovers spontaneously. The three major symptoms are (1) transient attacks of weakness, (2) myotonia (symptomatic only in potassium-sensitive periodic paralysis), and (3) interattack weakness, which may be progressive.

42. How are the different types of periodic paralysis classified?
According to proposed etiology (primary or secondary) or according to the change in serum potassium during attacks (hypo-, normo-, and hyperkalemic).
1. Primary: hypokalemic, hyperkalemic, or normokalemic.
2. Secondary: potassium depletion, potassium retention, thyrotoxic (hypokalemic), hypernatremia with defective thirst in hypothalamic lesions, or barium poisoning.

This and similar clinical classifications, however, are undergoing significant changes as the understanding of the genetic basis of these conditions is enhanced. For example, current evidence suggests that potassium-sensitive periodic paralyses and the myotonic disorder paramyotonia congenita are the result of single-base-pair changes in the alpha subunit of the skeletal muscle sodium channel gene. The gene abnormalities result in single amino acid substitutions in highly conserved regions of the sodium channel. The clinical variations of the diseases associated with the sodium channel gene, therefore, may be explained by a number of different allelic mutations. Hypokalemic periodic paralysis is associated with mutations in an alpha-subunit gene of a voltage-sensitive muscle calcium channel, the so-called dihydropyridine receptor.

43. What is the treatment for periodic paralysis?
Acetazolamide, a carbonic anhydrase inhibitor, is effective in some patients with each form of periodic paralysis. Its effect on the prevention of attacks of hypokalemic periodic paralysis, which is usually provoked by measures that lower the plasma potassium level, is particularly dramatic. Another carbonic anhydrase inhibitor, dichlorphenamide, may be more effective than acetazolamide in preventing the attacks and reducing interattack weakness. Patients who are intolerant of carbonic anhydrase inhibitors may benefit from potassium-sparing diuretics such as spironolactone and triamterene. A low-carbohydrate and low-sodium diet is generally recommended for patients with hypokalemic periodic paralysis. Inhalation of albuterol, a beta-adrenergic agonist, may prevent the attack in some patients with hyperkalemic periodic paralysis. Ingestion of a high-carbohydrate, low-potassium diet also may alleviate the attacks.

44. Which conditions may be associated with muscle hypertrophy?
• Some muscular dystrophies
  (Duchenne, Becker, limb-girdle)
• Myotonia congenita
• Chronic spinal muscular atrophy
• Cysticercosis
• Amyloidosis
• Childhood type of acid-maltase deficiency
• Myopathy of congenital hypothyroidism
  (Kocher-Debré-Sémélaigne syndrome)
• Hyperkalemic periodic paralysis
• Acromegaly
• Flier's syndrome (insulin resistance,
  acanthosis nigricans)
• Hereditary motor-sensory neuropathy
• Chronic relapsing inflammatory
  polyneuropathy
• Focal mononeuropathy (focal hyper-
  trophy)
• Radiculopathy (focal hypertrophy)
• Sarcoidosis (mostly focal)

45. Which myopathies cause respiratory failure?
- Some muscular dystrophies (Duchenne, Becker, limb-girdle, Emery-Dreifuss, myotonic,* congenital)
- Acid-maltase deficiency*
- Carnitine deficiency
- Nemaline myopathy*
- Mitochondrial myopathy
- Centronuclear myopathy*
- Polymyositis

* Respiratory failure may be the presenting feature.

46. Which myopathies are associated with dysphagia?
- Oculopharyngeal muscular dystrophy
- Inclusion body myositis
- Myotonic muscular dystrophy
- Mitochondrial myopathy
- Polymyositis and dermatomyositis
- Duchenne muscular dystrophy

47. Which myopathies are associated with cardiac disease?
- Myotonic dystrophy (arrhythmias, heart failure)
- Polymyositis (arrhythmias, heart failure)
- Limb-girdle dystrophy (arrhythmias, heart failure)
- Dystrophinopathy (heart failure, arrhythmia)
- Kearns-Sayre syndrome (arrhythmias)
- Emery-Dreifuss (arrhythmias)
- Acid-maltase deficiency (heart failure)
- Hyperkalemic periodic paralysis (arrhythmias)
- Carnitine deficiency (heart failure)

48. What is myokymia?
Myokymia is the continuous undulation of a group of muscle fibers caused by the successive spontaneous contraction of motor units. On EMG, they appear as groups of 2–10 potentials, firing at 5–60 Hz and recurring regularly at 0.2–1.0-second intervals. Myokymia, frequently observed in facial muscles, occurs in a number of brainstem diseases, especially multiple sclerosis, radiation-induced nerve damage, Guillain-Barré syndrome, chronic peripheral nerve disorders, timber rattlesnake envenomation, gold therapy, and Isaacs syndrome.

49. During an EMG study, the slightest movement of the needle evokes prolonged waxing-and-waning trains of high-frequency spikes and positive waves. What are these discharges called? In which conditions are they characteristically seen?
They are called myotonic discharges and occur because the muscle fibers continue to fire repetitively after stimulation. Myotonic discharges occur in myotonia congenita, paramyotonia congenita, myotonic dystrophy, Schwartz-Jampel syndrome, myopathy with infantile and adult forms of acid maltase deficiency, and hyperkalemic periodic paralysis. Myotonia congenita is due to abnormal chloride channel function, whereas paramyotonia congenita, hyperkalemic periodic paralysis, and Schwartz-Jampel syndrome are caused by abnormal sodium channel function. Myotonia in myotonic dystrophy and acid-maltase deficiency is caused by other, not fully understood, membrane defects.

50. What is neuromyotonia?
Neuromyotonia is the continuous muscle rippling and stiffness resulting from bursts of discharges from the peripheral nerve. It is neurogenic in origin and results from an unexplained hyperexcitability of the motor nerves. Myotonia differs from neuromyotonia in that myotonia is thought to be myogenic. This theory is supported by the failure of curare to inhibit myotonia.

51. What is Isaacs syndrome?

Isaacs syndrome has been described under several other names, including myokymia with impaired muscle relaxation, neuromyotonia, pseudomyotonia, quantal squander, armadillo disease, and continuous muscle fiber activity. The onset is typically during the second or third decade of life, and both sexes are affected equally. Complaints include muscle stiffness, intermittent cramping, and difficulty with chewing, speaking, and even breathing. The most remarkable feature of Isaacs syndrome is myokymia. Some patients display marked hyperhidrosis, muscle hypertrophy, or elevated CK. Detailed laboratory and cerebrospinal fluid evaluations typically are normal except for some nonspecific immunologic abnormalities.

The cause remains unknown. However, serum antibodies directed against voltage-dependent channels of presynaptic nerve terminals, resulting in hyperexcitability of the distal motor nerve or nerve terminals, have been identified in a number of patients. EMG studies of Isaacs syndrome show spontaneous and continuous long, irregularly occurring trains of variably formed discharges that originate in the proximal parts of nerves. Fasciculation, doublets, or multiplets, firing at intervals of about 20 msec, also may be present.

Successful symptomatic treatment has been achieved with phenytoin (300–400 mg/day) or carbamazepine (200 mg 3 or 4 times/day). Some patients may respond favorably to plasma exchange or intravenous immunoglobulin. Diazepam, clonazepam, and baclofen are of no benefit. Patients often remain well on therapy over many years, leading normal lives.

52. What is "stiff-person syndrome"?

Stiff-person or stiff-man syndrome is a fluctuating motor disturbance characterized by sudden muscular rigidity with superimposed spasms. It predominantly affects the axial and proximal limb muscles and is aggravated by emotional, somatosensory, or acoustic stimuli. Between the spasms the neurologic examination may be normal. Many patients have associated autoimmune endocrinopathies; the most common is insulin-dependent diabetes mellitus. Antibodies directed against the GABA-synthesizing enzyme glutamic acid decarboxylase (GAD) are present in the serum and CSF of some patients. EMG discloses a continuous low-frequency firing of normal motor unit potentials that persists at rest. In some patients the condition is associated with malignancies, but GAD antibodies are absent. Instead, they have autoantibodies directed against a 128-Kd antigen known as amphiphysin. A significant symptomatic improvement is achieved by oral administration of benzodiazepines, primarily diazepam (10–100 mg/day). Baclofen and valproic acid also may help the symptoms. Immune modulation by corticosteroids and plasmapheresis may result in improvement in some patients. There are increasing numbers of reports about the beneficial effects of intravenous gammaglobulin.

53. Which drugs cause an inflammatory myopathy?

A painful inflammatory myopathy develops in some patients treated with D-penicillamine or procainamide. In addition, phenylbutazone, niflumic acid, propylthiouracil, penicillin, sulphonamides, cimetidine (Tagamet), simvastatin, and cocaine have been reported to be associated with an inflammatory myopathy.

54. What are the most common myotoxic drugs?

1. Clofibrate and other lipid-lowering agents
2. Chloroquine
3. Emetine
4. Alcohol
5. Epsilon-aminocaproic acid
6. D-penicillamine
7. Phenformin
8. Zidovudine (AZT)

55. A patient with AIDS who is taking AZT complains of myalgia and weakness. What is wrong?

The exact diagnosis in this setting is often difficult. Myalgia and increased CK are frequently encountered in patients with AIDS, and some patients have a symmetric and predominantly proximal muscle weakness. EMG findings are those usually seen in polymyositis. Many patients have typical muscle biopsy findings of polymyositis (necrotic fibers with perimysial, endomysial, and perivascular lymphocytic inflation). AZT is also associated with myopathy, which is characterized chiefly by muscle wasting and proximal weakness and tends to occur in patients treated with high doses of the drug for more than 6 months. Muscle biopsy, however, may show changes suggestive of a mitochondrial disorder. Numerous "ragged red" fibers, indicative of abnormal mitochondria, may be seen. Rods (nemaline) and cytoplasmic bodies also may be seen. Both myopathy and biopsy abnormalities improve with discontinuation of AZT. It is thought that AZT inhibits mitochondrial DNA polymerase, which causes depletion of mitochondrial DNA and thus results in myopathy. Of interest, other antiretroviral agents used to treat HIV-infected patients, such as didanosine (ddI, Videx) and zalcitabine (ddC, Hivid), are more potent inhibitors of mitochondrial function but do not produce similar symptoms. Therefore, other unknown factors probably play a role.

56. What is steroid myopathy?

There are two forms of steroid myopathy. The more common form produces progressive, painless weakness. Typically the myopathy is related to chronic use, but inhaled corticosteroids can cause diaphragmatic weakness within 2 weeks of initial exposure. With long-term use of corticosteroids, patients typically have other systemic manifestations when the myopathy occurs. Chronic steroid myotoxicity can be prevented in part by exercise, and symptoms improve if the dose is reduced or discontinued. CK is not elevated, and EMG may be normal or show minimal myopathic changes.

The second form of steroid myopathy is related to high-dose exposure, usually in association with depolarizing neuromuscular blocking agents, sepsis, and/or malnutrition. It is characterized by acute, severe paralysis that can affect all muscles, including respiratory muscles. This syndrome has been given many names, including acute quadriplegic myopathy, thick filament myopathy, and critical illness myopathy. EMG often shows an acute axonal neuropathy in addition to myopathic changes, which can confound the diagnosis. Symmetric proximal weakness and atrophy develop over days. With supportive care, the patient may recover over months.

57. What is the neuroleptic malignant syndrome (NMS)?

NMS is a life-threatening complication of treatment with neuroleptic drugs such as phenothiazines, haloperidol, and clozapine; it has a mortality rate as high as 30%. Although it is most common early in therapy, symptoms may appear at any time during treatment. It is characterized by fever, muscle rigidity, elevated CK, and rhabdomyolysis. Patients may be delirious, and dysautonomia may occur. NMS may present initially with only one of the above symptoms. It is important the condition as soon as possible because early treatment can save lives.

58. What causes NMS? How is it treated?

The cause of NMS is poorly understood. It may result from blockade of dopamine receptors in the hypothalamus. Some experts postulate a direct effect on calcium influx into skeletal muscle, triggering intense contractions and a hypermetabolic state similar to malignant hyperthermia.

Treatment includes discontinuing the offending agent and initiating therapy with bromocriptine, 5 mg 3 times/day, or dantrolene, 0.5–3.0 mg IV once/day. Observation in an intensive care setting is usually prudent.

BIBLIOGRAPHY

1. Carpenter S, Karpati G: Pathology of Skeletal Muscles, 2nd ed. New York, Oxford University Press, 2001.
2. Engel AG, Franzini-Armstrong C: Myology, 2nd ed. New York, McGraw-Hill, 1994.
3. Griggs RC, Mendell JR, Miller RG: Evaluation and Treatment of Myopathies. Philadelphia, F.A. Davis, 1995.
4. Harati Y, Kolimas R: Cramps and myalgias. In Jankovic J, Tolosa E (eds): Movement Disorders. Baltimore, Williams & Wilkins, 1998.
5. Rolak LA, Harati Y (ed): Neuro-immunology for the Clinician. Boston, Butterworth-Heinemann, 1997.
6. Schapira AH, Griggs RC: Muscle Diseases. Boston, Butterworth-Heinemann, 1999.
Websites
http://enmc.spc.ox.ac.uk/dc/ndmppcrit
www.bio.unipd.ir/~telethon/muscle1.html
www.mdausa.org/disease

5. NEUROMUSCULAR JUNCTION DISEASES

Clifton L. Gooch, M.D., and Tetsuo Ashizawa, M.D.

ANATOMY AND PHYSIOLOGY

1. What are the presynaptic events of neuromuscular transmission?

When the action potential reaches the presynaptic nerve terminal, voltage-gated calcium channels open, allowing influx of calcium ions (Ca^{2+}). This triggers release of acetylcholine from presynaptic vesicles into the synaptic cleft.

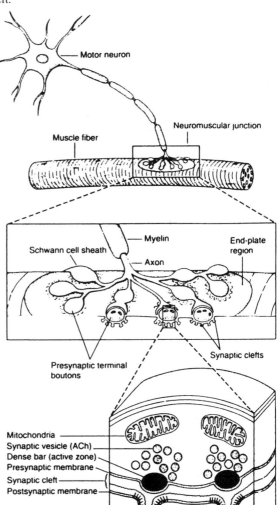

The neuromuscular junction. (From Kandel ER, Schwartz JH, Jessel TM (eds): Principles of Neural Science, 3rd ed. New York, Elsevier, 1991, p 136, with permission.)

2. What is the active zone?

The active zone is that specialized area of the presynaptic nerve terminal membrane visualized by freeze fracture electron microscopy that contains a series of particles aligned in two parallel rows. The particles are thought to represent the L-type voltage-gated Ca^{2+} channels (VGCCs) activated by motor nerve depolarization, which trigger the release of acetylcholine within the presynaptic vesicles into the synaptic cleft.

Maselli RA: Pathophysiology of myasthenia gravis and Lambert-Eaton syndrome. Neurol Clin North Am 12:387–399, 1994.

Engel AG, Fukuoka T, Lang B, et al: Lambert-Eaton myasthenic syndrome IgG: Early morphologic effects and immunolocalization at the motor endplate. Ann NY Acad Sci 505:333–345, 1987.

3. What are the postsynaptic events of neuromuscular transmission?

The binding of two acetylcholine molecules to each acetylcholine receptor opens a channel within the receptor, allowing Na^+ influx and generating small, subthreshold endplate potentials at the postsynaptic membrane known as miniature endplate potentials (MEPPs). The amplitude of the summated endplate potential (EPP) for each muscle fiber is proportional to the total number of MEPPs generated by the activation of many different acetylcholine receptors at the same time. When a sufficient number of receptors are activated simultaneously, the endplate potential becomes large enough to trigger an action potential. The action potential then propagates along the muscle sarcoplasmic membrane to the T-tubule system, leading to the release of Ca^{2+} from the sarcoplasmic reticulum, ultimately resulting in muscle contraction.

4. What are the events in the synaptic cleft during neuromuscular transmission?

After the acetylcholine molecules are released, they diffuse across the postsynaptic membrane and bind to acetylcholine receptors on the postsynaptic muscle endplate of a given muscle fiber. Acetylcholinesterase in the neuromuscular junction then catalyzes the hydrolysis of acetylcholine into choline and acetic acid within a fraction of a millisecond. Choline is subject to uptake by the presynaptic nerve terminal and is used for the synthesis of new acetylcholine via the enzyme choline acetyl transferase.

MYASTHENIA GRAVIS

5. What neuromuscular diseases demonstrate autoimmunity directed against constituents at the neuromuscular junction?

Myasthenia gravis (MG) and Lambert-Eaton myasthenic syndrome (LEMS) are the two diseases in which autoantibodies play a key pathogenic role at the neuromuscular junction. Studies have also suggested possible autoimmunity at the neuromuscular junction in amyotrophic lateral sclerosis (ALS), although further studies are needed to clarify this somewhat controversial observation.

Smith RG, Hamilton S, Hofmann F, et al: Serum antibodies to L-type calcium channels in patients with amyotrophic lateral sclerosis. N Engl J Med 327:1721–1728, 1992.

6. What are the neuromuscular manifestations of MG?

Patients with MG often have variable degrees of weakness and easy fatigability of skeletal muscles. Skeletal muscle weakness may or may not be present at rest but increases after sustained or repetitive exercise. The exercise-induced weakness improves rather dramatically after short rest. Extraocular muscles, bulbar muscles, and limb muscles often exhibit fatigability that is easily detectable on clinical examination. The most critical manifestation is respiratory weakness, which may result in death in a matter of hours.

7. What are the epidemiologic characteristics (incidence, sex differences, age of onset, familial occurrences, mortality, and remission rate) of MG?

The incidence of MG is approximately 1 in 20,000. The disease afflicts more women than men by a ratio of 3:2. Although the onset may be at any age from neonatal to late adult life, women in the third decade and men in the fifth decade have the peak incidence. Five to seven percent of cases are familial; however, no mendelian inheritance pattern is demonstrated. Studies in the era before effective immunotherapy and critical care revealed a mortality rate of 20–30% due to respiratory failure, with unchanged symptoms in 20%, improvement in 25%, and a later remission in the remaining 25%. Maximum symptoms usually appear within 3 years of disease onset. With contemporary immunologic therapy and respiratory and critical care, MG has become eminently treatable. Patients with MG seldom die when properly treated.

8. What are the HLA types associated with MG?

HLA-A1, B8, and DR3 and DR5 are frequently found in young Caucasian women with MG, whereas older men tend to have D2, A3, D7, and DRw2. In African-Americans, A1, B8, and DR5 are associated with MG. DR9 and DRw13 have been noted with increased frequency in pediatric Japanese and Bw46 in pediatric Chinese patients. Genetic susceptibility to experimental autoimmune myasthenia gravis (EAMG, see question 9) in animals has also been associated with certain histocompatibility types. Autoimmunity in MG may be subject to some genetic control via these major histocompatibility types.

DeBaets MH, Kuks JJ: Immunopathology of myasthenia gravis. In DeBaets MH, Oosterhuis HJGH (eds): Myasthenia Gravis. Boca Raton, FL, CRC Press, 1993, p 160.

9. What experimental evidence suggests that antibodies against the acetylcholine receptor cause MG?

Animals immunized with acetylcholine receptor develop serum antibodies against the receptor and exhibit clinical and electrophysiologic findings resembling human MG (experimental autoimmune myasthenia gravis, or EAMG). Passive transfer of human MG IgG to animals results in development of EAMG in the animals. Immunocytochemical studies have demonstrated IgG at the postsynaptic membrane of motor endplates in myasthenic skeletal muscles. In addition, the antibodies decrease the number of available acetylcholine receptors in cultured muscle cells in vitro.

10. What clinical evidence suggests that antibodies against the acetylcholine receptor cause MG?

More than 90% of patients with MG have circulating antibodies against the nicotinic acetylcholine receptor. Removal of the antibodies by plasmapheresis often improves the symptoms and signs of MG. In addition, mean antiacetylcholine antibody titers generally correlate with disease severity, whereas higher titers may be seen in early-onset disease and in patients with thymomas. Decreased titers after therapy also may correlate with improved symptoms in some patients. Favorable responses to immunotherapy are consistent with the antibody-mediated autoimmune pathogenesis of MG.

11. What are the immunopathologic mechanisms by which antiacetylcholine receptor antibodies cause MG?

The antibodies decrease the number of available nicotinic acetylcholine receptors in the postsynaptic membrane by several mechanisms:

1. The binding of the antibodies causes pharmacologic blockade of the cholinergic binding sites.

2. The antibodies cross-link adjacent receptors and increase the rate of internalization and subsequent degradation of the receptors.

3. The antibodies bound to the receptors activate the cascade of complement reactions. The resulting damage to the postsynaptic membrane leads not only to further receptor loss but also to widening of the synaptic cleft, which increases the diffusion of released acetylcholine and decreases the chance of acetylcholine molecules to reach the postsynaptic membrane.

4. The antibodies bound to the receptors also change the ion channel properties of the receptors.

12. Explain the concept of a safety margin in the context of synaptic transmission at the motor endplate.

Normally, the presynaptic nerve terminal releases a successively decreasing amount of acetylcholine on repetitive nerve stimulation at a slow rate, resulting in a successive decrease in the amplitude of endplate potentials at the postsynaptic membrane. At the normal neuromuscular junction, however, the endplate potentials are still large enough to trigger action potentials. Thus, the amplitude of compound muscle action potentials does not change with repetitive stimulation.

In MG, this safety margin is decreased because of the decreased number of acetylcholine receptors. Because fewer acetylcholine receptors are activated, the endplate potentials are smaller. These smaller potentials decline even further with repetitive stimulation, and an increasing number of endplate potentials fail to trigger an action potential in successive stimulations. This successive decrease in the total number of activated muscle fibers with repetitive nerve stimulation results in successively smaller compound muscle action potentials in patients with myasthenia.

13. What is the structure of the binding sites on the nicotinic acetylcholine receptor for acetylcholine and myasthenic autoantibodies?

The human acetylcholine receptor is a pentameric protein (molecular weight of 250,000) consisting of two alpha subunits and one each of beta, epsilon (or gamma in fetal form), and delta subunits. Acetylcholine binds to the main extracellular domain of the alpha subunit close to the N-terminal. Acetylcholine molecules must bind both alpha subunits of a receptor to open the channel within the receptor. The majority of myasthenic autoantibodies also bind to the main extracellular domain of the alpha subunit.

Ashizawa T, Oshima M, Ruan KH, Atassi MZ: Autoimmune recognition profile of the alpha chain of human acetylcholine receptor in myasthenia gravis. Adv Exp Med Biol 303:255–261, 1991.

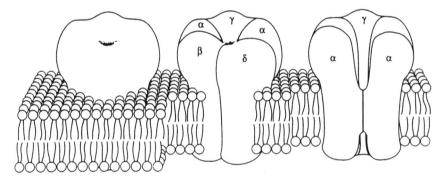

Diagram of the molecular structure of the acetylcholine receptor at the neuromuscular junction. (From Kandel ER, Schwartz JH, Jessel TM (eds): Principles of Neural Science, 3rd ed. New York, Elsevier, 1991, p 146, with permission.)

14. What is the Mary Walker phenomenon?

Fatigue and weakness of the forearm muscles develop in myasthenic patients during ischemic exercise testing when the forearm muscles are exercised with a cuff around the upper arm, inflated above systolic pressure. After the cuff is deflated, a dramatic myasthenic manifestation in the rest of the body may occur in some patients. This phenomenon, named after Mary Walker, who first described it in 1938, has been reproduced by several investigators and is also present in the myasthenic dog. Although some experts doubt that this is a true biologic phenomenon, others attribute it to the effect of released lactic acid from the exercised muscle. Lactic acid binds calcium and reduces ionized and total serum calcium. Lactate infusions increase weakness in patients with MG much more than in control patients.

Walker MB: Myasthenia gravis: A case in which fatigue of the forearm muscles could induce paralysis of the extraocular muscles. Proc Roy Soc Med 31:722:1938.

15. Which tumors are associated with MG?

Approximately 15% of patients with MG have a thymoma. Most thymomas are epithelial rather than lymphocytic in origin. Ninety percent are benign and easily treated with resection, whereas 10% are malignant with an average patient survival of 5–10 years. Thymic hyperplasia is seen in about 50% of patients with MG.

16. What are the diagnostic tests for thymoma?

Antiskeletal muscle antibodies, especially citric acid (CA)-extracted antigens, are detectable in most patients with MG and thymoma. Both sensitivity and specificity of anti-CA antibodies for thymoma in patients with MG are 94%. The sensitivity and specificity of CT scan of the chest for thymoma are 85% and 99%, respectively. Because most patients with MG undergo thymectomy, these tests may be most valuable in patients who have a marginal benefit/risk ratio for thymectomy or possible recurrence of thymoma.

Aarli JA, Gilhus NE, Matre R: Myasthenia gravis with thymoma is not associated with an increased incidence of non-muscle autoimmune disorders. Autoimmunity 11:159–182, 1992.

17. What data suggest that the thymus plays a major role in the pathogenesis of MG?

1. Most patients with MG have a histologic abnormality in the thymus, such as hyperplasia or thymoma.

2. Removal of the thymus improves MG.

3. Thymic B-lymphocytes produce antiacetylcholine receptor antibodies disproportionally more than other antibodies.

4. Addition of thymic cells to myasthenic B-lymphocytes in vitro enhances the production of antiacetylcholine antibodies but not other antibodies.

5. All subunits of the acetylcholine receptor, particularly the fetal type, are expressed in nonneoplastic MG thymuses. In contrast, MG thymomas do not appear to express any subunit but rather a protein epitope that cross-reacts with the alpha subunit.

6. Transplantation of MG thymus tissue to mice with severe combined immunodeficiency produces persistently elevated titers of antiacetylcholine receptor antibodies in serum and human IgG deposits at skeletal muscle endplates, whereas passive transfers of dissociated MG thymocytes show only a transient increase of antiacetylcholine receptor antibodies.

7. Myoid cells are present in the thymus, and the thymus is the site of T-lymphocyte maturation with acquisition of immunologic tolerance.

Geuder KI, Marx A, Witzemann V, et al: Pathogenetic significance of fetal-type acetylcholine receptors on thymic myoid cells in myasthenia gravis. Dev Immunol 2:69–75, 1992.

Schonbeck S, Padberg F, Hohlfeld R, Wekerle H: Transplantation of thymic autoimmune microenvironment to severe combined immunodeficiency mice: A new model of myasthenia gravis. J Clin Invest 90:245–250, 1992.

18. What is the myoid cell?

The myoid cells are musclelike cells found mainly within the medulla of the thymus. Although their number is few, they bear nicotinic acetylcholine receptors. Because antibodies against nicotinic acetylcholine receptors play the major pathogenic role in MG, the myoid cells may provide the primary antigens involved in the autoimmune response of MG. Myasthenic thymuses contain DR-positive lymphoid cells that may be able to present these antigens to T-lymphocytes, allowing sensitization.

19. What is the role of thymectomy in the treatment of MG?

Although prospective, randomized, controlled trials have not been conducted to evaluate the efficacy of thymectomy in MG, the beneficial effects appear overwhelming. Whether patients have thymoma, thymic hyperplasia, or an apparently normal thymus, early thymectomy frequently improves MG. Over 75% of patients benefit, and many eventually experience remission. Patients at high surgical risk (children and the elderly) may not benefit from resection. Congenital myasthenic syndromes do not respond to thymectomy, and neonatal MG improves without thymectomy. Thymectomy usually is not performed on patients with strictly ocular MG. Most experts prefer a transsternal approach over a transcervical approach because the chance of complete resection is better. Recently, thoracoscopic thymectomy, a less invasive procedure, has shown promising results.

20. What is neonatal myasthenia gravis?

Approximately 12% of neonates born to mothers with MG are "floppy" babies who have difficulty with breathing and sucking. The disease is transient, typically lasting for a few weeks and not exceeding 12 weeks. Passive transfer of maternal antibodies to the infant through the placenta is probably the major pathophysiologic mechanism. However, the severity and duration of maternal disease do not necessarily correlate with the occurrence of neonatal MG. Many infants born to severely affected mothers may have high antiacetylcholine antibody titers, but few develop neonatal myasthenia. In contrast, some infants of mothers in remission may develop the disease. The rate of destruction of the passively transferred antibodies in the child may influence the development of the illness. Analysis of the subclasses of antibodies suggests that infants with neonatal MG also may produce their own antibodies distinct from the maternal antibodies. Thus, elucidation of the exact pathophysiology of neonatal MG requires further investigation.

21. What are the congenital myasthenic disorders?

The congenital myasthenic disorders typically are characterized by the neonatal or infantile onset of extraocular, facial, bulbar, and limb weakness and fatigability that persist into adult life. Electrophysiologic findings suggest defective neuromuscular transmission. Unlike neonatal MG, however, the mother shows no evidence of the disease, acetylcholine receptor antibodies are not detectable in plasma, and the disease is not transient. Furthermore, patients do not respond to thymectomy or other treatments directed at the immune system.

The mechanisms for defective neuromuscular transmission are different in each of the congenital myasthenias. They are characterized by site of dysfunction within the neuromuscular junction. These disorders are the subject of ongoing investigation. New syndromes are described and existing syndromes are better defined each year. Other syndromes have been partially characterized but are not listed here.

Presynaptic	Defective acetylcholine packaging or synthesis (familial infantile MG: autosomal recessive)
	Reduced synaptic vesicles *and* reduced acetylcholine release (autosomal recessive in some)
Pre- and postsynaptic	Endplate acetylcholinesterase deficiency (autosomal recessive)
Postsynaptic	Acetylcholine receptor dysfunction with receptor deficiency
	• Classic slow channel syndrome (autosomal dominant)
	• Epsilon subunit mutation (autosomal recessive in some)
	• Acetylcholine receptor deficiency with short open time (autosomal recessive suspected)
	Acetylcholine receptor dysfunction alone
	• Fast channel syndrome (autosomal recessive)
	• Abnormal acetylcholine/acetylcholine receptor interaction (autosomal recessive suspected)

Engle AG: Congenital myasthenic syndromes. Neurol Clin North Am 12:273, 1994.

22. What are the diagnostic tests for MG?

The diagnosis of MG may be suspected from the clinical observation of skeletal muscle weakness increased by exercise and relieved by rest. To confirm the diagnosis of MG, the following features should be sought:

1. Improvement of weakness and fatigability by anticholinesterases (e.g., edrophonium [Tensilon] or neostigmine test)

2. Electrophysiologic evidence for defective neuromuscular transmission by repetitive stimulation or single-fiber EMG

3. The presence of circulating antibodies against acetylcholine receptors. Three major assays have been described, measuring binding, blocking, and modulating antiacetylcholine receptor antibodies. The binding antibody assay is 90% sensitive in generalized myasthenia and 70% sensitive in ocular myasthenia. The modulating antibody assay has a similar profile, with 90% sensitivity in generalized and a 27% sensitivity in ocular disease. The blocking antibody assay, however, is only 59% sensitive in generalized and only 30% sensitive in ocular MG, and is found in only 1% of patients whose binding antibody assay is negative. The specificity of each of these assays is similar at 99%.

Thymic pathology also may support the diagnosis.

23. What is the rationale for the edrophonium test?

Edrophonium (Tensilon) is a rapid- and short-acting anticholinesterase drug. The defective neuromuscular transmission in MG can be improved by anticholinesterase medications, which increase the concentration of acetylcholine in the synaptic cleft by inhibiting the breakdown of acetylcholine. The increased concentration of acetylcholine improves the chance that each acetylcholine receptor will encounter acetylcholine molecules, allowing activation of more receptors. Intravenous administration of edrophonium produces immediate and dramatic improvement in the signs of MG and therefore is a valuable diagnostic test.

24. How is the edrophonium test performed?

After noting the baseline degree of of weakness and fatigue, administer a test dose of 1 mg of edrophonium intravenously to verify that adverse effects do not occur. Keep a crash cart in the immediate vicinity in case of untoward cholinergic effects. Then inject up to 10 mg of edrophonium intravenously. Most people, including nonmyasthenic patients, may experience some degree of flushing, palpitation, and tearing. (In children, dosage depends on body weight, to a maximum of 10 mg). After administering the drug, document the level of weakness and fatigue again to determine any change. When ocular and bulbar signs are present, objective assessment is not difficult. However, when fatigue is demonstrable only in limb muscles, quantitative measurement of strength and fatigability is important, because relying on the patient's and examiner's impression can be misleading. Double-blind testing using normal saline as a control may be useful. A test that unequivocally demonstrates improvement of weakness and fatigability is strongly suggestive of MG.

25. Which electrophysiologic findings are diagnostic for MG?

A decrement of greater than 10–15% in the amplitude of the evoked compound action potential recorded from the skeletal muscle upon low-frequency (typically 3 per second) repetitive stimulation of the motor nerve is suggestive of MG. The first muscle response has normal amplitude, but subsequent responses show a reduction in amplitude before reaching a plateau in the fourth to sixth responses. This decrement may be transiently repaired by brief exercise of the tested muscle prior to repetitive stimulation (postexercise facilitation). The decrement may also be correctable in MG by administration of anticholinesterase medications such as edrophonium.

26. What is single-fiber electromyography (SFEMG)?

SFEMG involves simultaneous recordings of evoked responses from two muscle fibers belonging to the same motor unit. The motor unit discharge is elicited by either submaximal voluntary contractions of the muscle or repetitive submaximal stimulation of the nerve to that muscle. Recording from a normal muscle shows two evoked responses from the two muscle fibers firing with minimal fluctuation of the interval between the two. The fluctuation is called "jitter" and is due to the variable time required for neuromuscular transmission from discharge to discharge. In MG, the jitter is increased and may be associated with an occasional lack of response from one of the muscle fibers ("blocking"). Increased jitter also may occur in LEMS and diseases in which nerve sprouting exists.

27. What is pyridostigmine? Why is it the most widely used anticholinesterase medication in MG?

Pyridostigmine (Mestinon) is slightly longer-acting (with a half-life of 4 hours) and has fewer cholinergic side effects than neostigmine bromide and other anticholinesterase preparations. Unlike physostigmine, pyridostigmine has no unwanted CNS effects because it does not cross the blood-brain barrier. However, some cases of MG may be refractory to pyridostigmine but respond to other anticholinesterases.

28. What are the chronic adverse effects of anticholinesterases on the neuromuscular junction?

In addition to the acute event of cholinergic crisis, excessive acetylcholine may cause chronic changes at the postsynaptic membrane, resembling the endplate seen in MG. Postsynaptic junctional folds are simplified, and the number of acetylcholine receptors is decreased. The postsynaptic effects of excessive acetylcholine cause additional damage to the already existing changes due to MG antibodies.

29. What is Mestinon Timespan?

The bedtime dose of pyridostigmine may not last throughout the night. Patients with MG may complain of difficulty in swallowing medication the next morning. A slow-release tablet of 180 mg of pyridostigmine (Timespan) may alleviate this problem, although the release rate is somewhat unpredictable.

30. What dose of parenteral pyridostigmine is equivalent to the standard 60-mg oral pyridostigmine pill?

A parenteral dose of 2 mg is equivalent to an oral dose of 60 mg.

31. What are the drugs to be used with caution in MG?

Drugs that may adversely affect MG should be used with caution:

Antibiotics	**Neuromuscular blockers**	
Aminoglycosides	**Cardiac drugs**	
Neomycin	Quinine	
Streptomycin	Quinidine	
Kanamycin	Procainamide	
Gentamicin	Trimethaphan	
Tobramycin	Lidocaine	
Other peptide antibiotics	Beta-adrenergic blockers	
Polymyxin B	**Other drugs**	
Colistin	Phenytoin	Oxytocin
Other antibiotics	Chloroquine	Aprotinin
Oxytetracycline	Trimethadione	Propanidid
Rolitetracycline	Lithium carbonate	Diazepam
Lincomycin	Magnesium salts	Ketamine
Clindamycin	Meglumine diatrizoate	D-penicillamine
Erythromycin	Methoxyflurane	Carnitine
Ampicillin		

The aminoglycosides and two other peptide antibiotics, polymyxin B and colistin, may have adverse effects both pre- and postsynaptically. Other antibiotics (oxytetracycline, rolitetracycline, lincomycin, clindamycin, erythromycin, and ampicillin) and many drugs used for cardiac diseases also may exacerbate MG. Chloroquine and phenytoin may aggravate or unmask MG. Lithium carbonate may interfere with neuromuscular transmission by compromising pre- and postsynaptic Na^+ influx. Neuromuscular blocking agents, magnesium salts, and anticholinesterases require close monitoring when administered to patients with MG. Meglumine diatrizoate, a CT scan contrast material, has been reported to cause acute exacerbation in patients with MG. Methoxyflurane, an anesthetic, may unmask subclinical MG. Oxytocin, aprotinin, propanidid, diazepam, and ket-amine have been reported to prolong postoperative recovery in MG. Timoptic eyedrops may also worsen symptoms. Aminoglycosides, peptide antibiotics, oxprenolol, practolol, trimethaphan, phenytoin, trimethadione, D-penicillamine, and carnitine have been reported to induce MG in previously unaffected patients.

32. What precautions are necessary in treating MG with corticosteroids?

In addition to the usual side effects of corticosteroids, patients with MG may become weaker 1–3 weeks after initiation of oral prednisone therapy, usually followed by a gradual but marked improvement. Pretreatment with plasma exchange and/or IVIG or, alternatively, gradually in-creasing doses of oral prednisone, from 25 mg orally every other day to to 100 mg orally every other day, may alleviate this phenomenon. During the initial exacerbation associated with the in-troduction of prednisone, respiratory functions should be carefully monitored. With prednisone-induced improvement, the sensitivity of patients with MG to anticholinesterase drugs may increase, and the doses of anticholinesterase often need to be reduced or discontinued. Patients may require maintenance doses of prednisone for up to 2 years before its discontinuation, be-cause recurrences are common. Doses of prednisone must be reduced carefully, because relapses often result from reducing the doses too fast or too soon.

33. What causes drug-induced autoimmune myasthenia gravis?

Approximately 1% of patients taking D-penicillamine for the treatment of rheumatoid arthri-tis or Wilson's disease develop clinical myasthenia. The disease afflicts women six times more frequently than men and is associated with HLA-A1 and B8, which are frequent HLA types in spontaneous MG. The disease first strikes the ocular muscles and then becomes generalized. Patients with D-penicillamine–induced MG have autoantibodies against acetylcholine receptors. The disease and the autoantibodies slowly disappear after discontinuation of D-penicillamine. Trimethadone, an anticonvulsant, also may induce myasthenia, presumably via autoimmune mechanisms because the myasthenia is associated with high titers of antimuscle antibodies and antinuclear factor and clinically resembles systemic lupus erythematosus.

34. What is a myasthenic crisis?

Myasthenic crisis is an acute exacerbation of MG with respiratory and bulbar dysfunction. Respiratory care to maintain adequate ventilation is the most important factor in the treatment. Mortality of MG was drastically decreased with the introduction of ICUs even before the intro-duction of steroids as a treatment of MG. Life-threatening respiratory failure can be prevented by close monitoring of pulmonary functions, especially forced vital capacity and FEV_1, which de-cline before blood gases deteriorate. Early endotracheal intubation with mechanical ventilatory support is lifesaving in myasthenic crisis.

Reliance on anticholinesterase medications during a myasthenic crisis is controversial. When cholinergic crisis cannot be excluded as the cause of the clinical exacerbation, discontinuation of anticholinesterases under respiratory support is recommended. A few days later, an anticholin-esterase can be started at a low dose and the dose gradually increased as needed. High-dose oral prednisone therapy often provides improvement with time (whether high-dose IV steroids also have a role in myasthenic crisis is currently under investigation), and plasmapheresis and/or in-travenous gamma globulin also may be helpful during this acute phase. If the patient proves chronically refractory to steroids alone, immunosuppressive agents such as cyclophosphamide, cyclosporin-A, azathioprine, and methotrexate may be needed as adjunctive or alternate therapy. If thymectomy has not been performed, it should be done as soon as the patient can safely toler-ate the surgery.

35. What is a cholinergic crisis?

Overdosing with anticholinesterase may result in excessive acetylcholine in the synaptic cleft, causing depolarization block of acetylcholine receptors. The end result is defective neuromuscular transmission similar to a myasthenic crisis. Fasciculations are common. Establishing an airway, supporting respiration, and withholding anticholinesterase medications are the mainstays of treatment.

36. What is the value of the edrophonium test to differentiate myasthenic crisis from cholinergic crisis?

The edrophonium (Tensilon) test improves myasthenic crisis but aggravates cholinergic crisis. However, interpretation of the result is often difficult and misleading because one group of muscles may deteriorate while others improve. Securing the respiration and discontinuing all anticholinesterase drugs in a protected environment in the ICU offers a safer and more practical solution.

LAMBERT-EATON MYASTHENIC SYNDROME

37. What are the primary manifestations of Lambert-Eaton myasthenic syndrome (LEMS)?

In LEMS, weakness and fatigability of proximal muscles, especially in the thighs and pelvic girdle, with depressed or absent tendon reflexes are the primary manifestations. Muscle strength may increase for a short while after exercise (postexercise facilitation). Although ptosis may be present in LEMS, extraocular and bulbar muscles are otherwise spared as a rule. Mild autonomic dysfunction may be prominent in LEMS, manifesting primarily as dryness of the mouth.

38. What tumor is associated with LEMS?

About 50–66% of patients with LEMS have small-cell carcinoma of the lung at the time of presentation or will ultimately be diagnosed with it, usually within 2 years. Although immunologic evidence suggests that this tumor may play an important role in the pathogenesis of LEMS, a substantial minority of patients with LEMS never develop malignancy.

39. What experimental evidence suggests an autoimmune pathogenesis of LEMS?

Passive transfers of IgG from patients with LEMS to animals produce electrophysiologic defects characteristic of LEMS. The LEMS IgG contains autoantibodies against voltage-gated calcium channels.

40. Describe the autoimmune pathophysiology involved in LEMS.

The primary antigen for the LEMS antibodies appears to be present in the small-cell carcinoma of the lung that is often associated with LEMS. The LEMS antibodies cross-react with N type and L type voltage-gated Ca^{2+} channels and with synaptotagmin. The antibody action does not involve complement-mediated membrane lysis. The decreased number of the voltage-gated Ca^{2+} channels with the resulting decrease in miniature endplate potential (MEPP) frequency and the morphologic changes at the active zone have been attributed to the actions of LEMS antibodies.

41. Explain the mechanism of incremental response after high-frequency repetitive nerve stimulation in patients with LEMS.

In LEMS the decreased Ca^{2+} influx into the presynaptic nerve terminal upon depolarization of the presynaptic membrane results in insufficient release of acetylcholine from the presynaptic nerve terminal. With repetitive nerve stimulation, an accumulation of presynaptic calcium may facilitate the release of acetylcholine. This explains the incremental response of the compound muscle action potential to high-frequency repetitive stimulation of the nerve.

42. What are the morphologic changes at the neuromuscular junction in LEMS?

Light microscopy reveals proliferation and enlargement of the secondary synaptic clefts in LEMS in contrast to the widened and simplified postsynaptic folds in MG. The proliferative and hypertrophic postsynaptic membranes are considered to be a response to repeated degeneration and regeneration of presynaptic membranes. At the electron microscopic level, the freeze-fracture technique shows that the active zone protein particles are decreased in number and disorganized.

43. What is the treatment for LEMS?

Release of acetylcholine from the presynaptic nerve terminal is facilitated by guanidine hydrochloride, 4-aminopyridine, and 3,4-diaminopyridine. Because the latter two may decrease the seizure threshold, guanidine hydrochloride, 20–30 mg/day in divided doses, is the recommended treatment. Anticholinesterases also may improve symptoms. When an associated neoplasm is resectable, tumor removal may reverse the syndrome. Glucocorticoids and plasmapheresis have been useful, but other immunosuppressive agents may accelerate growth of the carcinoma. Improvement after intravenous gamma globulin treatment also has been reported.

44. What precautions must be taken for surgical procedures that require general anesthesia in MG and LEMS?

A thoracotomy for resection of the lung cancer in LEMS and a thymectomy in MG are often necessary procedures. Precautions include:

1. Delayed recovery from the effect of neuromuscular blocking agents must be anticipated in both LEMS and MG. Give a short-acting neuromuscular blocker in the minimal dose necessary for the surgical procedure.

2. If the patient has been taking glucocorticoids, give greater than equivalent doses intravenously before, during, and after surgery until the original oral glucocorticoid therapy can be reinstated.

3. Anticholinesterase therapy is usually unnecessary during surgery but is started postoperatively as needed when the patient regains consciousness. The differences between parenteral and oral doses of anticholinesterase should be recognized (see question 30).

4. Maintain normal serum electrolytes, calcium, and magnesium.

5. Avoid unnecessary medications to minimize drug-related complications.

6. Avoid medications that may worsen the defective synaptic transmission at the neuromuscular junction (see question 31).

OTHER NEUROMUSCULAR JUNCTION DISEASES

45. What are the clinical characteristics of botulism?

Two to 48 hours after ingesting improperly prepared canned or bottled foods contaminated with *Clostridium botulinum*, ocular and bulbar muscle paralysis begins, with difficulty in convergence of the eyes, diplopia, ptosis, weakness of the jaw muscles, dysphagia, and dysarthria. Nausea, vomiting, and diarrhea may precede these symptoms. Constipation, urinary retention, and nonreactive dilation of the pupils may occur because of autonomic dysfunction. Subsequently, the paralysis spreads and causes respiratory failure and total limb paralysis without abnormalities in mental status or sensation.

In infants, the initial manifestations are poor sucking and difficulty with feeding, weak cries, loss of head control, and bilateral ptosis, which subsequently result in generalized flaccid paralysis.

The course depends on the amount of toxin absorbed. In severe cases, death usually occurs within 4–8 days. If only a small amount of the toxin is absorbed, the symptoms are mild and recovery may be complete.

46. What is the infectious process in botulism?

Botulinum toxin is an exotoxin of *C. botulinum*. The presence of common bacteria inhibits the growth of *C. botulinum*, but infection occurs when the victim ingests improperly prepared canned or bottled foods in which the common bacteria are killed but the more resistant *Clostridium* spores are spared. In infants, the intestinal bacterial flora may not effectively inhibit the growth of *C. botulinum*. Human botulism is usually caused by exotoxin produced by types A, B, and E.

47. What is the pharmacologic action of black widow spider venom?

Black widow spider venom promotes release of acetylcholine from the presynaptic nerve terminal and depletes presynaptic acetylcholine. The venom also inhibits choline uptake. Clinically, this causes painful muscle spasm followed by weakness.

48. What is the pharmacologic action of curare?

Curare is a classic antagonist of nicotinic acetylcholine receptors and competes with acetylcholine for the binding site. Curare, therefore, has been used as a neuromuscular blocking agent (nondepolarizing blocker) for general anesthesia.

49. What snake venom causes a neuromuscular disorder? What is its importance in experimental studies of MG?

Pharmacologically, alpha-bungarotoxin blocks acetylcholine binding to the receptor, causing defective neuromuscular transmission similar to MG. This toxin comes from the binding of alpha-bungarotoxin to the receptor at multiple sites on the alpha subunit. Alpha-bungarotoxin has a high affinity for the alpha subunit of the nicotinic acetylcholine receptor, which makes this toxin a useful marker for acetylcholine receptors in both in vivo and in vitro experiments. All experiments on the purification, characterization, and localization of the receptor, as well as detection of serum autoantibodies against the receptor, have used alpha-bungarotoxin.

BIBLIOGRAPHY

1. Antel J, Birnbaum G, Hartung H-P (eds): Clinical Neuroimmunology. Malden, MA, Blackwell Science, 1998.
2. Rolak LA, Harati Y (eds): Neuroimmunology for the Clinician. Boston, Butterworth-Heinemann, 1997.
3. Vincent A, Wray D (eds): Neuromuscular Transmission: Basic and Applied Aspects. Manchester, England, Manchester University Press, 1990.

Websites
www.myasthenia.org
www.neuro.wustl.edu/neuromuscular/synmg.html

6. PERIPHERAL NEUROPATHIES

Yadollah Harati, M.D., F.A.C.P., and Robert J. Kolimas, M.D.

1. What are the most common diseases affecting the peripheral nerve?
The most important neuropathies can be classified by the mnemonic **DANG THE RAPIST**:

D Diabetes	**T** Trauma	**R** Rheumatic (collagen vascular)
A Alcohol	**H** Hereditary	**A** Amyloid
N Nutritional	**E** Environmental	**P** Paraneoplastic
G Guillain-Barré	toxins and	**I** Infections
	drugs	**S** Systemic disease
		T Tumors

2. What are the patterns of peripheral nerve damage?
The nerve can be damaged by injury to the myelin, axon, cell body, or vasa nervorum. Three basic pathologic mechanisms underlie nerve injury:

1. **Wallerian degeneration** develops after injury to the axon and myelin, as in transection of the nerve. Distal to the transection, the axon and then myelin degenerate, followed within 3–5 days by failure to generate and conduct a nerve action potential. The axon may regrow within the architecture provided by the basement membrane of Schwann cells, but the degree and efficiency of regrowth depend on good approximation of the nerve ends.

2. **Segmental demyelination** develops after damage to the myelin sheath or Schwann cell. Because the muscle is not denervated, no atrophy develops, whereas in wallerian degeneration the axon is also damaged and the muscle degenerates. Prognosis for complete recovery is good.

3. **Neuronal (axonal) degeneration** develops when damage to the cell body of the neuron results in distal dying of the axon and subsequent loss of myelin. Once the distal nerve dies, the muscle is denervated; hence, muscle atrophy develops. The denervated muscle is reinnervated by surrounding nerves, but recovery may not be complete.

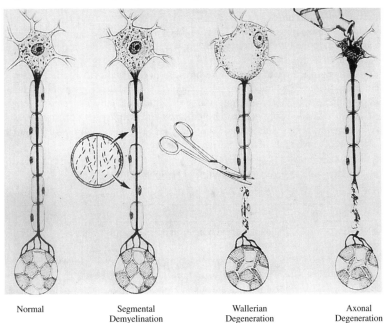

Normal   Segmental Demyelination   Wallerian Degeneration   Axonal Degeneration

83

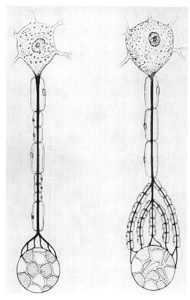

Segmental remyelination may follow segmental demyelination. The remyelinated segments are shorter and have a smaller diameter. Axonal regeneration is associated with the formation of clusters of small and thinly myelinated fibers.

Regeneration after   Regeneration after
Segmental Demyelination   Axonal Degeneration

3. What electrophysiologic mechanisms correlate with weakness in peripheral neuropathy?

Conduction block, denervation with loss of motor units, and failure of neuromuscular transmission. One or more of the above are needed. Slowing of motor conduction velocity in itself, even if severe, does not result in weakness.

4. What is conduction block?

A focal abnormality across a nerve segment that results in failure to conduct an action potential, although distal to the block conduction is preserved.

5. What is the significance of conduction block in peripheral neuropathy?

Conduction block occurs only in certain limited settings of acute reversible ischemic injury, compression-induced (paranodal or segmental) demyelination, and acquired demyelinative neuropathies. It generally does not occur in hereditary neuropathies with one major exception—hereditary neuropathy with liability to pressure palsy (HNPP). It is clinically important because it implies a potentially reversible defect causing weakness.

6. What are the clinical tests for the common root syndromes?

Clinical Tests for Common Root Syndromes

ROOT	MUSCLE TESTED	EXAMINATION	REFLEX
C5	Deltoid Biceps	Shoulder abduction: push down on arms abducted at 90°	Biceps
C6	Biceps Brachioradialis	Flexion at elbow: pull outward at wrist with elbows flexed at 90°	Brachioradialis
C7	Triceps Finger extensors	Extension at elbow: push down on elbow with arm in extension and supination	Triceps
C8	Finger flexors	Finger flexion: "squeeze my finger"	

(Table continued on following page.)

Clinical Tests for Common Root Syndromes (Continued)

ROOT	MUSCLE TESTED	EXAMINATION	REFLEX
T1	Intrinsic hand muscles	Finger abduction and adduction: fingers are spread out—try squeezing them inward	
L1–L3	Iliopsoas	Hip flexion: while sitting, patient flexes at hip. Push hip down with pressure at knee.	Cremasteric
L2–L3	Adductors	Hip adduction: try to push legs inward	
L3–L4	Quadriceps	Extension of leg at knee	Knee reflex
L4	Anterior tibial	Dorsiflexion of foot	Knee reflex
L5	Toe extensors Anterior tibial	Dorsiflexion of toes	
S1	Gastrocnemius Toe extensors	Plantarflexion of foot	Ankle jerk

7. Which peripheral neuropathies may have cranial nerve involvement?

Peripheral Neuropathies with Cranial Nerve Involvement

NEUROPATHY	MOST COMMONLY INVOLVED CRANIAL NERVES	LESS COMMONLY INVOLVED CRANIAL NERVES
Diphtheria	IX	II, III
Sarcoid	VII	I, III, IV, VI
Diabetes	III*	IV, VI, VII
Guillain-Barré syndrome (GBS)	VI, VII	
Miller-Fisher variant of GBS	III, IV	
Sjögren syndrome	V	
Polyarteritis nodosa	VII, III	VIII
Wegener granulomatosis	VIII	
Lyme disease	VII, V	All but I
Porphyria	VII, X	III, IV, V, XI, XII
Refsum's disease	I, VIII	
Primary amyloidosis	VII, V, III	VI, XII
Syphilis	III	IV, V, VII, VIII
Arsenic	V	

* Pupil is usually not affected.

8. Which neuropathies begin proximally rather than distally?
Most neuropathies begin distally, but a few may begin proximally:
1. Sensory neuropathies: porphyria and rare cases of Tangier disease.
2. Motor neuropathies: Guillain-Barré syndrome, chronic inflammatory demyelinating neuropathy, diabetes, and idiopathic acute brachial plexus neuropathy.

9. Which neuropathies begin in the arms rather than the legs?
Most neuropathies present with symptoms in the feet. Once the symptoms in the lower limbs proceed to the middle of the calf, the neuropathies begin to appear in the hands. Although this pattern generally holds, some neuropathies may start in the upper limbs:
1. Compression/entrapment syndromes
2. Diabetes
3. Vasculitic neuropathy
4. Guillain-Barré syndrome
5. Multifocal motor neuropathy
6. Lead toxicity
7. Porphyria
8. Sarcoidosis
9. Leprosy
10. Charcot-Marie-Tooth disease (rare)
11. Tangier disease
12. Inherited recurrent focal neuropathies
13. Some forms of familial amyloid polyneuropathy

10. Which neuropathies are often predominantly motor?
Guillain-Barré syndrome, diphtheric neuropathy, dapsone-induced neuropathy, porphyria, and multifocal motor neuropathy.

11. Which neuropathies are often predominantly sensory?
1. Drug toxicity: pyridoxine, doxorubicin, cisplatin
2. Autoimmune: Miller-Fisher syndrome, sensory variants of acute and chronic inflammatory demyelinating polyneuropathy, IgM paraproteinemia, paraneoplastic, Sjögren syndrome
3. Infectious: diphtheria, HIV, Lyme disease
4. Deficiency: vitamin E
5. Inherited: abetalipoproteinemia, spinocerebellar degeneration

12. What are the causes of multiple mononeuropathy (mononeuritis multiplex)?
1. Trauma or compression
2. Diabetes
3. Vasculitis, with or without connective tissue diseases; also virus-associated (HIV, hepatitis B and C)
4. Leprosy
5. Lyme disease
6. Sarcoidosis
7. Sensory perineuritis
8. Tumor infiltration
9. Lymphoid granulomatosis
10. Demyelinating idiopathic and paraproteinemic neuropathies (rare)
11. Hereditary neuropathy with liability to pressure palsies (HNPP)

13. In which conditions are the peripheral nerves palpably enlarged?
1. Hereditary motor and sensory neuropathies (HMSN) of Charcot-Marie-Tooth disease (demyelinative type) and Dejerine-Sottas syndrome (HMSNIII)
2. Amyloidosis
3. Refsum's disease
4. Leprosy
5. Acromegaly
6. Neurofibromatosis

14. What is an "onion-bulb" formation?
Onion-bulb formation is the pathologic hallmark of the hypertrophic neuropathies, in which repeated segmental demyelination and remyelination have occurred. As viewed in transverse sections, onion-bulb formations are multiple concentric layers of intertwined, attenuated Schwann cell processes surrounding the remaining nerve fibers. The Schwann cell processes are separated from each other by layers of collagen fibers. The onion-bulb formations may be seen in any condition with chronic segmental demyelination and remyelination but are frequently seen in Charcot-Marie-Tooth disease, Dejerine-Sottas syndrome, Refsum's disease, and chronic relapsing idiopathic (inflammatory) demyelinating neuropathy.

15. Which nerves are commonly used for biopsy?
The most common and best nerve to use is the sural nerve, a purely sensory nerve located lateral to the lateral malleolus. The nerve can be biopsied at this level or at a higher level between the heads of the gastrocnemius muscles. Superficial peroneal and radial cutaneous nerves offer advantages in certain situations; the radial cutaneous nerve is often biopsied in upper limb–predominant neuropathies (e.g., some cases of leprosy). The intermediate cutaneous nerve of the thigh also has been biopsied in patients with proximal diabetic neuropathy.

16. What are the indications for sural nerve biopsy?
Sural nerve biopsy is most helpful when the underlying condition is multifocal and asymmetric. Examples include many of the disorders associated with multiple mononeuropathies, especially vasculitis and leprosy. It may be obtained in chronic demyelinating neuropathies with the aim of confirming the diagnosis in patients who may be candidates for therapies with potentially harmful side effects. Nerve is one of a number of tissues useful in diagnosing amyloidosis. Genetic studies and enzyme assays have decreased the need for nerve biopsy in some inherited neuropathies, but it is still useful in unrecognized cases, for example, of HNPP and metachromatic leukodystrophy. Metabolic and toxic causes of peripheral neuropathies

are not usually diagnosed by sural nerve biopsy. Nerve biopsy may be of value as a final resort in patients with progressive, disabling peripheral neuropathy of undetermined etiology. With teased nerve fiber preparation, segmental demyelination, remyelination, or axonal degeneration is identified. In segmental demyelination, the diameter of demyelinated segments is reduced. In remyelination, the internodal length varies. Axonal degeneration causes breakdown of myelin into "ovoids and balls."

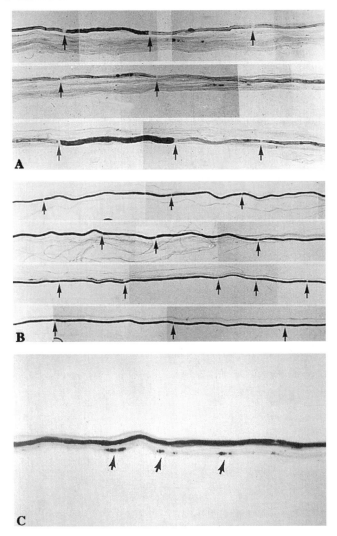

Teased nerve fiber preparation. *A,* Segmental demyelination. *B,* Remyelination. *C,* Axonal degeneration.

COMMON NEUROPATHIES

17. What is the most common cause of peripheral neuropathy in the world?

Diabetes. The most common cause used to be leprosy, but with implementation of aggressive World Health Organization (WHO) recommendations, its prevalence is declining; leprosy is now second to diabetes as a cause for peripheral neuropathy.

18. Which diabetic neuropathies are painful?
- Third cranial nerve neuropathy
- Acute thoracoabdominal neuropathy
- Acute distal sensory neuropathy
- Acute lumbar radiculoplexopathy
- Chronic distal small-fiber neuropathy

19. How does the global importance of leprous neuropathy compare to its importance in the U.S.?
Despite the 10-fold decline in the global prevalence of leprosy to about 1 million, it is still the most common cause of neuropathy in developing countries. In contrast, the prevalence of leprosy in the U.S. is low (< 10,000). The yearly incidence in the past decade (100–200) fluctuated in previous decades, depending on the extent to which immigrants and refugees from endemic areas entered the U.S. Leprous neuropathy should not be overlooked, however, because leprosy does occur in native U.S. citizens. Although they represent a minority of cases (10–20%) in most regions of the U.S., native citizens are affected more commonly in the endemic southern border areas of Texas, Louisiana, and Florida as well as Hawaii.

20. How does one recognize and diagnose hereditary neuropathy with liability to pressure palsy (HNPP)?
HNPP, also called recurrent pressure-sensitive neuropathy or tomaculous neuropathy, is readily identified in cases of recurrent compression-induced mononeuropathies and in patients with autosomal dominant familial patterns, demyelinative features, and "sausage-shaped" swellings or tomaculi on nerve biopsy. However, a traumatic mechanism is not always obvious, and the pathologic evidence of numerous tomaculi may be the only diagnostic clue in sporadic cases presenting with a generalized polyneuropathy. Demonstrating *PMP22* gene deletion confirms the diagnosis. Clinical heterogeneity is becoming apparent with increased use of this genetic study.

21. What clinical features aid in the early diagnosis of carpal tunnel syndrome?
1. Pain, paresthesias, or numbness worse at night or during activities that maintain wrist extension or flexion (e.g., driving) or require repetitive wrist motion.

2. Numbness often involving only partial median nerve innervation (e.g., thumb and index finger) rather than entire first three and one-half digits. Pain but not numbness may occur above the wrist.

3. Symptoms of intermittent hand weakness before overt weakness of thenar muscles and lateral lumbricals.

4. Rigorous study has demonstrated that provocative clinical tests, such as median nerve percussion (Tinel's sign) or wrist flexion (Phalen's test), are insufficiently specific to be diagnostically useful. Newer tests, such as direct external carpal tunnel compression, either over the transverse carpal ligament (carpal compression test [CCT]) or over the wrist (pressure provocative test [PPT]), are also not very accurate.
Kawl MP, Pagel KJ, Wheatley MJ, et al: Carpal compression test and pressure provocative test in veterans with median-distribution paresthesias. Muscle Nerve 24:107–111, 2001.

22. What are the three most common neurogenic causes of winging of the scapula?
1. **Long thoracic nerve palsy.** The long thoracic nerve innervates the serratus anterior muscle. Serratus anterior weakness leads to the most pronounced winging, which is accentuated with forward flexion of the arms and decreased with arm at rest. The superior (medial) angle of the scapula is displaced closer to the midline, whereas the inferior angle swings laterally and away from the thorax.

2. **Spinal accessory nerve palsy.** The spinal accessory nerve innervates the trapezius muscle. Trapezius muscle weakness leads to mild winging of the scapula at rest, which is accentuated by arm abduction to 90° and decreased by forward flexion to 90°. The superior (medial) angle of the scapula is displaced away from the midline, but the inferior angle is medially rotated. The shoulder is lower on the affected side because of atrophy of the trapezius muscle.

3. **Dorsal scapular nerve palsy.** The dorsal scapular nerve innervates the rhomboid muscle. Weakness of this muscle produces minimal winging at rest, which is accentuated by slowly lowering the arm from the forward overhead position and decreased by elevation of the arms overhead. The superior (medial) angle is displaced away from the midline, and the inferior angle is laterally displaced.

In addition, there are many nonneurogenic causes of winging of the scapula, including myopathies and muscular dystrophy.

23. What are the different types of Lyme neuropathies?

Lyme disease, a multisystem illness caused by a tick-borne spirochete, *Borrelia burgdorferi,* may cause many varieties of peripheral neuropathies, including cranial neuropathies (especially Bell's palsy), radiculitis, plexopathies, multiple mononeuropathies, a Guillain-Barré-like illness, and, more frequently, a symmetric sensory-motor neuropathy. In endemic areas, Lyme disease accounts for about two-thirds of pediatric cases of facial palsy and as many as one-fourth of adult cases. Involvement of other cranial nerves usually occurs in the setting of lymphocytic meningitis. Radiculitis may be indistinguishable from a compression-induced radiculopathy. Such radiculopathies usually occur in the lower limbs, and CSF pleocytosis is common. Unilateral or bilateral lumbosacral or brachial plexopathies are rarely observed. The symmetric distal sensory-motor neuropathy is usually mild and occurs in many patients with chronic Lyme disease.

24. Which kinds of peripheral neuropathies are associated with HIV infection?

Up to 50% of patients with HIV infection develop a peripheral neuropathy, which may take one or a combination of the following forms:

1. Distal symmetric neuropathy (most common form)
   • Painful sensory type
   • Sensory-motor type (mild or minimal motor involvement)
   • Diffuse inflammatory lymphocytosis syndrome (symmetric or asymmetric, sensorimotor)
2. Inflammatory demyelinating polyneuropathy (both acute and chronic forms, usually with elevated CSF cell counts)
3. Mononeuropathy multiplex
4. Polyradiculopathy (cytomegalovirus [CMV], herpes zoster, syphilis, lymphomatous)
5. Cranial neuropathy
6. Autonomic neuropathy
7. Nutritional, vitamin deficiency neuropathy
8. Drug-induced neuropathy

25. What are the most important industrial agents causing peripheral neuropathy?

1. **Acrylamide.** Only direct skin exposure to the monomer of acrylamide is neurotoxic to peripheral nerves, resulting in symptoms of numbness, gait unsteadiness, mild weakness, palmar hyperhidrosis, and skin peeling. The neuropathy is caused by impairment of axoplasmic transport mechanisms, particularly retrograde transport. Withdrawal from exposure to acrylamide usually results in slow recovery.

2. **Carbon disulfide.** Low-level prolonged inhalation of carbon disulfide, used in the production of cellophane films and rayon fibers, results in distal axonopathy. With higher levels or longer duration of exposure, encephalopathic, extrapyramidal, and psychotic abnormalities may develop. Removal of the agent causes slow and frequently incomplete recovery.

3. **Dimethylaminopropionitrile (DMAPN).** Inhalation of DMAPN, used in the manufacturing of polyurethane foam, results in urologic dysfunction (urinary hesitancy, decreased urine stream, incontinence, and sometimes impotence) followed by distal symmetric and predominantly sensory polyneuropathy, with a characteristic sensory loss in the sacral dermatomes. Removal from exposure results in gradual recovery.

4. **Ethylene oxide.** At high levels of exposure, ethylene oxide causes a symmetric, distal polyneuropathy, sometimes with encephalopathic symptoms. Prolonged low-level exposure

among hospital sterilizer workers and patients receiving long-term hemodialysis is claimed to cause a subclinical neuropathy. Withdrawal from exposure results in gradual improvement.

5. **Hexacarbons (n-hexane, methyl n-butyl ketone).** Industrial use of hexacarbon solvents in a poorly ventilated environment and the practice of inhalant abuse by teenagers (glue sniffing) are the major causes of hexacarbon neuropathy. Both n-hexane and methyl-n-butyl ketone (MBK) are metabolized to 2.5-hexanedione, the agent responsible for the neurotoxicity. The neurotoxic effect is caused by the interruption of the retrograde axoplasmic flow, resulting in symmetric distal sensory neuropathy with loss of ankle reflexes and focally swollen axons (giant axons) on nerve pathology. Some patients also may manifest symptoms of autonomic neuropathy. When the offending agent is stopped, the neuropathy characteristically progresses for another few months, but most patients with mild-to-moderate involvement recover completely.

6. **Methyl bromide.** Chronic exposure to high-to-moderate levels of methyl bromide results in the symptoms of distal sensorimotor neuropathy that gradually resolve after withdrawal from exposure. Pyramidal tract signs and cerebellar dysfunction also may be prominent. Whether the neuropathy is due to an axonopathy, myelin sheath disease, or both is not known. Methyl bromide has found use as a fumigant, fire extinguisher, refrigerant, and insecticide.

7. **Organophosphorus esters.** A number of organophosphorus esters, including tri-o-cresylphosphate (TOCP), leptophos, mipafox, chlorphos, and trichlorfon, cause a delayed, usually subacute motor-predominant distal axonopathy after a single or prolonged exposure. These esters are used as insecticides, petroleum additives, and modifiers of plastic. Their toxic effect on the peripheral nerves may involve inhibition of a neuropathy target esterase (NTE). The prognosis in mildly affected people is good, but severe cases have varying degrees of residual peripheral and central nervous system dysfunction.

8. **Trichlorethylene.** Industrial exposure to trichlorethylene results in a peculiar syndrome manifesting as sensorimotor trigeminal neuropathy, facial neuropathy, oculomotor dysfunction, and optic nerve dysfunction. The agent is used in dry cleaning, degreasing, and rubber production. The reason for its selective predilection for the cranial nerves is not known.

9. **Vacor.** When accidentally ingested, this rodenticide causes severe destruction of the pancreatic beta cells and severe acute axonal and autonomic neuropathy. Vacor is thought to impair fast anterograde axoplasmic flow.

26. What is critical-illness polyneuropathy?

Critical-illness polyneuropathy (CIP) develops in 50–70% of patients, usually in the critical care unit, who share not a specific illness or known cause but rather sepsis and/or trauma with associated organ failure. The condition leading to CIP is called systemic inflammatory response syndrome. Attention typically is brought to the neuropathy by difficulty in weaning the patient from the ventilator as a result of respiratory muscle weakness. Severe cases, with lengthy hospitalization, have limb weakness, sensory loss, and depressed stretch tendon reflexes. However, because clinical examination is often difficult in such patients, reliance on diagnostic interventions has increased. Electrophysiologic testing and nerve and muscle biopsies show findings consistent with axonal polyneuropathy and help to distinguish CIP from Guillain-Barré syndrome, disorders of neuromuscular transmission, and myopathy. Initially most patients who survived their critical illness were reported to recover from CIP, but more recent studies indicate that recovery may be slow and often incomplete, even after 1–2 years.

Zifko UA: Long-term outcome of critical illness polyneuropathy. Muscle Nerve 9(Suppl):S49–S52, 2000.

27. What is the outcome of the evaluation of patients with "peripheral neuropathy of undetermined etiology" when referred for a second opinion to a peripheral nerve expert at a tertiary referral center?

In 42% of such patients a hereditary neuropathy is found, in 21% an inflammatory neuropathy is identified by nerve biopsy, and in 13% other conditions are discovered. In 24% of cases, even after extensive evaluation, no etiology for the neuropathy is identified.

28. Genetic testing is currently available for which hereditary neuropathies?

Peripheral myelin protein 22 (PMP-22), myelin protein zero (P_0), and connexin (Cx32) are myelin proteins in which genetic defects have been identified in demyelinating hereditary motor and sensory neuropathies (HMSNs). Charcot-Marie-Tooth disease (HMSNIA/CMTIA) is associated most frequently with PMP-22 duplication, whereas HNPP is associated primarily with PMP-22 deletion. The X-linked form of CMTI can be identified by a point mutation of Cx32. It is not yet practical to identify all cases of these and other demyelinating HMSNs, which demonstrate genetic heterogeneity involving point mutations of PMP-22, P_0, and a regulatory protein. In one form of familial amyloid polyneuropathy (FAP) type I (Portuguese type), transthyretin protein (TTR) can be used to test for the most common point mutation (Val 30 Met). In the future new diagnostic procedures will allow genetic testing of other TTR variants.

Reilly MM: Classification of the hereditary motor and sensory neuropathies. Curr Opin Neurol 13:561–564, 2000.

IMMUNE-MEDIATED NEUROPATHIES

29. Where are immune-mediated peripheral neuropathies most likely to cause initial nerve damage?

In areas where the blood-nerve barrier is deficient, i.e., motor roots, dorsal root ganglion, and motor-nerve terminals. The blood-nerve barrier serves to protect nerve fibers and endoneurial content from the vascular compartment. Where that barrier is incomplete, circulating cellular and humoral immune components have access to the nerve.

30. What is the relationship between connective tissue disease and trigeminal sensory neuropathy?

Trigeminal sensory neuropathy, a slowly progressive cranial neuropathy with unilateral or bilateral facial numbness or paresthesia, may be the presenting manifestation of connective tissue disease. The trigeminal sensory neuropathy is thought to be caused by vasculitis or fibrosis of the gasserian ganglion. Alternatively, the previous blood-nerve barrier of this ganglion may allow autoantibodies access to react with peripheral nerve components.

31. What is POEMS syndrome?

P   Polyneuropathy
O   Organomegaly
E   Endocrinopathy
M   M-protein
S   Skin changes

POEMS is an expanded variant of osteosclerotic myeloma with peripheral neuropathy. Patients typically have a chronic progressive sensory-motor polyneuropathy, peripheral edema, ascites, hypertrichosis, diffuse hyperpigmentation and thickening of the skin, hepatomegaly, splenomegaly, lymphadenopathy, gynecomastia, impotence, amenorrhea, and digital clubbing.

32. What is the association between monoclonal gammopathy and neuropathy?

Approximately 10% of peripheral neuropathies are associated with serum monoclonal gammopathy (M-protein). Two-thirds of such cases are initially classified as monoclonal gammopathy of uncertain significance (MGUS), but the remaining third, in decreasing frequency, are identified as multiple myeloma, amyloidosis, macroglobulinemia, lymphoma, and leukemia. Only one-fourth of cases of MGUS neuropathy are still found to be idiopathic with long-term follow-up. The risk of developing an identifiable cause is 17% at 10 years and 33% at 20 years. Hence, it is important to follow patients indefinitely. Clinically, patients with idiopathic monoclonal gammopathy and neuropathy are generally over 50 years of age with a 2:1 male-to-female predominance and develop a symmetric sensory (early) and motor (late) neuropathy or polyradiculopathy that affects the legs more than arms. Cranial nerves are not involved, and autonomic features generally do not occur. CSF protein levels are elevated in 83% of patients.

33. What is the significance of the type of M-protein and the presence of peripheral nerve antibodies in MGUS neuropathy?

IgM is the most commonly found M-protein and is more likely than IgG or IgA to be related to the neuropathy. Patients with IgM are more likely to have a demyelinating neuropathy that is more rapidly progressive and severe. Autoantibodies recognizing various peripheral nerve glycoconjugates are present in 50–82% of such patients with IgM. Although a number of autoantibody tests are commercially available, their value is debatable; the pathogenic role is best established for IgM directed against myelin-associated glycoprotein (MAG). The treatment of patients with MGUS neuropathy is difficult. Patients with IgG or IgA as opposed to IgM respond more satisfactorily to corticosteroids or cytotoxic immunosuppressive agents, and plasma exchange in controlled trials has proved effective in patients with IgG and IgA but not IgM gammopathy. Uncontrolled trials suggest a beneficial effect of high-dose intravenous gammaglobulin, and in a control study with IgM-associated neuropathy, a modest short-lived benefit was shown in a small percentage of patients.

Chassande B, Léger J-M, Younes-Chennoufi AB, et al: Peripheral neuropathy associated with IgM monoclonal gammopathy: Correlations between M-protein antibody activity and clinical/electrophysiological features in 40 cases. Muscle Nerve 21:55–62, 1998.

Notermans NC: Monoclonal gammopathy and neuropathy. Curr Opin Neurol 9:334–337, 1996.

Dyck PJ, Low PA, Windebank AJ, et al: Plasma exchange in polyneuropathy associated with monoclonal gammopathy of uncertain significance. N Engl J Med 325:1482–1486, 1991.

CHRONIC IMMUNE-RELATED DEMYELINATING POLYRADICULONEUROPATHY

34. What are the major criteria for the diagnosis of chronic immune-related demyelinating polyradiculoneuropathy (CIDP)?

The diagnosis of CIDP depends on the subacute onset of progressive limb muscle weakness and sensory dysfunction with hypo- or areflexia, elevated CSF protein with no more than minimal mononuclear pleocytosis, and demyelinative features on nerve conduction studies and nerve biopsy.

35. What immunosuppressive therapies are used in CIDP?

Immunosuppression has long been a mainstay of CIDP treatment, which is often challenging because of partial or no response, relapses, and treatment side effects. **Corticosteroids** are considered the treatment of first choice. Most patients who respond to prednisone demonstrate a positive effect within 8 weeks of therapy. Intermittent high-dose (1,000 mg) intravenous methylprednisolone has been used successfully in some patients and is probably a safer alternative to chronic oral corticosteroids. Patients who require prolonged treatment with high doses (1–1.5 mg/kg/day) of prednisone and patients who either fail to respond to corticosteroids or develop complications from such therapy are candidates for alternate or additional therapies. **Azathioprine** has shown benefit anecdotally in several small studies, but its efficacy is disputed. It may be useful in patients who fail to respond to corticosteroids or are intolerant to their side effects. **Cyclophosphamide** may be used in patients unresponsive to initial therapies; further studies are necessary before final conclusions about risk-benefit ratios can be made. An uncontrolled study of a small number of patients with CIDP refractory to corticosteroids, azathioprine, and plasma exchange has shown an excellent-to-moderate response to cyclosporine A. IVIG is also of benefit in some patients with CIDP and may be used when other treatments are contraindicated or as a first-line therapy.

Harati Y: Chronic immune-related demyelinating polyradiculoneuropathy. In Rolak LA, Harati Y (eds): Neuro-immunology for the Clinician. Boston, Butterworth-Heinemann, 1997, pp 229–235.

36. Many neuropathies are treated with corticosteroids. What are the risks of oral steroids? How can the risks be prevented?

Generally, patients are started on 60–100 mg/day for 2–3 weeks and then switched to 60–100 mg alternate-day therapy over 6–8 weeks. Patients are kept on this dose until maximal therapeutic effect is achieved (usually 4–6 months). The physician must discuss the side effects of steroids with the patient and take steps to prevent them. The following recommendations are helpful:

1. **Ulcers.** Patients should be started on antacids (e.g., Maalox, Amphojel) and a histamine receptor blocker (Pepcid, 20 mg orally at bedtime). Maalox, which contains aluminum and magnesium, may lead to loose stools, whereas Amphogel may lead to constipation.

2. **Hypokalemia** may be prevented by having the patient take 30 mEq/day of oral potassium supplement or eat one or two bananas a day.

3. **Glucose intolerance** may occur in patients with latent diabetes or with a family history of diabetes. Efforts should be made to control the problem with dietary modification, but hypoglycemic agents may be required.

4. **Hypertension.** A low-sodium diet is essential. Patients may need antihypertensive drugs such as diuretics.

5. **Osteopenia.** Older women are particularly susceptible to osteopenia. Patients should be started on calcium carbonate (Os-Cal, 500 mg orally 2 times/day). Tums may be used as a source of calcium (300 mg/tablet) and as an antacid.

6. **Weight gain.** Patients must be placed on a low-calorie, low-carbohydrate, low-salt, and high-protein diet.

7. **Cataracts and glaucoma.** Ophthalmologic evaluations need to be done every few months.

8. **Myopathy.** Steroid myopathy is suspected if the patient's weakness seems to increase while muscle enzymes and EMG remain unchanged. Women seem to be more susceptible to steroid myopathy. It is usually sufficient to reduce the dose of steroid therapy; if improvement follows, one can assume that weakness was due to the drug. A muscle biopsy shows type II fiber atrophy. The onset of steroid-induced myopathy partly depends on the dosage and duration of the steroid; however, individual susceptibility varies considerably and the onset may occur in weeks rather than months.

37. Discuss the role of plasma exchange (PE) in CIDP.

Initial reports of significant short-term improvement of some patients with CIDP have been confirmed by controlled studies. With careful monitoring, benefit usually can be demonstrated within 6 weeks. Approximately 20–30% of patients with CIDP become refractory to all other therapies and dependent on long-term intermittent PE or intravenous gammaglobulin. At present, PE is most commonly used (1) in the subgroup of patients with disability requiring treatment with immediate effectiveness while prednisone therapy is initiated; (2) in patients with intermittent acute exacerbations; and (3) as alternative therapy in patients who are refractory or intolerant of other immunosuppressive therapies or in whom such therapies present substantial risks (e.g., diabetic or immunocompromised patients).

Hahn AF, Bolton CF, Pillay N, et al: Plasma exchange therapy in chronic inflammatory demyelinating polyneuropathy: A double-blind, sham-controlled, cross-over study. Brain 119:1055–1066, 1996.

38. Discuss the roles of intravenous immunoglobulin (IVIG) and interferon in CIDP.

The usefulness of IVIG in refractory and untreated CIDP has been confirmed by controlled studies. IVIG usually is administered intravenously in a dose of 0.4 gm/kg of body weight per day for 3–5 days or 1 gm/kg/day for 2 days. Half or less of this dose as an initial treatment may be less effective, although a single-day induction dose appears sufficient as a pulse treatment. Benefits can be remarkable but are often short-lived (2–9 weeks), and stabilization of CIDP has been shown with regularly pulsed therapy. The best response is observed in patients with active symptoms of recent onset (less than 1 year). IVIG may offer advantages over chronic immunosuppressive or chronic plasmapheresis therapy in ease of use and relative safety. In a controlled, crossover study of 20 patients with CIDP, IVIG proved to be as effective as PE for short-term therapy. Refractory cases continue to drive the search for newer treatments, such as interferon α2a and interferon β1a. Preliminary studies indicate some benefit.

Dyck PJ, Litchy WJ, Kratz KM, et al: A plasma exchange versus immunoglobulin infusion trial in chronic inflammatory demyelinating polyradiculoneuropathy. Ann Neurol 36:838–845, 1994.

Gorson KC, Ropper AH, Clark BD, et al: Treatment of chronic inflammatory demyelinating polyneuropathy with interferon-α2a. Neurology 50:84–87, 1998.

Hahn AF, Bolton CF, Zochodne D, et al: Intravenous immunoglobulin treatment in chronic inflamma-tory demyelinating polyneuropathy: A double-blind, placebo-controlled, crossover study. Brain 119:1067–1077, 1996.

Mendell JR, Barohn RJ, Kissel JT, et al: Intravenous immunoglobulin (IVIg) in untreated patients with chronic inflammatory demyelinating polyradiculoneuropathy (CIDP). Neurology 54:A212, 2000.

39. What distinguishes multifocal motor neuropathy (MMN) with conduction block (CB) from CIDP and motor neuron disease?

MMN with CB is a presumed immune-mediated, chronic asymmetric motor neuropathy. The presence of weakness, atrophy, and fasciculations with sparing of sensation and asymmetric loss of reflexes identifies it as a lower motor neuron syndrome. Hyperreflexia does not occur, and bulbar involvement is rare. It is identified as a neuropathy primarily on the basis of the electrophysiologic findings of conduction block with a distinct predilection for more restricted and multifocal in-volvement of motor nerves. As opposed to CIDP, it usually starts and predominates in the upper limbs with a greater degree of asymmetry. Recognized treatments include high-dose IVIG (first choice) and cyclophosphamide. IVIG may result in fairly rapid, although temporary improve-ment in association with partial resolution of CB. Long-term management usually requires re-treatment at intervals immediately before expected relapse. The frequent association with elevated anti-GMI antibodies does not correlate with responsiveness to IVIG. Early studies with interferon β1a have shown encouraging results in refractory cases.

Frederico P, Zochodne DW, Hahn AF, et al: Multifocal motor neuropathy improved by IVIG. Randomized, double-blind, placebo-controlled study. Neurology 55:1256–1262, 2000.

Léger J-M, Chassande B, Musset L, et al: Intravenous immunoglobulin therapy in multifocal motor neu-ropathy. A double-blind, placebo-controlled study. Brain 124:145–153, 2001.

Martina IS, van Doorn PA, Schmitz PI, et al: Chronic motor neuropathies: Response to interferon-beta 1a after failure of conventional therapies. J Neurol Neurosurg Psychiatry 66:197–201, 1999.

Van den Berg LH, Franssen H, Wokke JHJ: The long-term effect of intravenous immunoglobulin treat-ment in multifocal motor neuropathy. Brain 121:421–428, 1998.

GUILLAIN-BARRÉ SYNDROME

40. Describe the typical presentation of Guillain-Barré syndrome (GBS).

A typical patient with GBS reports a numb or tingling sensation in the arms and legs, fol-lowed by rapidly progressive ascending symmetric muscle weakness. Symptoms often begin 1–3 weeks after a viral upper respiratory or gastrointestinal infection, immunization, or surgery. Paralysis is maximal by 2 weeks in more than 50% of patients and by 1 month in more than 90%. A patient with a severe case of GBS may present with flaccid quadriplegia and an inability to breathe, swallow, or speak (due to oropharyngeal and respiratory paresis). Ten to 20% of patients require artificial respiration. Over 50% of patients develop facial weakness, and 10% have ex-traocular muscular paralysis. Hyporeflexia or areflexia is invariably present. Preservation of re-flexes in a severely weakened patient should seriously challenge the diagnosis of GBS. The patient may have mild impairment of distal sensation, but significant sensory loss is not seen. Many patients also have symptoms of autonomic dysfunction.

41. What are the two main pathologically distinct presentations of GBS?

1. Acute inflammatory demyelinating polyradiculoneuropathy (AIDP) due to an immune attack on Schwann cell membrane or myelin sheath.

2. Acute (motor or motor-sensory) axonal neuropathy (AMAN or AMSAN) due to an immune attack against the axolemma/axoplasm. This presentation is distinguished from severe cases of AIDP, in which secondary axonal damage may occur.

42. What are the early immunopathologic events in AIDP?

Recent pathologic studies indicate that binding of complement-fixing antibodies to target antigen may be the primary event leading to complement activation and disruption of compact myelin. What previously had been observed as early lymphocytic infiltration of roots and nerves with macrophage-mediated myelin stripping and finally segmental demyelination may actually be a secondary event.

Griffin JW, Li CY, Ho TW, et al: Guillain-Barré syndrome in Northern China. The spectrum of neuropathological changes in clinically defined cases. Brain 118:577–595, 1995.

43. What are the typical laboratory findings in GBS?

About 1 week after the onset of symptoms, CSF protein content begins to rise in most patients and peaks in 4–6 weeks. The CSF cell count does not increase. Nerve conduction velocities are slowed in AIDP but may be normal early in the course of the disease (first 2 weeks). Conduction block accounts for most of the initial weakness, but after 2–3 weeks axonal damage may contribute to weakness with EMG evidence of muscle denervation.

44. What is the significance of *Campylobacter jejuni* infection in GBS?

In the U.S., most patients (75%) with GBS and a preceding *C. jejuni* infection present with AIDP and are at increased risk of developing the more severe axonal form of the disease. Not all patients with serologic evidence of *C. jejuni* have GI symptoms before the onset of GBS. Cross-reactivity between antigens from *C. jejuni* and various peripheral nerve gangliosides may explain the pathogenetic connection between the infection and GBS.

45. What are the predictors of severe disease and poorer outcome in patients with GBS?

1. Old age
2. Rapid onset of severe tetraparesis
3. Need for early artificial ventilation
4. Severely decreased compound muscle action potentials (< 20% of normal)
5. Acute motor-sensory axonal form of the disease

There are conflicting data as to whether evidence of preceding *C. jejuni* infection or presence of anti-GM1 antibodies is a predictor of disease severity or outcome. The vast majority of patients with poor outcome required mechanical ventilation, and among this group predictors of poor outcome include increased age (highly predictive), upper limb paralysis, duration of ventilation, presence of inexcitable nerves, and delayed transfer to a tertiary center. Recovery in ventilated patients with GBS may be prolonged, and final judgment about outcome may require 2 or more years of follow-up.

Fletcher DD, Lawn ND, Wolter TD, et al: Long-term outcome in patients with Guillain-Barré syndrome requiring mechanical ventilation. Neurology 54:2311–2315, 2000.

46. What percent of patients with GBS suffer a relapse or second episode?

Over the past 25 years, most large series of patients with GBS report a 2–3% incidence of relapse, which may occur months to years after the initial episode.

47. How is GBS treated?

Plasma exchange (PE) and IVIG started within 2 weeks of the illness equally improve the degree and rate of recovery. Although PE initially was studied in moderate-to-severe disease, for which at least four exchanges are needed, the French Cooperative Group suggests that mild disease also benefits from at least two exchanges. Despite initial concerns about early relapse in about 10% of patients treated with IVIG, such patients responded to retreatment; furthermore, similar fluctuations and relapses have been reported with PE. Efficacy of the two treatments appears to be equal in all subsets of GBS, except perhaps IgG anti-GMI-positive patients, who usually present with AMAN. Findings of greater efficacy with IVIG than with PE await confirmation by large prospective studies. Because IVIG offers the advantages of greater ease and convenience as well as greater safety of administration at similar costs, it is now considered the treatment of first choice. There is no added benefit from combining the two treatments. Corticosteroids are *not* indicated.

French Cooperative Group on Plasma Exchange in Guillain-Barré Syndrome. Ann Neurol 41:298–306, 1997.

Hadden RD, Cornblath DR, Hughes RA, et al: Electrophysiological classifications of Guillain-Barré syndrome: Clinical association and outcome. Plasma Exchange/Sandoglobulin Guillain-Barré Syndrome Trial Group. Ann Neurol 44:780–788, 1998.

Kuwabara S, Mori M, Ogawara K, et al: Intravenous immunoglobulin therapy for Guillain-Barré syndrome with IgG anti-GMI antibody. Muscle Nerve 24:54–58, 2001.

Plasma Exchange/Sandoglobulin Guillain-Barré Syndrome Trial Group: Randomized trial of plasma exchange, intravenous immunoglobulin, and combined treatments on Guillain-Barré syndrome. Lancet 349:225–230, 1997.

Visser LH, van der Meche FGA, Meulstee J, et al: Risk factors for treatment related clinical fluctuations in Guillain-Barré syndrome. J Neurol Neurosurg Psychiatry 64:242–244, 1998.

MOTOR NEURON DISEASES

48. What is the most common condition affecting the motor neurons?

Amyotrophic lateral sclerosis (ALS) is a progressive degenerative disorder of the upper and lower motor neurons. It produces muscular weakness, spasticity, Babinski sign, and hyperreflexia (upper motor neurons) as well as flaccidity, atrophy, fasciculations, and hyporeflexia (lower motor neurons). The deficits are strictly motor without significant signs of sensory loss, dementia, or cerebellar or extrapyramidal disease. Motor neurons controlling eye movements and sphincter function are usually spared as well. The reason for this selectivity is uncertain, although evidence suggests that cell-specific differences in protective regulatory calcium-binding proteins may be important. The disease, which usually begins in the sixth decade of life with a range spanning most of adulthood, generally progresses to death within 3–5 years from aspiration or respiratory paralysis.

49. How can the diagnosis of ALS be confirmed?

The diagnosis depends on recognizing the characteristic clinical picture. Efforts to identify a biochemical marker have been unsuccessful; advances in treatment will further drive the need for a method of earlier diagnosis. At present, the most useful test is EMG, which shows widespread denervation and reinnervation (fasciculations and polyphasic, high-amplitude muscle potentials). Muscle biopsy shows neurogenic atrophy (small, angular fibers and possibly fiber type grouping). Although serum CK levels may be mildly elevated, other tests are usually normal.

50. What causes ALS?

Approximately 8–10% of patients have a family history of the disease, usually in an autosomal dominant pattern. A genetic defect in an enzyme involved in free-radical metabolism, superoxide dismutase type 1 (SOD1), localized to chromosome 21, accounts for 15–20% of familial ALS. Although this gene is not implicated in the great majority of sporadic ALS cases, impaired free-radical catabolism may play a role. Neuronal cytoskeletal abnormalities are a pathologic feature of ALS, and alterations in neurofilaments have been speculated to affect motor neuron integrity or even trigger oxidative damage. Toxins also have been implicated in the etiology of ALS, following the discovery of glutamate-like substances capable of selectively damaging motor neurons, such as BOAA in chickpeas (cause of lathyrism) and BMAA in cycad seeds (linked to Western Pacific ALS). These observations led to theories of endogenous excitotoxins such as glutamate. Other observations, such as the association of ALS and other autoimmune diseases with findings of T-cell lymphocytes and deposits of IgG and complement in the spinal cord, motor cortex, and neuromuscular junction, have led investigators to search unsuccessfully for evidence of a primary autoimmune mechanism. Whatever the cause, increased intracellular calcium may be a unifying factor among various mechanisms involved in the motor neuron death associated with ALS.

Rosen DR, Siddique T, Patterson D, et al: Mutations in Cu/Zn superoxide dismutase gene are associated with familial amyotrophic lateral sclerosis. Nature 362:59–62, 1993.

Siklos L, Engelhardt J, Harati Y, et al: Ultrastructural evidence for altered calcium in motor nerve terminals in amyotrophic lateral sclerosis. Ann Neurol 39:203–216, 1996.

51. What is the differential diagnosis of ALS?

Other conditions that may affect the pyramidal tract and lower motor neurons or mimic some of their clinical features include cervical cord/foramen magnum lesions (tumor, syringomyelia, syringobulbia, spondylosis), thyrotoxicosis, hyperparathyroidism, dysproteinemia, paraneoplastic conditions, and hexosaminidase A deficiency.

52. What treatments for ALS have shown efficacy in controlled studies?

Riluzole, which may inhibit glutamate release, among other effects, shows a modest improvement in survival rate and is the first drug approved for use in ALS. Numerous clinical trials over the past 10–15 years have failed to demonstrate the efficacy of various growth and neurotrophic factors as well as a variety of immunosuppressive-immunomodulating therapies.

Lacomblez L, Bensimon G, Leigh PN, et al: Dose-ranging study of riluzole in amyotrophic lateral sclerosis. ALS/Riluzole Study Group III. Lancet 347:1425–1431, 1996.

Lai EC: Therapeutic developments in amyotrophic lateral sclerosis (ALS). Exp Opin Invest Drugs 8:347–361, 1999.

53. What other conditions primarily affect the lower motor neuron (anterior horn cell)?

The differential diagnosis of deficits primarily confined to the anterior horn cell (AHC) includes several inherited diseases such as X-linked bulbospinal muscular atrophy and proximal spinal muscular atrophy. The latter includes infantile (Werdnig-Hoffmann disease), juvenile (Kugelberg-Welander disease), and adult forms. Acquired lower motor neuron syndromes include poliomyelitis, postpolio syndrome, progressive muscular atrophy, MMN with CB, and AHC degeneration in other conditions (e.g., Creutzfeldt-Jakob disease).

54. What is primary lateral sclerosis? Does it really exist?

It is a form of slowly progressive acquired motor neuron disease in which only signs of corticospinal tract disease are seen. Patients rarely develop bulbar or lower motor neuron signs. Modern laboratory evaluation has allowed the exclusion of other upper motor neuron syndromes, giving support that primary lateral sclerosis is a distinct entity.

Hudson AJ, Kiernan JA, Munoz DG, et al: Clinico-pathological features of primary lateral sclerosis are different from amyotrophic lateral sclerosis. Brain Res Bull 30:359–364, 1993.

55. Who was Lou Gehrig?

Lou Gehrig, whose name has been given to ALS, played first base for the New York Yankees from 1923–1939, usually batting after Babe Ruth in the line-up. He had a lifetime batting average of .340 with 23 grand slams (a record) and was the first modern player to hit four home runs in one game. He is best known as "Ironman"—a name undiminished despite the recent breaking of his record of playing 2,130 consecutive games. A kind, conscientious, thoughtful, hard-working, shy, and courteous man, Lou Gehrig, who died of ALS, was a true sports hero.

56. Name eight other famous people who suffer(ed) from ALS.

1. David Niven, actor
2. Jacob Javits, senator
3. Henry Wallace, U.S. vice president
4. Ezzard Charles, heavyweight boxer
5. Bob Waters, football player and coach
6. Stephen Hawking, physicist
7. Eliot Porter, photographer
8. Dmitri Shostakovich, composer

BIBLIOGRAPHY

1. Aminoff MJ: Electromyography in Clinical Practice: Clinical and Electrodiagnostic Aspects of Neuromuscular Disease, 3rd ed. New York, Churchill Livingstone, 1998.
2. Brown RH, Swash M, Meininger V: Amyotrophic Lateral Sclerosis. London, Martin Dunitz, 1999.
3. Mendell JR, Cornblath DR, Kissell JT: Diagnosis and Management of Peripheral Nerve Disorders. Oxford, Oxford University Presss, 2000.
4. Mitsumoto H, Chad DA, Pioro EP: Amyotrophic Lateral Sclerosis. Philadelphia, F.A. Davis, 1998.
5. Rolak LA, Harati Y (eds): Neuro-immunology for the Clinician. Boston, Butterworth-Heinemann, 1997.

Websites

www.neuro.wustl.edu/neuromuscular
www.neuropathy.org

7. RADICULOPATHY AND DEGENERATIVE SPINE DISEASE

Steven B. Inbody, M.D.

1. What is the likelihood that you will experience at least one functionally disabling episode of back or neck pain during your lifetime?

Approximately 80% of Americans experience back pain during their lifetime. However, the duration of pain is usually self-limited, and 80–90% of attacks resolve within 6 weeks.

The socioeconomic impact of neck and back pain related to disorders of the spine is enormous. Neck and back pain continues to be the most common cause of disability in patients under the age of 45. Except for the common cold, low back pain and neck pain are the second and third leading causes, respectively, of absenteeism at the work place. Currently, 6–8 million people in the U.S. claim total disability due to back pain. The health care costs for its evaluation and treatment are currently estimated to approach $40 billion dollars per year, with 8–10 million people seeking treatment annually. Back pain is the third most frequent reason for surgical procedures, and the fifth most frequent cause for hospitalization.

Anderson GBJ: The epidemiology of spinal disorders. In Frymoyer JW (ed): The Adult Spine: Principles and Practice. Philadelphia, Lippincott-Raven, 1997, pp 93–141.

2. Discuss the significance of the AHCPR Guidelines for the diagnosis of "nonspecific spinal pain."

Despite the magnitude of the problem, medical science remains unable to identify the precise cause(s) of acute spine-related pain. Instead, physicians commonly use nonspecific diagnoses, such as neck or back strain, even though the injury may have affected any of the pain-sensitive structures, including the disc, facet joints, spinal nerve root, paraspinal musculature, and ligamentous support. The causes of chronic spinal pain are equally uncertain, although often it is attributed to degenerative conditions of the spine, despite contrary scientific evidence that fails to correlate symptoms to radiologic signs of degeneration. Similarly, disc herniation has been popularized as a cause of spinal and radicular pain, despite the fact that MRI or CT commonly demonstrates disc herniations in asymptomatic people. Although many clinicians expect the underlying causes of neck or back pain to be elucidated through the diagnostic process, the specific tissue responsible for spine-related pain can be identified in less than 20% of cases.

As a result of this diagnostic confusion and its secondary impact on treatment with spiraling health care costs, "back problems" became an early target of the federally mandated Agency for Health Care Policy and Research (AHCPR). In 1994, evidence-based guidelines for the diagnosis and treatment of spinal pain were published. After a comprehensive investigation, the AHCPR abandoned its attempts to define the origin of nonspecific spinal pain and instead resorted to classifying patients into the categories of nonspecific spinal pain with or without leg symptoms.

Agency for Health Care Poalicy and Research: Guidelines No. 14, Clinical Practice Guidelines 95-0642. Washington, DC, U.S. Department of Health and Human Services, Public Health Service, 1994.

3. What are the presumed mechanisms of spinal pain?

The current but limited understanding of the pathophysiology of spinal pain involves the interplay among four distinct mechanisms: (1) the multiple pain-sensitive tissues of the spine; (2) the functional anatomy and complex biomechanics of the spine and its susceptibility to trauma; (3) the biochemical or inflammatory response of injured spinal tissues, which initiates a cascade of neurochemical changes that activate the sensory nerve endings; and (4) the peripheral and central nervous system processing of the nociceptive information, leading to the sensation of pain.

4. Which anatomic structures are potential pain generators?

Essential to identification of the potential pain generators within the spine is an understanding of the functional anatomy of the spinal motion segment. The fundamental components of the motion segment include the intervertebral disc and the two paired synovial joints, the posterior zygapophyseal joints (facets). Each posterior joint is composed of a superior facet that articulates with the inferior facet of the suprajacent vertebra. These three joints function as articulating supports between all of the vertebrae and are called the **three-joint complex**. The functions of these three supports or joints are so intimately linked that change in any one affects the other two.

Pain-sensitive structures within the three-joint complex include (1) the **intervertebral disc**, which once was thought to be inert but is pain-sensitive along the posterior one-third of its fibrous shell, the outer annular fibers; (2) the **posterior longitudinal ligament**, which restrains the disc from protruding into the spinal canal, and (3) the **ventral dura matter**, which envelopes the exiting spinal root. These structures derive their nociceptive innervation from the sinuvertebral nerve. The other structures with independent nociceptive innervation include (1) the **posterior facet joints**, which are thought to monitor excessive joint movement and to mediate protective muscular reflex; (2) the **periostum** of the vertebral body; (3) the **spinal nerve roots and dorsal root ganglia;** and (4) the **paraspinal musculature, tendons, fascia, and ligaments,** which insert on the spine and represent the primary defense against trauma.

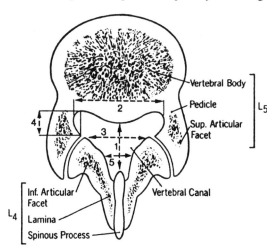

L4–L5 vertebral bodies. (From Yong-Hing K, Kirkaldy-Willis WH: The pathophysiology of degenerative disease of the lumbar spine. Orthop Clin North Am 14:491–504, 1983, with permission.)

5. Describe the pathophysiologic process of spinal spondylosis.

The cascade of degenerative osteoarthritic changes, often affecting the three-joint complex, is the basis of spinal spondylosis (degenerative spine disease). This degenerative cascade can be divided into three stages of variable duration: dysfunction, instability, and restabilization. The process often begins with the normal age-related desiccation of the intervertebral disc, which may be accelerated by repetitive trauma. Initially 80–90% of the weight of the three-joint complex is borne across the posterior third of the disc, but as disc height declines, the center of biomechanical loading shifts posteriorly, redistributing the weight toward the facet joints. The stage of **dysfunction** usually includes annular tears of the disc, synovial inflammation, and cartilage destruction at the facets. Radiographic findings at this stage are usually minimal. The stage of **instability** is characterized by loss of disc space height and capsular laxity at the facet joints, which permits increased intersegmental motion. Clinical and radiographic findings are more apparent and severe. In the **restabilization** stage, the increasing stress on the facets, is accommodated by osteophytic bone growth to stabilize the trijoint complex.Often pathologic change starts in one support (such as a disc or posterior joint) and by itself may cause symptoms. Later the interplay between the changes in the three supports results in combined three-joint complex degeneration. Pathologic changes in the three-joint complex at one intervertebral level lead to mechanical changes that affect the levels above and below, resulting in multilevel spondylosis.

6. What is the distinction among spondylosis, spondylolysis, and spondylolisthesis?

Spondylosis refers to osteoarthritis involving the articular surfaces (joints and discs) of the spine, often with osteophyte formation and cord or root compression. **Spondylolysis** refers to a separation at the pars articularis, which permits the vertebrae to slip. The pars defect may be unilateral or bilateral. **Spondylolisthesis** may result from bilateral pars defects or degenerative disc disease. Spondylolisthesis is defined as the anterior subluxation of the suprajacent vertebra, often producing central canal stenosis; it is the slipping forward of one vertebra on the vertebra below. When symptomatic, all three conditions cause pain in the lower back after motion or lifting. Splinting with contraction of the lumbar paraspinal muscles is frequent. The three disorders are confirmed radiographically; flexion/extension spine films often demonstrate segmental instability.

7. What spondytic changes of the intervertebral disc and posterior joints give rise to spinal stenosis?

The earliest changes in the nucleus pulposus and annulus fibrosus are probably biochemical and may be part of aging. Trauma superimposed on these changes accelerates the degeneration. The layers of the annulus separate and form circumferential tears. Several of these circumferential tears may coalesce to form a radial tear, through which nuclear material may extrude, producing the typical disc herniation or prolapse. Even if a disc herniation does not occur, the multiple tears produce weakening and circumferential bulging of the annulus with loss of disc height. Further disc narrowing results from aging of the nucleus pulposus, which changes from a gelatinous consistency in childhood to a fibrotic consistency in adulthood.

Synovitis is the earliest demonstrable change in the posterior joints, which are composed of articular cartilage, a synovial membrane, and a capsule. Articular cartilage destruction occurs later. The joint capsule becomes lax as a result of the thinning of the articular cartilage, producing instability and eventual subluxation in the joints. The two posterior joints may be unequally affected, resulting in a rotatory component. Eventually, osteophytes form around the articular processes, narrowing both the lateral recess and the central canal. These severe degenerative changes, characterized by bony overgrowth of the vertebral endplates (osteophyte formation) and facet hypertrophy, often result in progressive foraminal and central canal stenosis.

8. What is the difference between a disc bulge, protrusion, and herniation?

The radiologic and pathologic terminology commonly used to describe the changing profile of the intervertebral disc is not uniformly defined. A **bulging disc** occurs when dehydration leads to gradual flattening of the disc and increases the circumference of the intact annular ring, which then extends beyond and overhangs the margins of the vertebral body. The smooth contour of the benign bulge contrasts with **disc protrusion**, in which the gelatinous disc material protrudes focally into tears or fissures within the intact annular shell, causing a focal outpouching of the still intact annular fibers. **Disc herniation** refers to extrusion of nuclear material through the disrupted annular shell and may be subcategorized as **subligamentous** or **transligamentous**, depending on the integrity of the posterior longitudinal ligament.

9. List and describe the most common causes of spinal stenosis.

Although more than 25 causes of spinal stenosis have been identified, four conditions account for the majority of cases:

1. Idiopathic (developmental) spinal stenosis is the result of shorter-than-normal pedicles, thickened convergent lamina, and a convex posterior vertebral body. Idiopathic spinal stenosis

rarely becomes symptomatic on its own but rather predisposes to normal degenerative changes, eventually becoming symptomatic.

2. Degenerative spinal stenosis accounts for approximately one-half of all cases. Degenerative changes affect the facets posteriorly and the disc anteriorly. As the facets become lax, allowing instability and subluxation, osteophytes form and narrow both the nerve root and central canals. Simultaneously, disc degeneration, characterized by tears in the circumferential anular fibers, allows the disc to bulge into the nerve root and central canals.

3. Degenerative spondylolisthesis occurs when the facets degenerate, allowing slippage of the upper vertebra forward over the lower vertebra.

4. Postoperative spinal stenosis occurs after laminectomy or spinal fusion. Stenosis is produced by bone formation and scar tissue.

10. What are the differences between radicular and referred pain?

The features of radiculopathy include pain, weakness, reflex change, and sensory loss. **Radicular pain** usually is described as electrical, stinging, burning, searing, shooting, or sharp. It is distributed uniquely within the territory of the affected root and may radiate down (but never up) the limb. The pain may be constant but worsens instantaneously from any act that abruptly increases intraspinal pressure, such as coughing or sneezing. Sensory loss is usually incomplete with respect to density and extent within the root territory.

Referred pain is a phenomena that historically has been well described with myocardial ischemia or visceral pathology. Recently referred pain associated with somatic tissues has been appreciated as a cause of regional pain, independent of localized nociceptive pain. The quality of referred pain may be shooting, but it is not electrical like radicular pain and does not radiate the same distances. Irritated or injured tissues such as muscle, facet joint, and the periosteum of the spine can cause referred pain in a distribution that resembles the dermatomal pattern of the spinal segment innervating the affected tissue.

11. Describe the clinical features of mechanical pain and its association with intersegmental instability.

As much as 98% of neck or back pain has been reported to be caused by the various mechanical disorders of the spine, which have many features in common. In most cases, the symptoms are strongly dependent on position. Postures that load the spine, such as sitting, typically worsen the pain. In addition, static loading is often the worst; thus, tolerance for remaining in one position for prolonged periods is decreased.

The potential causes of mechanical spine pain include all of the pain-sensitive tissues and structures of the spine that possess nociceptor innervation. Depending on the tissue, patients often describe the nociceptive pain as dull or aching, usually localized near the site of injury. Many tissues also produce a referred pain pattern remote from the site of injury.

12. Which spinal disorders cause both axial pain (back or neck) and disturbances in neurologic function of the limb (leg or arm)?

Three syndromes are recognized in which spinal disorders cause both back or neck pain and neurologic dysfunction. Examples are from the lumbar spine:

1. **Herniated disc causing a single nerve root compression** (leg pain > back pain). Clinical features include positive straight leg-raising test and radicular pain in the limb disproportionate to pain in the spine. Loss of strength, reflex, and sensation occurs in the territory of the compressed root.

2. **Lateral recess syndrome** (leg pain ≥ back pain). Single or multiple nerve roots on one or both sides become compressed. Pain in the limb is usually equal to or greater than that in the spine. Symptoms are brought on by either walking or standing and are relieved with sitting. Testing by straight leg raising may be negative.

3. **Spinal stenosis** (leg pain < back pain). Multiple nerve roots are involved, and the pain in the spine is significantly greater than that in the limb. Symptoms develop with standing or walking. Impairment in bowel, bladder, and sexual function may occur.

LUMBAR SPINE DISEASE

13. What are the clinical features of lumbar disc disease?

Acute lumbosacral disc herniation may cause a continuum of pain ranging from an isolated dull ache to severe radicular pain due neurocompression in the foramen or lateral recess. A rare complication is cauda equina syndrome due to a massive central herniation. Pain is often sudden in onset and exacerbated with the Valsalva maneuver. Concomitant paraspinal spasm is often present. The L5–S1 disc is involved most frequently; a posterolateral herniation entraps the S1 nerve root, causing posterolateral leg, lateral heel, and sole pain; weakness of planterflexion; and a diminished Achilles reflex. A lateral herniation at the L5–S1 level may entrap the L5 nerve root. Less commonly, the L4–L5 disc is involved; herniations at higher levels are infrequent.

14. What are the differentiating signs and symptoms of an L4, L5, and S1 radiculopathy?

Compression of the L4 root produces pain radiating to the hip, anterior thigh, knee, and medial calf. Sensation is impaired over the medial calf and the territory of the saphenous nerve. L5 root compression produces pain radiating to the posterolateral buttock, lateral posterior thigh, and lateral leg. Sensory loss is most likely in a triangular wedge involving the great toe, second toe, and adjacent skin on the dorsum of the foot. S1 root compression causes pain to radiate to the posterior buttock, posterior calf, and lateral foot. Sensory loss occurs along the lateral aspect of the foot, especially the third, fourth, and fifth toes.

Weakness is rarely complete in unoperated patients. Muscle weakness due to L4 root compression is difficult to establish owing to the heavy overlap of root innervation. The quadriceps, abductor longus, gluteus medius, and tibialis anterior muscles may be weak. Weakness from an L5 root compression is most commonly found in the extensor hallucis longus, extensor digitorum brevis, and peroneus longus muscles. It is most easily identified in the extensor hallucis longus. It is difficult to identify weakness from involvement of the first sacral root. It is most easily found in the flexor hallucis brevis, but the hamstrings and gastrocnemius may also be affected.

The reflex changes may be relative or absolute. A reduced patellar reflex is seen in an L4 root compression, but because of overlapping innervation, there may be minimal change. Ordinarily no reflex change is associated with L5 root compression. The angle jerk is consistently reduced or absent in an S1 root compression, as are the hamstring reflexes, especially in the semimembranosus.

15. What are the clinical features of lumbar stenosis?

Most patients are older than 50 years and have had symptoms referable to lumbar spinal stenosis for 1 or more years. Neurogenic intermittent claudication or pseudoclaudication is the most common presenting and constant symptom in lumbar spinal stenosis. Symptoms are usually bilateral, with one leg more involved than the other, but they may be unilateral. Although most patients describeleg symptoms as painful, the pain is distinctively different from the radicular type of pain seen with an acutely and laterally herniated intervertebral disc. The pain is usually of a dull, aching quality. The whole lower extremity is generally affected. The pain is provoked by walking and, in many patients, merely by standing. It is quickly relieved by sitting or leaning forward. In some patients the pain is accompanied by numbness of the affected leg that is usually described as a sensation of deadness rather than a tingling sensation. About one-half of patients report weakness in the affected leg "as though it might at any moment give way." Low back pain with various degrees of severity is present in about 65% of patients with lumbar spinal stenosis.

16. What is the mechanism for neurogenic claudication in lumbar spinal stenosis?

Symptoms are related to the increase in lordotic posture provoked by standing or walking. Myelographic studies have shown that in lordosis the cross-sectional area of the spinal canal narrows because of anterior encroachment by bulging discs, posterior encroachment by shortening and thickening of the ligamentum flavum, and lateral approximation of the articular facets. In flexion (as in sitting), all of these encroachments reverse, with a resultant increase in the cross-sectional area of the spinal canal. The comparatively unique features of lower extremety weakness suggest a vascular component to the neurapraxis. The documented increase in epidural pressure has been postulated to cause venous congestion from multilevel compression and then secondary arterial insufficiency.

17. What are the diagnostic findings in the straight leg-raising test?
    A straight leg-raising test suggests lumbosacral root or sciatic nerve involvement if passive hip flexion with the leg extended at the knee reproduces the patient's usual back or leg pain. These findings, although not specific for discogenic disease, are absent in patients with symptomatic lumbar stenosis.

18 What is the differential diagnosis of low back pain?
    The most common alternate diagnoses include focal hip pathology, vertebal compression fractures, metastasis from malignancy, anklylosising spondylitis, and vertebral osteomyelitis. Rare causes of low back pain include abdominal aortic aneurysm, pelvic disorders, abdominal visceral pathology, and other neuropathic disorders (e.g., inflammatory poly- or mono-neuropathies).

THORACIC SPINE DISEASE

19. What are the clinical features of thoracic disc disease?
    Pain is the most common initial symptom in thoracic disc herniation, occurring in approximately 60% of cases. The pain usually occurs near the midline, unilaterally or bilaterally, and may have a characteristic radicular distribution. The second most common symptom is numbness. Motor weakness involving the lower extremities is an initial symptom in 28% of patients. Bladder involvement is a rare initial symptom but may be seen in 30% of patients at presentation.

20. Describe the clinical presentation of a thoracic disc herniation.
    Less than 1% of protruded discs occur in the thoracic spine. Over 75% of herniated thoracic discs develop below T8, with the highest incidence at the T11–T12 level. The protrusion is usually central. Most patients have a degenerative process as the main causative factor; trauma accountis for only 10–20% of protruded discs.

21. What is the differential diagnosis of thoracic pain?

Malignant or benign tumors of the spine	Thoracic compression fractures
Ankylosing spondylosis	Intraabdominal processes (gallbladder disease,
Thoracoabdominal neuropathy	gastric ulcer, pancreatitis)
(diabetes)	Cardiac causes
Intercostal neuralgia	Intramedullary lesion such as a demyelinating
Herpes zoster	process

CERVICAL SPINE DISEASE

22. Describe the clinical features of cervical disc disease.
    The hallmark of radiculopathy is ipsilateral arm pain, weakness, and sensory changes in a dermatomal distribution. The most frequent levels for cervical disc disease are C5–C6 and C6–C7; C4–C5 and C7–T1 are less common; and C3–C4 is rare. In addition to the root symptoms, patients may have limited range of neck motion and complain of neck pain with movement, especially with hyperextension or the Valsalva maneuver. Radicular symptoms are the same whether due to compression by an acute disc herniation or mechanical irritation by a chronic foraminal spondylotic spur.

23. What are the differentiating signs and symptoms between a C6 and C7 radiculopathy?
Compression of the sixth cervical root (from either osteophytes or disc herniation at the C5–C6 level) produces weakness of the deltoid and biceps muscles, a diminished biceps reflex, and diminished skin sensation in the thumb and index finger. Compression of the seventh cervical nerve root (from either osteophytes or disc herniation at the C6–C7 level) produces weakness of the triceps muscle, a diminished triceps reflex, and diminished skin sensation in the index and middle fingers.

24. What is Spurling's maneuver?
Named for the neurosurgeon who popularized the posterior approach for cervical disc surgery, this maneuver is the cervical equivalent to the lumbar straight leg raise. Reproduction of the patient's pain on extension and ipsilateral rotation of the head is pathognomonic for cervical root irritation.

25. List the four clinical syndromes associated with cervical spondylitic and describe the neurologic dysfunction in each.
Neurologic dysfunction from cervical spondylosis can be separated into four distinct but overlapping groups:
1. The **lateral or radicular syndrome** occurs when disc material, osteophytes, or hypertrophic facets impinge on nerve roots. Pain in the neck is often lateralized and radiates into the occiput or scapula. The pain is often aggravated by neck movement, and the cervical spine is often tender to percussion. Radicular pain and paresthesia in the upper limb are frequent features of the syndrome and are sometimes precipitated or aggravated by neck movement, coughing, sneezing, or straining. Objective neurologic findings follow dermatomal patterns and include weakness, fasciculations, atrophy, loss of reflexes, and a decrease in pain or temperature sensation. In the pure lateral syndrome, long tract signs are absent.
2. The **medial or spinal syndrome** produces pure myelopathy without root symptoms or signs. Neck pain is variable, but most patients have some limitation of neck mobility. The earliest symptoms are usually stiffness and weakness of the lower extremities, which can be asymmetric. Gait ataxia and paresthesia of the feet are also common. Examination reveals spasticity with exaggerated reflexes and extensor plantar responses.
3. The **combined medial and lateral syndrome** accounts for the largest group of patients. Symptoms or signs of root disease in the upper extremities accompany long tract signs in the lower limbs.
4. A **vascular syndrome** represents a fourth group of patients with spondylosis and symptoms distinct from those already described. They characteristically have little or no pain or root symptoms. The acute or subacute onset of the myelopathy differentiates this group from the more common spondylitic myelopathy, which is insidious in onset. This syndrome develops quickly; some patients awaken with the deficit.

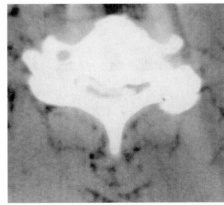

CT scan shows compression of the cervical spinal cord caused by severe cervical spondylosis.

26. What is the differential diagnosis for cervical pain?

Diseases that most closely mimic cervical disc disease include brachial plexus lesions and shoulder dysfunction due to tendinitis, subacromial bursitis, or rotator cuff disease. Neoplastic or infectious processes also need to be excluded.

DIAGNOSTIC EVALUATION

27. What are the relative strengths and limitations of the four primary radiologic procedures currently indicated for evaluation of the spine?

A combination of imaging modalities may be necessary to adequately evaluate spinal disorders and nerve root compression.

Plain radiographs provide important information about alignment, degenerative bony changes, and deformities.

Dynamic flexion/extension films are important to determine sagittal balance and presence of osseous instability.

Magnetic resonance imaging (MRI) provides images in multiple planes and is noninvasive; it is not subject to bony artifact, and is excellent for studying intrinsic cord disease, annular fissures or tears, the integrity of the posterior longitudinal ligament, and compromised spinal roots. It also is useful for ruling out other possibilities such as Chiari malformation, spinal cord tumors, and injury to surrounding soft tissues. With gadolinium enhancement, MRI is unmatched for the evaluation of the postoperative spine when postsurgical scarring must be differentiated from a recurrent disc fragment.

Myelography with postmyelogram computed tomography (CT) is excellent for evaluating nerve root compression and visualizes the lateral recess and intervertebral foramen far more laterally than MRI. It provides excellent details of the anatomy, in multiple planes with reconstructions, and remains the gold standard for evaluating nerve root compression.

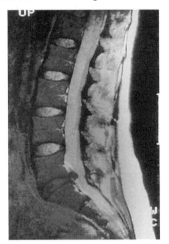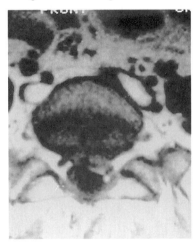

MRI scan shows a herniated disc at L5 on sagittal *(left)* and axial *(right)* views.

28. What is the false-positive rate for MRI of the spine?

MRI of asymptomatic young adults shows a significantly abnormal disc in approximately one of four cases. In people older than 60, disc abnormalities are present in 57% of scans and herniated discs in 36%.

Matsumoto M, Fujimura Y, Suzuki N, et al: MRI of cervical intervertevral discs in asymptomatic subjects. J Bone Joint Surg 80B:19–24, 1998.

29. Discuss the role of electromyography (EMG) in the evaluation of radiculopathy.

In light of studies suggesting spine MRI abnormalities in 25–55% of the normal population, EMG provides neurophysiologic confirmation of the radiographic lesion. EMG evidence of altered innervation suggests significant nerve root compromise. The most widely accepted EMG evidence of radiculopathy is the presence of positive sharp waves and fibrillation potentials. EMG changes are first seen in muscles closest to the site of nerve injury, underscoring the importance of examination of the paraspinous muscles. A disadvantage of EMG is the delay in appearance of reliable abnormalities until 7–10 days after a root injury. The sequence of EMG changes begins with positive sharp waves in paraspinal muscles between days 7 and 10, followed by paraspinous fibrillation potentials and positive sharp waves in limb muscles between days 17 and 21.

Preston DC, Shapiro BE: Electromyography and Neuromuscular Disorders. Boston, Butterworth-Heinemann, 1998.

30. What is the role of the H-reflex in an S1 radiculopathy?

The H-reflex is an evoked potential study performed by electrically stimulating the S1 root and measuring the nerve conduction velocity proximally. It complements the routine nerve conduction and EMG analysis of muscles and is routinely performed during the same evaluation. Unlike EMG, the H-reflex may demonstrate abnormalities within 1 or 2 days after nerve root injury.

31. What is the diagnostic role of selective nerve root blocks or provocative discography?

Although these procedures are rarely indicated for acute pain, they may have a role in patients with chronic pain and equivocal MRI or EMG findings. Selective nerve root blocks should be done with fluoroscopic guidance to avoid spread to the next nerve root level. Discography, when followed by CT, is positive when it provokes concordant pain and demonstrates internal annular pathology of the disc.

NONOPERATIVE TREATMENT OF SPINAL PAIN

32. What is the rationale for nonoperative treatment of spine-related pain?

The natural history of nonspecific spine pain has been demonstrated to be benign. Approximately 90% of patients experience improvement within 3 months. Recent studies temper these results by suggesting that 75% of patients have one or more relapses, and 72% continue to have pain at 1 year.

Patients with radiculopathy, whether due to soft disc herniation or spondylitic compression, usually improve with time. Acute radiculopathies from soft disc herniation resolve spontaneously in more than 90% of cases. Further support for nonoperative management comes from multiple studies demonstrating resorption of protruded or extruded disc material over time. Recent uncontrolled studies have shown that patients with radiculopathy due to herniated discs who satisfied criteria for surgical intervention but declined the procedure were successfully treated nonoperatively. Good-to-excellent results were achieved in 83% of patients with cervical pain and 90% of patients with lumbar pain.

Mochida K, Komori H, Okawa A, et al: Regression of cervical disc herniation observed on magnetic resonance images. Spine 23:990–995,1998.

33. Discuss the roles of bed rest, cervical collars, and lumbar bracing.

Although bed rest has been shown to be beneficial for acute spinal pain for periods up to 1 week, it should be limited to 2 days at most, with modified activities thereafter. Immobilization with a cervical soft collar or lumbar bracing may provide modest benefit during the acute phase of pain. The patient must take great care to avoid deconditioning.

Malanga GA, Nadler SF: Nonoperative treatment of low back pain. Mayo Clin Proc 74:1135–1148, 1999.

34. What is the role of physical therapy in patients with neck and back pain?

The goal of physical therapy is to alleviate pain, restore function, teach and train the patient to compensate for deteriorated function, and, if possible, prevent further deterioration and recurrence.

Physical therapy for nonspecific spine pain, may be divided into passive (physical modalities) and active (therapeutic exercise) therapies. Alleviation of pain may be obtained through the use of physical modalities, and function may be restored through exercise. Passive therapies include modalities such as ultrasound, electric stimulation, traction, heat and ice, and manual therapy, which use physical energy to modulate pain as well as reduce inflammation, muscular symptoms, and joint stiffness. Passive modalities are most appropriate for short-term use with acute injury or an exacerbation of a chronic problem. Active therapies involve prescribed comprehensive therapeutic exercise, such as the McKenzie program. Dynamic lumbar stabilization is used to facilitate muscular control and protect the patient from biomechanical stresses, including tension, compression, torsion, and shear. Functional restoration is perhaps the most important goal because it makes the patient self-sufficient and autonomous.

Tan JC: Practice Manual of Physical Medicine and Rehabilitation. Diagnostics, Therapeutics and Basic Problems. St. Louis, Mosby, 1998, pp 133–155.

35. Which categories of medication may be of help during acute phases of pain?

Nonsteroidal anti-inflammatory drugs typically are helpful for acute musculoskeletal inflammation, but in patients with severe inflammation or nerve root swelling, a brief, tapering schedule of glucocorticoids is often most beneficial.

Muscle relaxants are of doubtful benefit for reactive or reflexive muscular spasm, but they often are of significant benefit in facilitating sleep when sleep cycles are disrupted by pain.

Adjuvant analgesics are indicated primarily for concurrent neuropathic pain, although their sedative side effects (e.g., tricyclics) can improve sleep as well as provide antidepressant benefit.

Short-term pain relief with **opiate-based medications** can be beneficial with appropriate indications. Tolerance issues often limit their general use.

36. What are the indications for therapeutic injections?

Therapeutic injections of local anesthetics, corticosteroids, or other substances may be administered directly into painful soft tissues, facet joints, nerve roots, the epidural space, or intrathecally. They have been advocated to alleviate acute pain or an exacerbation of chronic pain and to help the patient maintain an ambulatory outpatient status, participate in a rehabilitation program, decrease the need for analgesics, or avoid surgery.

OPERATIVE TREATMENT OF THE SPINE

37. What are the common indications for operative treatment of the spine?

General indications for surgery include (1) persistent and intolerable pain that has been refractory to several months of comprehensive treatment; (2) functional limitations of activities of daily living, including walking distance or standing endurance, to a degree that compromises necessary activities; or (3) severe or progressive muscle weakness or disturbed bladder or sexual function. In addition, confirmatory evidence identifying the symptom-generating spinal structure is assumed.

38. Which surgical procedures are recommended for cervical radiculopathy?

The goal of surgery for cervical radiculopathy is adequate decompression of the nerve roots, using either an anterior or posterior approach. The anterior approach is recommended for medial or central disc herniation or when fusion is contemplated. A posterior approach is necessitated by a posterolateral disc or osteophytes that are otherwise inaccessible. The options are as follows:

1. **Anterior cervical disectomy (ACD)** is indicated when patients have minimal neck pain, normal cervical lordosis, and single-level pathology to avoid the potential complications of fusion.

2. **Anterior cervical disectomy and fusion (ACDF)** is indicated for patients with symptoms of instability or more than one operative level. The risk of developing kyphosis from disc space collapse is also reduced.

3. **ACDF with internal fixation.** Plating is recommended for multilevel fusions with documented instability or history of prior fusion failure. It allows early mobilization without bracing.

4. **Posterior foraminotomy** involves removing one or more hemilaminae to remove osteophytes or lateral disc fragment. When it is used for soft disc herniation, the need for fusion is obviated.

Narayan P, Haid RW: Treatment of degenerative cervical disc disease. Neurol Clin 19:217–229, 2001.

39. Which surgical procedures are recommended for cervical spondylotic myelopathy?

The goal of surgery for cervical spondylotic myelopathy is adequate decompression of the spinal cord. Options include the following:

1. **Single- or multiple-level ACDFs** are performed when the pathology is limited to the disc space and does not involve the vertebral body.

2. **Single- or multiple-level corpectomy with fusion** is indicated for multiple levels of spondylotic compression.

3. **Laminectomy with or without fusion** is indicated for patients with congenital cervical stenosis or a disease processthat involves more than three levels or multiple discontiguous levels.

Narayan P, Haid RW: Treatment of degenerative cervical disc disease. Neurol Clin 19:217–229, 2001.

40. Which surgical procedures are recommended for lumbar spine disease?

The surgical options for decompression of the neural elements within the spinal canal and exit foramina include the following:

1. In **partial laminectomy or laminotomy**, a hole in the lamina is created to allow the removal of a free disc fragment.

2. **Decompressive laminectomy** is indicated for central canal and lateral recess stenosis and often includes a medial facetectomy. If foraminal narrowing is present or the procedure is bilateral, foraminotomy and fusion may be necessary.

3. **Microdisectomy** is essentially the equivalent to the hemilaminectomy for removal of a disc fragment but requires less soft tissue dissection. Potential disadvantages are the limited field of vision and the possibility of not recognizing adjacent pathology, such as lateral recess stenosis.

4. In **percutaneous discectomy**, disc material is removed through a trocar inserted percutaneously into the disc. Concern about the inabilitly to address local pathology may be obviated with a recent modification using an arthroscope.

Hall H: Surgery: Indications and options. Neurol Clin 17:113–130, 1999.

41. What is the most common postoperative complication of spinal surgery?

Arachnoiditis, which refers to adhesive fibrosis of the lumbosacral roots, presumably from an inflammatory etiology. Although it has been associated with various inflammatory conditions (e.g., oil-based myelogram dye, intrathecal injections), its occurrence in the postoperative period has been related to bleeding, trauma, infection, or the use of hemostatic agents such as Gelfoam at the operative site. Symptoms typically emerge long after the inciting event and include low back pain radiating to the buttocks and legs, followed by regional weakness and atrophy implicating multiroot involvement. Diagnosis is by MRI, which can demonstrate thickening and clumping of the roots of the cauda equina and adherence with enhancement of the thecal sac dura.

42. What are the most common causes of the failed (surgical) back?

1. The diagnosis was wrong. Therefore, even if the surgical treatment was technically flawless, the patient must be regarded as having never been treated and requires a thorough reassessment with generation of a new treatment plan.

2. The diagnosis was correct, but the treatment was technically flawed, inappropriate, or incompetent.

3. Whether or not the diagnosis was correct, something new has happened—perhaps an immediate or late consequence of treatment or an unrelated but intercurrent complication. This situation usually occurs when two or more pain-generating mechanisms coexist. For example, in disc herniation removal of disc material improves radicular symptoms but fails to address the me-

chanical pain produced by spinal instability after the herniation.

4. A complication of diagnosis or treatment has arisen; for example, development of arachnoiditis, injury to a nerve root, or disc space infection.

5. No counseling has been given. Physicians must negotiate a plan of postsurgical treatment, stressing patient participation in functional restoration and dispelling unrealistic expectations of complete restoration to normal.

BIBLIOGRAPHY

1. Anderson GBJ: The epidemiology of spinal disorders. In Frymoyer JW (ed): The Adult Spine: Principles and Practice. Philadelphia, Lippincott-Raven , 1997, pp 93–141.
2. Argoff CE, Wheeler AE: Spinal and radicular pain disorders. Neurol Clin 16:833–849, 1998.
3. Hall H: Surgey: Indications and options. Neurol Clin 17:113–130, 1999.
4. Malanga GA, Nadler SF: Nonoperative treatment of low back pain. Mayo Clin Proc. 74:1135–1148; 1999.
5. Matsumoto M, Fujimura Y, Suzuki N, et al: MRI of cervical intervertevral discs in asymptomatic subjects. J Bone Joint Surg 80B:19–24, 1998.
6. Mochida K Komori H, Okawa A, et al: Regression of cervical disc herniation observed on magnetic resonance images. Spine 23:990–995, 1998.
7. Narayan, P, Haid RW: Treatment of degenerative cervical disc disease. Neurol Clin 19:217–229, 2001.
8. Preston DC, Shapiro BE: Electromyography and Neuromuscular Disorders. Boston, Butterworth-Heinemann, 1998.
9. Tan JC: Practice Manual of Physical Medicine and Rehabilitation. Diagnostics, Therapeutics and Basic Problems. St. Louis, Mosby, 1998, pp133–155.
Websites
mcns10.med.nyu.edu/spine/spine-surgery-p5.html
www.backandbodycare.com

8. MYELOPATHIES

Richard M. Armstrong, M.D., F.R.C.P.C.

1. What is the anatomic organization of the spinal cord?

The gray matter forms a butterfly-shaped column in the center of the cord, containing the cell bodies of many of the motor, sensory, and autonomic neurons. These neurons are grouped into various zones (Rexed's laminae), depending on their function. Surrounding the gray matter are the white matter pathways, or long tracts, which carry ascending and descending information throughout the cord.

2. What are the most important long tracts in the spinal cord? Where in the cord is each located?

Long Tracts in the Spinal Cord

TRACT	LOCATION	FUNCTION
Gracile	Medial dorsal column	Proprioception from the leg
Cuneate	Lateral dorsal column	Proprioception from the arm
Spinocerebellar	Superficial lateral column	Muscular position and tone
Pyramidal	Deep lateral column	Upper motor neuron
Lateral spinothalamic	Ventrolateral column	Pain and thermal sensation

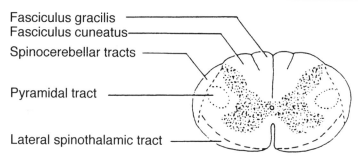

The major long tracts of the spinal cord. (From Joynt R: Clinical Neurology. Philadelphia, J.B. Lippincott, 1992, with permission.)

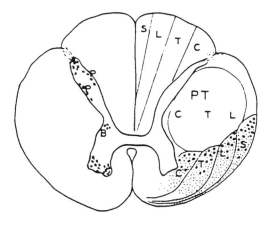

The somatotropic organization of the major long tracts of the spinal cord. The dorsal columns have lower-extremity fibers (sacral and lumbar) lying medially, whereas the pyramidal and spinocerebellar tracts have lower-extremity fibers lying laterally. C = cervical, T = thoracic, L = lumbar, S = sacral, PT = pyramidal tract. (From Joynt R: Clinical Neurology. Philadelphia, J.B. Lippincott, 1992, with permission.)

3. What is the pyramidal tract?

The pyramidal tract is made up of axons arising from the posterior frontal and anterior parietal cortex that terminate in the cord after passing through the pyramid of the medulla. It helps to control motor function.

4. What is pyramidal decussation?

At the level of the lower medulla, 80% of the fibers derived from one hemisphere cross the midline and innervate cells in the cord contralateral to the side of origin.

5. What results from nondecussation of the pyramids?

Nondecussation may occur in association with an anomaly of the medullary cord junction. Clinically, it may be expressed as mirror movements.

6. Where are the long tracts that regulate bladder function?

The pathways for micturition lie in the lateral columns of the cord.

7. What are the fasciculi proprii?

The fasciculi proprii, or ground bundles, are short fiber connections between segments of the cord. They help to control spinal reflex patterns.

8. What is the intermediolateral cell column?

The intermediolateral cell column is composed of neurons that lie in a column in the lateral horn of the gray matter of the cord from T1 to L3 segments. These neurons give rise to sympathetic efferent nerves.

9. Where are the neurons that innervate the axial musculature located?

Axial musculature axons are found in the ventral horn of the gray matter in the cord and lie medially to neurons innervating the limb musculature.

10. What are myotomes and dermatomes?

The spinal cord is organized segmentally, with a pair of spinal nerves exiting from each of its 29 segments. Each pair supplies a specific group of muscles (the myotome) and a specific area of skin (the dermatome).

11. What are the dermatomes at the umbilicus? At the nipple line?

The umbilicus is at T10. The nipple line is at T5.

12. What is the relationship of the cord segment and its spinal nerves to the vertebral body?

The spinal cord extends from the medullary cervical junction at the foramen magnum to the level of the body of the first lumbar vertebra. The spinal roots exit in relation to their corresponding vertebral body. The first seven cervical nerves exit above the vertebral body, and the eighth exists below C7. The remainder of the spinal roots exit below their corresponding vertebral body.

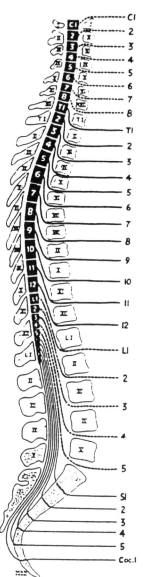

Sagittal section of the spinal cord and vertebral column showing the relationship of the nerve roots to the intervertebral foramina. (From Joynt R: Clinical Neurology. Philadelphia, J.B. Lippincott, 1992, with permission.)

13. Describe the origin and distribution of the anterior spinal artery.

The anterior spinal artery lies along the median ventral plane of the cervical cord. It receives 6–8 major radicular branches, and other branches of the ascending cervical and vertebral arteries help to supply the cervical and upper thoracic cord. The anterior spinal cord artery gives rise to small central arteries that enter the ventral fissure and penetrate the cord to supply the anterior columns and ventral gray matter. Circumferential branches supply the anterolateral two-thirds of the cord.

14. What is the artery of Adamkiewicz?

The artery of Adamkiewicz is a major radicular branch that arises from the aorta and enters the cord between T10 and L3. It supplies the lumbar and lower thoracic segments, anastomosing with anterior spinal artery in the lower thoracic region, which is thus the watershed area of the cord. The lumbar radicular artery is commonly called the artery of Adamkiewicz.

15. What is the arterial supply of the posterior third of the cord?

Paired dorsolateral arteries extend the length of the cord and supply the posterior third of the cord through circumflex and penetrating vessels.

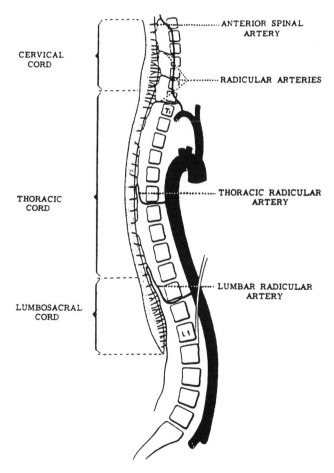

Blood supply of the spinal cord. (From Joynt R: Clinical Neurology. Philadelphia, J.B. Lippincott, 1992, with permission.)

16. What is a myelopathy?

A myelopathy is any pathologic process that affects primarily the spinal cord and causes neurologic dysfunction. The most common causes of myelopathies are:

1. Congenital and developmental defects
   - Syringomyelia
   - Neural tube formation defects
2. Trauma
3. Compromise of the spinal cord
   - Cervical spondylosis
   - Inflammatory arthritis
   - Acute disc herniation
4. Spinal neoplasms
5. Physical agents
   - Decompression sickness
   - Electrical injury
   - Radiation
6. Toxins
   - Nitrous oxide
   - Triorthocresyl phosphate
7. Metabolic and nutritional disorders
   - Pernicious anemia
   - Chronic liver disease
8. Remote effect of cancer
9. Arachnoiditis
10. Postinfectious autoimmune disorders
    - Acute transverse myelitis
    - Connective tissue disease
11. Multiple sclerosis
12. Epidural infections
13. Primary infections
14. Vascular causes
    - Epidural hematoma
    - Atherosclerotic, abdominal aneurysm
    - Malformation

17. What clinical findings suggest a myelopathy?

Myelopathies usually have a triad of clinical findings:

1. Bilateral upper motor neuron weakness of the legs (paraparesis, paraplegia) or legs and arms (quadriparesis, quadriplegia)

2. Bilateral impairment of sensation with a "level" that separates a region of normal sensation from a region of impaired sensation

3. Bowel or bladder sphincter dysfunction

18. What is Lhermitte's sign?

Lhermitte's sign is present when the patient reports an electric shocklike sensation down the spine with neck flexion. The symptom is produced by stretching and irritation of damaged fibers in the dorsal columns of the cervical cord. It may occur in cervical spondylogenic myelopathy or with intramedullary lesions such as a demyelinating plaque.

Goldblatt D, Levy J: The electric sign and the incandescent lamp. Semin Neurol 5:191–193, 1985.

19. What is Brown-Sequard syndrome?

Brown-Sequard syndrome is caused by a lateral hemisection of the spinal cord, usually at or below the cervical enlargement, that severs the pyramidal tract (which has already crossed in the medulla), the uncrossed dorsal columns, and the crossed spinothalamic tract. The region ipsilateral and below the level of the lesion demonstrates upper motor neuron weakness or paralysis and loss of tactile discrimination and position and vibration sense. The tendon reflexes become hyperactive with subsequent spasticity and an extensor plantar response. Contralateral to the lesion there is loss of sense of pain and temperature to a dermatome one or two levels below the lesion.

20. What is spinal shock?

If the cord is transected suddenly by mechanical trauma, ischemia, or compression, there is an initial period when reflex activity begins to function autonomously and hyporeflexia with flaccidity may occur. Development of upper motor neuron signs may take several weeks. There also may be autonomic dysfunction with diffuse sweating and hypotension.

21. What are the signs of anterior spinal artery occlusion?

Anterior spinal ischemia causes bilateral impairment of pain and temperature below the lesion, accompanied by weakness and bladder dysfunction. The reflexes may be hyperactive below the level of the lesion. Dorsal column function (position and vibration) is spared.

22. What is transverse myelitis?

Transverse myelitis is an inflammatory process that is localized over several segments of the cord and functionally transects the cord. It may occur as an infectious or parainfectious illness or as a manifestation of multiple sclerosis, vasculitis, or an autoimmune process. In a significant number of cases (40%), no specific etiology is ever identified.

Rolak LA: Transverse myelitis. In Gilchrist JM (ed): Prognosis in Neurology. Boston, Butterworth-Heinemann, 1998, pp 563–570.

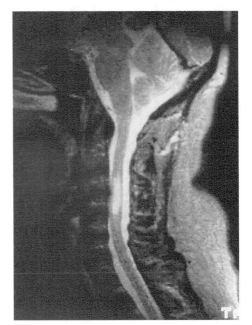

Sagittal T2-weighted MRI shows increased signal within the cervical cord caused by acute inflammatory transverse myelitis.

23. What are the clinical features of acute transverse myelitis?

The sudden onset of weakness and sensory disturbance in the legs and trunk is the usual presenting feature. Ultimately, sphincter dysfunction is common. Pain and temperature are usually affected, but proprioception and vibration are often spared. The tendon jerks below the lesion may be initially depressed and then hyperactive. A sensory level indicates the level of the lesion.

24. Describe the management of patients with transverse myelitis.

Appropriate imaging studies of the cord and spinal column should be obtained to exclude a compressive lesion. Diagnostic studies (hematologic, CSF analysis) should exclude, if possible, multiple sclerosis vasculitis or an infectious process (e.g., zoster, HIV, HTLV-1). Supportive nursing care and careful management of bladder and bowel function are essential. A trial of high-dose intravenous corticosteroids may be tried if infectious causes and compressive lesions have been excluded.

If the MRI of the brain also shows inflammatory lesions, there is a greater than 50% chance that the transverse myelitis is due to a first attack of multiple sclerosis (MS). Patients with abnormal MRI may benefit from treatment with interferon beta-1a to delay the onset of new MS lesions.

Jacobs LD, Beck RW, Simon JH, et al: Intramuscular interferon beta-1a therapy initiated during a first demyelinating event in multiple sclerosis. N Engl J Med 343:898–904, 2000.

25. What is syringomyelia?

Syringomyelia is a longitudinal cystic cavity that develops within the substance of the cord. It may extend over a few or many segments of the cord and even into the medulla (syringobulbia). The cavity is irregular and tends to intrude into the anterior horns of the gray matter and the gray matter dorsal to the central canal. The cavity wall is unremarkable; only gliosis is present.

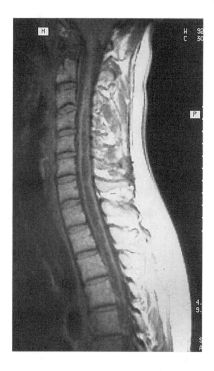

Sagittal MRI shows an extensive syrinx cavity in the cervical and thoracic spinal cord. This syrinx is associated with a developmental defect—an Arnold-Chiari malformation at the base of the skull (protrusion of the cerebellar tonsils down through the foramen magnum).

26. What are the clinical features of syringomyelia?

The classic clinical features are dissociated sensory loss (loss of temperature and pain with intact proprioception) and lower motor neuron weakness (flaccid paralysis, atrophy, fasciculations) that result from cavity extension and destruction of central spinal gray matter. Syringomyelia most commonly occurs in the lower cervical and upper thoracic segments in a capelike distribution. Long tract signs may be evident below the level of the lesion, and sphincter abnormalities and sympathetic dysfunction (Horner's syndrome) also may develop.

27. What causes syringomyelia?

The formation of the syrinx cavity is not fully understood. **Primary syringomyelia** is presumed to be a developmental abnormality. It has been suggested that it is a form of dysraphism resulting from incomplete closure of the neural tube or that it results from an intramedullary vascular anomaly that causes tissue necrosis and cavitation. Another theory proposes that it results from pulsing pressure waves transmitted from the fourth ventricle because of anomalies in the fourth ventricle foramina. **Secondary syringomyelia** is recognized as a cavity formed in relation to an acquired injury, such as an intramedullary tumor, traumatic damage, or central necrosis resulting from ischemia.

28. What is the treatment for syringomyelia?

The standard therapy for progressive syringomyelia is surgical decompression and shunting of the cavity. Unfortunately, results are seldom impressive, and symptoms often continue to progress.

29. What is cervical spondylosis?

Cervical disc narrowing and osteophytic proliferation are common (> 50%) in persons 40 years or older. These changes may result in cord compression if the canal diameter is small and also may compromise circulation to the cord. Spondylitic changes also may compress the spinal nerves that exit through the foramen.

30. What is spondylogenic myelopathy?

Spondylogenic myelopathy is caused by spondylitic changes compressing the cord. It occurs in middle to late age and is more common in men than women. Long tract involvement resulting from cord compromise may be associated with radicular features. Upper motor neuron weakness (paresis, hypertonia, hyperreflexia) may appear before sensory impairment. When sensory loss does develop, dorsal columns tend to be more affected than lateral spinothalamic tracts. Bladder and bowel dysfunction is less common.

31. How is spondylogenic myelopathy best managed?

The management of spondylogenic myelopathy is controversial. In a patient with severe disease, a significantly narrowed canal, and severe neurologic compromise, surgical treatment is probably indicated to prevent further deterioration. Many patients with features of myelopathy and radicular pain are managed conservatively with a cervical collar and antiinflammatory medication. The course tends to be chronic; there may be intermittent exacerbations, improvement, or long periods of stable symptoms.

32. What are the other common causes of cord compression?

Causes of spinal cord compression are best conceptualized in terms of their anatomic location, either inside or outside the cord (medulla) and surrounding meninges (especially the dura).
1. Intramedullary and intradural
   • Primary cord neoplasms
   • Syringomyelia
   • Metastasis or abscess within the substance of the cord (rare)
2. Extramedullary and intradural
   • Neurofibroma and schwannoma
   • Meningioma
3. Extramedullary and extradural
   • Epidural metastases from a remote primary neoplasm. The most common metastases that compress the cord arise from the breast, lung, GI tract, lymphoma/myeloma, and prostate.
   • Epidural abscess
   • Epidural hematoma

33. What are the most common neoplasms arising with the spinal cord?

Most primary spinal cord tumors are either astrocytomas or ependymomas.

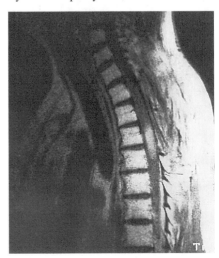

Sagittal T1-weighted MRI, after gadolinium enhancement, shows an astrocytoma arising within the thoracic spinal cord (an intramedullary, intradural lesion).

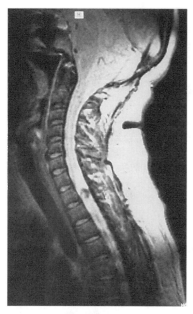

Sagittal T2-weighted MRI shows a neurofibroma displacing the thoracic spinal cord (an extramedullary, intradural lesion).

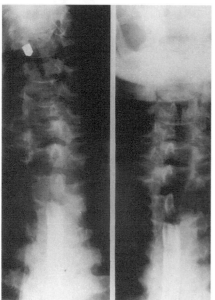

Myelogram shows a block of the column of dye at T2 caused by spinal cord compression from metastatic prostate cancer (an extramedullary, extradural lesion).

34. What is tropical spastic paraparesis?

This disorder has been recognized clinically for many years in tropical areas and Japan. It is characterized by a chronic course in which mild-to-severe leg weakness develops with increased muscle tone and extensor plantar responses. One-half of patients have posterior column sensory signs, and 15% have optic nerve involvement. The condition is caused by infection with a retrovirus, HTLV-1; thus, it is sometimes called HTLV-1-associated myelopathy (HAM).

McKendall RR: HTLV-1 infection. In Samuels M, Feske S (eds): Office practice of Neurology. New York, Churchill Livingstone, 1996, pp 435–438.

35. What is subacute combined degeneration of the spinal cord?

This condition, which results from vitamin B12 deficiency, is characterized by demyelination and vacuolar degeneration of the posterior columns and corticospinal tracts. Frequently an associated peripheral neuropathy presents clinically with accentuated tendon jerks and extensor plantar responses (because of the corticospinal tract involvement). The sensory impairment resulting from posterior column damage may be much more severe than the loss of spinothalamic modalities. Nitrous oxide exposure may produce a similar pathologic picture.

36. Does myelopathy occur as part of acquired immunodeficiency syndrome (AIDS)?

HIV infection may affect the spinal cord and produce a picture of acute or subacute myelitis. Myelopathy is found in approximately 25% of AIDS autopsies. The pathologic picture is vacuolar degeneration similar to that seen in vitamin B12 deficiency.

BIBLIOGRAPHY

1. Mihai C, Mattson DH: Myelitis and myelopathy. In Joynt RJ, Griggs RC (eds): Clinical Neurology. Philadelphia, J.B. Lippincott, 1997, pp 1–31.
2. Victor M, Ropper AH: Principles of Neurology, 7th ed. New York, McGraw-Hill, 2000.
Websites
www.spinalinjury.net
www2.spinewire.com

9. BRAINSTEM DISEASE

Eugene C. Lai, M.D., Ph.D.

CLINICAL ANATOMY OF THE BRAINSTEM

1. What is the functional importance of the brainstem?

The brainstem is a small, narrow region connecting the spinal cord with the diencephalon and cerebrum. It lies ventral to the cerebellum, which it links via the cerebellar peduncles. Its functions are critical to survival. The brainstem is densely packed with many vital structures such as long ascending and descending pathways that carry sensory and motor information to and from higher brain regions. It contains the nuclei of cranial nerves III through XII and their intramedullary fibers. It also possesses groups of neurons that are the major source of noradrenergic, dopaminergic, and serotonergic inputs to most parts of the brain. In addition, other specific nuclear groups, such as the reticular formation, olivary bodies, and red nucleus, lie within the brainstem. In short, it is a complicated but highly organized structure that controls motor and sensory activities, respiration, cardiovascular functions, and mechanisms related to sleep and consciousness. Consequently, a small lesion in the brainstem can affect contiguous structures and cause disastrous neurologic deficits.

2. What are the three main divisions of the brainstem?

Medulla, pons, and midbrain.

3. Describe the function of the medulla.

The medulla (bulb) is the direct rostral extension of the spinal cord. It contains the nuclei of the lower cranial nerves (mainly IX, X, XI, and XII) and the inferior olivary nucleus. The dorsal column pathways decussate in its central region to form the medial lemniscus, whereas the corticospinal tracts cross on the ventral side as they descend caudally. Together with the pons, the medulla also participates in vital autonomic functions such as digestion, respiration, and regulation of heart rate and blood pressure.

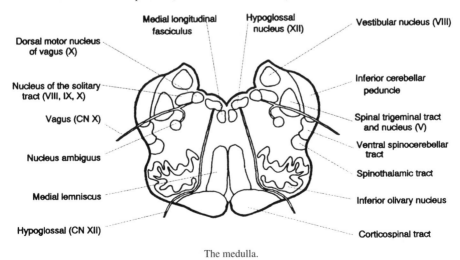

The medulla.

4. Describe the function of the pons.

The pons (bridge) lies rostral to the medulla and appears as a bulge mounting from the ventral surface of the brainstem. The pons contains nuclei for cranial nerves V, VI, VII, and VIII as well as a large number of neurons that relay information about movement from the frontal cerebral hemispheres to the cerebellum (frontopontocerebellar pathway). Other clinically pertinent pathways in the pons are those for the control of saccadic eye movements (medial longitudinal fasciculus) and the auditory connections.

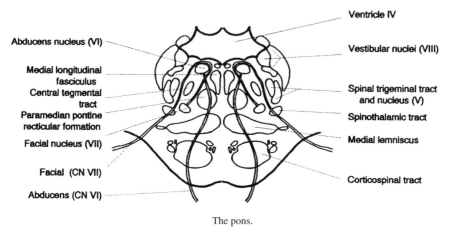

The pons.

5. Describe the function of the midbrain.

The midbrain, the smallest and most rostral component of the brainstem, plays an important role in the control of eye movements and coordination of visual and auditory reflexes. It contains the nuclei for cranial nerves III and IV. Other important structures are the red nuclei and substantia nigra. The periaqueduct area has an important but poorly understood influence on consciousness and pain perception.

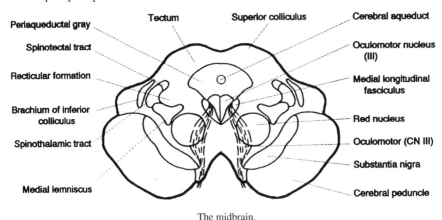

The midbrain.

6. Which cranial nerves are not found in the brainstem?

The twelve pairs of cranial nerves are numbered in rostral-caudal sequence. The brainstem contains the nuclei of all cranial nerves except two: the optic (II) nerve, which terminates in the thalamus, and the olfactory (I) nerve, which synapses in the olfactory bulb.

7. What are the main functions of the cranial nerves?

The cranial nerves have three main functions: (1) to provide motor or general sensory functions; (2) to mediate special senses such as vision, hearing, olfaction, and taste; and (3) to carry the parasympathetic innervation that controls visceral functions.

8. What are the locations and functions of the individual cranial nerves?

Location and Function of Cranial Nerves

NERVE	LOCATION OF NUCLEI	FUNCTION
Olfactory (I)	Olfactory bulb	Sensory: smell and olfactory reflex
Optic (II)	Thalamus	Sensory: vision and visual reflexes
Oculomotor (III)	Midbrain	Motor: eye movement, eyelids, pupillary constriction, accommodation of lens
Trochlear (IV)	Midbrain	Motor: eye movement (superior oblique)
Trigeminal (V)	Midbrain Pons Medulla	Sensory: proprioception for chewing Sensory: from face and cornea. Motor: to masticatory muscles and tensor tympani muscle Sensory: from face and mouth
Abducens (VI)	Pons	Motor: eye movement (lateral rectus)
Facial (VII)	Pons	Sensory: from skin of external ear, taste from anterior tongue. Motor: facial expression, stapedius muscle movement, salivation, and lacrimation
Vestibulocochlear (VIII)	Pons and medulla	Sensory: equilibrium and hearing
Glossopharyngeal (IX)	Medulla	Sensory: from middle ear, palate, pharynx, and posterior tongue, taste from posterior tongue. Motor: swallowing, parotid gland salivation
Vagus (X)	Medulla	Sensory: from pharynx, larynx, thorax, and abdomen, taste from epiglottis. Motor: swallowing and phonation. Autonomic: parasympathetics to thoracic and abdominal viscera
Spinal accessory (XI)	Medulla	Motor: sternocleidomastoid and upper trapezius muscles
Hypoglossal (XII)	Medulla	Motor: tongue

9. How can understanding the anatomy and function of individual cranial nerves assist in localizing brainstem lesions?

The relatively compact positioning of the cranial nerve nuclei and their intramedullary nerve fibers at specific levels, as well as their proximity to certain vertically directed fiber tracts, creates a series of anatomic patterns that provide a basis for the localization of brainstem lesions. Generally speaking, the motor nuclei of the cranial nerves are situated medially, the spinothalamic fibers run along the dorsal lateral portion, and the corticospinal fibers run along the ventral portion of the brainstem.

10. What is the approach to localizing a brainstem lesion?

As a consequence of the unique anatomic arrangements in the brainstem, a unilateral lesion within this structure often causes "crossed syndromes," in which ipsilateral dysfunction of one or more cranial nerves is accompanied by hemiplegia and/or hemisensory loss on the contralateral body. Exquisite localization of a brainstem lesion depends on signs of long-tract (corticospinal and spinothalamic pathways) dysfunction to identify the lesion in the longitudinal (or sagittal) plane and on signs of cranial nerve dysfunction to establish its position in the cross-sectional (or axial) plane. Localization of disorders of the brainstem can be simplified by summarizing the patient's neurologic deficits to answer the following questions: Is the lesion affecting unilateral or bilateral structures of the brainstem? What is the level of the lesion? If the lesion is unilateral, is it medial or lateral in the brainstem?

11. What are the common symptoms and signs of brainstem lesions?
Symptoms

1. Double vision
2. Vertigo
3. Nausea
4. Incoordination

5. Gait imbalance
6. Numbness of the face
7. Hoarseness
8. Difficulties with swallowing and speaking

Signs

1. Multiple cranial nerve dysfunctions
3. Gaze palsies
3. Nystagmus
4. Sympathetic dysfunction (Horner's syndrome)
6. Hearing loss
6. Dysphagia
7. Dysarthria

8. Dysphonia
9. Tongue deviation or atrophy
10. Paresis or dysesthesia of the face with contralateral motor or sensory deficits in the body (crossed symptoms)
11. Unilateral hemiparesis with ataxia
12. Significant bilateral brainstem lesions produce altered mental status or coma

12. What is the approach to localizing an isolated cranial nerve deficit?

An isolated cranial nerve defect, especially of VI and VII, is most often due to a peripheral and not a brainstem lesion.

13. How do the presentations of intra-axial and extra-axial lesions of the brainstem differ?

A lesion that directly affects the tissues of the brainstem is called intra-axial or intramedullary. It usually presents with simultaneous cranial nerve and long-tract symptoms and signs. A lesion outside the brainstem is called extra-axial. It affects the brainstem by initially compressing and interfering with the functions of individual cranial nerves. Later, as it enlarges, neighboring structures within the brainstem may be affected, causing additional long-tract signs.

14. What is the differential diagnosis for a brainstem lesion?

Intra-axial lesions	Extra-axial lesions
Neoplasm	Acoustic neuroma
Ischemia/infarct	Meningioma
Hemorrhage	Chordoma
Vascular malformation	Aneurysms
Demyelinating disease	Epidermoid
Inflammatory lesion	Arachnoid cyst

15. What is the radiographic examination of choice for brainstem lesions?

Magnetic resonance imaging (MRI) is the examination of choice for suspected brainstem lesions. It provides a highly sensitive and noninvasive method of evaluating the posterior fossa, unhampered by skull base artifact. Enhancement with gadolinium may be useful to characterize breakdown of the blood-brain barrier. MR angiography also may be helpful to investigate further the major branches of the vertebrobasilar system in brainstem ischemia or infarction.

16. Outline a practical approach to characterizing intra-axial brainstem lesions by MRI.

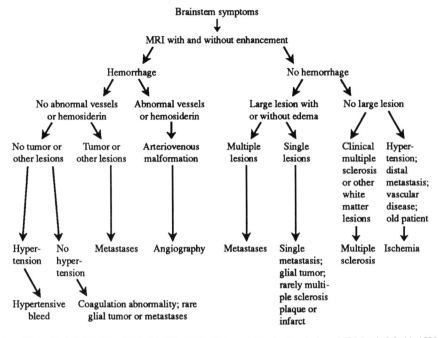

Adapted from Gaskill MF, Wiot JG, Lukin RR: MRI of intra-axial brain stem lesions. MRI Decis 3:2–11, 1989.

BRAINSTEM VASCULAR DISEASES

17. What is the vascular supply of the brainstem?

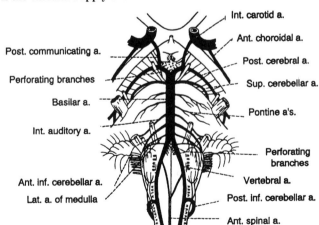

The blood supply of the brainstem is derived from the vertebrobasilar system of the posterior circulation. The paired **vertebral arteries** arise from the subclavian artery on each side and join at the pontomedullary junction to form the **basilar artery**. The main branches of the vertebral artery are the **anterior spinal, posterior spinal,** and **posterior inferior cerebellar** (PICA) arteries. Branches of the basilar artery include the **anterior inferior cerebellar** (AICA), **internal auditory,** and **superior cerebellar arteries**. The basilar artery then terminates by dividing into the two posterior cerebral arteries at the midbrain level. (From Baker AB, Joynt RJ: Clinical Neurology, vol 3. Philadelphia, J.B. Lippincott, 1988, with permission.)

18. Describe the vascular supply of the medulla.

The medulla is supplied by the vertebral arteries and their branches. Its blood supply may be further subdivided into two groups, the **paramedian bulbar** and the **lateral bulbar arteries**. The paramedian bulbar arteries are penetrating branches, mainly from the vertebral artery, that supply the midline structures of the medulla. At the lower medulla, branches from the anterior spinal artery also contribute to this paramedian zone. The lateral portion of the medulla is supplied by the lateral bulbar branches of the vertebral artery or the posterior inferior cerebellar artery.

19. Describe the vascular supply of the pons.

The basilar artery is the principal supplier of the pons. It gives off three types of branches. The **paramedian arteries** supply the medial basal pons, including the pontine nuclei, corticospinal fibers, and medial lemniscus. The **short circumferential arteries** supply the lateral aspect of the pons and the middle and superior cerebellar peduncles. The **long circumferential arteries** together with branches from the anterior inferior cerebellar and superior cerebellar arteries supply the pontine tegmentum and the dorsolateral quadrant of the pons.

20. Describe the vascular supply of the midbrain.

Arteries supplying the midbrain include branches of the superior cerebellar artery, posterior cerebral artery, posterior communicating artery, and anterior choroidal artery. Branches of these arteries, like those of the pons, can be grouped into **paramedian arteries**, which supply the midline structures, and the **long and short circumferential arteries**, which supply the dorsal and lateral midbrain.

Because the blood supply to the brainstem at each level is divided into several territories (usually medial and lateral), occlusion of specific arteries manifests clinical features that reflect their vascular distribution.

21. What is the medial medullary syndrome?

The medial medullary (Dejerine's) syndrome is caused by occlusion of the anterior spinal artery or its parent vertebral artery, resulting in the following signs:

1. Ipsilateral paresis of the tongue (damage to cranial nerve XII), which deviates toward the lesion
2. Contralateral hemiplegia (damage to corticospinal tract) with sparing of the face
3. Contralateral loss of position and vibratory sensation (damage to medial lemniscus)

22. What is the consequence of occlusion of a dominant anterior spinal artery?

The central medullary area may be supplied by a single dominant anterior spinal artery. Occlusion of this vessel then leads to bilateral infarction of the medial medulla, resulting in quadriplegia (with face sparing), complete paralysis of the tongue, and complete loss of position and vibratory sensation. The patient will be mute although fully conscious.

23. What is the lateral medullary syndrome?

The lateral medullary (Wallenberg's) syndrome is often due to vertebral artery or posterior inferior cerebellar artery occlusion. Vertebral artery dissection can also be a cause. Damage to the dorsolateral medulla and the inferior cerebellar peduncle results in the following signs:

1. Ipsilateral loss of pain and temperature sensation of the face (damage to descending spinal tract and nucleus of cranial nerve V)
2. Ipsilateral paralysis of palate, pharynx, and vocal cord (damage to nuclei or fibers of IX and X) with dysphagia and dysarthria
3. Ipsilateral Horner's syndrome (damage to descending sympathetic fibers)
4. Ipsilateral ataxia and dysmetria (damage to inferior cerebellar peduncle and cerebellum)
5. Contralateral loss of pain and temperature on the body (damage to spinothalamic tract)
6. Vertigo, nausea, vomiting, and nystagmus (damage to vestibular nuclei)
7. Other signs and symptoms may include hiccups, diplopia, or unilateral posterior headache.

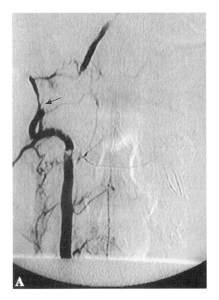 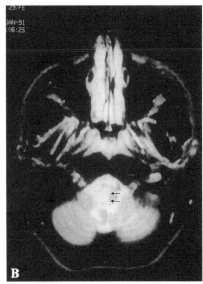

Dissection of the right vertebral artery (*A*, arrow) causing a lateral medullary infarct (Wallenberg's syndrome), seen as an area of increased signal (*B*, arrows) on a T2-weighted MRI of the brainstem.

24. What is the ventral pontine syndrome?

The ventral pontine (Millard-Gubler) syndrome is caused by paramedian infarction of the pons and results in the following signs:
1. Ipsilateral paresis of the lateral rectus (damage to cranial nerve VI) with diplopia
2. Ipsilateral paresis of the upper and lower face (damage to cranial nerve VII)
3. Contralateral hemiplegia (damage to corticospinal tract) with sparing of the face

25. What is the lower dorsal pontine syndrome?

The lower dorsal pontine (Foville's) syndrome is caused by lesions in the dorsal tegmentum of the lower pons, resulting in the following signs:
1. Ipsilateral paresis of the whole face (damage to nucleus and fibers of VII)
2. Ipsilateral horizontal gaze palsy (damage to paramedian pontine reticular formation and/or VI nucleus)
3. Contralateral hemiplegia (damage to corticospinal tract) with sparing of the face

26. What is the upper dorsal pontine syndrome?

The upper dorsal pontine (Raymond-Cestan) syndrome is caused by obstruction of the long circumferential branches of the basilar artery and results in:
1. Ipsilateral ataxia and coarse intention tremor (damage to the superior and middle cerebellar peduncles)
2. Ipsilateral paralysis of muscles of mastication and sensory loss in face (damage to sensory and motor nuclei and tracts of V)
3. Contralateral loss of all sensory modalities in the body (damage to medial lemniscus and spinothalamic tract)
4. Contralateral hemiparesis of the face and body (damage to corticospinal tract) may occur with ventral extension of the lesion.
5. Horizontal gaze palsy may occur, as in the lower dorsal pontine syndrome.

27. What is the ventral midbrain syndrome?

The ventral midbrain (Weber's) syndrome is caused by occlusion of median and paramedian perforating branches and may result in:

1. Ipsilateral oculomotor paresis, ptosis, and dilated pupil (damage to fascicle of cranial nerve III, including parasympathetic fibers)

2. Contralateral hemiplegia, including the lower face (damage to corticospinal and cortico-bulbar tracts)

28. What is the dorsal midbrain syndrome?

The dorsal midbrain (Benedikt's) syndrome results from a lesion in the midbrain tegmentum caused by occlusion of paramedian branches of the basilar or posterior cerebral arteries or both. Its signs are:

1. Ipsilateral oculomotor paresis, ptosis, and dilated pupil (damage to fascicle of cranial nerve III, including parasympathetic fibers as in Weber's syndrome)

2. Contralateral involuntary movements, such as intention tremor, ataxia, and chorea (damage to red nucleus)

3. Contralateral hemiparesis may be present if the lesion extends ventrally.

4. Contralateral hemianesthesia may be present if the lesion extends laterally, affecting the spinothalamic tract and medial lemniscus.

29. What is the dorsolateral midbrain syndrome?

The dorsolateral midbrain syndrome is caused by infarction of the circumferential arteries and results in:

1. Ipsilateral Horner's syndrome (damage to sympathetic tract)

2. Ipsilateral severe tremor that may be present at rest and grossly worsened by attempted movement (damage to superior cerebellar peduncle prior to crossing to the opposite red nucleus). Tremor and ataxia can be present bilaterally if both the superior and cerebellar peduncle and red nucleus are affected.

3. Contralateral loss of all sensory modalities (damage to spinothalamic tract and medial lemniscus that now ascend together)

30. What are the symptoms of brainstem transient ischemic attacks?

Transient circulatory insufficiency in the vertebrobasilar distribution causes brief episodes of brainstem dysfunction characterized by a more patchy and variable presentation. The symptoms of the recurrent attacks may be identical or vary in detail. In basilar artery disease, each side of the body may be affected alternately. All of the structures in the same ischemic distribution may be affected simultaneously, or symptoms of brainstem dysfunction may spread from one region to another. The symptoms may then end abruptly or fade gradually. They are often premonitory symptoms of impending brainstem strokes that may result in devastating consequences.

Transient brainstem ischemic attacks affecting the medulla occur particularly often. Vertigo, dysarthria, dysphagia, and tingling around the mouth suggest dysfunction in this region. At pontine levels frequent symptoms are vertigo; imbalance; hearing abnormalities; tingling, numbness, or weakness of the limbs; and diplopia. Midbrain ischemia may cause diplopia, ataxia, sudden loss of consciousness, and weakness of limbs. Symptoms of brainstem ischemia are usually multiple, and isolated findings (such as vertigo or diplopia) are more often caused by peripheral lesions affecting individual cranial nerves.

31. What are the most common causes of brainstem transient ischemic attacks?

Causes of transient brainstem ischemia include atherosclerotic stenosis of vessels in the vertebrobasilar system, embolization from the heart or ulcerated plaques, recurrent hypotension, vertebral steal syndrome, and cervical spondylosis compromising the vertebral circulation. Transient brainstem ischemic episodes also may occur in the prodromal phase of migraine (especially in basilar migraine in which the entire attack may be dominated by a prolonged is-chemic event in the brainstem).

32. What is the "top of the basilar" syndrome?

Occlusion of the rostral basilar artery, usually embolic, often results in the "top of the basi-lar" syndrome caused by infarction of the midbrain, thalamus, and portions of the temporal and occipital lobes. This syndrome should be suspected in a patient with sudden onset of unrespon-siveness, confusion, amnesia, abnormal eye movement, and visual defect. The neurologic signs may be variable, but the most common include:

1. **Impairments of ocular movements**—unilateral or bilateral vertical (upgaze, downgaze, or complete) gaze palsy, skew deviation, hyperconvergence or convergence spasms causing pseudo-VI-nerve palsy, convergence-retraction nystagmus, and retraction of the upper eyelids.

2. **Abnormalities in pupils**—small with incomplete light reactivity (diencephalic dysfunc-tion), large or mid-position and fixed (midbrain dysfunction), ectopic pupils (corectopia), oval pupils.

3. **Alterations of consciousness and behavior**—stupor, somnolence, apathy, lack of atten-tion, memory deficits, agitated delirium.

4. **Defects in vision**—homonymous hemiopsia, cortical blindness, Balint's syndrome (im-paired visual form discrimination and color dysnomia), and abnormal color vision.

5. **Motor weakness, sensory deficits, and reflex abnormalities** are usually variable and subtle and due to the involvement of long tracts at the infarcted region.

This syndrome may be reversible in patients who are younger and do not have significant risks for cerebrovascular disease.

Caplan LR: "Top of the basilar" syndrome. Neurology 30:72–79, 1980.

33. What is the locked-in syndrome?

Locked-in syndrome occurs in patients with bilateral ventral pontine lesions. Its most common cause is pontine infarction. Other common causes include pontine hemorrhage, trauma, central pontine myelinolysis, tumor, and encephalitis. The patient is quadriplegic because of bi-lateral damage of the corticospinal tracts in the ventral pons. He or she is unable to speak and in-capable of facial movement because of involvement of the corticobulbar tracts. Horizontal eye movements are also limited by the bilateral involvement of the nuclei and fibers of cranial nerve VI. Consciousness is preserved because the reticular formation is not damaged. The patient has intact vertical eye movements and blinking because the supranuclear ocular motor pathways that run dorsally are spared. The patient is able to communicate by movement of the eyelids, but otherwise is completely immobile. Sometimes an incomplete state of this syndrome may occur when the patient retains some horizontal gaze and facial movement. The locked-in syndrome must be distinguished from the persistent neurovegetative state (such as coma vigil or akinetic mutism), in which the patient appears awake but does not react to environmental stimuli and is unable to communicate in any form (thought to be due to a lesion in the rostral midbrain, basal-medial frontal region, or limbic lobes).

Bauby J-D: The Diving Bell and the Butterfly. New York, Alfred A. Knopf, 1997.

34. What are the common causes of brainstem hemorrhage?

Pontine hemorrhage is usually caused by uncontrolled systemic hypertension, resulting in a sudden loss of consciousness, quadriparesis, and pinpoint pupils. Progressive central herniation from supratentorial mass lesions can compress the brainstem and cause hemorrhage in the mid-line of the midbrain (Duret hemorrhage), producing coma and bilateral large and fixed pupils. Diencephalic bleeding, such as thalamic hemorrhage, can dissect into the cerebral peduncles and midbrain, producing acute severe headache, hemiparesis, and III nerve palsy. Small petechial hemorrhages occur in the brainstem of patients with head injuries, blood dyscrasias, or hemor-rhagic disorders. Ruptured aneurysms or arteriovenous malformations of the vertebrobasilar system may result in subarachnoid hemorrhage that injures the brainstem.

OTHER BRAINSTEM SYNDROMES

35. What is Parinaud syndrome?

Parinaud syndrome is also known as the dorsal midbrain or collicular syndrome. The lesion is in the rostral dorsal midbrain, damaging the superior colliculi and pretectal structures. Patients report difficulty in looking up and blurring of distant vision. The common tetrad of findings is:

1. Paralysis of upgaze and accommodation, but sparing of other eye movements
2. Normal-to-large pupils with light-near dissociation (loss of pupillary reflex to light with preservation of pupilloconstriction in response to convergence)
3. Eyelid retraction
4. Convergence-retraction nystagmus (eyes make convergent and retracting oscillations following an upward saccade)

Causes include tumors of the pineal gland, stroke, hemorrhage, trauma, hydrocephalus, or multiple sclerosis. The upgaze palsy can be mimicked by progressive supranuclear palsy, thyroid ophthalmopathy, myasthenia gravis, Guillain-Barré syndrome, or congenital upgaze limitation.

36. What is internuclear ophthalmoplegia?

Internuclear ophthalmoplegia (INO) is a disorder of horizontal ocular movement due to a lesion in the brainstem (usually in the pons, specifically along the medial longitudinal fasciculus between the VI and III nuclei). Horizontal gaze requires the coordinated activity of the lateral rectus muscle of the abducting eye (innervated by the VI nerve) and the medial rectus muscle of the adducting eye (innervated by the III nerve). This integrated function is regulated by the paramedian pontine reticular formation (or pontine gaze center), which receives inputs from the contralateral occipital and frontal eyefields and sends fibers to the ipsilateral abducens (VI) nucleus and the contralateral oculomotor (III) nucleus. Fibers from the pontine gaze center run rostrally together with vestibular and other fibers to make up the medial longitudinal fasciculus (MLF).

The cause is commonly multiple sclerosis in young adults, especially when the syndrome is bilateral. In older people the syndrome is often unilateral and caused by occlusion of the basilar artery or its paramedian branches. Occasionally INO can be caused by lupus erythematosus and drug overdose (e.g., barbiturates, phenytoin, amitriptyline). Pseudo-INO occurs rarely as a feature of myasthenia gravis, Wernicke's encephalopathy, and Guillain-Barré syndrome.

Many patients with INO have no symptoms, but some have diplopia or blurred vision. On lateral gaze, the signs of INO include:

1. Impaired or paralyzed adduction of the eye ipsilateral to the lesion. The deficit can range from complete medial rectus paralysis to slight slowing of an adducting saccade.
2. Horizontal nystagmus of the abducting eye contralateral to the lesion.
3. Bilateral INO results in defective adduction to the right and left, and nystagmus of the abducting eye on both directions of gaze.
4. Convergence is usually preserved. Skew deviation and vertical gaze nystagmus are sometimes present.

37. What is the "one-and-a-half" syndrome?

This disorder of horizontal ocular movement is characterized by a lateral gaze palsy on looking toward the side of the lesion and INO on looking in the other direction. The location of the lesion is the paramedian pontine reticular formation or VI nerve nucleus. MLF fibers crossing from the contralateral VI nucleus are also involved, causing INO. The common causes of this syndrome are similar to those of INO (e.g., multiple sclerosis, stroke). Hemorrhage or tumor in the lower pons is also in the differential diagnosis. Pseudo-one-and-a-half syndromes may occur with myasthenia gravis, Wernicke's encephalopathy, or Guillain-Barré syndrome. Clinical signs include:

1. Horizontal gaze palsy on looking toward the size of the lesion ("one").
2. INO on looking away from the side of the lesion ("half"). This paralyzes adduction and causes nystagmus on abduction. As a result, the ipsilateral eye has no horizontal movement, and the only lateral ocular movement that remains is abduction and nystagmus of the contralateral eye.

3. Associated signs include skew deviation, gaze-invoked nystagmus on vertical gaze, and exotropia of the eye contralateral to the lesion.

4. Vertical ocular movements and convergence are usually intact.

38. What is bulbar palsy?

The bulb is the medulla, and the term bulbar palsy refers to a syndrome of lower motor neuron paralysis, affecting muscles innervated by cranial nerves (mainly IX to XII) that have their nuclei closely approximated in the lower brainstem. Muscles of the face, palate, pharynx, larynx, sternocleidomastoid, upper trapezius, and tongue are usually affected. Patients may present clinically with dysarthria, dysphagia, hoarseness, nasal voice, palatal deviation, diminished gag reflex, or weakness of the sternocleidomastoid, upper trapezius, or tongue. Atrophy and fasciculations may be evident. Bulbar palsy may result from various conditions involving the motor nuclei of the lower brainstem or their intramedullary fibers, the corresponding peripheral nerves, the myoneural junction, or the musculature. Causes of intra-axial lesions include brainstem infarct, syringobulbia, glioma, poliomyelitis, encephalitis, and motor neuron disease (amyotrophic lateral sclerosis or progressive bulbar palsy). Extra-axial causes are neoplasms (meningioma or neurofibroma), chronic meningitis, aneurysms, neck trauma, and congenital abnormalities (Chiari malformation or basilar impression). Myasthenia gravis, Guillain-Barré syndrome, myositis, and diphtheria also may present with similar signs and symptoms.

39. What is pseudobulbar palsy?

Pseudobulbar palsy is a syndrome of upper motor neuron paralysis that affects the corticobulbar system above the brainstem bilaterally. Although it presents with most of the signs and symptoms of bulbar palsy, the causative lesion is not in the brainstem. This condition causes dysphagia, dysarthria, and paresis of the tongue (without atrophy or fasciculations). In contrast to bulbar palsy, the reflex movements of the soft palate and pharynx are frequently hyperactive. The jaw jerk is brisk. Frontal signs (grasp, snout, suck, and glabellar reflex) may be present. Emotional incontinence with exaggerated crying (or, less often, laughing) is also common and may be due to disruption of frontal efferents subserving emotional expression. Multiple lacunar infarcts or chronic ischemia in the hemispheres affecting bilateral corticobulbar fibers usually causes this syndrome. Other causes are amyotrophic lateral sclerosis (ALS) and multiple sclerosis. In ALS a combination of upper and lower motor neuron disease often results in coexisting bulbar and pseudobulbar palsies (wasting and fasciculations of the tongue associated with brisk jaw jerk).

OTHER BRAINSTEM DISEASES

40. What is a brainstem glioma?

Brainstem glioma is the most frequent neoplasm affecting the brainstem. It occurs mostly in children and adolescents and is often associated with neurofibromatosis. The tumor arises in the region of the VI nerve nucleus and gradually enlarges to involve the VI and VII nerves and adjacent vestibular structures. Vestibular, cerebellar, and lower cranial nerve symptoms may be present and slowly progressive over a period of months or years before the diagnosis is made because motor and sensory symptoms in the body are usually absent.

41. What other neoplasms affect the brainstem?

Ependymomas occur in the fourth ventricle and may cause obstruction, resulting in intermittent noncommunicating hydrocephalus accompanied by headache and protracted vomiting from involvement of the chemoreceptor trigger zone on the floor of the fourth ventricle. **Metastatic lesions** of the brainstem may arise from malignant melanoma or neoplasms of the lung and breast, but are relatively rare.

42. What are the common metabolic causes of brainstem dysfunction?

Extraocular movements and cerebellar pathways are vulnerable to damage by metabolic insults because they are highly metabolically active. These dysfunctions are usually acute and reversible.

The common presentations are ataxia, vertigo, nausea, vomiting, dysarthria, nystagmus, and gaze palsies such as INO. Common causes are alcohol intoxication and overdose of sedative drugs (e.g., barbiturates) and anticonvulsants (e.g., phenytoin).

43. How does thiamine deficiency affect the brainstem?

Wernicke's encephalopathy is a complication of alcoholism and malnutrition resulting in thiamine deficiency. It usually presents with characteristic mental changes of gross confusion, ataxia, extraocular movement abnormalities, and other signs of brainstem dysfunction. The brainstem signs can be readily reversed by parenteral thiamine therapy, but the confusional state may resolve more slowly.

44. How does demyelinating disease affect the brainstem?

Multiple sclerosis often results in demyelination of the fast-conducting, heavily myelinated nerve fibers traveling along the brainstem. These include the cerebellar-vestibular pathways, medial longitudinal fasciculus, and pyramidal pathways. Bilateral INO is almost pathognomonic of multiple sclerosis. Another hallmark of brainstem multiple sclerosis is the combination of bilateral cerebellar and pyramidal signs producing ataxia and pathologically brisk reflexes.

45. What is central pontine myelinolysis?

Central pontine myelinolysis is another demyelinating disease that affects the brainstem white matter, mostly in the central pons and occasionally the cerebral hemispheres. It occurs primarily in patients suffering from malnutrition or alcoholism complicated by hyponatremia. Rapid correction of the hyponatremia has been implicated as a cause of the demyelination. This disorder develops as a subacute progressive quadriparesis with lower cranial nerve involvement. It is usually fatal, but survival with recovered neurologic function is possible. It can be prevented by correcting the electrolyte disturbance gradually rather than rapidly.

Karp BI, Laurend R: Pontine and extrapontine myelinolysis: A neurologic disorder following rapid correction of hyponatremia. Medicine 72:369–371, 1993.

VERTIGO

46. Define vertigo.

Vertigo is a false sense of movement, either of oneself or of the environment. The feeling may involve the whole body or be limited to the head. It should be distinguished from dizziness or giddiness resulting from near syncope, postural hypotension, hyperventilation, multiple sensory deficits, ataxia, or other etiologies. The spinning or swirling sensations of vertigo are related to disturbances of the vestibular system.

47. What are the common causes of vertigo?

The causes of vertigo are central (due to a brainstem lesion) or peripheral (due to an inner ear or vestibular nerve lesion). Central vertigo is almost always accompanied by other signs of brainstem dysfunction, such as double vision, weakness or numbness of the face, dysarthria, or dysphagia. Peripheral vertigo is usually accompanied by tinnitus or hearing loss but no other neurologic abnormalities.

Common Causes of Vertigo

CENTRAL	PERIPHERAL
Brainstem stroke or transient ischemic attack	Vestibular neuronitis
Multiple sclerosis	Benign positional vertigo
Neoplasms	Ménière's disease
Syringobulbia	Local trauma or posttraumatic
Arnold-Chiari deformity	Physiologic (e.g., motion sickness)
Basilar migraine	Drugs/toxins (e.g., antibiotics, diuretics, antineoplastics, or anticonvulsants)
Cerebellar hemorrhage	Posterior fossa tumors/masses (e.g., acoustic neuroma)

48. What signs and symptoms help to distinguish central from peripheral vertigo?

Central vs. Peripheral Vertigo

SIGNS AND SYMPTOMS	CENTRAL VERTIGO	PERIPHERAL VERTIGO
Nystagmus	Often vertical or rotatory; may change with direction of gaze; increases with looking toward side of lesion	Mostly horizontal or sometimes rotatory; unidirectional and conjugate; increases with looking away from side of lesion
Latency of onset and duration of nystagmus	No latency after head motion; persistent and lasts > 60 sec	Latency after head motion; fatigable and lasts < 60 sec
Caloric test	May be normal	Abnormal on side of lesion
Brainstem or cranial nerve signs	Often present	Absent
Hearing loss, tinnitus	Absent	Often present
Nausea and vomiting	Usually absent	Usually present
Vertigo	Usually mild	Severe, often rotational
Falling	Often falls toward side of lesion	Often falls to side opposite nystagmus
Visual fixation or eye closing	No change or increase of symptoms	Inhibits nystagmus and vertigo

49. What is vestibular neuronitis?

Vestibular neuronitis is a condition affecting primarily young adults, causing a sudden attack of vertigo without tinnitus or hearing loss. This benign disorder usually resolves within several days. The etiology is presumed to be a viral infection.

50. What is Ménière's disease?

Ménière's disease causes the symptomatic triad of episodic vertigo, tinnitus, and hearing loss. It is caused by an increased amount of endolymph in the scala media. Pathologically, hair cells degenerate in the macula and vestibule.

51. What is benign positional vertigo? How is it diagnosed?

Benign positional vertigo is a disorder characterized by paroxysms of vertigo and nystagmus on assumption of certain positions of the head. Hearing tests are normal. The diagnosis is made by performing head maneuvers that elicit the patient's symptoms and nystagmus. The cause is calcification and dislocation of otoliths, which move freely in the semicircular canal, thus abnormally stimulating the hair cells within the semicircular canals.

52. What are canalith repositioning (Epley) maneuvers?

Epley maneuvers are performed as a treatment for benign positional vertigo. While lying supine, the patient's head is rotated through a series of positions that rolls the otoliths out of the semicircular canals and thus removes the cause of the positional vertigo.

Epley JM: The canalith repositioning procedure for treatment of benign paroxysmal positional vertigo. Otolaryngol Head Neck Surg 107:399–406, 1992.

CONSCIOUSNESS

53. What are the functions of the reticular formation in the brainstem?

The reticular formation is composed of a network of diffuse aggregations of neurons distributed throughout the central parts of the medulla, pons, and midbrain. It fills the spaces between cranial nerve nuclei and olivary bodies and intermixes between ascending and descending fiber tracts. Its neurons receive afferent information from the spinal cord, cranial nerve nuclei, cerebellum, and cerebrum and send efferent impulses to the same structures. Their widespread connections give them extensive influence over many neuronal activities. The main functions of the reticular formation are:

1. Activation of the brain for behavioral arousal and different levels of awareness
2. Modulation of segmental stretch reflexes and muscle tone for control of motor function
3. Coordination of autonomic functions, such as control of breathing and cardiovascular activities
4. Modulation of the perception of pain

Steriade M: Arousal: Revisiting the reticular activating system. Science 272:225–227, 1996.

54. How do you examine for brainstem dysfunction in a comatose patient?

When examining a comatose patient, one should be aware of signs and symptoms indicating that the coma is due to brainstem (reticular formation) dysfunction. This is especially true of impending brainstem failure from increased intracranial pressure causing herniation into the posterior fossa. This dysfunction travels in a rostral-caudad direction, ending in death with medullary involvement. Emergency management to reduce the intracranial pressure should be implemented immediately. The following observations are used to monitor the patient's condition:

- Mental status
- Breathing pattern
- Pupillary size and light response
- Spontaneous eye movement or deviation
- Oculocephalic reflex on head turning (doll's eye movement)
- Oculovestibular test of gaze response to ice-water calorics
- Motor response to supraorbital nerve pressure (noxious stimulus)
- Presence of other brainstem reflexes (corneal, gag, and ciliospinal)

55. How does the clinical examination localize the level of brainstem dysfunction in a comatose patient?

Localization of Level of Brainstem Dysfunction

SIGNS AND SYMPTOMS	SUBCORTICAL	MIDBRAIN	PONS	MEDULLA
Consciousness	Lethargy or stupor	Coma	Coma	Coma
Breathing	Cheynes-Stokes	Central hyperventilation	Apneustic or cluster	Atactic
Pupils	Small and reactive	Midposition and fixed (III nucleus); unilateral dilated and fixed (III nerve); large and fixed (pretectal)	Pinpoint	Midposition and fixed, often irregular in shape
Oculocephalic and oculovestibular responses	Present	Absent or abnormal	Absent or abnormal	Absent
Motor response to stimulation	Decortication	Decerebration	Decerebration or no response	No response

56. How do you test for irreversible loss of brainstem function?

Brain death is a clinical diagnosis of irreversible cessation of all cerebral and brainstem function. Complete loss of brainstem function begins with apneic coma. On examination, all brainstem reflexes (corneal, pupillary, gag, ciliospinal) are absent. The pupils are midposition or large and fixed. Oculocephalic and oculovestibular reflexes are absent. Muscle tone is flaccid, with no spontaneous facial movement and no motor response to noxious stimuli. This condition should be present for 6–24 hours in adults. Metabolic causes (hypothermia, hypotension) and drug effects (neuromuscular blockers, sedative drugs) need to be ruled out. Many local institutions have developed their own, slightly modified criteria for brain death.

57. What is the apnea test?

The apnea test is an essential test for the cessation of brainstem function. It stimulates the respiratory centers in the brainstem by inducing hypercarbia. One technique is ventilation of the patient with 100% oxygen for 10–30 minutes (depending on the severity of any underlying lung injury) followed by disconnection from the respirator and administration of 100% oxygen through a catheter in the trachea or via T-piece at a flow rate of 6 L/min. Absence of spontaneous respiratory effort with a $PaCO_2$ of above 60 mmHg confirms clinical apnea. Arterial blood gas should be checked before and after the withdrawal of ventilation. Sometimes the test cannot be completed because of ventricular arrhythmias or hypotension. In that situation, the diagnosis of irreversible brainstem dysfunction is made by clinical judgment.

BIBLIOGRAPHY

1. Baloh RW: Dizziness, Hearing Loss, and Tinnitus. Philadelphia, F.A. Davis, 1998.
2. Kandel ER, Schwartz JH, Jessell TM: Principles of Neural Science, 3rd ed. New York, Elsevier, 1991.
3. Leigh RJ, Zee DS: The Neurology of Eye Movements, 4th ed. Philadelphia, F.A. Davis, 2001.
4. Patten J: Neurological Differential Diagnosis. London, Springer, 1996.
5. Plum F, Posner JB: The Diagnosis of Stupor and Coma, 3rd ed. Philadelphia, F.A. Davis, 1982.
6. Victor M, Ropper AH: Principles of Neurology, 7th ed. New York, McGraw-Hill, 2001.

Websites
www.lib.uchicago.edu/hw/neuroanatomy
www.wfubmc.edu/neurology/vertigo/vergito1.html

10. CEREBELLAR DISEASE

Eugene C. Lai, M.D., Ph.D.

1. What is the functional importance of the cerebellum?

The cerebellum coordinates movement and maintains equilibrium and muscle tone through a complex regulatory and feedback system. It receives somatosensory input from the spinal cord, motor information from the cerebral cortex, and input about balance from the vestibular organs of the inner ears. It integrates all this information and aids in organizing the range, velocity, direction, and force of muscular contractions to produce steady volitional movements and posture. It does so by constantly screening its sensory inputs and modulating its motor outputs. The cerebellum also plays an important role in the coordination of the planning of limb movements. In addition, it participates in learning motor tasks, as its function can be modified by experience.

Damage to the cerebellum alone does not impair sensory perception or muscle strength. Rather, it disrupts coordination of limb and eye movements, impairs balance, and decreases muscle tone.

2. What is the basic anatomy of the cerebellum?

The cerebellum can be divided into three major lobes by transverse fissures. The primary fissure, located on the upper surface of the cerebellum, divides the cerebellum into an **anterior lobe** and a **posterior lobe**. The posterolateral fissure on the underside of the cerebellum separates the large posterior lobe from the small **flocculonodular lobe**. The cerebellar cortex consists of three layers based on its microscopic anatomy: the molecular cell layer, the Purkinje cell layer, and the granule cell layer. Three pairs of deep nuclei are present within the cerebellum. From medial to lateral these are the fastigial, interposed (may be separated into globose and emboliform), and dentate nuclei. A more functionally useful method of describing the cerebellum is based on its longitudinal zonal patterns and their different connections. A midline zone, known as the **vermis**, separates the two cerebellar hemispheres on each side. Each hemisphere in turn is composed of an **intermediate zone** and a **lateral zone**. These three zones, together with the flocculonodular lobe, represent the major functional subdivisions of the cerebellum by virtue of their distinct input and output pathways.

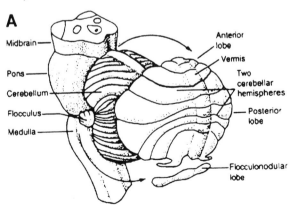

A

Midbrain

Pons

Cerebellum

Flocculus

Medulla

Anterior lobe

Vermis

Two cerebellar hemispheres

Posterior lobe

Flocculonodular lobe

The cerebellum is divided into anatomically distinct lobes. *A*, The cerebellum is unfolded to reveal the lobes normally hidden from view.

(Continued on following page.)

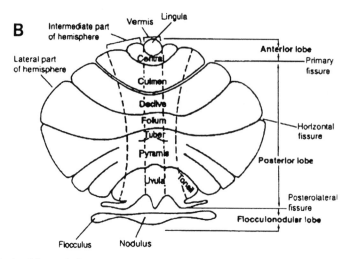

B, The main body of the cerebellum is divided by the primary fissure into anterior and posterior lobes. The posterolateral fissure separates the flocculonodular lobe. Shallower fissures divide the anterior and posterior lobes into nine lobules. The cerebellum has three functional regions: the central vermis and the lateral and intermediate zones in each hemisphere. (From Ghez C: The cerebellum. In Kandel ER, et al (eds): Principles of Neural Science. New York, Elsevier, 1991, with permission.)

3. What are the connections and functions of the major divisions of the cerebellum?

Connections and Functions of Major Divisions of the Cerebellum

FUNCTIONAL DIVISION	MAJOR INPUT	MAJOR OUTPUT	FUNCTION
Flocculonodular lobe (vestibulocerebellum)	Vestibular nuclei, labyrinth, visual system	Vestibular nuclei, medial and lateral vestibular tracts	Equilibrium (axial), eye movements, vestibular reflexes
Vermis (spinocerebellum)	Vestibular, visual, and auditory systems, face, proximal body parts	Vestibular nucleus, reticular formation, contralateral motor cortex, and medial descending system via the **fastigial** nucleus	Axial and proximal muscle control and execution, progressive movement
Intermediate zone (spinocerebellum)	Spinal cord (distal body parts)	Contralateral red nucleus, motor cortex, and lateral descending system via the **interposed** nucleus	Distal muscle control and execution, progressive movement
Lateral zone (cerebrocerebellum)	Contralateral cerebral cortex via pontine nuclei	Contralateral red nucleus, thalamus, motor and premotor cortex via **dentate** nucleus	Motor planning initiation and timing

4. What are the principal afferent and efferent pathways of the cerebellum?

The afferent and efferent pathways to and from the cerebellum course through three pairs of tracts (cerebellar peduncles) that connect the cerebellum to the brainstem:

1. The **inferior cerebellar peduncle** (restiform body) consists of mainly afferent fibers. A single efferent tract, the fatigiobulbar tract, goes to the vestibular nucleus from the flocculonodular lobe. Afferent fibers enter the inferior cerebellar peduncle from at least five sources, including

(1) the vestibulocerebellar tract, (2) the olivocerebellar tract, (3) the dorsal spinocerebellar tract, (4) the cuneocerebellar tract, and (5) the reticulocerebellar tract.

2. The **middle cerebellar peduncle** (brachium pontis) consists almost entirely of crossed afferent fibers from the pontine nuclei that transmit impulses from the cerebral cortex to the intermediate and lateral zones of the cerebellum (corticopontocerebellar tract).

3. The **superior cerebellar peduncle** (brachium conjunctivum) consists principally of efferent projections from the cerebellum. Rubral, thalamic, and reticular projections arise from the dentate and interposed nuclei. The fastigiobulbar tracts run with this peduncle for a short distance before it enters the inferior cerebellar peduncle. Afferent fibers include the ventral spinocerebellar tract and the trigeminocerebellar and tectocerebellar projections.

5. What are the blood supplies to the cerebellum?

The vertebral and basilar arteries give off three paired branches to the cerebellum: the superior, the anterior inferior, and the posterior inferior cerebellar arteries, which are interconnected by anastomoses. The superior cerebellar artery runs over the superior surface of the cerebellum, while the other arteries supply the inferior surface.

The **superior cerebellar artery** arises from the rostral part of the basilar artery and supplies the lateral midbrain and pontine tegmentum, superior cerebellar peduncle, upper segment of the middle cerebellar peduncle, dentate nucleus, rostral vermis, and superior portion of of the rostral cerebellar hemisphere.

The **anterior inferior cerebellar artery** arises from the caudal basilar artery and supplies the smallest territory of all the cerebellar arteries. It provides supply to the lateral pontomedullary tegmentum, lower segment of the middle cerebellar peduncle, flocculus, and adjacent inferior surface of the cerebellar hemispheres. Penetrating branches supply part of the dentate nucleus and nearby white matter.

The **posterior inferior cerebellar artery** derives from the vertebral artery and supplies the lateral medullary tegmentum, inferior cerebellar peduncle, and caudal portions of the cerebellar nuclei, inferior vermis, and inferior cerebellar hemisphere, including the tonsils.

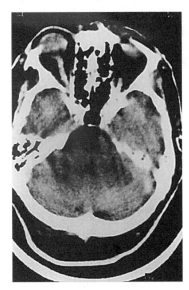 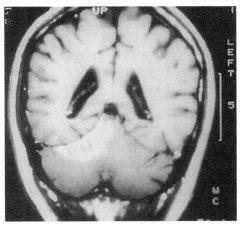

Above, T1-weighted MRI shows a hemorrhagic infarction of the right superior cerebellar artery territory.
Left, CT scan shows an infarction of both anterior inferior cerebellar arteries.

6. What are the main clinical features of cerebellar diseases?

Cerebellar diseases comprise a disturbance of equilibrium, muscle tone, and execution of movement. The following findings may be present: hypotonia, ataxia, dysmetria, dysdiadochokinesia, nystagmus, rebound phenomenon, postural instability, scanning speech, and intention tremor. These findings vary in severity depending on whether the lesion is acute or chronic, bilateral or unilateral, hemispheric or midline. The common findings of cerebellar dysfunction can be remembered by the mnemonic **HANDS Tremor**:

H = **H**ypotonia (loss of muscle tone)
A = **A**synergy (lack of coordination)
N = **N**ystagmus (ocular oscillation)
D = **D**ysarthria (speech abnormalities)
S = **S**tation and gait (imbalance, gait ataxia)
Tremor = **Tremor** (coarse intention tremor)

7. What are the clinical tests for cerebellar dysfunction?

Tests for Cerebellar Dysfunction

ABNORMALITY	METHODS OF EXAMINATION
Hypotonia	Passive movement of extremities to check muscle tone; pendular patellar reflexes; rebound phenomenon; inspect for rag doll (flaccid) posture
Asynergy	Finger-nose-finger, heel-to-shin, and rapid-alternating supernation-pronation tests to evaluate rate, range, force, and accuracy of voluntary movement
Nystagmus	Ocular oscillations through the fields of gaze
Dysarthria	Abnormalities in articulation and prosody (scanning or explosive speech, altered accent)
Stance and gait	Broad-based stance and gait, difficulty with tandem walk, and postural instability
Tremor	Limb tremor at rest, with sustained posture, and during action

Because most of the tests of cerebellar functions require the cooperation and volitional movement of the patient, clinical features of cerebellar dysfunction cannot be elicited from a paralyzed or comatose patient.

8. How do you differentiate cerebellar and sensory ataxia?

The cerebellum can coordinate and equilibrate movement only if it receives the proper proprioceptive information. Therefore, if the proprioceptive system is defective, the patient has imbalance and ataxia. The proprioceptive defect can be compensated by visual guidance; therefore, the patient with sensory loss exhibits worsening of movement with the eyes closed.

Cerebellar vs. Sensory Ataxia

CLINICAL FINDING	CEREBELLAR ATAXIA	SENSORY ATAXIA
Hypotonia	Present	Absent
Asynergy, dysmetria	Present	Absent
Nystagmus	Present	Absent
Dysarthria	Present	Absent
Tremor	Present	Absent
Loss of vibration and position sense	Absent	Present
Areflexia	Absent	Present
Dystaxia much worse with eyes closed (Romberg test)	Absent	Present

9. What are the general principles in localizing a cerebellar lesion?

Specific cerebellar regions possess distinct functions. There is also a topical representation of individual body parts in the cerebellum. Thus, signs of cerebellar dysfunction may have localizing significance. Some general principles include:

• Lesions of the rostral midline impair coordination involving stance and gait.
• Lesions of the caudal midline impair axial truncal posture and equilibrium.
• Lateral lesions impair the limbs ipsilateral to the cerebellar lesion.

- Lesions of the cerebellar hemisphere ultimately impair movement on the ipsilateral side of the body because of a doublecrossing of the pathways. The ascending cerebellocortical fibers cross in the midbrain and project to the contralateral cortex, and then the descending corticospinal fibers cross back in the medulla to project to the contralateral body.
- Lesions of the afferent or efferent pathways to the cerebellum may cause signs similar to lesions of the cerebellum itself.
- Lesions of the superior cerebellar peduncle and the deep nuclei usually produce the most severe disturbance of cerebellar dysfunction.

10. What are the major cerebellar syndromes?

There are four major cerebellar syndromes: rostral vermis syndrome, caudal vermis syndrome, hemispheric syndrome, and pancerebellar syndrome. They are distinguished by their presentations and the anatomic regions affected. Recognition of these syndromes may help to narrow the differential diagnosis of cerebellar lesions.

Cerebellar Syndromes

CLINICAL SYNDROMES	REGION(S) INVOLVED	DISTRIBU-TION OF DEFICITS	COMMON CAUSES	HYPO-TONIA	INCOORDINATION OF			NYSTAGMUS	DYS-ARTHRIA
					Arms	Legs	Gait and Trunk		
Cerebellar hemisphere syndrome	Unilateral intermediate and lateral zones	Ipsilateral head and body	Infarct, neoplasm, abscess, demyelination	+	+	+	+	+ (bidirectional, coarser, slower on gaze to side of lesion; faster, finer on gaze to other side)	+
Rostral vermis syndrome	Anterior and superior vermis	Gait and trunk	Alcoholism, thiamine deficiency	+	+ −	+	+	−	−
Caudal vermis syndrome	Flocculo-nodular and posterior vermis	Axial disequi-librium	Midline neoplasm	+ −	−	+ −	+	+ (variable)	−
Pancerebellar syndrome	All regions	Bilateral signs of cerebellar dysfunction	Toxic/metabolic, infectious/postinfectious, paraneoplastic, degenerative disorders	+	+	+	+	+ (variable type)	+

11. What are the common acquired diseases of the cerebellum?

Acquired cerebellar diseases frequently present as acute ataxia with or without other cerebellar signs. They are often treatable if recognized early. Therefore, one should be astute with the differential diagnosis of acute ataxia so that the disorder can be identified and management plans initiated as early as possible. Cerebellar diseases have a broad differential diagnosis. Initially, they may be divided by etiology into acquired or inherited disorders. Some common acquired cerebellar diseases are as follows:

1. **Vascular diseases**
   Infarction (mostly thrombotic, sometimes embolic)
   Hemorrhage (from hypertension, vascular malformation, or tumor)
   Transient ischemic attacks
   Basilar migraine (usually in children)
   Vascular malformation
   Systemic vasculitides (systemic lupus erythematosus)

2. **Neoplasms**
   Primitive neuroectodermal tumor (PNET or medulloblastoma; in children)
   Astrocytoma (often cystic; midline in children and hemispheric in adults)
   Hemangioblastoma (may be associated with von Hippel-Lindau disease)
   Metastatic tumor (may be multiple)
3. **Infections**
   Acute cerebellar ataxia of childhood (possible viral etiology)
   Tuberculosis or tuberculoma
   Cysticercosis
   Bacterial infection and abscess (through direct extension of mastoid infection)
   Chronic panencephalitis of congenital rubella infection
   Viral encephalitis (involving cerebellum or brainstem)
4. **Inflammatory or autoimmune disorders**
   Multiple sclerosis
   Acute postinfectious cerebellitis
   Postinfectious disseminated encephalomyelitis
   Miller-Fisher variant of acute inflammatory polyneuropathy
5. **Paraneoplastic syndromes**
   Paraneoplastic cerebellar degeneration (commonly associated with lung, ovarian, or
      breast carcinomas)
   Opsoclonus-myoclonus (secondary to neuroblastoma)
6. **Metabolic disorders**
   Hypothyroidism
   Hyperthermia
   Hypoxia
   Deficiencies of thiamine (in alcoholics), niacin (pellagra), vitamin E, essential amino
      acids, and zinc
7. **Drugs and toxins**
   Anticonvulsants: phenytoin, carbamazepine, barbiturates
   Chemotherapeutic agents: 5-fluorouracil, cytosine arabinoside
   Heavy metals: thallium, lead, organic mercury
   Alcohol (may be indirectly due to malnutrition)
   Toluene
8. **Developmental abnormalities**
   Chiari malformations
   Dandy-Walker syndrome
   Cerebellar aplasia
   Basilar impression
9. **Trauma**
   Postconcussion
   Hematoma or contusion

12. What are some of the major inherited cerebellar diseases?

The classification of inherited cerebellar diseases is confusing and nonuniform. These diseases usually cause progressive degeneration and atrophy of the cerebellum. They are also known as hereditary ataxias because their common major neurologic sign is ataxia, or clumsiness and incoordination of movement. Inherited diseases can be classified according to time of onset, inheritance pattern, known or unknown etiology, and clinical features.The more common ones are listed below:

1. **Friedreich's ataxia.** This autosomal recessive disorder is listed separately because it is relatively common, with a prevalence of about 1 in 100,000.
2. **Syndromes associated with defective DNA repair** (autosomal recessive)
   Ataxia-telangiectasia (low IgA and IgE levels)
   Xeroderma pigmentosum

3. **Mitochondrial encephalopathies**
   Leigh's disease
   Kearns-Sayre syndrome
4. **Syndromes of known metabolic etiology**
   Abetalipoproteinemia or hypobetalipoproteinemia (deficient apolipoprotein B)
   Wilson's disease (low or absent copper ceruloplasmin)
   Refsum's disease (deficient phytanic acid hydroxylase)
   Aminoacidurias (Hartnup disease)
   Disorders of pyruvate and lactate metabolism (metabolic acidosis)
   Urea cycle enzyme defects (hyperammonemia)
   Biotinase deficiency (metabolic acidosis)
   Hexosaminidase deficiency
   Leukodystrophies (metachromatic, Krabbe's)
   Ceroid lipofuscinosis
   Niemann-Pick disease
5. **Other inherited syndromes**
   Autosomal dominant diseases
      Olivopontocerebellar atrophy (ataxia, ophthalmoplegia, optic atrophy)
      Spinocerebellar ataxia (ataxia, dysarthria, sensory loss)
      Machado-Joseph disease (variable cerebellar, extrapyramidal, and pyramidal
      involvement)
   Autosomal recessive diseases
      Ramsay-Hunt syndrome (ataxia and myoclonus)
      Behr's syndrome (ataxia, optic atrophy, mental retardation)
   X-linked spinocerebellar ataxia (rare)

13. Summarize the current classification of autosomal dominant spinocerebellar ataxias (SCAs).

Type 1 (SCA1)	CAG repeat in ataxin-1 gene on chromosome 6p
Type 2 (SCA2)	CAG repeat in ataxin-2 gene on chromosome 12q
Type 3 (SCA3)	CAG repeat in ataxin-3 gene on chromosome 14q; also known as Machado-Joseph disease (MJD)
Type 4 (SCA4)	Locus on chromosome 16q
Type 5 (SCA5)	Locus on chromosome 11p
Type 6 (SCA6)	CAG repeat in human alpha-1a calcium channel subunit gene on chromosome 19p
Type 7 (SCA7)	CAG repeat in ataxin-7 gene on chromosome 3q
Type 8 (SCA8)	CTG repeat on chromosome 13q
Type 9 (SCA9)	Locus not yet characterized
Type 10 (SCA10)	Locus on chromosome 22q
Type 11 (SCA11)	Locus on chromosome 15q
Type 12 (SCA12)	CAG repeat on chromosome 5q
Type 13 (SCA13)	Locus on chromosome 19q
Type 14 (SCA14)	Locus on chromosome 19q

14. Describe the common clinical features of autosomal dominant SCAs.

Dominant SCA syndromes have many overlapping signs that are often difficult to distinguish on clinical grounds. Most of the disorders affect the cerebellum and its pathways, resulting in progressive deterioration of cerebellar function manifested by increasing unsteadiness of gait, incoordination of lilmb movements, and dysarthria.

15. What are the clinical features of Friedreich's ataxia?

Friedreich's ataxia is an autosomal recessive disease affecting the cerebellum, spinal cord, peripheral nerve, and heart. Carbohydrate metabolism is also altered. It has an early onset, before age 20, and a rapidly progressive course. The initial presentation is frequently gait ataxia, but arm ataxia also may be significant. Scoliosis and dysarthria are common. Loss of all tendon reflexes, loss of vibration and position sense, and extensor plantar responses are typical. Other associated features include muscle weakness and atrophy, hypertrophic cardiomyopathy, pes cavus, abnormal ocular motility, diabetes, and deafness. Most patients are confined to a wheelchair by early adulthood. The etiology of Friedreich's ataxia is unknown, but recently the genetic defect was localized to an expanded GAA triplet repeat on chromosome 9. There is presently no effective treatment. Symptomatic treatment of scoliosis by orthopedic intervention and cardiac abnormalities by appropriate medication may prolong survival.

Campuzano V, Montermini L, Molto MD, et al: Friedreich's ataxia: Autosomal recessive disease caused by an intronic GAA triplet repeat expansion. Science 271:1423–1425, 1996.

16. What is the difference in the diagnosis of posterior fossa neoplasm in children vs. adults?

Posterior fossa neoplasms account for approximately 50% of the total number of neoplasms in children. The four major types are cerebellar astrocytoma, medulloblastoma (primitive neuroectodermal tumor), ependymoma of the fourth ventricle, and brainstem glioma. In adults, posterior fossa neoplasms are much rarer. They consist mainly of hemangioblastoma, metastatic tumor, acoustic neuroma (schwannoma), and meningioma.

Albright L: Posterior fossa tumors. Neurosurg Clin North Am 3:881–891, 1992.

17. Describe the presentations of cerebellar infarction or hemorrhage. What are the management concerns?

The presentations of cerebellar infarction and hemorrhage may be indistinguishable. Abrupt onset of headache, vomiting, vertigo, and ataxia, especially in a hypertensive patient, should be considered a neurologic emergency, and vascular etiology should be ruled out. A high index of suspicion may lead to the proper diagnosis with CT or MRI scanning. Expanding hematoma or edema may rapidly lead to brainstem compression and cerebellar herniation accompanied by signs such as hemiparesis, pontine gaze abnormalities, depressed consciousness, irregular breathing, or coma. Prompt surgical evacuation of the hematoma or removal of necrotic cerebellar tissue may be life-saving.

Amarenco P: The spectrum of cerebellar infarctions. Neurology 41:973–979, 1991.

18. What are the clinical features and causes of the cerebellopontine angle syndrome?

Lesions at the space between the cerebellum and the pons often present by compressing and interfering with the functions of the nearby cranial nerves, namely V, VII, and VIII. Involvement of cranial nerve V is often detected by depression or absence of the ipsilateral corneal reflex. Later other sensory and motor functions may be affected, as manifested by numbness of the face and weakness of the mastication muscles. Involvement of cranial nerve VII may produce facial myokymia (involuntary contraction of the facial musculature) or a lower motor neuron paralysis of the ipsilateral face. Hearing loss, tinnitus, and vertigo are features of damage to cranial nerve VIII. As the lesion enlarges, distortion of the brainstem may occur, producing bilateral long-tract signs or obstruction of the aqueduct to cause hydrocephalus and symptoms of increased intracranial pressure. Compression of the cerebellar hemisphere adjacent to the cerebellopontine angle presents with ipsilateral limb ataxia and intention tremor or nystagmus.

19. What is an acoustic neuroma?

The acoustic neuroma (or schwannoma) is the most common extraaxial lesion that causes the cerebellopontine angle syndrome. It originates from schwann cells in the sheath of cranial nerve VIII, close to the attachment of the nerve to the brainstem. It can be distinguished from other lesions of the cerebellopontine angle by the fact that it involves cranial nerve VIII early; the functions of cranial nerve VII are usually resistant to this tumor and are not affected until much later. The early involvement of cranial nerve VII is sufficient cause to consider the possibility of other lesions, such as meningioma, epidermoidoma, craniopharyngioma, glomus jugulare tumor, and aneurysm of the basilar artery. Intraaxial masses of the brainstem and cerebellum also may cause the syndrome if they are sufficiently large and extend into the cerebellopontine space.

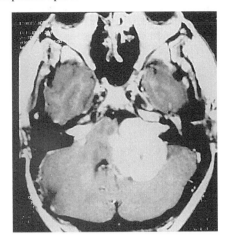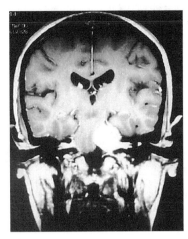

Gadolinium-enhanced T1-weighted MRIs show bilateral acoustic neuromas (especially large on the left) in a patient with neurofibromatosis.

20. What are the clinical features of the cerebellar herniation syndromes?

Mass lesions in the cerebellum, particularly neoplasms and hematomas, often initially present as nonspecific symptoms such as headache. As the lesions enlarge, the increased pressure causes the cerebellum to herniate in one of two directions, downward or upward.

Downward herniation of the cerebellum is most common. Increased pressure in the posterior fossa pushes the cerebellar tonsils downward through the foramen magnum to compress the medulla. It is characterized by progressive vomiting, stiff neck, skew deviation of the eyes, coma, ataxic breathing, apnea, and death. There are no pupillary changes until the patient is terminal. This condition is fatal if not anticipated and prevented early.

Upward herniation occurs when the cerebellar mass pushes the cerebellum and upper brainstem through the tentorial opening. The clinical features are caused by progressive compression of the pons and midbrain. The patient is usually obtunded or comatose with small pupils (reactive at first) or anisocoria. Oculocephalic and oculovestibular responses are abnormal. Hemiparesis may progress to quadriparesis and decorticate posturing. Abnormal breathing (central hyperventilation or apneustic breathing) can be observed.

21. What is the treatment for cerebellar herniation?

Osmotic agents and hyperventilation may provide temporary relief, but definitive treatment for cerebellar herniations consists of surgical decompression and removal of the mass, if possible.

22. What is paraneoplastic cerebellar degeneration?

Paraneoplastic cerebellar degeneration (PCD) is the most common remote effect of neoplasm affecting the brain. It is associated with lung (especially small cell), ovarian, and breast neoplasms and Hodgkin's disease. Cerebellar signs usually begin with gait ataxia, developing over a few weeks to months. The symptoms may progress rapidly to severe and symmetric truncal and limb ataxia with dysarthria and nystagmus. Thus, when an adult develops a rapidly progressing and symmetric cerebellar syndrome, PCD should be promptly considered. Pathologically, severe loss of Purkinje cells affects all parts of the cerebellum. Early neuroimaging studies are typically normal, but later studies show signs of progressive cerebellar atrophy. Cerebellar symptoms may improve in some patients when the causative neoplasms are removed, but they are not improved by plasmapheresis.

23. What is the cause of PCD?

An autoimmune process may be the cause of PCD, and antibodies to cerebellar Purkinje cells are observed in patients' sera and spinal fluid. The two main antibodies may be used as markers for patients with PCD. The Yo antibodies (or anti-Purkinje cell cytoplasmic antibodies) are found in gynecologic cancer patients with PCD, whereas the Hu antibodies (antineuronal nuclear antibodies) are present in some patients with small-cell lung cancer with PCD. The pathogenic basis of these antibodies is still uncertain.

Lai EC: Paraneoplastic syndromes. In Rolak LA, Harati Y (eds): Neuroimmunology for the Clinician. Boston, Butterworth-Heinemann, 1997.

BIBLIOGRAPHY

1. Adams RD, Victor M, Ropper AH: Principles of Neurology, 6th ed. New York, McGraw-Hill, 1997.
2. Kandel ER, Schwartz JH, Jessell TM: Principles of Neural Science, 3rd ed. New York, Elsevier, 1991.
3. Rolak LA, Harati Y: Neuroimmunology for the Clinician. Boston, Butterworth-Heinemann, 1997.
Websites
www.anatomy.wisc.edu
www.icondata.com/health/pedbase/files/spinocer.htm
www.ataxia.org

11. BASAL GANGLIA AND MOVEMENT DISORDERS

Philip A. Hanna, M.D., Francisco Cardoso, M.D., and Joseph Jankovic, M.D.

ANATOMY AND PHYSIOLOGY

1. What are the components of the basal ganglia?

The basal ganglia are a group of nuclei situated in the deep part of the cerebrum and upper part of the brainstem. Included among these nuclei are the striatum, which is composed of the caudate, putamen, and ventral striatum; the pallidum, which is composed of the internal (medial) and external (lateral) parts of the globus pallidus (GP); the subthalamic nucleus (STN); and the substantia nigra (SN), with the pars compacta (SNc) and pars reticulata (SNr). The putamen and GP are combined to form the lenticular (or lentiform) nucleus because of their lenslike appearance. These interrelated structures are primarily responsible for control of motor functions.

Obeso JA, et al: Pathophysiology of the basal ganglia in Parkinson's disease. Trends Neurosci 23(10 Suppl):S8–S19, 2000.

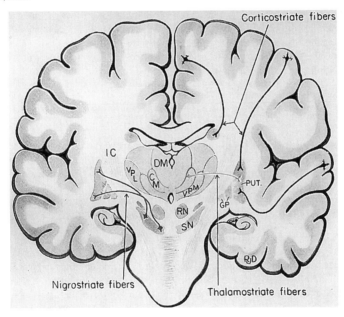

The basal ganglia and thalamus. PUT = putamen, GP = globus pallidus, SN = substantia nigra, RN = red nucleus, IC = internal capsule, VPL = ventral posterior lateral nucleus, VPM = ventral posterior medial nucleus, CM = centromedian nucleus, DM = dorsomedian nucleus.

2. How are the basal ganglia organized?

There are three levels of organization within the basal ganglia. The first level consists of the two major striatal outputs: (1) the indirect pathway to the external segment of the GP (GPe) and (2) the direct pathway to the SNr and internal segment of the GP (GPi). The second level of organization consists of pathways from the cerebral cortex (sublaminae of layer V) to the patch (striosome) and matrix compartments of the striatum (which are organized in a mosaic pattern). The third level of organization is related to the topography of cortical projections to other regions of the striatum.

Gerfen CR:Molecular effects of dopamine on striatal-projection pathways. Trends Neurosci 23(10 Suppl):S64–S70, 2000.

3. How can the matrix and patch compartments of the striatum be distinguished?

These two subpopulations of striatal medium spiny neurons have distinct neurochemical properties as well as distinct afferents and efferents. Neurochemically, the patches are enriched in opiate receptors and display weak acetylcholinesterase staining. The limbic-related allocortex projects predominantly to the patches. The output from the patches is directed at cholinergic neurons mainly situated in the ventral GP and dopaminergic neurons in the SNc. On the other hand, the neurons of the matrix mainly receive fibers from the neocortical areas, such as sensorimotor cortex, which project chiefly to the GABAergic neurons of the SNr and GPe.

In summary, the patches are more related to limbic and nonspecific functions, and the matrix is involved with more specific, sensorimotor tasks. However, these distinctions are not absolute because of transitional areas in which the above features overlap.

Canales JJ, Graybiel AM: A measure of striatal function predicts motor stereotypy. Nat Neurosci 3:377–383, 2000.

4. What are the neurotransmitters of the two major striatal output pathways?

The majority of the neurons in the striatum are GABAergic medium spiny cells that project to the GPe and SNr. Approximately 50% of these cells also contain substance P and dynorphin and project to the SNr and GPi. The other half of the neurons express enkephalin and project their axons to the GPe. These pathways are respectively called striatonigral or direct and striatopallidal or indirect pathways.

Chase TN, Oh JD: Striatal dopamine- and glutamate-mediated dysregulation in experimental parkinsonism. Trends Neurosci 12(10 Suppl):S86–S91, 2000.

Kawaguchi Y, et al: Striatal interneurons: Chemical, physiological, and morphological characterization. Trends Neurosci 18:527, 1995.

5. What is the role of the STN in the neurophysiology of the basal ganglia?

The STN receives inhibitory input from the striatopallidal (indirect) pathway. The STN has strong excitatory (glutaminergic) projections to the GPi/SNr, which in turn provide inhibitory projections (GABAergic) to the ventral thalamic nuclei.

Levy R, et al: Re-evaluation of the functional anatomy of the basal ganglia in normal and parkinsonian states. Neuroscience 76:335, 1997.

6. What is the source of the major output of the basal ganglia?

The GABAergic neurons of the SNr and the GPi, which may be considered as a single neuronal complex, innervate the mediodorsal and ventral tier thalamic nuclei (which provide feedback to the frontal cortex), the intralaminar thalamic nuclei (which provide feedback to the striatum), the superior colliculus (important in the control of the ocular movements), and the pedunculopontine nucleus (seemingly involved in the maintenance of posture).

7. What is the neurotransmitter of the nigrostriatal system?

The nigrostriatal system is composed of the dopaminergic neurons in the SNc, which project to the medium spiny neurons of the striatum.

8. How many types of dopamine receptors have been identified?

Five dopamine receptors, D1–D5, have now been pharmacologically characterized and cloned. The activation of D1 and D5 receptors increases the intracellular level of cyclic adenosine monophosphate (cAMP); these receptors have been mapped, respectively, to chromosomes 5 and 4. The D1 receptor is localized chiefly in the caudate, putamen, nucleus accumbens, and olfactory tubercle, whereas the D5 receptor is predominantly expressed in the hippocampus and hypothalamus. The D2 and D4 receptors have been linked to chromosome 11, and the gene for the D3 receptor has been identified on chromosome 3. The D2 receptor, expressed in two isoforms (D2S and D2L), decreases the intracellular level of cAMP and has the same distribution as the D1 receptor. The D3 receptor, which apparently also acts by decreasing the cAMP level, has been identified in the olfactory tubercle, hypothalamus, and nucleus accumbens. A similar mechanism of action has been proposed for the D4 receptor, found in the frontal cortex, medulla, and midbrain.

The functional significance of this multitude of receptors is not clearly understood. The role of the D1 and D2 receptors in the motor systems has been studied more extensively; activation of the D1 receptors appears to be important in mediating dystonic movements, whereas activation of the D2 receptors may result in chorea. Clozapine, a specific blocker for the D4 receptor, is an effective dibenzodiazepine antipsychotic agent. Akathisia, acute dystonic reaction and tardive dyskinesia have been reported with clozapine, which appears also to have D2-blocking activity.

Dave M: Clozapine-related tardive dyskinesia. Biol Psychiatry 35:886, 1994.
Khan ZU, et al: Dopamine D5 receptors of rat and human brain. Neuroscience 100:689–699, 2000.

9. How are the D1 and D2 dopamine receptors expressed in the striatum?

The D1 dopamine receptor is predominantly expressed on the striatonigral neurons, whereas the D2 receptors are primarily found on the striatopallidal neurons. Evidence suggests that in the striatum the D1 and D2 receptors have an excitatory and inhibitory action, respectively.

PARKINSONISM

10. What are the neurophysiologic changes in the basal ganglia in Parkinson's disease (PD)?

Neuronal loss in the SNc with consequent dopamine depletion in the striatum is the neuro-chemical-pathologic hallmark of PD. This dopaminergic deafferentation produces an imbalance in the striatal activity, with hypoactivity of the striatonigral pathway and hyperactivity of striatopallidal pathways. This imbalance results in decreased inhibition (disinhibition) of the STN and increased activity of the GPi/SNr neurons, causing increased inhibition of the thalamic ventral tier nuclei. Because these thalamic nuclei are responsible for the activation of the cortical areas involved in the generation of movements, the final effect of dopamine deficiency is poverty or slowness of movements (hypokinesia). In fact, in monkeys with parkinsonism induced by 1-methyl-4-phenyl-1,2,3,6-tetrahydropyridine (MPTP), akinesia was reversed by subthalamotomy.

Braak H, Braak E: Pathoanatomy of Parkinson's disease. J Neurol 247(Suppl 2):II3–II10, 2000.

11. What are the cardinal symptoms and signs of parkinsonism?

Tremor at rest is one of the most typical signs of parkinsonism. It is characterized by an oscillatory pronation-supination at a 3–5 Hz frequency. In addition to the hands, where it assumes an appearance of pill rolling, this type of tremor is commonly observed in the facial musculature (lips and chin) as well as in the legs. Head tremor, however, is rare in parkinsonism, and its presence should suggest the diagnosis of essential tremor (ET).

The term **bradykinesia** is used to describe slowness of movements that often causes difficulties for the patients in getting dressed, feeding, and maintaining personal hygiene. Bradykinesia is evident when a patient performs rapid alternating movements, such as pronation and supination of the forearms.

Rigidity, often associated with the cogwheel phenomenon, is another hallmark of parkinsonism. Impairment of the postural reflexes is responsible for the falls that are frequently experienced by parkinsonian patients. Parkinsonian gait often reflects a combination of bradykinesia, rigidity, and postural instability.

In addition to the above features, there are other important symptoms and signs in parkinsonism. Approximately 50% of patients with PD experience pain, which may be their presenting symptom. Micrographia, or small-sized handwriting, is another frequent and precocious sign of PD. The co-existence of rigidity and bradykinesia in the facial musculature accounts for decreased blinking rate and facial expression (hypomimia or mask facies). Seborrhea, weight loss, and various signs of autonomic dysfunction are also often found in patients with PD. Involvement of the upper and lower gastrointestinal tract in PD is evidenced respectively by dysphagia and constipation.

The chronology of appearance and the pattern of combination of clinical features depend on the cause of the parkinsonism. For example, in progressive supranuclear palsy (PSP), postural reflex impairment occurs early in the course of the disease, whereas prominent rest tremor at onset suggests the diagnosis of PD.

Gelb DJ, Oliver E, Gilman S: Diagnostic criteria for Parkinson's disease. Arch Neurol 56:33–39, 1999.

12. What are the most common causes of parkinsonism?

In a highly selected population, such as that attending a movement disorders clinic, PD is responsible for 77.7% of the cases of parkinsonism. The other most frequent causes are parkinsonism-plus syndrome (12.2%), secondary parkinsonism (8.2%), and heredodegenerative parkinsonism (0.6%).

Riley DE: Secondary parkinsonism. In Jankovic J, Tolosa E: Parkinson's disease and movement disorders. Baltimore, Williams & Wilkins, 1999.

Causes of Parkinsonism

I. Idiopathic parkinsonism
    Parkinson's disease (PD)
      Sporadic form
      Familial form

II. Secondary parkinsonism
    Drug-induced
      Dopamine receptor blockers (neuroleptics, including antiemetics such as metoclopramide)
      Dopamine depleters (reserpine, tetrabenazine)
      Calcium channel blockers (flunarizine, cinnarizine, diltiazem)
      Lithium
      Methyldopa
    Hemiatrophy-hemiparkinsonism
    Hydrocephalus
      Normal pressure hydrocephalus
      Noncommunicating hydrocephalus
    Hypoxia
    Infectious diseases
      AIDS   Intracytoplasmic hyaline inclusion disease
      Creutzfeldt-Jakob disease   Postencephalitic parkinsonism
      Fungus   Subacute sclerosing panencephalitis
    Metabolic
      Acquired hepatocerebral degeneration (chronic liver insufficiency)
      Hypocalcemic parkinsonism
    Paraneoplastic parkinsonism
    Syringomesencephalia
    Toxin
      Carbon disulfide   Ethanol
      Carbon monoxide   Manganese
      Cyanide   Methanol
      Disulfiram   1-Methyl-4-phenyl-1,2,3,6-tetrahydropyridine (MPTP)
    Trauma
    Tumor
    Vascular
      Multiinfarcts
      Binswanger's disease
      Lower body parkinsonism

(Table continued on following page.)

Causes of Parkinsonism (Continued)

III. **Parkinsonism-plus syndromes**
   Alzheimer's disease-parkinsonism
   Cortical basal ganglionic degeneration (CBGD)
   Diffuse Lewy body disease
   Multiple system atrophy (MSA)
     Shy-Drager syndrome
     Sporadic olivopontocerebellar atrophy (OPCA)
     Striatonigral degeneration
   Parkinsonism-dementia-amyotrophic lateral sclerosis
   Progressive pallidal atrophy
   Progressive supranuclear palsy (PSP)

IV. **Heredodegenerative diseases**

Ceroid-lipofuscinosis	X-linked dystonia-parkinsonism
Gerstmann-Strausler-Scheinker disease	Disinhibition–dementia–parkinsonism–
Familial OPCA	dementia complex
Hallervorden-Spatz disease	Autosomal dominant Lewy body disease
Huntington's disease	Hereditary ceruloplasmin deficiency
Levodopa-responsiveness (fluctuating) dystonia	Familial progressive subcortical gliosis
Machado-Joseph disease (Azorean heredoataxia)	Familial basal ganglia calcification
Mitochondrial cytopathies with striatal necrosis	Familial parkinsonism with peripheral
Neuroacanthocytosis	neuropathy
Thalamic dementia syndrome	Parkinsonian–pyramidal syndrome
Wilson's disease	

13. What causes PD?

Although PD was first described in 1817, its cause is still unknown. The recognition that MPTP can produce in humans and nonhuman primates a parkinsonian syndrome very similar to PD led to the hypothesis that an MPTP-like substance in the environment could cause PD. This theory was strengthened by the finding that people living in rural areas and exposed to pesticides that are structurally related to MPTP, such as paraquat, had a relatively high risk for developing PD. MPTP exerts its neurotoxic action by inhibiting complex I of the respiratory chain of the inner mitochondrial membrane. This group of enzymes has been reported to be impaired in patients with PD. Despite these striking similarities, there are definite differences between MPTP-induced parkinsonism (MPTP-P) and PD. Rest tremor is less frequently found in humans with MPTP-P and virtually absent in monkeys exposed to MPTP. PD is a progressive disease, but there is no evidence of progression of MPTP-P. Typical Lewy bodies (LB) found in the brains of patients with PD have not been demonstrated in MPTP-P.

One of the theories about the cause of PD is that a defective antioxidant system leads to increased formation of highly reactive and toxic free-oxygen radicals (oxidative stress). Indeed, the findings of increased nigral basal lipid peroxidation, reduced glutathione levels, increased total iron, and decreased ferritin in the SN suggest increased generation of free radicals. Despite this evidence, the precise role of oxidative mechanisms in the pathogenesis of PD remains to be established.

A growing body of evidence supports the notion that genetic factors play an important role in the etiology of PD. Families with an autosomal dominant transmission of otherwise typical PD have been described, as have monozygotic twins concordant for the disease. Recently, a mutation in the alpha-synuclein gene (long arm of chromosome 4) was identified in a large Italian kindred and in three unrelated Greek families with autosomal-dominant inheritance, although this mutation does not appear to play a major role in familial PD (Scott et al). Autosomal recessive juvenile parkinsonism (AR-JP) maps to the long arm of chromosome 6 (6q25.2–q27), called the "parkin gene," in Japanese and European kindreds (in which various mutations are implicated). Investigators recently reported an Italian family with apparent autosomal dominant transmission with compound deletions in the parkin gene. In addition, a susceptibility locus for PD was mapped to chromosome 2 by other investigators.

The possibility of involvement of maternal transmission has been raised by several reports of mutations of mitochondrial DNA in the SN. Other areas of the brain of patients with PD, such as the striatum, and the SN of patients with multiple system atrophy (MSA), do not display this abnormality.

The etiology of PD is still speculative, but a combination of environmental factors may be associated with a genetic predisposition.

Abbas N, et al: A susceptibility locus for Parkinson's disease maps to chromosome 2p13. Nat Genet 18:262–265, 1998.

Kuopio AM, et al: Environmental risk factors in Parkinson's disease. Mov Disord 14:928–939, 1999.

Polymeropoulos MH, et al: Mutation in the alpha-synuclein gene identified in families with Parkinson's disease. Science 276:2045, 1997.

Scott WK, et al: The alpha-synuclein gene is not a major risk factor in familial Parkinson disease. Neurogenetics 2(3):191–192, 1999.

14. What are the clinical and pathologic hallmarks of PD?

Patients with PD may have several combinations of parkinsonian symptoms. Typically, the onset is insidious in the sixth decade of life, and the symptoms usually begin unilaterally or predominate on one side of the body. It is possible to recognize two clinical types of PD: a **tremor-dominant** form with earlier age of onset, slower progression, and relatively preserved cognition and a **postural instability and gait difficulty** (PIGD) form with more bradykinesia, more rapid progression, and dementia. Furthermore, essential tremor is more likely to coexist in the tremor-dominant form. Pathologically, there is loss of dopaminergic neurons in the SNc, and the surviving neurons contain LB. Although to a lesser degree than the SNc, other pigmented nuclei of the brainstem, such as the locus ceruleus and tegmental ventral area, are also involved by a similar process. A recent clinicopathologic study showed that the presence of a resting tremor is more likely to be associated with LB at autopsy.

Jankovic J, et al: Variable expression of Parkinson's disease: A base-line analysis of the DATATOP cohort. Neurology 40:1529, 1990.

Jankovic J, et al: Tremor and longevity in relatives of patients with Parkinson's disease, essential tremor and control subjects. Neurology 45:645, 1995.

15. How specific is the clinical diagnosis of PD?

Two clinicopathologic studies (Rajput et al., 1991; Hughes et al., 1992a) addressed this question. In both series, 24% of the patients with the clinical diagnosis of PD were found to have another diagnosis at necropsy. These studies show that patients with typical symptoms may have variable pathologic findings; conversely, typical pathologic findings can be expressed by dissimilar signs. Findings of asymmetric onset, no evidence for other causes of parkinsonism, and no atypical features of PD increased the specificity of the clinical diagnosis in the London series to 92%, but 32% of the PD cases did not satisfy these criteria, indicating a low sensitivity.

Hughes AJ, et al: Diagnosis of idiopathic Parkinson's disease: A clinico-pathological study of 100 cases. J Neurol Neurosurg Psychiatry 55:181, 1992a.

Hughes AJ, et al: What features improve the accuracy of clinical diagnosis in Parkinson's disease: A clinicopathologic study. Neurology 42:1142, 1992b.

Jankovic J, et al: The evolution of diagnosis in early Parkinson disease. Parkinson Study Group. Arch Neurol 57(3):369–372, 2000.

16. Do any tests support an antemortem diagnosis of PD?

Currently, no biologic marker allows an in vivo diagnosis of PD. However, some tests may be helpful in supporting the diagnosis of PD. The values of homovanillic acid, a metabolite of dopamine, in the cerebrospinal fluid (CSF) are usually low, but computed tomography (CT) scans and magnetic resonance imaging (MRI) of the head are usually normal.

Positron emission tomography (PET) scanning with 18F-fluorodopa, a radioactive isomer of levodopa, provides an index of the nigrostriatal integrity. PD is associated with reduction of

18F-fluorodopa uptake, particularly in the putamen. Dopamine D2 receptor ligands, such as raclopride and spiperone, can be imaged with PET to demonstrate increased density of these receptors in patients with PD not exposed to dopaminergic drugs. This receptor upregulation probably reflects denervation hypersensitivity secondary to the loss of nigrostriatal axons. Despite its usefulness, PET scanning is a cumbersome and expensive method of assessing the integrity of striatal dopaminergic terminals. It is not a practical diagnostic test for PD.

Single-photon emission tomography (SPECT) may be more practical and less expensive than PET, but its spatial resolution is limited. Preliminary studies using IBZM, a ligand of D2 receptors, and iodine-123-labeled RTI-55 to image presynaptic dopamine uptake sites suggest that eventually SPECT may be useful for early diagnosis of PD. The presynaptic dopamine uptake sites are impaired in early PD as a result of the loss of dopaminergic terminals; therefore, the RTI SPECT could be helpful in the early detection of PD. Furthermore, SPECT imaging of presynaptic vesicles with C-11 dihydrotetrabenazine may assist in differentiating PD from atypical parkinsonism.

Brooks DJ: Morphological and functional imaging studies in the diagnosis and progression of Parkinson's disease. J Neurol 247(Suppl 2):II11–II18, 2000.

Gilman S, et al: Decreased striatal monoaminergic terminals in olivopontocerebellar atrophy and multiple system atrophy demonstrated with positron emission tomography. Ann Neurol 40:885, 1996.

Staffen W, et al: Measuring the progression of idiopathic Parkinson's disease with [123I] beta-CIT SPECT. Neural Transm 107:543–552, 2000.

17. What is the rationale for using deprenyl in PD?

Deprenyl is an inhibitor of the enzyme monoamine oxidase B (MAOB). The conversion of MPTP to MPP+, the active substance that produces parkinsonism, is catalyzed by MAOB. In nonhuman primates inhibitors of MAOB prevent the formation of MPP+ and so prevent the development of MPTP-P. If PD is caused by an MPTP-like substance, antioxidant therapy may be a rational protective treatment. Yet recent studies have demonstrated that deprenyl can partially "rescue" neurons even after MPTP is converted to MPP+; thus, deprenyl may provide benefit through means other than MAO inhibition. Three double-blind studies assessed the role of deprenyl in the treatment of PD and showed that MAOB inhibitors delayed the need for levodopa (although this initial benefit is not sustained). However, the interpretation of this result is still disputed, and some authors argue that instead of changing the rate of neurodegeneration, deprenyl exerts a minimal symptomatic effect. For example, deprenyl is metabolized to L-methamphetamine and L-amphetamine and may have a mild CNS stimulatory effect. Because deprenyl may provide a neuroprotective effect and is well tolerated by most patients, it is recommended during early therapy of PD. Patients are usually started on one 5-mg tablet after breakfast in the first week and one tablet after breakfast and lunch thereafter. The most common untoward effects of the 10-mg dose are headache and nausea. Dosages higher than 10 mg/day should be avoided because both MAOA and B may be inhibited. Inhibition of MAOA may be associated with cardiovascular side effects.

Parkinson Study Group: Effects of tocopherol and deprenyl on the progression of disability in early Parkinson's disease. N Engl J Med 328:176, 1993.

Parkinson Study Group: Impact of deprenyl and tocopherol treatment on Parkinson's disease in DATATOP patients not requiring levodopa. Ann Neurol 39:29, 1996.

Magyar K, Haberle D: Neuroprotective and neuronal rescue effects of selegiline: Review. Neurobiology 7(2):175–190, 1999.

18. What is the role of anticholinergic drugs and amantadine in the treatment of PD?

In the early stages of PD, anticholinergic drugs, combined with deprenyl, may be used as the primary treatment. With progression of disease, patients require the addition of levodopa. Even in this circumstance, some patients still benefit from using anticholinergics and amantadine. Tremor is occasionally resistant to dopaminergic therapy and may be better controlled with the use of levodopa in association with ancillary medications. In contrast to the anticholinergics, amantadine, a drug that has mild anticholinergic effects and increases the release of dopamine, also improves rigidity and bradykinesia. Furthermore, recent studies have revealed the utility of amantadine in reducing levodopa-induced dyskinesias.

The anticholinergic medications must be used cautiously because, in addition to causing dryness of the mouth and bladder retention, they may produce disorientation, confusion, and memory loss, particularly in the elderly. Amantadine in some patients also may cause cognitive side effects as well as livedo reticularis, ankle swelling, and worsening of congestive heart failure.

Jankovic J, Marsden CD: Therapeutic strategies in Parkinson's disease. In Jankovic J, Tolosa E (eds): Parkinson's Disease and Movement Disorders, 3rd ed. Baltimore, William & Wilkins, 1998.

Luginger E, et al: Beneficial effects of amantadine on L-dopa–induced dyskinesias in Parkinson's diseaes. Mov Disord 15:873–878, 2000.

19. When should levodopa therapy be started in the treatment of PD?

The mainstay in the treatment of PD is the replacement of dopamine. This therapy was introduced in the 1960s. Instead of using dopamine, which does not cross the blood-brain barrier, the current approach consists of combining levodopa and carbidopa. Levodopa is transformed into dopamine, and carbidopa is a peripheral inhibitor of the enzyme dopa-decarboxylase. The inhibition of this enzyme in the periphery, but not in the brain, decreases substantially the required levodopa dosage and the occurrence of gastrointestinal side effects (nausea and vomiting). In Europe and other countries, benseraside is available as an inhibitor of dopa-decarboxylase.

The controversy about the best timing for introducing levodopa is not yet settled. One argument for early use is that levodopa is the most effective treatment for PD; therefore, there is no reason to deprive patients of its benefits. The proponents of early levodopa therapy also argue that the occurrence of central side effects of levodopa (e.g., dyskinesias and clinical fluctuations) are related to progression of the disease and not to the duration or cumulative dosage of levodopa. Conversely, those who prefer postponing the use of levodopa argue that levodopa is neurotoxic and contributes directly to the development of complications such as the wearing-off effect and dyskinesia.

A rational strategy is to start levodopa when the parkinsonian symptoms begin to impair activities of daily living or to interfere with social and occupational functioning. Sinemet CR (a continuous-release preparation) may be the preferred starting formulation because constant activation of receptors provides a more predictable and longer response than the intermittent dopaminergic input of regular Sinemet. A typical starting dose is Sinemet CR 25/100 2 or 3 times/day. Maintenance doses of 200–600 mg/day of levodopa may be needed in patients with moderately advanced Parkinson's disease. Other formulations include Sinemet 10/100, Sinemet 25/250, and Sinemet CR 50/200. The dosage of carbidopa should be kept at less than 150 mg/day because it may penetrate the blood-brain barrier and inhibit central dopa-decarboxylase at higher levels. Thus, use of the 25/250 tablets may be preferred over the 25/100 tablets if sufficiently high levodopa doses are needed.

Agid Y: Levodopa: Is toxicity a myth? Neurology 50:858–863, 1998.

Camp DM, Loeffler DA, LeWitt PA: L-Dopa does not enhance hydroxyl radical formation in the nigrostriatal dopamine system of rats with a unilateral 6-hydroxydopamine lesion. J Neurochem 74:1229–1240, 2000.

Shulman LM: Levodopa toxicity in Parkinson disease: Reality or myth? Reality—practice patterns should change. Arch Neurol 57(3):406–407; discussion, 410, 2000.

20. What are the most common peripheral side effects of levodopa therapy? How are they managed?

Nausea and vomiting are common side effects in the beginning of the use of levodopa. Most of the patients overcome this difficulty by taking the medication after meals. In some patients extra amounts of carbidopa (typically, one 25-mg tablet with each dose of Sinemet) may be necessary. A small proportion of patients have nausea and vomiting despite these measures. Treatment of the GI side effects should not include dopamine blockers, such as metoclopramide, because they may cause worsening of PD. Diphenidol and cyclizine are useful alternatives.

The most common cardiovascular side effect is orthostatic hypotension. The management of this complication involves adding salt to the diet, wearing elastic stockings, and using medications such as fluodrocortisone, indomethacin, or midodrine.

Jankovic J, et al: Neurogenic orthostatic hypotension: A double-blind placebo controlled study with midodrine. Am J Med 95:38, 1993.

21. What clinical fluctuations are recognized in PD?

Although the most dramatic fluctuations in patients with PD are related to levodopa therapy, some who have not been previously treated with dopaminergic drugs exhibit fluctuations in severity of their symptoms and signs. Fluctuations are not exclusively motor phenomena. Mood and autonomic functions also fluctuate. For example, some patients display depression when they are "off" and euphoria when they are "on." Fatigue and stress usually make these symptoms more prominent. The most dramatic example of spontaneous fluctuations is paradoxical dyskinesia: under extreme stress, patients completely immobilized by parkinsonism are suddenly able to stand up and run.

Levodopa-induced fluctuations are the most important motor fluctuations because of their potential to cause significant disability. The most common type of clinical fluctuation is the shortening of the response to levodopa (wearing-off phenomenon); as a consequence, anti-parkinsonian benefits ("on" period) are lost after 2–3 hours (or even less) and the parkinsonian symptoms reemerge ("off" period). Occasionally, the action of levodopa ends suddenly, the so-called "on-off" effect. Motor fluctuations are probably caused by a loss of dopaminergic terminals in the striatum, with consequent impairment of the brain's ability to buffer the shifts in levodopa availability. Among the most challenging problems in the treatment of PD are motor blocks, or freezing, which are sudden episodes of inability to move the legs, usually triggered by being in crowded places and walking through narrow passages. Attempts at overcoming such episodes by moving the upper part of the body are common causes of falls. This symptom is probably not related to dopaminergic changes. Therefore, use of levodopa or dopamine agonists is usually ineffective. Although desipramine may benefit a few patients, the most effective treatment consists of using sensory, especially visual, cues to guide the motor planning. An inverted L-shaped cane has been shown to be helpful to many patients, who can overcome freezings by stepping over the handle of the cane.

Nutt JG, et al: Motor fluctuations during continuous levodopa infusions in patients with Parkinson's disease. Mov Disord 12:285–292, 1997.

Olanow CW, Obeso JA: Preventing levodopa-induced dyskinesias. Ann Neurol 47(4 Suppl 1):S167–S176, 2000.

Schrag A, Quinn N: Dyskinesias and motor fluctuations in Parkinson's disease: A community-based study. Brain 123(Pt 11):2297–2305, 2000.

Clinical Fluctuations in Parkinson's Disease

FLUCTUATION	MANAGEMENT
End-of-dose deterioration ("wearing off")	Increase frequency of levodopa doses Sinemet CR Dopamine agonists Deprenyl Amantadine Infusions of levodopa or dopamine agonists
Delayed onset of response	Give before meals Reduce protein Antacids Infusions of levodopa or dopamine agonists
Drug-resistant "offs"	Increase levodopa dose and frequency Give before meals Infusions of levodopa or dopamine agonists
Random oscillation ("on-off")	Dopamine agonists Deprenyl Infusions of levodopa or dopamine agonists Levodopa withdrawal
Freezing*	Increase dose Dopamine agonists Desipramine Inverted L-shaped cane

* May not be related to levodopa therapy.

22. How can Sinemet CR be useful to the management of fluctuations in PD?

The controlled-release preparation of carbidopa/levodopa, Sinemet CR (25/100 or 50/200 mg tablets), is a useful alternative to standard Sinemet (10/100, 25/100, 25/250). The transition from the regular to the controlled preparation of Sinemet has to be carefully planned. Because of lower bioavailability of the CR preparation, the authors usually increase the daily dosage of levodopa by 30%; many patients require a 50% increase in the final dose of Sinemet CR compared with the baseline dosage of standard Sinemet. A potential problem of the CR preparation is the long latency. This difficulty is usually overcome by adding one-half or one tablet of Sinemet 25/100 to the first morning dose of Sinemet CR. Unfortunately, many patients have coexisting clinical fluctuations and peak-dose dyskinesias. Peak-dose dyskinesias tend to deteriorate with the increased dopaminergic stimulation provided by Sinemet CR.

23. What are the most common types of levodopa-induced dyskinesias (LID)? How are they treated?

After 3 years of treatment, approximately 50% of patients with PD display some degree of involuntary movements related to levodopa. Phenomenologically, LID may be classified into three main categories:

1. **Peak-dose dyskinesias** (improvement–dyskinesia–improvement or I–D–I) coincide with the time of maximal clinical improvement and usually consist of choreatic movements.

2. **Diphasic dyskinesias** (dyskinesia–improvement–dyskinesia or D–I–D) occur at the onset and/or at the end of the "on" period and usually consist of dystonia and repetitive stereotypic movements of the legs. Some patients display a combination of the two types and have dyskinesia the entire "on" period (square-wave dyskinesias).

3. **"Off" dyskinesias**, typically painful dystonias, coincide with the period of decreased mobility. The most common example is early morning dystonia. Dopaminergic stimulation increases "on" dyskinesias and decreases the other two types. Conversely, antidopaminergic drugs improve all forms of LID, although they worsen the PD. Dystonia induced by levodopa may improve significantly with the use of baclofen, an agonist of gamma-aminobutyric acid (GABA) receptors. Clozapine has been reported to reduce dopa-induced dyskinesias.

Bennett JP, et al: Suppression of dyskinesias in advanced Parkinson's disease: Moderate daily clozapine doses provide long-term dyskinesia reduction. Mov Disord 9:409, 1994.

Ferreira JJ, Rascol O: Prevention and therapeutic strategies for levodopa-induced dyskinesias in Parkinson's disease. Curr Opin Neurol 13(4):431–436, 2000.

Stacy M: Pharmacotherapy for advanced Parkinson's disease. Pharmacotherapy 20(1 Pt 2):8S–16S, 2000.

Levodopa-induced Dyskinesias

PATTERN	PHENOMENON	MANAGEMENT
Peak-dose (I–D–I)	Chorea	Reduce each dose of levodopa
		Add dopamine agonists
	Dystonia	Reduce each dose of levodopa
		Clonazepam
		Baclofen
		Anticholinergics
	Pharyngeal dystonia	Reduce each dose of levodopa
		Add anticholinergics
	Respiratory dyskinesia	Reduce each dose of levodopa
		Add dopamine agonists
	Myoclonus	Clonazepam
		Valproate
		Methysergide
	Akathisia*	Anxiolytics
		Propranolol
		Opioids

(Table continued on following page.)

Levodopa-induced Dyskinesias (Continued)

PATTERN	PHENOMENON	MANAGEMENT
Diphasic (D–I–D)	Dystonia	Increase each dose of levodopa Baclofen Sinemet CR
	Stereotypies	Increase each dose of levodopa Baclofen
Off dyskinesia	Dystonia	Baclofen Dopamine agonists Anticholinergics Sinemet CR Tricyclics Lithium Botulinum toxin
	Akathisia*	Anxiolytics Propranolol Opioids
Striatal posture*	Dystonia	Increase levodopa Anticholinergics Thalamotomy Botulinum toxin

I–D–I= improvement-dyskinesia-improvement, D–I–D = dyskinesia-improvement-dyskinesia.
* May be unrelated to levodopa therapy.

24. What is the role of dopamine agonists in the treatment of PD?

Dopamine agonists directly stimulate dopamine receptors and, in contrast to levodopa, do not require enzymatic transformation into metabolites. Because dopamine agonists bypass the presynaptic elements of the nigrostriatal system, they have some advantages in relation to levodopa. For example, they cause dyskinesias and clinical fluctuations less frequently and usually have a levodopa-sparing effect. The most established use of dopamine agonists is as an adjunct to levodopa, especially in patients with clinical fluctuations and dyskinesias. Evidence indicates that early introduction of dopamine agonists decreases the possibility of development of complications of long-term levodopa therapy, by maintaining the doses of levodopa at low levels.

25. What dopamine agonists are available to treat PD? What are their most common side effects?

Until 1997 only two dopamine (DA) agonists (bromocriptine and pergolide) were clinically used in PD. Since then, pramipexole and ropinirole have become commercially available. Cabergoline (a potent D2 agonist marketed in the U.S. for treatment of galactorrhea) is too expensive for use in PD. Apomorphine, another DA agonist, may be given intravenously, intranasally, sublingually or subcutaneously.

Both bromocriptine and pergolide are ergot derivatives and have the risk of complications such as vasoconstriction (with acroparesthesias and angina), exacerbation of peptic ulcer disease, erythromelalgia, and pulmonary and retroperitoneal fibrosis. Pramipexole and ropinirole are nonergoline agonists and should have a lower risk of such complications.

Dopamine agonists act on the various DA receptors in different ways. Bromocriptine stimulates dopamine D2 receptors and inhibits D1 receptors, whereas pergolide stimulates both D1 and D2 receptors. The difference in the mechanism of action between the two drugs suggests that pergolide has more efficacy than bromocriptine. Pramipexole has D2 stimulatory activity with preferential affinity (stimulation) for the D3 receptor, whereas ropinirole is a relatively pure D2 agonist. DA agonists provide some benefit as monotherapy, but they are most often used as adjunctive therapy in patients with levodopa-induced fluctuations. Studies with pergolide demonstrate that it reduces the daily requirement of levodopa. Furthermore, DA agonists have been shown to enhance survival and growth of dopaminergic neurons in culture as well as to reduce oxidative stress by decreasing DA turnover. Pramipexole may be neuroprotective and possibly improves neurotrophic activity in mesencephalic dopaminergic cultures. A recent study concluded that initial treatment with ropinirole monotherapy (supplemented with levodopa if necessary) results in successful management of early Parkinson's disease for up to 5 years with a reduced risk of dyskinesia.

Although dopamine agonists display fewer side effects than levodopa, they may exacerbate peak-dose dyskinesias, and other undesired dopaminergic effects, such as nausea, vomiting, anorexia, malaise, orthostatic hypotension, confusion, and hallucinations, may occur.

Hanna PA, et al: Switching from pergolide to pramipexole in Parkinson's disease: An open study. J Neural Transm [in press].

Jankovic J, Marsden CD: Therapeutic strategies in Parkinson's disease. In Jankovic J, Tolosa E (eds): Parkinson's Disease and Movement Disorders, 3rd ed. Baltimore, William & Wilkins, 1998.

Le WD, et al: Neuroprotection of pramipexole against dopamine and levodopa-induced cytotoxicity. Mov Disord 12:840, 1997.

Leiberman A, et al: Clinical evaluation of pramipexole in advanced Parkinson's disease: Results of a double-blind, placebo-controlled, parallel-group study. Neurology 49:162, 1997.

Rascol O, et al: A five-year study of the incidence of dyskinesia in patients with early Parkinson's disease who were treated with ropinirole or levodopa. 056 Study Group. N Engl J Med 342:1484–1491, 2000.

26. What other medications are under evaluation for use in Parkinson's disease?

Inhibition of carechol-o-methyl transferase (COMT), which degrades dopamine, by drugs such as entacapone and tolcapone serves to prolong dopamine release. Entacapone inhibits only peripheral COMT, whereas tolcapone inhibits both central and peripheral COMT. Other MAO inhibitors, such as rasagiline, which also appears to have a dopaminergic effect, are under study. There is a growing interest in the use of antiglutaminergic drugs, particularly for putative neuroprotection. One such drug, riluzole (used in amyotrophic lateral sclerosis), may provide such an effect in PD. Intraventricular use of glial-derived neurotrophic factor (GDNF) in monkeys resulted in diminished parkinsonism and is undergoing a pilot human trial.

Chong BS, Mersfelder TL: Entacapone. Ann Pharmacother 34:1056–1065, 2000.

Finberg JP, et al: Pharmacology and neuroprotective properties of rasagiline. J Neural Transm 48:S95, 1996.

Gash DM, et al: Functional recovery in parkinsonian monkeys treated with GDNF. Nature 380:252, 1996.

Jankovic J: New and emerging therapies for Parkinson disease. Arch Neurol 56:785–790, 1999.

Kurth MC, et al: Tolcapone improves motor function and reduces levodopa requirement in patients with Parkinson's disease experiencing motor fluctuations: A multicenter, double-blind, randomized, placebo-controlled trial. Neurology 48:81, 1997.

27. What is the role of surgery in the treatment of PD?

Thalamotomy, the most established neurosurgical procedure for treatment of PD, consists of lesioning the ventral inferior medial (VIM) nucleus of the thalamus, which is involved in the generation of parkinsonian tremor. Thalamotomy is reserved for patients with predominantly unilateral parkinsonism who fail to respond to conservative therapy. Approximately 80% of patients with PD who undergo this procedure show improvement of the tremor without significant side effects. Bilateral surgery is not recommended, however, because of the complication of dysarthria.

More recently, the use of deep brain stimulation (DBS) of the VIM has been shown to be of marked benefit, primarily for tremor, and is able to suppress dyskinesias. DBS involves implanting an electrode in the VIM and delivering high-frequency chronic stimulation via an implantable pulse generator located subcutaneously in the subclavicular area. Patients can turn the device on and off via an external magnet. DBS can be done bilaterally with a lower risk of dysarthria than thalamotomy.

The recognition that PD is associated with hyperactivity of the subthalamic nucleus (STN) led to a successful treatment of MPTP monkeys by subthalamotomy. Some human patients, inadvertently treated with subthalamotomy instead of thalamotomy, noted improvement not only in tremor but also in bradykinesia. Recent use of STN DBS has demonstrated benefit for contralateral bradykinesia and other parkinsonian signs.

The pallidum, particularly the posteroventral part of the internal segment of the globus pallidus (GPi), has increasingly become a surgical target in Parkinson's disease. The main benefit of pallidotomy is the marked reduction of contralateral LIDs, with some ipsilateral benefit. Tremor, bradykinesia, and rigidity are also reduced but more variably. After pallidotomy, patients typically have a lower levodopa requirement. DBS into the GPi is receiving increased attention.

Benabid AL, et al: Chronic electrical stimulation of the ventralis intermedius nucleus of the thalamus as a treatment of movement disorders. J Neurosurg 84:203, 1996.

Hallett M, Litvan I: Scientific position paper of the Movement Disorder Society evaluation of surgery for Parkinson's disease. Task Force on Surgery for Parkinson's Disease of the American Academy of Neurology Therapeutic and Technology Assessment Committee. Mov Disord 15(3):436–438, 2000.

Jankovic J, et al: Outcome after stereotactic thalamotomy for Parkinsonian, essential and other types of tremor. Neurosurgery 37:680, 1995.

Jankovic J, et al: Levopa-induced dyskinesias treated by pallidotomy. J Neurol Sci 167:62–67, 1999.

Limousin P, et al: Bilateral subthalamic nucleus stimulation for severe Parkinson's disease. Mov Disord 10:672, 1995.

28. What is the role of transplant surgery in the treatment of PD?

Interest in the transplantation of adrenal medulla into the basal ganglia was sparked by the hypothesis that the adrenal chromaffin cells produce dopamine when implanted into parkinsonian striatum. After initial encouraging reports, this procedure has been virtually abandoned in the United States because of its modest benefits and high risk of morbidity. Human fetal mesencephalic transplantation has undergone a great deal of study. A recent double-blind, placebo-controlled trial (real and sham surgery) demonstrated some improvement in clinical measures of PD in patients younger than 60 years receiving real surgery. There was no significant improvement in reaction time after real or sham surgery, but there was a trend toward improvement in movement time for implanted patients under 60 years of age. The authors found a placebo effect at 4 months. Recent porcine transplantation has shown promise as an alternative source of dopaminergic cells.

Fink JS, et al: Porcine xenografts in Parkinson's disease and Huntington's disease patients: Preliminary results. Cell Transplant 9:273–278, 2000.

Kordower JH, et al: Neuropathological evidence of graft survival and striatal reinnervation after the transplantation of fetal mesencephalic tissue in a patient with Parkinson's disease. N Engl J Med 332:1118, 1995.

Pullman SL, et al: Computerized analysis of reaction and movement times after fetal cell tissue transplantation in Parkinson disease patients. Neurology 54(Suppl 3):A49, 2000.

29. Is there any relationship between Alzheimer's disease (AD) and PD?

Currently available data do not support the existence of a common etiology for AD and PD. However, approximately 20% of patients with PD have troublesome dementia. AD accounts for an unknown proportion of these cases. Unlike AD, the pattern of dementia in PD is characterized by lack of cortical signs, such as aphasia and apraxia, and the presence of forgetfulness, bradyphrenia, and depression. The different patterns suggest that different mechanisms are responsible for cognitive dysfunction in the two diseases, and pathologic studies support this distinction. PD is characterized by relative sparing of the cortex and by neuronal loss in the SN and other subcortical structures, such as the locus ceruleus. LBs are found in the remaining cells. On the other hand, the cerebral cortex is primarily involved in AD; neurofibrillary tangles and deposits of amyloid are the most important lesions. However, a recent study shows that over 50% of patients with AD display parkinsonism and myoclonus during the course of the disease.

Wilson RS, et al: Progression of parkinsonism and loss of cognitive function in Alzheimer disease. Arch Neurol 57:855–860, 2000.

30. What are the main clinical features of progressive supranuclear palsy (PSP)?

PSP is the second most common cause of idiopathic parkinsonism. Typically, the onset is in the seventh decade, with no family history. Patients have ophthalmoparesis of downgaze, parkinsonism, pseudobulbar palsy, and frontal lobe signs. Eyelid abnormalities are common. For example, patients with eyelid freezing have difficulty with either opening or closing the eyes due to inhibition of levator palpebrae or orbicularis oculi muscles, respectively. The presence of dementia in PSP is controversial. The prevalence of dystonia in patients with pathologically proven PSP is about 13%.

Jankovic J: Progressive supranuclear palsy. In Griffin JW, Johnson RT (eds): Current Therapy in Neurological Diseases, 5th ed. St. Louis, Mosby, 1997, pp 279–282.

31. What is the cause of PSP?

The cause of PSP is unknown. Radiologic and pathologic evidence indicates that a multiinfarct state can cause a picture identical to PSP. Idiopathic PSP is pathologically characterized by marked neuronal cell loss in subcortical structures, such as the nucleus basalis of Meynert, pallidum, subthalamic nucleus, substantia nigra, locus ceruleus, and superior colliculi. Other pathologic features include neurofibrillary tangles, granulovacuolar degeneration, and gliosis. Atrophy, generalized or focal (midbrain or cerebellum), is the most common neuroradiologic finding in idiopathic PSP. However, up to 25% of the patients with PSP have no abnormality on CT and/or MRI of the brain. Growing evidence suggests linkage disequilibrium between a PSP gene and allelic variants of the tau gene.

Higgins JJ, et al: An extended 5'-tau susceptibility haplotype in progressive supranuclear palsy. Neurology 55:1364–1367, 2000.

Litvan I, et al: Accuracy of clinical criteria for the diagnosis of progressive supranuclear palsy (Steele-Richardson-Olszewski syndrome). Neurology 46:922, 1996.

Winikates J, Jankovic J: Vascular progressive supranuclear palsy. J Neural Transm 42:S189, 1994.

32. How can PSP be distinguished from PD?

The most distinctive feature of PSP is the supranuclear downgaze palsy, which is not found in PD, the most common misdiagnosis of PSP. The differentiation is particularly difficult when the characteristic supranuclear ophthalmoparesis is not evident, as may be the case in early stages of PSP. Some patients who never develop this finding are found at autopsy to have PSP. The difficulty in establishing the diagnosis of PSP is suggested by an average delay in making the diagnosis of 3.6 years after onset of symptoms. Computerized posturography is a useful tool in reliably differentiating early PSP from PD and age-matched controls.

Cardoso F, Jankovic J: Progressive supranuclear palsy. In Calne DB (ed): Neurodegenerative Diseases. Philadelphia, W.B. Saunders, 1993.

Ondo W, et al: Computerized posturography analysis of progressive supranuclear palsy: A case-control comparison with Parkinson's disease and healthy controls. Arch Neurol 57(10):1464–1469, 2000.

Differential Diagnosis of Progressive Supranuclear Palsy (PSP) and Parkinson's Disease (PD)

CLINICAL FEATURES	PSP	PD
Age at onset (decade)	7th	6th
Initial symptoms	Postural and gait disorder	Tremor and bradykinesia
Family history	–	±
Multi-infarct state	±	–
Dementia	± (visual/motor)	±
Downgaze ophthalmoparesis	+	–
Eyelid abnormalities	+	±
Pseudobulbar palsy	+	±
Gait	Wide, stiff, unsteady	Slow, shuffling, narrow, festinating
Rigidity	Axial (neck)	Generalized
Facial expression	Astonished, worried	Hypomimia
Tremor at rest	–	+
Dystonia	+	±
Corticobulbospinal signs	±	–
Symmetry of findings	+	–
Weight loss	–	+
Improvement with DA drugs	–	+
Levodopa-induced dyskinesias	–	+

+ = yes or present, – = no or absent, DA = dopamine.

33. What is the treatment of PSP?

Levodopa and dopamine agonists are the most frequently used agents in the treatment of PSP. However, even with high doses, they usually provide only a transient and slight improvement of parkinsonian symptoms. The loss of dopamine receptors in the striatum and the presence of extensive lesions involving other neurotransmitters, such as acetylcholine, probably account for the failure of pharmacologic therapy. Currently no drug provides sustained relief in patients with PSP. With progression of disease, patients usually become bedridden, unable to swallow or talk. Gastrostomy is necessary in advanced stages. Death, usually related to respiratory complications, occurs after a mean disease duration of 7–8 years.

Kompoliti K, et al: Pharmacological therapy in progressive supranuclear palsy. Arch Neurol 55:1099–1102, 1998.

Tolosa E, Valldeoriola F: Progressive supranuclear palsy. In Jankovic J, Tolosa E (eds): Parkinson's Disease and Movement Disorders, 3rd ed. Philadelphia, Lippincott Williams & Wilkins, 1998.

34. What are the most important characteristics of vascular parkinsonism?

Multiple vascular lesions in the basal ganglia may be associated with parkinsonism. Tremor at rest is not a common finding, and bradykinesia and rigidity tend to be more significant in the legs. In some patients the findings are virtually limited to the lower extremities; hence the designation lower body parkinsonism. Unlike PD, the gait in patients with vascular parkinsonism is characterized by a broad base. Some patients show stepwise progression. Associated findings, such as dementia, spasticity, weakness, and Babinski signs, are commonly observed. Neuroradiologic studies, especially MRI, show a multiinfarct state. The response to dopaminergic therapy is usually poor.

Winikrates J, Jankovic J: Clinical correlates of vascular parkinsonism. Arch Neurol 56:98–102, 1999.

35. Is it possible to distinguish drug-induced parkinsonism from PD on clinical grounds?

Drugs are one of the most common causes of parkinsonism in the general population. Drugs that block postsynaptic dopamine receptors and/or deplete presynaptic dopamine may cause parkinsonism. The table in question 12 lists some of these medications. Clinical studies indicate that drug-induced parkinsonism is indistinguishable from PD. Discontinuation of the offending drug promotes remission of the syndrome in most cases, although sometimes the parkinsonism persists. Such patients may have subclinical PD and require dopaminergic therapy.

Chabolla DR, et al: Drug-induced parkinsonism as a risk factor for Parkinson's disease: A historical cohort study in Olmsted County, Minnesota. Mayo Clin Proc 73:724–727, 1998.

36. What is multiple system atrophy (MSA)?

MSA is a neuropathologic term that includes Shy-Drager syndrome (SDS), sporadic forms of olivopontocerebellar atrophy (OPCA), and striatonigral degeneration (SND). SDS is characterized by parkinsonism, which occasionally responds to dopaminergic therapy, and dysautonomia. Although cerebellar findings dominate in OPCA, mild parkinsonism and pyramidal signs are also usually recognized. Patients with SND typically have parkinsonism and pyramidal signs with laryngeal stridor, although in some cases SND is indistinguishable from PD. The division of MSA into SDS, OPCA, and SND is controversial. Although usually clinically distinct at onset, with progression symptoms overlap substantially. The three syndromes have a common pathologic substratum consisting of cell loss and gliosis in the striatum, substantia nigra, locus ceruleus, inferior olive, pontine nuclei, dorsal vagal nuclei, cerebellar Purkinje cells, and intermediolateral cell columns of the spinal cord. The characteristic histologic marker—glial cytoplasmic inclusions, which are seen particularly in oligodendrocytes—has helped to distinguish MSA as a clinicopathologic entity.

Hanna PA, Jankovic J, Kirkpatrick JB: Multiple system atrophy: The putative causative role of environmental toxins. Arch Neurol 56:90–94, 1999.

Litvan I, et al. What is the accuracy of the clinical diagnosis of multiple system atrophy? A clinicopathologic study. Arch Neurol 54:937, 1997.

37. What is the treatment of MSA?

Dopaminergic drugs are the mainstay of the treatment of MSA. However, despite the use of high doses of levodopa, no significant improvement is usually observed. The loss of cells in the striatum and widespread lesions of other neurotransmitters probably accounts for the failure of treatment.

Hughes AJ, et al: The dopaminergic response in multiple system atrophy. J Neurol Neurosurg Psychiatry 55:1009, 1992.

Litvan I: Recent advances in atypical parkinsonian disorders. Curr Opin Neruol 12:441–446, 1999.

38. What is cortical-basal ganglionic degeneration (CBGD)?

Patients with CBGD display a combination of cortical (pyramidal signs, myoclonus, and apraxia) and subcortical findings (rigidity and dystonia) as well as a distinctive alien limb sign. CBGD is virtually the only disease that causes this constellation of symptoms and signs. Until late stages of the disease, patients do not experience cognitive decline or dysautonomia. Convergence disturbances and oculomotor apraxia are common neuroophthalmic signs. The neuropathologic hallmarks are swollen achromatic neurons, neuronal loss, and gliosis in the cerebral cortex, SN, lateral nuclei of the thalamus, striatum, locus ceruleus, and Purkinje layer of the cerebellum. The cause is entirely obscure. No familial forms have been reported. The disease progresses relentlessly until death, usually within 10 years after onset. Response to dopaminergic therapy is usually poor.

Hanna PA, Doody RS: Alien limb sign. In Litvan J, Goetz CG, Lang AE (eds): Corticobasal Degeneration and Related Disorders. Advances in Neurology Series, vol. 82 Philadelphia, Lippincott Williams & Wilkins, 2000.

TREMORS

39. What is essential tremor (ET)?

ET is a neurologic disease characterized by action tremor of the hands in the absence of any identifiable causes, such as drugs or toxins. Other types of tremor, such as isolated head and voice tremor, are also expressions of ET. It is estimated that at least 5 million Americans are affected by ET. Characterized by action-postural tremor of the hands and arms, ET may be asymmetric at onset and have a kinetic component. Patients with severe forms of ET may display tremor at rest. The postural component is observed during maintenance of postures, such as holding the arms outstretched in front of the body. The kinetic component, often more severe than the postural component, is apparent during the performance of certain tasks, such as handwriting or the finger-to-nose maneuver. Although sometimes labeled as benign, ET may be a source of marked disability and embarrassment. ET is presumably transmitted by an autosomal dominant gene with variable expression. Recently a familial essential tremor gene (in Icelandic families) was mapped to chromosome 13. However, about 35% of patients with ET have a negative family history. Supportive criteria for diagnosis of ET include improvement with alcohol, propranolol, and primidone. The table below summarizes the findings of a survey of 350 patients with ET at the Baylor College of Medicine Parkinson's Disease Center and Movement Disorders Clinic.

Lou JS, Jankovic J: Essential tremor: Clinical correlates in 350 patients. Neurology 41:234, 1991.

Gulcher JR: Mapping of a familial essential tremor gene, FET1, to chromosome 3q13. Nature Genet 17:84, 1997.

Higgins JJ, Pho LT, Nee LE: A gene *(ETM)* for essential tremor maps to chromosome *2p22-p25*. Mov Disord 12:859–864, 1997.

Essential Tremor: Clinical Correlates

VARIABLE	RESULT	N
Gender	179 M/171 F	350
Age at evaluation (yr)	58.4 ± 16.4	350
Duration of symptoms (yr)	18.7 ± 17.5	326
Family history		350
First-degree relative	219 (62.5%)	
Other relatives	25 (7.1%)	
Anatomic distribution		350
Hands	314 (89.7%)	
Head	143 (40.8%)	
Voice	62 (17.4%)	
Leg	48 (13.7%)	
Jaw	25 (7.1%)	

Table continued on following page

Essential Tremor: Clinical Correlates (Continued)

VARIABLE	RESULT	N
Anatomic distribution (cont.)		
Face	8 (2.9%)	
Trunk	6 (1.7%)	
Tongue	5 (1.4%)	
Orthostatic	2 (0.6%)	
Associated disorders		350
Dystonia	165 (47.1%)	
Cervical dystonia	94 (26.8%)	
Writer's cramp	48 (13.7%)	
Blepharospasm	26 (7.4%)	
Laryngeal dystonia	14 (4.0%)	
Others	21 (6.0%)	
Parkinsonism	72 (20.2%)	
Myoclonus	8 (2.2%)	
Improvement with drugs		
Alcohol	96 (66.7%)	144
Propranolol	22 (68.0%)	32
Primidone	8 (72.1%)	13

From Lou JS, Jankovic J: Essential tremor: Clinical correlates in 350 patients. Neurology 41:234, 1991, with permission.

40. How can enhanced physiologic tremor be differentiated from ET?

Physiologic tremor is a rhythmic oscillation with a frequency of 8–12 Hz, determined largely by the mechanical properties of the oscillating limb. Under several circumstances the tremor may be enhanced and appears identical to ET. Enhanced physiologic tremor is the most common cause of postural tremor. However, unlike ET, its frequency can be reduced by mass loading.

Jankovic J: Essential tremor: Clinical characteristics. Neurology 54(11 Suppl 4):S21–S23, 2000.

Causes of Enhanced Physiologic Tremor

Stress-induced	Drugs
Anxiety	Beta agonists (e.g., theophylline, terbutaline, epinephrine)
Emotion	Cyclosporine
Exercise	Dopaminergic drugs (levodopa, dopamine agonists)
Fatigue	Methylxanthines (coffee, tea)
Fever	Psychiatric drugs (lithium, neuroleptics, tricyclics)
	Stimulants (amphetamines, cocaine)
Endocrine	Valproic acid
Adrenocorticosteroids	
Hypoglycemia	Toxins (arsenic, bismuth, bromine, ethanol withdrawal,
Pheochromocytoma	mercury, lead)
Thyrotoxicosis	

41. What physiopathologic mechanisms underlie ET?

Only 14 patients with ET have had a thorough pathologic examination, and no specific abnormality was found. It has been suggested that the postural tremor of ET arises from spontaneous firing of the inferior olivary nucleus, which drives the cerebellum and its outflow pathways via the thalamus to the cerebral cortex and then to the spinal cord. Functional MRI (fMRI) studies have demonstrated increased activation of the cerebellum and red nucleus in ET. Most PET and fMRI evidence indicates that the inferior olive is not likely to be the tremor generator in ET; instead, the generator is probably in the cerebellum. This theory is supported by bilateral overactivity of cerebellar connections by PET in patients with primary writing and primary orthostatic tremor. Clinical data also support a cerebellar role in the pathogenesis of ET: over 50% of patients with ET have difficulty in performing tandem gait, which is considered an indicator of cerebellar function, and hemispheric cerebellar stroke may abolish ipsilateral ET.

Bucher SF, et al: Activation mapping in essential tremor with functional magnetic resonance imaging. Ann Neurol 41:32, 1997.

Wills AJ, et al: A positron emission tomography study of primary orthostatic tremor. Neurology 46:747, 1996.

42. Is there an association between ET and PD?

According to different sources, the prevalence of ET in patients with PD ranges from 3–8.5%. The prevalence of PD in ET is debated (4.5–21.8%). The relatively high frequency of familial tremor (15–23%) among patients with PD supports the existence of an etiologic link between PD and ET. In a large family with levodopa-responsive Lewy-body parkinsonism studied by Ferrar et al., certain members of the pedigree had postural tremor without parkinsonism. Furthermore, an allele (263bp) of the nonamyloid component of plaques (NACP)-Rep1 polymorphism has been associated with sporadic PD in a German and more recently in an American population of patients with PD. The authors conclude that the association of this allele with PD and ET "suggests a possible etiologic link between these two conditions." Further epidemiologic and genetic studies are needed before the controversy about the relationship between PD and ET can be resolved.

Benamer TS, et al: Accurate differentiation of parkinsonism and essential tremor using visual assessment of [123I]-FP-CIT SPECT imaging: The [123I]-FP-CIT Study Group. Mov Disord 15:503–510, 2000.

Farrer M, et al: A chromosome 4p haplotype segregating with Parkinson's disease and postural tremor. Hum Mol Genet 8:81–85, 1999.

Tan EK, et al: Polymorphism of NACP-Rep1 in Parkinson's disease: An etiologic link with essential tremor? Neurology 54:1195–1198, 2000.

43. What is the relationship between ET and dystonia?

Although tremor is frequently found in patients with dystonia, it is not always clear whether the oscillatory movement is a form of dystonia (hence a dystonic tremor) or whether it represents coexistent ET. Postural hand tremor, phenomenologically identical to ET, may precede or be the initial manifestation of dystonia. The lack of demographic and other differences between patients with ET and ET-dystonia supports the notion that ET is a single disease entity with a clinical spectrum that often includes dystonia. Some investigators argue, however, that the postural tremor in patients with dystonia has different clinical characteristics—such as irregularity and a broader range of frequencies, asymmetry of contractions, and associated myoclonus—that distinguish it from ET.

Jankovic J, et al: Cervical dystonia: Clinical findings and associated movement disorders. Neurology 41:1088, 1991.

Jedynak CP, Bonnet AM, Agid Y: Tremor and idiopathic dystonia. Mov Disord 6:230, 1991.

Pal PK: Head tremor in cervical dystonia. Can J Neurol Sci 27:137–142, 2000.

44. What is orthostatic tremor?

Orthostatic tremor (OT) is a relatively rare but frequently misdiagnosed disorder. It is more common in women, and the onset is typically in the sixth decade. It consists of a rapid (13–14 Hz) tremor of the legs triggered by standing. Postural tremor of the hands and a family history of ET are frequent features, suggesting that OT is a variant of ET. Clonazepam is the treatment of choice; other less effective options are propranolol, primidone, and phenobarbital.

FitzGerald PM, Jankovic J: Orthostatic tremor: An association with essential tremor. Mov Disord 6:60, 1991.

Wills AJ, et al: Levodopa may improve orthostatic tremor: Case report and trial of treatment. J Neurol Neurosurg Psychiatry 66:681–684, 1999.

45. What other tremors are variants of ET?

Besides OT, other types of tremor are also considered to be variants of ET. However, some authors argue that the pharmacologic differences between these tremors and ET support the notion that they represent distinct entities. There is evidence, for example, that some isolated site (head tremor) and task-specific tremors, such as primary handwriting tremor, actually represent forms of dystonic tremor. This controversy will not be settled until biologic markers for ET and for dystonia are available.

Louis ED, Ford B, Barnes LF: Subtypes of essential tremor. Arch Neurol 57:1194–1198, 2000.

Variants of Essential Tremor

VARIANT	TREATMENT
Chin tremor	Propranolol, primidone
Facial tremor	Clonazepam, propranolol, primidone
Head tremor	Clonazepam, primidone, propranolol, trihexyphenidyl
Orthostatic tremor	Clonazepam, propranolol, primidone, phenobarbital
Shuddering attacks (childhood)	Propranolol
Task-specific tremor (writing)	Propranolol, primidone, trihexyphenidyl, botulinum toxin
Tongue tremor	Propranolol, primidone
Truncal tremor	Clonazepam, propranolol, primidone
Voice tremor	Propranolol, ethanol, botulinum toxin

46. Discuss the treatment of ET.

Propranolol remains the most effective medication for ET, although other beta blockers also have an antitremor activity. Daily doses of up to 360 mg may be necessary to control tremor. Fatigability, depression, bradycardia, hypotension, weight gain, and sexual impotence are potential side effects of propranolol and, to a lesser degree, the other beta blockers. Contraindications for their use include chronic obstructive pulmonary disease, asthma, congestive heart failure, and insulin-dependent diabetes mellitus.

Primidone, an anticonvulsant medication, also has been shown to be highly effective for the treatment of ET in both open and controlled studies. It should be started at low doses (25 mg at bedtime) to avoid the occasional, acute, idiosyncratic toxic reaction characterized by severe nausea, vomiting, sedation, confusion, and ataxia. The daily dosage may be increased to 300 mg. If the patient does not improve on this dosage, further increments are usually useless. Fewer side effects occur with the long-term use of primidone than with propranolol.

Less effective but occasionally useful medications are lorazepam, clonazepam, alprazolam, and diazepam. Alcohol, although effective in approximately two-thirds of patients with ET, is not recommended because of the possibility of addiction, although ET does not appear to increase the risk of alcoholism. Gabapentin "may be effective in some cases of ET," according to a recent double-blind study.

Pilot trials have demonstrated that **botulinum toxin** injected into the affected musculature is a useful alternative in the treatment of patients who are unresponsive to other measures. As a last resort in clinically intractable ET, contralateral thalamotomy is efficient and well tolerated. More recently, chronic high-frequency thalamic stimulation has been shown to suppress completely disabling ET. Unlike thalamotomy, this procedure can be performed bilaterally.

Jankovic J, et al: A randomized, double-blind, placebo-controlled study to evaluate botulinum toxin type A in essential hand tremor. Mov Disord 11:250, 1996.

Ondo W, et al: Gabapentin for essential tremor: A multiple-dose, double-blind, placebo-controlled trial Mov Disord 15:678–682, 2000.

Ondo W, Almaguer M, Jankovic J, Simpson RK: Thalamic deep brain stimulation: Comparison between unilateral and bilateral placement. Neurology 2000 [in press].

47. What are the characteristics and most common causes of kinetic tremor?

Kinetic tremors result from lesions of the cerebellar outflow pathways. The tremor has a 3–4 Hz frequency and is typically observed on the finger-to-nose test. In patients with cerebellar lesions, titubation (anterior/posterior oscillation of the trunk and head) and postural tremor of the hands are often seen in addition to the kinetic tremor. Patients who have lesions in the midbrain, involving the superior cerebellar peduncle and nigrostriatal system, also display tremor at rest (midbrain tremor).

Multiple sclerosis, trauma, stroke, Wilson's disease, phenytoin intoxication, acute alcoholic intoxication, cerebellar parenchymatous alcoholic degeneration, and tumor are the most important causes of kinetic tremor.

The treatment of kinetic tremors remains unsatisfactory. Drugs useful in the treatment of ET, such as propranolol and primidone, are ineffective in the treatment of kinetic tremors. Isoniazid, carbamazepine, and glutethimide may control kinetic tremor in some patients. Attaching weights to the wrist also may be modestly helpful. Injections of botulinum toxin or thalamotomy may benefit selected patients. Buspirone has been reported to help some patients with mild cerebellar tremor.

Lou JS, et al: Use of buspirone for treatment of cerebellar ataxia. An open-label study. Arch Neurol 52:982, 1995.

Schulder M, et al: Thalamic stimulation in patients with multiple sclerosis. Stereotact Funct Neurosurg 72(2–4):196–201, 1999.

48. What is neuropathic tremor?

Tremor has been associated with several neuropathies. Approximately 40% of patients with hereditary motor and sensory neuropathy (Charcot-Marie-Tooth disease) display action tremor. There is no relationship between tremor and severity of neuropathy. Certain features of the tremor (age at onset, anatomic distribution, response to alcohol, and family history of tremor) overlap with ET, suggesting an association between the two conditions. Patients with chronic relapsing and dysgamma-globulinemic neuropathies also have been reported to display tremor. One study showed that, like ET, the tremor in patients with chronic relapsing radiculoneuropathies is associated with activation of both cerebellar hemispheres.

Bain PG, et al: Tremor associated with benign IgM paraproteinaemic neuropathy. Brain 119(Pt 3):789–799, 1996.

Brooks DJ, et al: A comparison of the abnormal patterns of cerebral activation associated with essential and neuropathic tremor. Neurology 42(Suppl 3):423, 1992.

Cardoso FC, Jankovic J: Hereditary motor-sensory neuropathy and movement disorders. Muscle Nerve 16: 904, 1993.

49. What is the relationship between tremor and peripheral trauma?

The occurrence of tremor and other movement disorders, especially dystonia and myoclonus, after peripheral trauma is well established. Typically, peripherally induced tremors have rest and action components. Some patients develop a typical picture of parkinsonism, with rest tremor, bradykinesia, hypomimia, and response to levodopa. The physiopathology of this movement disorder is unknown. Although conventional neurophysiologic studies show abnormalities of the peripheral nerves in less than one-half of patients, it is reasonable to speculate that damage to the peripheral nervous system causes sustained changes in the central nervous system, which account for the movement disorders. The common association with reflex sympathetic dystrophy suggests that dysautonomia plays a role in the generation of posttraumatic movement disorders. About 60% of patients have predisposing factors such as personal and family history of ET and exposure to neuroleptics.

Treatment is difficult. Anticholinergic agents and antitremor medications, such as propranolol and primidone, are usually ineffective. Clonazepam may provide moderate relief in some patients. Some authors have successfully used injections of botulinum toxin into the affected musculature to control posttraumatic movement disorders. Thalamotomy is another consideration when conservative treatment fails.

Cardoso FC, Jankovic J: Post-traumatic peripherally-induced tremor and parkinsonism. Arch Neurol 52:263, 1995.

Deuschl G, et al: Tremor in reflex sympathetic dystrophy. Arch Neurol 48:1247, 1991.

Ellis SJ: Tremor and other movement disorders after whiplash type injuries. J Neurol Neurosurg Psychiatry 63:110–112, 1997.

DYSTONIA

50. What is torsion dystonia?

Torsion dystonia is a neurologic condition characterized by sustained contractions of both agonist and antagonist muscles, frequently causing twisting and repetitive movements or abnormal postures. Because there is no biochemical, pathologic, or radiologic marker for dystonia, the diagnosis is based on the recognition of clinical features. A characteristic feature of dystonia that helps to differentiate it from other hyperkinetic movement disorders is that dystonic movements are repetitive and patterned. For reasons that are poorly understood, patients with dystonia have the ability to suppress or decrease the involuntary movements by gently touching the affected area (sensory trick or **geste antagonistique**). Stress and fatigue make dystonia worse, whereas sleep and relaxation improve it.

Jankovic J, Fahn S: Dystonic disorders. In Jankovic J, Tolosa E (eds): Parkinson's Disease and Movement Disorders, 3rd ed. Baltimore, Williams & Wilkins, 1998.

Classification of Dystonia

1. **Etiology**
   Idiopathic
     Familial
     Sporadic
   Symptomatic
2. **Age at onset**
   Childhood onset   0–12 years
   Adolescent-onset   13–20 years
   Adult-onset   > 20 years
3. **Distribution**
   Focal   Single body part
   Segmental   One or more contiguous body parts
   Multifocal   Two or more noncontiguous body parts
   Generalized   Segmental crural dystonia and dystonia in at least one additional body part
   Hemidystonia   One-half of the body

51. What features suggest the diagnosis of secondary dystonia?

Secondary forms of dystonia, which account for 25% of cases, are suspected in patients with a history of head trauma, peripheral trauma, encephalitis, toxin exposure, drug exposure, perinatal anoxia, kernicterus, and seizures. Abnormal findings such as dementia, ocular motility abnormalities, ataxia, spasticity, weakness, or amyotrophy are often present in patients with secondary dystonia. Furthermore, onset of dystonia at rest instead of with action, early onset of speech involvement, hemidystonia, abnormal laboratory tests, and abnormal brain imaging suggest the diagnosis of secondary dystonia. The list of causes of secondary dystonia is long, but it is important to try to identify those that are potentially treatable, especially Wilson's disease and tardive dystonia.

Causes of Secondary Dystonia

Metabolic disorders	**Miscellaneous**
Aminoacid disorders	Arteriovenous malformation
Glutaric aciduria	Atlantoaxial dislocation or subluxation
Hartnup's disease	Brain tumor
Homocystinuria	Cerebellar ectopia and syringomyelia
Methylmalonic acidemia	Central pontine myelinolysis
Tyrosinosis	Cerebral vascular or ischemic injury
Lipid disorders	Drugs
Ceroid lipofuscinosis	Anticonvulsants
GM1-gangliosidose	Antipsychotics
GM2-gangliosidose	Bromocriptine
Metachromatic leukodystrophy	Ergot
Miscellaneous metabolic disorders	Fenfluramine
Leber's disease	Levodopa
Leigh's disease	Metoclopramide

Table continued on following page

Causes of Secondary Dystonia (Continued)

Miscellaneous metabolic disorders *(cont.)*	Miscellaneous causes *(cont.)*
Lesch-Nyhan syndrome	Head trauma
Mitochondrial encephalopathies	Infection
Triosephosphate isomerase deficiency	Acute infectious torticollis
Vitamin E deficiency	AIDS
	Creutzfeldt-Jacob disease
Neurodegenerative disorders	Encephalitis lethargica
Ataxia telangiectasia	Reye's syndrome
Azorean heredoataxia (Machado-Joseph disease)	Subacute sclerosing panencephalitis
Familial basal ganglia calcifications	Syphilis
Hallervorden-Spatz disease	Tuberculosis
Huntington's disease	Paraneoplastic brainstem encephalitis
Infantile bilateral striatal necrosis	Perinatal cerebral injury and kernicterus
Intraneuronal inclusion disease	Peripheral trauma
Multiple sclerosis	Plagiocephaly
Neuroacanthocytosis	Psychogenic dystonia
Parkinson's disease	Toxins
Progressive pallidal degeneration	Carbon monoxide
Progressive supranuclear palsy	Carbon disulfide
Rett syndrome	Methane
Wilson's disease	Wasp sting

52. What are the most common types of idiopathic dystonia?

The classic idiopathic dystonia, much more common among Ashkenazi Jews, is transmitted by an autosomal dominant gene whose expression is extremely variable. Phenocopies (sporadic cases) account for at least 20% of the cases of idiopathic dystonia. At the onset, the dystonic movements occur during performance of voluntary movements (action dystonia). Occasionally, dystonia is triggered by specific actions, such as playing a particular musical instrument or handwriting (task-specific dystonia). With progression of disease, the movements are brought about by less specific actions of the affected body part. With further deterioration, actions in other areas activate the dystonia (for example, torticollis worsened by handwriting). The latter phenomenon is called overflow. Dystonia at rest, with abnormal postures, is usually indicative of severe forms of idiopathic dystonia. Idiopathic dystonia starting in childhood usually has a focal onset in the feet and tends to generalize, whereas most focal dystonias in adults remain restricted to the part of the body initially involved. Because axial involvement is prominent in childhood-onset forms of dystonia, this diagnosis should be entertained in children and teenagers with kyphoscoliosis.

Paroxysmal dystonia encompasses a heterogenous and relatively rare group of conditions. Although psychogenic dystonia accounts for some cases, the majority are thought to be of neurologic origin, possibly representing a form of subcortical epilepsy, arising from the basal ganglia. The organic forms, sporadic or autosomal dominant, can be categorized as either kinesiogenic or nonkinesiogenic. In the kinesiogenic variety, the attacks are precipitated by sudden movements, lasting less than 5 minutes and recurring up to 100 times/day. Anticonvulsants, such as carbamazepine and phenytoin, are usually effective in preventing the episodes. In the nonkinesiogenic paroxysmal dystonia the attacks are less frequent (3/day), last longer (minutes to hour), and often are triggered by alcohol, coffee, and fatigue. Clonazepam is partially effective in most patients. Secondary paroxysmal dystonias may be caused by strokes, multiple sclerosis, and trauma to the peripheral and central nervous system.

Hwu WL, et al: Dopa-responsive dystonia induced by a recessive GTP cyclohydrolase I mutation. Hum Genet 105:226–230, 1999.

Segawa M: Hereditary progressive dystonia with marked diurnal fluctuation. Brain Dev 22(Suppl 1):65–80, 2000.

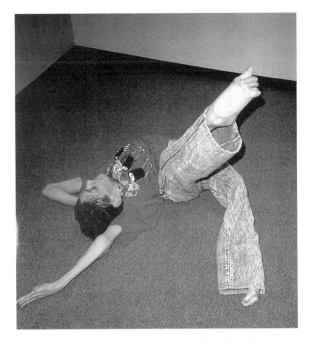

Patient with childhood-onset generalized dystonia.

53. Where is the gene for classical dystonia located?

Molecular genetic techniques link the dystonia (DYT1) gene to chromosome 9 (9q34). Recently, the mutation in the DYT1 gene has been characterized as a GAG deletion in the carboxy terminal of the gene that codes for an adenosine triphosphate-binding protein called torsin A. Evidence that adult-onset forms of focal dystonia are also related to the same gene awaits confirmation.

Brassat D, et al: Frequency of the DYT1 mutation in primary torsion dystonia without family history. Arch Neurol 57:333–335, 2000.

Kramer PL, et al: The DYT1 gene on 9q34 is responsible for most cases of early limb-onset idiopathic torsion dystonia in non-Jews. Am J Hum Genet 55:468, 1994.

Ozelius LJ, et al: The early-onset torsion dystonia gene (DYT1) encodes an ATP-binding protein. Nat Genet 17:40, 1997.

54. What is the most common form of focal dystonia?

The cervical region is the area most frequently affected by dystonia. Among 1000 patients with dystonia at the Baylor College of Medicine Parkinson's Disease Center and Movement Disorders Clinic, 76% have cervical dystonia, alone (33% patients) or associated with involvement of other areas. It is slightly more common in women (61%). Depending on the muscles involved, different types of postures are observed. Most patients with cervical dystonia have a combination of abnormal postures, such as torticollis, laterocollis, and anterocollis. Pain is a feature in about 70% of the patients with neck dystonia, whereas tremor, either dystonic or essential-type, is observed in 60% (see figure at top of following page).

55. What are the other forms of focal dystonia?

Blepharospasm, either isolated (11%) or combined with oromandibular dystonia (23%), is the second most common form of focal dystonia. It is defined as an involuntary, bilateral eye closure produced by dystonic contractions of the orbicularis oculi muscles. Blepharospasm is three times more common in women than men. Onset is usually gradual; often, before the onset of sustained

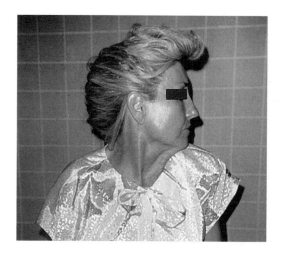

Patient with cervical dystonia manifested chiefly by torticollis to the left and marked contraction and hypertrophy of the right sternocleidomastoid muscle.

eyelid closure, patients experience excessive blinking triggered by bright light, wind, and stress. With progression, most patients develop dystonia involving other facial muscles as well as the masticatory and cervical musculature. Sensory tricks that help to maintain the eyes open include pulling on the upper eyelids, talking, and yawning. Up to 15% of patients with blepharospasm become legally blind because of inability to keep their eyes open.

Dystonic writer's cramp is a form of task-specific dystonia associated with handwriting. Although able to use their hands for performing daily chores, after a few seconds or minutes of writing patients develop dystonic, usually painful, spasms of the forearm musculature, which prevent them from writing further. With progression of disease, the dystonia becomes less task-specific, occurs during other activities, and may spread to involve more proximal muscles. Approximately 50% of patients develop similar symptoms contralaterally. Other task-specific dystonias occur among musicians (piano player's cramp, guitar player's cramp) and others whose recreational or occupational activities require fine motor coordination. The actual prevalence of these task-specific dystonias is unknown because only a few patients seek medical attention.

Cardoso F, Jankovic J: Dystonia and dyskinesia. Psychiatr Clin North Am 20:821–838, 1997.

Ibanez V, et al: Deficient activation of the motor cortical network in patients with writer's cramp. Neurology 53:96–105, 1999.

56. What are the most effective medications for the treatment of generalized or segmental dystonias?

Levodopa, effective in about 10% of children with dystonia, should be tried in all childhood-onset dystonias. If there is no significant improvement in 2 months, levodopa is replaced by anticholinergics. The initial dose of trihexyphenidyl (Artane) is 2 mg twice daily. High doses, sometimes up to 100 mg/day, may be necessary. The benefits may not be appreciated for 3–4 months after initiation of therapy. Moderate-to-dramatic improvement is observed in up to 70% of patients, but the efficacy may decrease with chronic use. The usefulness of these medications, especially in adults, is limited by the occurrence of peripheral (dry mouth and blurred vision) and central (forgetfulness, confusion, hallucinations) side effects. Other drugs that should be tried are baclofen, carbamazepine, benzodiazepines, and antidopaminergics. Extreme caution should be used with dopamine receptor-blocking drugs because of their potential to cause tardive dyskinesia.

Levodopa (in children) and anticholinergics (in adults) are the first options among the systemic drugs. Clonazepam is occasionally highly effective in blepharospasm, whereas baclofen may be particularly useful in cranial dystonia. Systemic treatment of focal dystonias is disappointing, however. If oral medications are ineffective, local injections of botulinum toxin should be considered in patients with focal dystonia. Injections of botulinum toxin into the affected musculature is now considered the first choice of treatment.

Jankovic J, Fahn S: Dystonic syndromes. In Jankovic J, Tolosa E (eds): Parkinson's Disease and Movement Disorders, 3rd ed. Baltimore, Williams & Wilkins, 1998.

57. What surgical procedure is available for the treatment of dystonia?

There has been a growing resurgence of interest in the use of thalamotomy for the treatment of dystonia. Ideal candidates are patients with severe unilateral dystonia (hemidystonia) who are not responsive to medical therapy.

Another procedure that was used more extensively before the widespread application of botulinum toxin injections is peripheral denervation surgery. Three types of procedures are used for cervical dystonia: (1) extradural sectioning of dorsal (posterior) rami with or without myotomy, (2) intradural sectioning of anterior cervical roots (anterior cervical rhizotomy), and (3) microvascular decompression of the spinal accessory nerve. No studies have compared the various procedures.

Intrathecal baclofen has recently been investigated for use in dystonia. Pallidotomy has been shown to be a safe and effective treatment in medically refractory cases of generalized dystonia.

Cardoso F, et al: Outcome after stereotactic thalamotomy for dystonia and hemiballismus. Neurosurgery 36:501, 1995.

Krauss JK, et al: Symptomatic and functional outcome of surgical treatment of cervical dystonia. J Neurol Neurosurg Psychiatry 63:642–648, 1997.

Kumar R, et al: Globus pallidus deep brain stimulation for generalized dystonia: Clinical and PET investigation. Neurology 53:871–874, 1999.

Ondo WG, et al: Pallidotomy for generalized dystonia. Mov Disord 13:693–698, 1998.

58. What is the role of botulinum toxin in the treatment of dystonia?

Botulinum toxin, one of the most lethal biologic toxins, is produced by the bacteria *Clostridium botulinum*. It acts at the neuromuscular junction, where it binds to the presynaptic cholinergic terminal and inhibits the release of acetylcholine. This functional denervation causes weakness and atrophy. After 3–4 months, sprouting and regrowth of the nerve terminals occur.

Botulinum toxin has been found to be effective in 95% of patients with blepharospasm, 90% of patients with spasmodic dysphonia, 85% of patients with cervical dystonia, and a majority of patients with oromandibular and hand dystonia. Patients with generalized dystonia displaying prominent disability in a single region may benefit from application of botulinum toxin to the involved area. The complications of botulinum toxin treatment are limited to local weakness; different consequences depend on the area. For example, patients with blepharospasm may have ptosis, whereas dysphagia is a potential complication of treatment for cervical dystonia. Most complications, however, resolve spontaneously after 2–4 weeks. A small percentage (3–5% in some series) of patients develop antibodies directed against botulinum toxin.

Hanna PA, Jankovic J, Vincent A: Comparison of mouse bioassay and immunoprecipitation assay for botulinum toxin antibodies. J Neurol Neurosurg Psychiatry 66:612–616, 1999.

Hanna PA, Jankovic J: Mouse bioassay versus Western blot assay for botulinum toxin antibodies: Correlation with clinical response. Neurology 50:1624–1629, 1998.

Jankovic J, Hallett M (eds): Therapy with Botulinum Toxin. New York, Marcel Dekker, 1994.

59. What other conditions may be treated with botulinum toxin?

Conditions other than dystonia also have been successfully treated with botulinum toxin. Strabismus was the first disease to be treated with botulinum toxin. Ninety percent of patients with hemifacial spasm, a form of segmental myoclonus, improve with injections of the toxin. Over 50% of patients with tremor of the hand and/or head improve with botulinum toxin. Reports also describe efficacy of this treatment in patients with various disorders associated with abnormal or inappropriate muscle contractions, including tics.

Jankovic J, Brin M: Therapeutic uses of botulinum toxin. N Engl J Med 324:1186, 1991.

Kwak CH, Hanna PA, Jankovic J: Botulinum toxin in the treatment of tics. Arch Neurol 57:1190–1193, 2000.

Scott BL, Jankovic J, Donovan DT: Botulinum toxin injection into vocal cord in the treatment of malignant coprolalia associated with Tourette's syndrome. Mov Disord 11:431, 1996.

TIC DISORDERS

60. What are tics?

Tics are relatively brief, sudden, rapid, and intermittent movements (motor tics) or sounds (vocal tics). They may be repetitive and stereotypic. Tics are usually abrupt in onset and brief (clonic tics) but may be slow and sustained (dystonic tics). Examples of even more prolonged tics (tonic tics) include abdominal or limb tensing. Simple tics are caused by contractions of only one group of muscles and result in a brief, jerklike movement or single, meaningless sound. Motor tics may also be complex, consisting of coordinated sequenced movements that resemble normal motor acts but are inappropriately intense and timed. Complex vocal tics include linguistically meaningful utterances and verbalizations. Tics, especially if dystonic, are associated with premonitory feelings that are relieved by performing the tics. Unlike other hyperkinetic dyskinesias, tics may be temporarily suppressed, leading some authors to suggest that in many patients they are purposefully, albeit irresistibly, performed.

Phenomenologic Classification of Tics

MOTOR TICS	VOCAL TICS
Simple tics	Simple tics
Clonic tics	Blowing
Blinking	Coughing
Head jerking	Grunting
Nose twitching	Screaming
Dystonic tics	Sneezing
Abdominal tensing	Squeaking
Blepharospasm	Sucking
Bruxism	Throat clearing
Oculogyric movements	Complex tics
Shoulder rotation	Coprolalia (shouting of obscenities)
Sustained mouth opening	Echolalia (repetition of someone else's phrases)
Torticollis	Palilalia (repetition of one's own utterances or
Complex tics	phrases)
Copropraxia (obscene gestures)	
Ecopraxia (imitating gestures)	
Head shaking	
Hitting	
Jumping	
Kicking	
Throwing	
Touching	

61. What are the most common causes of tic disorders?

Tourette's syndrome and related disorders are the most important and common causes of tics. However, these dyskinesias may accompany other hereditary disorders or follow acquired diseases.

Jankovic J: Tourette syndrome: Phenomenology and classification of tics. Neurol Clin 15:267–275, 1997.

Etiologic Classification of Tics

Physiologic tics	
Mannerisms	Gestures
Pathologic tics	
Primary	
Transient tic disorder	Torsion dystonia
Chronic tic disorder	Huntington's disease
Chronic motor tic disorder	Neuroacanthocytosis
Chronic phonic tic disorder	
Tourette's syndrome	*Table continued on following page*

Secondary (tourettism)

Chromosomal abnormalities
   Down syndrome
   Fragile X syndrome
   XYY syndrome
   XXX + 9p mosaicism
Drugs
   Anticonvulsants
   Dopamine receptor-blocking drugs
   Levodopa
   Stimulants
     Amphetamine
     Cocaine
     Methylphenidate
     Pemoline
Head trauma

Infections
   Creutzfeldt-Jacob disease
   Encephalitis
   Postencephalitic parkinsonism
   Sydenham's chorea
Mental retardation
   Autism
   Pervasive developmental disorders
   Rett's syndrome
   Rubella syndrome
   Static encephalopathy
Others
   Carbon monoxide poisoning
   Schizophrenia
   Stroke

62. What features are necessary to make the diagnosis of Tourette's syndrome (TS)?

According to currently established criteria, the diagnosis of TS requires all of the following features: onset before age 21, multiple motor tics, one or more vocal tics, fluctuating course, and presence of tics for more than 1 year. Tics that last less than 1 year are categorized as transient tic disorder (TTD). TTD is estimated to occur in 5–24% of school children; there is no accurate way to predict whether TTD will evolve into TS. Chronic motor tic disorder (CMTD) or chronic phonic tic disorder (CPTD) have the same criteria as TS, but patients display only either motor or phonic (vocal) tics.

TS, defined by the motor manifestations, is three times more frequent in males, but when obsessive compulsive disorder (OCD) is included, the male preponderance becomes much less significant. The onset is around age 7 years for facial tics with gradual progression in a rostrocaudal fashion. The diagnosis is often delayed because of a tendency to misinterpret or not recognize the tics or behavioral problems as abnormal. Behavioral problems usually precede the onset of tics by 2–3 years.

Jankovic J: Phenomenology and classification of tics. Neurol Clin 15:267, 1997.

63. What is the clinical spectrum of tic disorders and Tourette's syndrome?

A growing body of evidence supports the notion that primary tic disorders represent a clinical spectrum, ranging from the mild TTD to TS. Several studies show that TTD, CMTD, CPTD, and TS are transmitted as inherited traits in the same families, suggesting that they may represent an expression of the same genetic defect. One problem with the current criteria of TS is that they do not take into account the extensive range of psychopathology and academic problems. For example, OCD is encountered in at least 50% of patients and is related to the same gene responsible for the expression of tics. Attention-deficit hyperactivity disorder (ADHD) is also quite frequent (50–60%) among patients with TS, but the genetic association between the two conditions is less well understood. Other behavioral disturbances frequently observed in TS are aggressiveness, anxiety, conduct disorders, depression, learning difficulties, panic attacks, and sleep abnormalities.

64. How is TS genetically transmitted?

TS displays a sex-influenced, autosomal dominant mode of inheritance with variable expressivity as TS, CMTD, or OCD. A male offspring who inherits the TS gene has a 100% chance of expressing the gene either as TS, CMTD, or OCD; a 99% chance of having either TS or CMTD; and a 45% chance of having TS alone. A female offspring inheriting the same gene has a 71% chance of having the TS, CMTD, or OCD phenotype; a 56% chance of having either TS or CMTD; and a 17% chance of having TS alone. Other authors, however, suggest that the inheritance in TS is semirecessive semidominant; patients with mild-to-moderate forms are heterozygous, whereas more severe forms represent a homozygous state.

A recent study of 76 affected sib-pair families with a total of 110 sib-pairs revealed two regions, 4q and 8p, with lod scores of 2.38 and 2.09, respectively. Four other regions, on chromosomes 1, 10, 13, and 19, had a lod score greater than one. Another recent study found evidence for bilineal transmission (both parents having one or more of the following: attention deficit disorder, obsessive-compulsive behavior, or tics) in one-fourth of TS families.

Hanna PA, Janjua FN, Contant CF, Jankovic J: Bilineal transmission in Tourette syndrome. Neurology 53:813–818, 1999.

Tourette Syndrome Association International Consortium for Genetics: A complete genome screen in sib pairs affected by Gilles de la Tourette syndrome. Am J Hum Genet 65:1428–1436, 1999.

65. How is Tourette's syndrome treated?

Tics require treatment when they are socially embarrassing, painful (dystonic tics often cause pain), and severe enough to interfere with functioning. Their management relies on the use of dopamine blockers such as fluphenazine, which is more effective and associated with less sedation than other antidopaminergic drugs. Typically, a daily dose of 3–6 mg is sufficient to provide adequate relief. These drugs should be used cautiously because of the potential for causing tardive dyskinesia.

The behavioral problems present in TS usually cause more disabilities than tics. Clonidine is considered the first option in the management of ADHD. A significant number of patients experience drowsiness at the beginning of treatment. Once they are stabilized on the medication, they are switched to a clonidine patch. Deprenyl, a specific inhibitor of the enzyme monoamine oxidase type B, the metabolites of which share some properties with amphetamines, was recently shown in an open study to represent an effective alternative for treatment of ADHD without causing tics. Clomipramine is the first option to treat OCD, but imipramine, fluoxetine, and sertraline also may be useful. Carbamazepine and lithium are sometime used in patients with impulse control problems.

Kurlan R: Treatment of tics. Neurol Clin. 15:403–410, 1997.

Guidelines for the Treatment of Tourette's Syndrome

FEATURE	TREATMENT	
Tics	1. Fluphenazine 2. Pimozide 3. Haloperidol 4. Trifluoperazine	5. Molindone 6. Tetrabenazine 7. Botox
Attention deficit hyperactivity disorder	1. Clonidine 2. Deprenyl	3. Methylphenidate 4. Dextroamphetamine
Obsessive compulsive disorder	1. Clomipramine 2. Fluoxetine	3. Imipramine 4. Sertraline
Low impulse control	1. Carbamazepine	2. Lithium

CHOREA

66. What is Huntington's disease (HD)?

HD is clinically characterized by the presence of a triad composed of chorea, cognitive decline, and a positive family history. Chorea consists of involuntary, continuous, abrupt, rapid, brief, unsustained, irregular movements that flow randomly from one body part to another. Patients can suppress chorea partially and temporarily and frequently incorporate movements into semipurposeful activities (parakinesia). Affected patients have a peculiar, irregular gait. Besides chorea, other motor symptoms include dysarthria, dysphagia, postural instability, ataxia, myoclonus, and dystonia. The tone is decreased, and the deep reflexes are often hung up and pendular. All patients eventually develop dementia, mainly characterized by loss of recent memory, impairment of judgment, concentration, and acquisition. Neurobehavioral disturbances occasionally precede motor symptoms and consist of personality changes, apathy, social withdrawal, agitation, impulsiveness, depression, mania, paranoia, delusions, hostility, hallucinations, and psychosis.

Virtually all patients have a family history of a similar condition transmitted in an autosomal dominant fashion. Caudate and putamen atrophy on neuroimaging studies is another feature supportive of the diagnosis of HD.

67. What is the Westphal variant?

In 10% of cases of HD, the onset is before age 20 (Westphal variant). The disease is then characterized by the combination of progressive parkinsonism, dementia, ataxia, and seizures.

68. What are other common causes of chorea?

It is probable that levodopa-induced chorea in parkinsonism is the most common cause of chorea. Usually this diagnosis is not difficult once the history is available.

The combination of chorea and psychiatric symptoms can be found in Wilson's disease. However, the diagnosis is easily made by finding a Kayser-Fleischer ring, low plasma ceruloplasmin, and evidence of hepatic dysfunction. Sydenham's chorea is a form of autoimmune chorea, preceded by a group A streptococcal infection. Rarely encountered in the United States, this condition is one of the most common causes of chorea in underdeveloped areas. Systemic lupus erythematosus and primary antiphospholipid antibody syndrome are other causes of autoimmune chorea. Senile chorea is a condition in which chorea is the only feature; no family history of HD is present.

Penney KB, et al: Huntington's disease in Venezuela: 7 years of follow-up on symptomatic and asymptomatic individuals. Mov Disord 5:93, 1990.

Stracciari A, et al: Effect of liver transplantation on neurological manifestations in Wilson disease. Arch Neurol 57:384–386, 2000.

69. Is it possible to make a diagnosis of HD in asymptomatic individuals?

The HD gene (designated IT15) has been identified near the tip of the short arm of chromosome 4 (4p16.3). An unstable expansion of the *CAG* repeat sequence is present at the 5' end of this large (210 kb) gene. The HD gene encodes a 348-kDa protein called huntingtin. Recent studies suggest that the aggregation of mutant huntingtin may be part of the pathogenesis of HD. All patients with HD studied to date have had > 36 *CAG* repeats. HD families also display "anticipation," or progressively earlier onset of disease in successive generations, typically with increasing *CAG* repeat size. Such findings allow genetic testing of at-risk individuals before the onset of symptoms. However, until effective treatment is available for HD, many ethical and legal dilemmas associated with genetic testing remain to be solved.

Ashizawa T, Gasser T: Genetics of movement disorders. In Jankovic J, Tolosa E (eds): Parkinson's Disease and Movement Disorders, 3rd ed. Baltimore, William & Wilkins, 1998.

DiFiglia M, Sapp E, Chase K: Aggregation of huntingtin in neuronal intranuclear inclusions and dystrophic neurites in brain. Science 277:1990, 1997.

70. What are the neuropathologic findings in HD?

The most important pathologic findings in HD are neuronal loss and gliosis in the cortex and striatum, particularly the caudate nucleus. Chorea seems to be primarily related to loss of medium spiny striatal neurons projecting to the lateral pallidum. This results in functional hypoactivity of the subthalamic nucleus with consequent hyperactivity of the thalamic tier.

71. Is there any protective treatment for HD?

Unfortunately, to date no therapeutic intervention has been capable of halting the relentless progression of HD. In the adult form, death occurs after a mean duration of 15 years, whereas in the juvenile variant the mean survival is 9 years. Current treatment relies on neuroleptics, which temporarily relieve chorea and psychosis by interfering with dopaminergic transmission. However, these drugs cause several side effects, including tardive dyskinesia. An alternative approach is to use medications that deplete presynaptic dopamine (e.g, reserpine), which have not been reported to cause tardive dyskinesia. Benzodiazepines and antidepressants are also commonly used for anxiety and depression associated with HD. Fetal transplantation has shown no beneficial results.

DRUG-INDUCED MOVEMENT DISORDERS

72. What is an acute dystonic reaction (ADR)?

ADR is an abrupt, drug-induced dystonia, especially of the head and neck. About 2.5% of patients treated with neuroleptics develop ADR within the first 48 hours of treatment. Cocaine use increases the likelihood of ADR. Although it is one of the first described neuroleptic in-duced-movement disorders, the pathophysiology of ADR remains unknown. Because it fol-lows the use of dopamine receptor-blocking drugs and improves with anticholinergics, it is presumed that changes in the striatal dopamine and acetylcholine are important in the genesis of ADR.

73. What is tardive dyskinesia (TD)?

TD is a hyperkinetic movement disorder caused by dopamine receptor-blocking drugs. According to current criteria, it is possible to make the diagnosis of TD when the hyperkinesia develops during treatment with neuroleptics or within 6 months of their discontinuation and per-sists for at least 1 month after stopping all neuroleptic agents. It is estimated that 20% of patients exposed to neuroleptics develop TD, but the values range from 13–49%. Severe TD seems to be more common in young males and elderly females.

DeLeon ML, Jankovic J: Clinical features and management of tardive dyskinesias, tardive myoclonus, tardive tremor, and tardive tourettism. In Sethi K (ed): Drug Induced Movement Disorders. New York, Marcel Dekker, 2000.

74. What is the importance of recognizing stereotypy in an adult patient?

Stereotypy is defined as a seemingly purposeful, coordinated, but involuntary, repetitive, rit-ualistic gesture, mannerism, posture, or utterance. Examples of stereotypies include repetitive grimacing, lip smacking, tongue protruding, and chewing movements. The tongue also may move laterally in the mouth ("bon-bon sign"). In addition, patients with tardive dyskinesias, the most common form of adult-onset stereotypy, often exhibit head bobbing, body rocking, leg crossing and uncrossing, picking at clothing, shifting weight, and marching in place.

Stereotypy is the most common form of TD (78% of cases). The second most common form of TD is dystonia (75% of patients). The presence of stereotypies in an adult without mental retar-dation or untreated schizophrenia strongly suggests the diagnosis of TD, especially in association with other movement disorders commonly present in TD (akathisia, tremor, myoclonus, chorea, and tics).

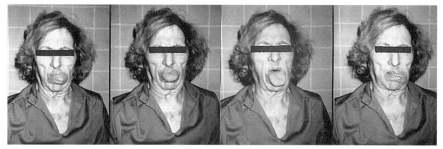

Patient with tardive dyskinesias manifesting stereotypic orolingual movements.

75. What is the pathogenesis of TD?

Because medications that cause TD block the dopamine receptors, dysfunction of striatal dopaminergic systems has been implicated in the pathogenesis. However, the mechanism of pro-duction of TD is still not understood. Clinical and experimental evidence suggests that TD and lev-odopa-induced dyskinesias share a common pathogenetic mechanism. These studies suggest that TD ultimately results from disruption of the lateral pallidal-subthalamic GABAergic projection,

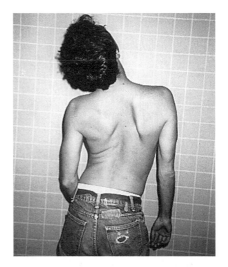

Patient with axial tardive dystonia.

leading to inhibition of the subthalamic nucleus. Recent evidence supports the notion that dopamine receptor-blocking drugs exert a neurotoxic effect, resulting in neuronal damage. There is no explanation, however, for the diversity of movement disorders in TD. The relatively specific pharmacologic profile of each of these dyskinesias suggests that different mechanisms are involved in their generation.

DiMonte DA, et al: Relationship among nigrostriatal denervation, parkinsonism, and dyskinesias in the MPTP primate model. Mov Disord 15:459–466, 2000.

76. How is TD treated?

The first step in the treatment of TD is to stop the offending drug, which results in spontaneous remission in approximately 60% of cases. Drugs that deplete dopamine, such as reserpine, are the most effective agents for treatment of TD. Tardive dystonia has a less satisfactory response to systemic treatment than other forms of TD. Tardive dystonia may improve with anticholinergic agents, whereas the other types, including stereotypy, may worsen. In patients with focal forms of dystonia, such as cranial and cervical dystonia, injection of botulinum toxin into the affected musculature is a useful and safe alternative.

Jankovic J, Beach J: Long-term effects of tetrabenazine in hyperkinetic movement disorders. Neurology 48:358, 1997.

Ondo WG, Hanna PA, Jankovic J: Tetrabenazine treatment for tardive dyskinesia: Assessment by randomized videotape protocol. Am J Psychiatry 156:1279–1281, 1999.

OTHER MOVEMENT DISORDERS

77. How can myoclonus be distinguished from chorea and tics?

Myoclonus is defined as a brief, sudden, shocklike jerk that may be caused not only by active muscle contractions (positive myoclonus) but also by lapses of muscle contraction (negative myoclonus). Many of the individual movements of chorea are myoclonic, but, unlike myoclonus, they are continuous, occurring in a constant flow. Tics may resemble myoclonus, but they are usually preceded by premonitory feelings, and patients usually have some degree of control over them.

78. How is myoclonus classified?

Myoclonus may be classified by etiology, pathophysiology, and distribution (see table on following page).

Classification of Myoclonus

Etiology

Physiologic myoclonus
  Anxiety
  Benign infantile myoclonus with feeding
  Exercise
  Hiccup
  Nocturnal myoclonus
Essential myoclonus
  Autosomal dominant
  Sporadic
Epileptic myoclonus
  Benign familial myoclonic epilepsy
  Childhood myoclonic epilepsies
    Cryptogenic myoclonus epilepsy
    Infantile spasms
    Juvenile myoclonus epilepsy
    Myoclonic astatic epilepsy
  Fragments of epilepsy
    Epilepsia partialis continua
    Isolated myoclonic epileptic myoclonic jerks
    Myoclonic absences in petit mal
    Photosensitive myoclonus
  Progressive myoclonus epilepsy
Symptomatic myoclonus
  Basal ganglia degenerations
    Cortical basal ganglionic degeneration
    Hallervorden-Spatz disease
    Huntington's disease
    Myoclonic dystonia
    Parkinson's disease
    Progressive supranuclear palsy
  Dementias
    Alzheimer's disease
    Creutzfeldt-Jacob disease
    Gerstmann-Sträussler-Schenker disease
  Focal lesions
    Dentato-olivary lesions
    Stroke
    Thalamotomy
    Trauma (central or peripheral nervous system)
    Tumor

Symptomatic myoclonus (continued)
  Metabolic and toxic encephalopathies
    Biotin deficiency
    Bismuth
    DDT
    Drugs, including levodopa
    Dialysis syndrome
    Heavy metal poisoning
    Hepatic failure
    Hypoglycemia
    Hyponatremia
    Infantile myoclonic encephalopathy
    Methyl bromide
    Mitochondrial encephalopathy
    Multiple carboxylase deficiency
    Nonketotic hyperglycemia
  Physical encephalopathies
    Decompression injury
    Electric shock
    Heat stroke
    Posthypoxia
  Spinocerebellar degeneration
  Storage disease
    Ceroid lipofuscinosis
    Lafora body disease
    Lipidoses
      GM1-gangliosidosis
      GM2-gangliosidosis
      Krabbe's disease
      Tay-Sachs disease
  Viral encephalopathies
    Arbor virus encephalitis
    Encephalitis lethargica
    Herpes simplex encephalitis
    Postinfectious encephalitis
    Subacute sclerosing panencephalitis

Pathophysiology

Cortical	*Brainstem*	*Spinal*
Epilepsia partialis continua	Palatal	Propriospinal
Focal	Essential	Segmental
Generalized	Symptomatic	*Peripheral*
Multifocal	Reticular	
Thalamic	Startle	

Distribution

Axial	Generalized	Segmental
Focal	Multifocal	

Adapted from Marsden CD: Myoclonus: Classification and treatment. Syllabus for the Movement Disorders Course, AAN, p 93, 1992.

79. How is myoclonus treated?

Recognition of the different types of myoclonus has practical implications, because each of the categories has a unique pathophysiologic mechanism and specific treatment. Myoclonus related to metabolic encephalopathies improves with treatment of the metabolic disturbance.

Epileptic myoclonus is initially treated with sodium valproate. If toxic reactions occur or the patient is still symptomatic, either clonazepam or primidone may be added. Clonazepam is the first choice in myoclonus arising from the brainstem, but 5-hydroxy-tryptophan, clomipramine, and fluoxetine are useful alternatives. Spinal and other segmental myoclonus also may respond to clonazepam or drugs that enhance serotoninergic transmission, but injections of botulinum toxin in the affected musculature has been the most useful treatment.

80. What is asterixis?

Asterixis is a form of negative myoclonus mainly associated with metabolic encephalopathies; electrophysiologically it is characterized by the presence of brief silences of electric muscular activity. Although originally described in patients with hepatic encephalopathy, asterixis may be caused by many other conditions. The early stages of metabolic dysfunction assume a rhythmic aspect, resembling tremor. With progression of the underlying cause, when patients hold their arms outstretched, the wrists display a characteristic flexion (caused by electric silence in the antigravity muscles).

Causes of Asterixis

Hepatic failure	Drugs	Lesions in the CNS
Respiratory failure	Anticonvulsants	Medial frontal cortex
Renal failure	Salicylates	Parietal lobe
Cardiac failure	Levodopa	Internal capsule
Chronic hemodialysis		Thalamus
Polycythemia		Rostral midbrain

81. What is the stiff person syndrome (SPS)?

Patients with this rare disorder have progressive, usually symmetric, rigidity of the axial muscles that may fluctuate in intensity. Motion, tactile stimulation, emotion, and startle are common triggering factors of the spasms. EMG shows continuous normal motor unit potentials in the affected muscles despite the patient's attempts to relax. The diagnosis is supported by relief of the rigidity with general and spinal anesthesia, peripheral nerve blocks, and diazepam, which is still the first-line treatment of SPS.

An insight into the pathophysiology of SPS was provided by the finding that 20 of 33 patients had autoantibodies against glutamic acid dehydoxylase (GAD). The hypothesis of an autoimmune etiology of SPS is further supported by the presence of other autoantibodies (to islet cells and gastric parietal cells, for example), coexistent autoimmune diseases such as insulin-dependent diabetes mellitus, vitiligo, thyroid disease, family history of presumed autoimmune conditions, and improvement with plasmapheresis and corticosteroid drugs.

Blum P, Jankovic J: Stiff-person syndrome: An autoimmune disease. Mov Disord 6:12, 1990.

82. What is Wilson's disease?

Wilson's disease is an autosomal recessive disease; the gene is linked to markers located in the q14-21 region on chromosome 13. The prevalence of the disease is estimated to be 1 in 30,000. It is associated with impaired incorporation of copper into ceruloplasmin as well as impaired biliary excretion of copper. The result is copper overloading in the liver, cornea, and brain, particularly in the basal ganglia. Virtually all patients display laboratory and/or clinical evidence of liver insufficiency. The most useful laboratory screening test is plasma ceruloplasmin, which usually is less than 20 mg/dl (normal: 24–45 mg/dl).

The most common neurologic findings are parkinsonism, bulbar signs (e.g., dysarthria and dysphagia), dystonia, postural tremor, and ataxia. Psychiatric symptoms, such as depression and psychosis, are particularly common among adults.

MRI of the head may display either decreased or increased signal intensity in the striatum on T2-weighted images. MRI of the midbrain may show a specific "face of a giant panda" appearance, which is produced by reversal of the normal hypointensity of the substantia nigra, midbrain tegmentum, and hypointensity in the superior colliculi.

83. What is the treatment for Wilson's disease?

Early diagnosis is essential, because treatment with copper-chelating agents often completely reverses the neurologic and hepatic symptoms. All siblings and cousins should be screened because presymptomatic patients require treatment to prevent development of symptoms. Penicillamine is the drug of choice for Wilson's disease; the typical dose is 250 mg 4 times/day in combination with pyridoxine (25 mg/day). Side effects are initial exacerbation of symptoms, rash, optic neuritis, thrombocytopenia, leukopenia, and nephrotoxicity. Other options to decrease copper overload are triethylene tetramine dihydrochloride, zinc sulphate, and tetrathiomolybdate. Symptomatic treatment of neurologic symptoms includes levodopa, anticholinergics, and injections of botulinum toxin. Liver transplant may be necessary in terminal cases of hepatic insufficiency.

Stracciari A, et al: Effect of liver transplantation on neurological manifestations in Wilson disease. Arch Neurol 57:384–386, 2000.

Stremmel W, et al: Wilson disease: Clinical presentation, treatment, and survival. Ann Intern Med 115:720, 1991.

84. What are the paraneoplastic movement disorders?

Opsoclonus-myoclonus designates a combination of rapid, erratic, involuntary movements of the eyes, with multifocal myoclonus (dancing eyes–dancing feet syndrome). Most cases occur between ages 6 and 18 months. Fifty percent of cases are related to an underlying neoplasm, especially neuroblastoma. This syndrome also occurs in adults with brainstem encephalitis, either paraneoplastic or infectious (Whipple's disease). Steroids dramatically improve this form of myoclonus. A few cases have been reported in patients with SPS, breast cancer, and autoantibodies against amphiphysin.

Ataxia is another well-established paraneoplastic movement disorder. The mechanism is cerebellar degeneration related to anti-Purkinje cell antibodies. There are also reports of parkinsonism, chorea, dystonia, segmental rigidity, and action and segmental myoclonus as remote effects of neoplasm.

Posner JB: Autoantibodies in childhood opsoclonus-myoclonus syndrome. J Pediatr 130:855–857, 1997.

Rosin L, et al: Stiff-man syndrome in a woman with breast cancer: An uncommon central nervous system paraneoplastic syndrome. Neurology 50:94–98, 1998.

BIBLIOGRAPHY

1. Jankovic J: The extrapyramidal disorders. In Goldman L, Bennett JC (eds): Cecil Textbook of Medicine, 21st ed. Philadelphia, W.B. Saunders, 2000, pp 2077–2087.
2. Jankovic J, Tolosa E (eds): Parkinson's Disease and Movement Disorders, 3rd ed. Baltimore, Williams & Wilkins, 1998.
3. Marsden CD, Fahn S (eds): Movement Disorders 3. London, Butterworths, 1993.
Websites
www.apdaparkinson.com
www.psp.org
www.dystonia-foundation.org
tsa.mgh.harvard.edu

12. AUTONOMIC NERVOUS SYSTEM

Yadollah Harati, M.D., F.A.C.P., and Hazem Machkhas, M.D.

1. What are the physiologic responses to stimulation of the sympathetic and parasympathetic systems?

Sympathetic Stimulation	*Parasympathetic Stimulation*
Tachycardia	Bradycardia
Hypertension	Hypotension
Bronchodilation	Bronchoconstriction
Mydriasis	Miosis
Vasoconstriction	Lacrimal secretion
Decreased peristalsis	Salivary secretion
Decreased kidney output	Palmar sweating
Piloerection	Vasodilation
Sphincter constriction	Increased peristalsis
Ejaculation	Exocrine gland secretion
Glycogenolysis	Bladder contraction
	Penile erection

Diagram of the sympathetic nervous system. (From Low PA (ed): Clinical Autonomic Disorders, 2nd ed. Philadelphia, Lippincott-Raven, 1997, with permission.)

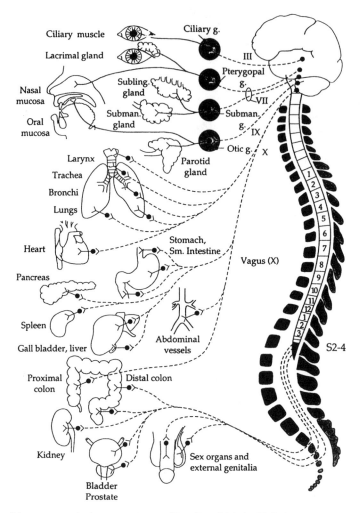

Ciliary muscle
Lacrimal gland
Ciliary g.
III
Pterygopal. g.
Nasal mucosa
Subling. gland
VII
Oral mucosa
Subman. gland
Subman. g.
IX
Larynx
Trachea
Bronchi
Lungs
Otic g.
X
Parotid gland
Heart
Stomach, Sm. Intestine
Pancreas
Vagus (X)
Spleen
Gall bladder, liver
Abdominal vessels
Proximal colon
Distal colon
Kidney
Sex organs and external genitalia
Bladder
Prostate
S2-4

Diagram of the parasympathetic nervous system. (From Low PA (ed): Clinical Autonomic Disorders, 2nd ed. Philadelphia, Lippincott-Raven, 1997, with permission.)

2. What features of the history must be explored in all patients with suspected autonomic dysfunction?

Some cardinal symptoms of autonomic dysfunction may be drug-induced or have a psychogenic etiology. With this caveat in mind, special attention to symptoms involving the following systems is essential when obtaining a history:

1. **Cardiovascular**—Orthostatic lightheadedness, dizziness, blurred vision, syncope or near-syncope, fatigue, headache and neck ache after prolonged standing, postprandial-postexercise lightheadedness or angina pectoris, fainting after alcohol ingestion or insulin injection, palpitations, resting tachycardia, orthostatic cerebral transient ischemic attack symptoms, angina pectoris.

2. **Sudomotor and vasomotor**—Partial or complete loss of sweating, heat intolerance (hot, flush, dizzy, and weak without sweating), excessive sweating (partial or total), facial and upper trunk gustatory sweating (especially when food incites salivation or with ingestion of cheese), nocturnal sweating, skin cracks on distal extremity, dry and shiny skin, unusually cold or warm feet, reduced skin wrinkling, and peripheral edema.

3. **Secretomotor**—Dry mouth and eyes.

4. **Genitourinary**—History of urinary tract infections, lengthened interval between micturition, increased volume of first morning void, need for straining to initiate and maintain voiding, weakness of stream, postvoid dribbling, sensation of incomplete emptying and overflow incontinence, frequency and urgency with or without dysuria (with superimposed infection), impotence (difficulty in initiating and/or maintaining erection), reduced or absent waking erection, diminished libido, retrograde ejaculation, decreased volume of ejaculation, reduced vaginal lubrication.

5. **Respiratory**—Irregular breathing or apnea during sleep.

6. **Gastrointestinal**—Dysphagia, retrosternal discomfort, heartburn, anorexia, epigastric fullness during or after meals, recurrent episodes of nausea and vomiting (fasting and/or postprandial) associated with upper abdominal pain, constipation, diarrhea (especially nocturnal), or fecal incontinence (especially at night), weight loss.

7. **Ocular**—Blurring of vision, photophobia, asymmetric pupils, drooping of eyelids.

8. **Factors aggravating symptoms**—Alcohol, hot temperature (environmental, hot bath, fever), exercise, bed rest, food ingestion, and hyperventilation.

3. What physical examination must be performed in all patients with suspected autonomic dysfunction?

A careful examination of the skin provides valuable clues to the presence of autonomic dysfunction. Particular attention should be given to acral vasomotor and trophic changes of the skin, abnormal sweating patterns, and the presence of allodynia or hyperalgesia. Examination of the eyes (ptosis) and pupillary shape, size, and response to light and accommodation is essential. Cardiovascular examination includes measurement of the heart rate at rest in response to deep breathing and Valsalva maneuver. Supine blood pressure (BP) and heart rate after 5–10 minutes of rest followed by measurement after active standing for 3 minutes should be checked in every patient with suspected dysautonomia. If orthostatic hypotension (systolic and diastolic drop > 20 mmHg or mean arterial BP drop > 20 mmHg) is not noted in a patient who nevertheless has symptoms of orthostatic hypotension, the patient should be asked to do 12 squats (orthostatic stress test), after which the standing BP is repeated.

4. What are the main clinical features that differentiate autonomic failure from autonomic hyperactivity?

Autonomic failure	Autonomic hyperactivity
Orthostatic hypotension	Neurogenic hypertension
Impotence	Hyperventilation
Hypohidrosis	Hyperhidrosis
Bladder dysfunction	Tachyarrhythmias
GI dysmotility	Diaphoresis
Horner's syndrome	Neurogenic pulmonary edema
Visual disturbances	Hyperthermia or hypothermia

5. What are the major anatomic differences between the sympathetic and parasympathetic nervous systems?

Because of the close proximity of sympathetic ganglia to the primary efferent sympathetic neurons (interomediolateral and interomediomedial columns), the sympathetic preganglionic fibers are short, whereas the postganglionic fibers may extend a long way to their target organs. The parasympathetic preganglionic neurons, on the other hand, are relatively long myelinated fibers that synapse with parasympathetic relay ganglia located near or within the wall of individual innervated organs. The postganglionic parasympathetic fibers are therefore short (1 mm to several cm).

The ratio of preganglionic to postganglionic neurons is usually much smaller in the parasympathetic nervous system, where it is 1:15 to 1:20. The large number of postganglionic neurons in the sympathetic system explains the wide range of sympathetic autonomic effects and the massive sympathetic outflow that occurs during strenuous and stressful situations. Many simultaneous diverse responses may occur as a result of sympathetic activation, including raised arterial blood pressure, increased blood flow to active muscles, increased muscle glycolysis and blood glucose level, enhanced mental activity and muscular strength, increased sphincter contraction, and decreased gastrointestinal peristalsis. A disorder that predominantly affects the sympathetic nervous system may therefore render the body incapable of dealing appropriately with strenuous physical or emotional stimulation. In contrast, the small proportion between the number of preganglionic and postganglionic neurons in the parasympathetic system promotes a more localized response and allows highly specific, controlled function of the parasympathetic system.

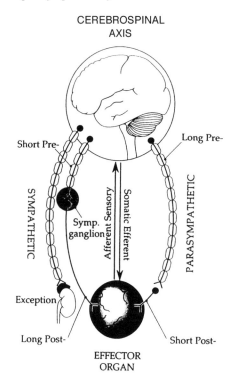

Schematic diagram comparing the sympathetic and parasympathetic nervous systems. (From Low PA (ed): Clinical Autonomic Disorders, 2nd ed. Philadelphia, Lippincott-Raven, 1997, with permission.)

6. Discuss the major neurotransmitters and their receptors in the autonomic nervous system.

Acetylcholine (ACh) is the neurotransmitter for all preganglionic neurons and for the parasympathetic postganglionic neurons. Its receptors in the autonomic nervous system are divided into nicotinic and muscarinic types. Nicotinic receptors, of which there are two subtypes, are ligand-gate sodium channels that mediate fast responses and are found mainly in the ganglia. Muscarinic receptors mediate slower responses and are found mostly throughout autonomic effector tissues. Five subtypes (M_1–M_5) have been identified and cloned.

Norepinephrine (NE) is the neurotransmitter for most sympathetic postganglionic fibers. Adrenergic receptors are divided into alpha (α_1 and α_2) and beta (β_1, β_2, and β_3) types and are localized in various autonomic effector tissues.

7. What other neurotransmitters play a role in the autonomic nervous system?

Researchers have identified a plethora of neuropeptides that act as neuromodulators or cotransmitters in autonomic signaling. Examples include substance P, somatostatin, vasoactive intestinal peptide, oxytocin, and enkephalins. Less conventional neurotransmitters, such as nitric oxide and carbon monoxide, have recently been implicated in autonomic transmission. The colocalization of more than one neurotransmitter to a single nerve terminal is well documented.

8. How useful is measurement of plasma catecholamines in the evaluation of dysautonomia?
Measurement of plasma NE is a useful, though crude, index of postganglionic sympathetic activity. The origin of plasma NE is primarily a spillover from postganglionic sympathetic junctional clefts. The measured NE, however, is a small portion of the released sympathetic nerve terminal NE that has escaped the enzymatic catabolism or reuptake and diffuses out of the junctional cleft into the bloodstream. The plasma level is determined by various processes that affect release, reuptake, or metabolism and removal from the plasma, such as emotion, exercise, eating, smoking, caffeine, time of day, blood volume, and hypoglycemia. Because NE is relatively unstable in plasma, care must be taken during sample collection, storage, and processing. The accuracy of plasma NE levels, therefore, greatly depends on rigorous attention to numerous factors capable of influencing plasma catecholamine levels.

9. What is the normal catecholamine response?
In normal subjects, the plasma level of NE is 150–170 pg/ml after 30 minutes in the supine position, increases 50–100% above supine values after 5 minutes of standing, and remains constant after 10 minutes of standing.

10. How does age affect catecholamine measurements?
Because plasma NE increases with age, the value must be corrected for age. The mechanism for increase with age is controversial; both reduced clearance and increased release have been suggested. Microneurographic recordings show an increase in muscle sympathetic activity with age, supporting the hypothesis of increased NE release.

11. Can catecholamine measurements localize the site of autonomic dysfunction?
Patients with a neuropathy causing a primarily postganglionic autonomic abnormality have a subnormal plasma level of NE in the supine position that fails to increase normally during standing. Because of considerable overlap between preganglionic and postganglionic abnormalities in individual patients with autonomic dysfunction, however, plasma NE values alone are usually not sufficiently diagnostic for the site of the lesion.

12. What is the role of the nucleus tractus solitarius (NTS) in the central autonomic network?
This important nucleus, situated at the dorsomedial medulla, receives inputs from neocortical regions and from nuclei of the forebrain, higher brainstem, and diencephalon (see figure on following page). The autonomic afferents, which convey information important to the control of cardiac rhythm and motility, peripheral vascular tone, respiration, and gastrointestinal motility and secretion, terminate at different parts of this nucleus. Axons that originate from the NTS end on the neurons of the reticular formation of the ventrolateral medulla, which in turn project to the interomediolateral (IML) cell column of the lateral horn of the spinal cord. The descending fibers projecting to the IML are diffusely dispersed in the spinal cord. Attempts to identify a group of degenerating fibers in the spinal cord following lesions of the brainstem or hypothalamus have generally been unsuccessful. NTS neurons also send efferent fibers to higher brainstem, hypothalamic and limbic structures, the vagus nerves, and neuronal groups of the spinal cord subserving respiration. In addition to autonomic afferent and efferent fibers, the NTS also receives somatic afferents from the spinal cord (dorsolateral horn) and spinal trigeminal lemniscus. This allows the NTS to serve as an integration station for the autonomic and somatic information, playing a vital role in the maintenance of body homeostasis.

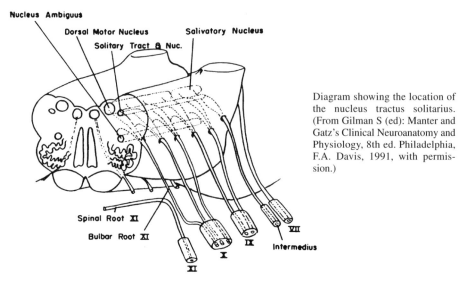

Diagram showing the location of the nucleus tractus solitarius. (From Gilman S (ed): Manter and Gatz's Clinical Neuroanatomy and Physiology, 8th ed. Philadelphia, F.A. Davis, 1991, with permission.)

13. What are the characteristics of the interomediolateral (IML) and interomediomedial (IMM) columns of the spinal cord?

The neurons of the IML and IMM are located in the spinal lateral gray column of the thoracic and upper lumbar regions of the spinal cord. They form the **primary efferent sympathetic neurons** or preganglionic neurons. Their axons, which precede the autonomic ganglia (hence preganglionic fibers), project onto a ganglionic neuron (**secondary efferent sympathetic neurons**) with its cell body in one of the paravertebral sympathetic trunk ganglia or related ganglia. The preganglionic fibers are finely myelinated, contributing to the whitish appearance of the white rami and ventral spinal roots through which they reach the ganglionic neurons. The number of neurons of the human IML and IMM and their axons diminish with age at a rate of 8% per decade. The main neurotransmitter of these neurons is ACh, but they also contain several important neuropeptides.

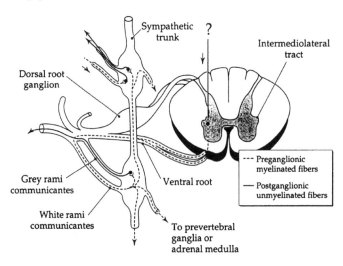

Diagram of the efferent sympathetic connections from the spinal cord, including the IML columns. (From Low PA (ed): Clinical Autonomic Disorders, 2nd ed. Philadelphia, Lippincott-Raven, 1997, with permission.)

14. What are the most important peripheral neuropathies associated with autonomic dysfunction?

Peripheral Neuropathies Associated with Autonomic Dysfunction

Inherited peripheral neuropathies with dysautonomia
- Hereditary sensory and autonomic neuropathy (HSAN) I, II, III* (Riley-Day syndrome), IV, and V
- Hereditary motor-sensory neuropathies (HMSN) I and II
- Fabry's disease*
- Multiple endocrine neoplasia, type 2b (MEN 2b)
- Amyloidosis* (familial amyloid polyneuropathy types I, II, and III)
- Porphyria*
- Some spinocerebellar degenerations

Infectious, parainfectious, and immune-mediated peripheral neuropathies with dysautonomia
- Leprosy
- AIDS
- Chagas' disease
- Systemic lupus erythematosus
- Systemic sclerosis
- Sjögren syndrome
- Rheumatoid arthritis
- Mixed connective tissue disease
- Guillain-Barré syndrome*
- Chronic inflammatory neuropathy
- Acute pandysautonomia*
- Pure cholinergic dysautonomia*

Autonomic neuropathies associated with systemic metabolic disease
- Diabetes*
- Chronic renal failure
- Alcoholism
- Nonalcoholic liver disease
- Vitamin B12 deficiency
- Paraneoplastic syndrome
- Primary amyloidosis*

Autonomic neuropathies associated with industrial agents, metals, toxins, and drugs
- Organic solvents
- Organophosphates
- Acrylamide
- Vacor
- Heavy metals
- Botulism*
- Vincristine*
- Cisplatinum

* Autonomic dysfunction is prominent and clinically important.

15. What are the salient manifestations of diabetic autonomic neuropathies?

Cardiovascular
Postural hypotension
Resting tachycardia
Painless myocardial infarction
Sudden death

Gastrointestinal
Esophageal motor incoordination
Gastric dysrhythmia, hypomotility (gastroparesis diabeticorum)
Pylorospasm
Uncoordinated intestinal motility ("diabetic diarrhea," spasm)
Intestinal hypomobility (constipation)
Gallbladder hypocontraction (diabetic cholecystopathy)
Anorectal dysfunction (fecal dysfunction)

Genitourinary
Diabetic cystopathy (atonic bladder, postmicturition dribbling)
Male impotence
Ejaculatory disorders
Reduced vaginal lubrication, dyspareunia

Respiratory
Impaired breathing control
Sleep apnea

Thermoregulatory
Sudomotor (diminished, excessive, or gustatory sweating)
Vasomotor (vasoconstriction, vasodilation, neuropathic edema)

Pupillary abnormalities
Miosis
Disturbances of dilation
"Argyll-Robertson"-like pupils

Neuroendocrine abnormalities
Reduced pancreatic polypeptide release
Reduced somatostatin release
Reduced motilin and gastric inhibitory peptide release
Enhanced gastrin release
Reduced norepinephrine release (orthostatic-, exercise-, and hypoglycemia-induced)
Reduced parathyroid hormone secretion (hypercalcemia induced)
Elevated atrial natriuretic hormone
Impaired glucose counterregulation (hypoglycemia unawareness)
Impaired norepinephrine release in response to hypoglycemia

16. What autonomic dysfunction is seen in Guillain-Barré syndrome (GBS)?

About 65% of patients with GBS have some dysautonomia. The incidence is higher when there is more sensory involvement or when axonal damage is extensive. Dysautonomias are important causes of complications, and death due to cardiovascular collapse in the setting of autonomic dysfunction occurs in approximately 3–14% of patients. Afferent baroreflex abnormalities may cause intermittent hypertension and hypotension associated with orthostatic hypotension. Abrupt fluctuations of blood pressure may precede fatal arrhythmias. Urine and plasma levels of catecholamines and vanillylmandelic acid may be elevated, and fluctuations in blood pressure may correlate with the rise and fall of circulating atrial natriuretic factor in some, but not all, patients.

Less frequent and less severe symptoms of autonomic dysfunction include urinary incontinence or retention, constipation, fecal incontinence, gastroparesis, and pupillary abnormalities.

17. Describe the appropriate management for the blood pressure fluctuations seen in GBS.

Blood pressure fluctuations in GBS are best monitored in a medical ICU setting. The ICU staff should be alerted for potential severe and fluctuating episodes of hypotension, hypertension, bradycardia, and tachycardia. Adequate administration of isotonic intravenous fluids should be started, a bladder catheter should be placed, fluid intake and output should be carefully monitored, and blood pressure should be measured frequently. Most importantly, continuous EKG monitoring is mandatory. In addition, other coexisting causes of cardiovascular instability should be assessed with arterial blood gases, serum electrolytes and glucose measurements, urine osmolality and electrolyte concentration, and evaluation for infection.

Treatment of autonomic hypotension is aimed at improving venous return to the heart, minimizing vagal reflex slowing of the heart rate, and lessening orthostatic positional changes. Venous return is optimized by the use of isotonic replacement fluids, at times with the aid of Swan-Ganz monitoring of pulmonary capillary wedge pressure, and by mechanical measures to reduce venous distention and edema in the lower extremities (e.g., leg wraps, elastic stockings). Vagal stimulation is minimized by reducing positive pressure during artificial ventilation, avoiding sudden postural changes, reducing tracheal stimulation during suctioning, and hyperoxygenating prior to suctioning. If hypotension does not respond to these measures, pressor drugs may be necessary. These must be used with **extreme caution**, because hypersensitivity responses are common. The use of short-acting agents such as dopamine or phenylephrine is recommended. There is often a delay of several minutes in blood pressure responses to pressor drugs. For prolonged hypertensive episodes, it is best to use short-acting agents (preferably beta-blockers) that can be titrated to the blood pressure response. Again, hypersensitivity with resultant hypotension is a potential complication. There may be an exaggerated hypotensive response to even small doses of intravenous drugs (e.g., morphine, furosemide, nitroglycerin, edrophonium chloride, thiopental).

18. How long does the cardiovascular instability persist in GBS?

There is no strong correlation between the severity of peripheral weakness and the risk or severity of dysautonomia. Cardiovascular instability may be seen in otherwise minimally disabled patients. As a rule, severely affected patients (especially if they require mechanical ventilation) have significant autonomic fluctuations, which resolve when ambulation is regained. The duration of cardiovascular instability ranges from a few days to a few weeks.

19. Describe the appropriate management for the arrhythmias seen in GBS.

Bradycardia of nonsinus origin is probably best treated with a transvenous pacemaker. Sinus tachycardia due to vagal damage occurs in about 50% of patients and usually responds to fluid replacement therapy. Its occurrence in a patient **without infection or circulatory cause** indicates vagal denervation. Absence of beat-to-beat (R-R) variation of heart rate during normal and deep breathing in a patient with early GBS is an important and reliable index of impending cardiovascular dysautonomia due to vagal nerve dysfunction. Acute atrial fibrillation and ventricular tachycardia are best managed by ICU experts, but if beta blockers are used, they must have a rapid onset and offset of action.

20. **What is the appropriate management for the other dysautonomias seen in GBS?**

Adynamic ileus and atonic bladder may occur. Adynamic ileus requires upper GI tract decompression via a nasogastric tube and maintenance of NPO status. Urinary retention is treated with an indwelling catheter while the patient is on IV fluids; if present in the rehabilitation phase of GBS, it is treated with sterile intermittent catheterization.

21. **Describe the clinical features of acute pandysautonomia.**

The heterogeneous and usually monophasic and self-limiting syndrome of acute pandysautonomia (acute autonomic neuropathy, acute panautonomic neuropathy) is rare. Pandysautonomia refers to concomitant involvement of both sympathetic and parasympathetic components of the autonomic nervous system, with relative or complete sparing of the somatic nerve fibers. The disorder may be preceded by viral or other febrile illnesses. The typical patient has orthostatic hypotension, anhidrosis, cold or heat intolerance, reduced lacrimation and salivation, disturbances of the bowel (ileus and abdominal colic, diarrhea, and constipation) and bladder (atony), impotence, a fixed heart rate, and fixed pupils. Symptoms evolve over a few days to a few months. People of all ages and of both sexes may be affected, and there is usually no family history. There are usually minimal or no motor, sensory, or coordination abnormalities, but tendon reflexes may be diminished or absent. Occasionally loss of sensation and sensory nerve action potentials, myelopathy, or abnormal electroencephalograms are reported. Cerebrospinal fluid (CSF) protein may be modestly elevated, which has led some experts to suggest that this entity may be a variant of GBS. Recovery is usually prolonged. One-third of patients do well, one-third remain severely disabled, and one-third make partial recovery with significant persistent deficits. The syndrome may be indistinguishable from the more severe forms of paraneoplastic autonomic neuropathy. No convincingly effective treatment for this condition exists other than supportive therapy for orthostatic hypotension and bowel and bladder symptoms. Anecdotal evidence, consisting of a few case reports, suggests that high-dose intravenous gamma-globulin may enhance recovery.

22. **What are the autonomic abnormalities seen in Sjögren's syndrome?**

This autoimmune exocrinopathy, which affects women nine times as frequently as men, is estimated to be second in frequency only to rheumatoid arthritis among collagen vascular diseases. In addition to the clinical presentation, the determination of highly specific autoantibodies, Ro (SS-A) and La (SS-B), directed against low–molecular-weight ribonuclear proteins, aids in the diagnosis of Sjögren's syndrome. All forms of peripheral neuropathy (sensory neuropathy, sensorimotor neuropathy, multiple mononeuropathies, sensory neuronopathy, cranial neuropathy, and entrapment syndromes) may be seen in association with Sjögren's syndrome. Autonomic dysfunction, including Adie's pupil, anhidrosis, orthostatic hypotension, and impaired cardiac parasympathetic function, may be superimposed on a generalized neuropathy in about 25% of patients. In most patients, sural nerve biopsy shows axonal degeneration, periarteriolar and perivenular inflammatory cell infiltration, and necrotizing vasculitis. Autonomic neuropathy also may be a prominent feature of other autoimmune diseases or mixed connective tissue diseases.

23. **Name the four most common paraneoplastic autonomic syndromes.**

Lambert-Eaton myasthenic syndrome (LEMS), autonomic neuropathy, intestinal pseudo-obstruction, and subacute sensory neuropathy.

24. **What is LEMS?**

LEMS is an antibody-mediated autoimmune disease. The target of the aberrant immune response is the presynaptic voltage-gated calcium channel at the neuromuscular junction. In 90% of patients, antibodies can be detected by radioimmunoassay. The cardinal symptom of LEMS is weakness, which usually spares the extraocular muscles. In about 60% of cases, the syndrome is paraneoplastic, associated almost exclusively with small-cell lung cancer. Onset of symptoms may precede detection of tumor by 1–4 years. LEMS is frequently associated with autonomic symptoms, including dry mouth (74%), impotence (41%), constipation (18%), blurred vision (8%), and impaired sweating (4%). Some patients also may have orthostatic light-headedness, difficulty with micturition, or tonic pupils. About 57% of patients demonstrate cholinergic and adrenergic supersensitivity of pupils when tested with 2.5% methacholine and 0.5% phenylephrine. Tear production is also reduced. Variations in heart rate and blood pressure may occur with the Valsalva maneuver or deep breathing, and sweat tests also may be abnormal.

25. How is LEMS treated?

When an underlying neoplasm is identified, removal or treatment of the tumor usually results in substantial improvement in all symptoms, including those of autonomic dysfunction. In patients who do not have an underlying malignancy, the treatment is directed toward the enhancement of cholinergic function and immunosuppression. Antiacetylcholinesterase agents, guanidine hydrochloride, 4-aminopyridine, and 3-4 diaminopyridine have been used to enhance neuromuscular transmission and improve autonomic dysfunction. Of these, 3-4 diaminopyridine is most effective and causes the fewest side effects. It increases the quantal release of acetylcholine by blocking voltage-dependent potassium conductance, prolonging the nerve terminal depolarization, and enhancing voltage-gated calcium influx. Guanidine inhibits the binding and uptake of calcium into mitochondria, thereby increasing the free intracellular calcium level and facilitating acetylcholine release; however, this drug has a number of hematologic (neutropenia, aplastic anemia) and CNS side effects that limit its use. Pyridostigmine and prostigmine provide limited symptomatic relief. Immunosuppression with corticosteroids, plasma exchange, or intravenous gamma-globulin may prove beneficial in patients with either the nonneoplastic or neoplastic forms of LEMS. A combination of 3-4 diaminopyridine and intravenous gamma-globulin may produce the highest likelihood of improvement. Drugs that adversely affect neuromuscular transmission, particularly those with calcium channel-blocking properties, should be avoided in patients with LEMS.

26. What is paraneoplastic autonomic neuropathy?

Some patients with small-cell lung cancer, pancreatic adenocarcinoma, or Hodgkin's disease may develop autonomic symptoms (orthostatic dizziness, impotence, dry mouth, urinary retention, or GI symptoms) that may improve with treatment of the tumor. Patients with autonomic neuropathy may have antineuronal (anti-Hu) autoantibodies. Approximately 40% of patients have the newly identified antibodies directed against the nicotinic ACh receptors in the autonomic ganglia. The presentation of autonomic neuropathy may precede or follow the diagnosis of malignancy.

27. What is paraneoplastic intestinal pseudoobstruction?

Pseudoobstruction of the bowel, with or without other symptoms of autonomic dysfunction, may be seen in association with small-cell lung cancer, pulmonary carcinoid, undifferentiated epithelioma, and malignant thymoma. These patients also may have gastroparesis and esophageal peristaltic abnormalities. They may subsequently develop other dysautonomic symptoms. The motility disorder may resolve with the treatment of the underlying tumor. The salient GI pathologic features include loss of myenteric plexus neurons, fragmentation and degeneration of axons, and plasma cell and lymphocytic infiltrations. Some patients have elevated titers of antineuronal nuclear antibody (anna-1 or anti-Hu), which reacts with antigens shared by the tumor cells and the myenteric plexus neurons.

28. What is paraneoplastic subacute sensory neuropathy?

Some patients with this syndrome, which usually occurs in association with small-cell lung cancer, may have one or several of the following autonomic dysfunctions: orthostatic hypotension, tonic pupils, hypohidrosis, dry mouth, diminished lacrimation, impotence, urinary retention, and constipation. Serum and CSF of patients with this syndrome frequently contain antineuronal nuclear (anti-HU) antibody, a polyclonal complement-fixing IgG that also reacts against a 35–40 kda protein of small-cell lung cancer cells. The neuronal nuclear antigen has the same molecular weight but lacks the 38 kda band. Treatment of the underlying tumor may result in the partial alleviation of autonomic and somatic symptoms.

29. What is the differential diagnosis of nonpsychogenic causes of male sexual impotence?

1. Penile arterial insufficiency
2. Excessive venous leakage
3. Spinal cord damage
4. Conus medullaris damage
5. Cauda equina damage
6. Sacral plexus damage
7. Peripheral neuropathies
8. Central and peripheral autonomic disorders
9. Drugs
10. Alcohol
11. Hyperprolactinemia
12. Peyronie's disease

30. What are the most common cardiovascular disturbances associated with CNS disease?
Cardiac arrhythmias, myocardial injury, and changes in blood pressure.

31. What cardiac arrhythmias are associated with CNS disease?
A number of CNS disorders, including subarachnoid hemorrhage, cerebral infarction and hemorrhage, brain tumors, and head injury, may cause a variety of supraventricular and ventricular arrhythmias unrelated to the any underlying cardiac disease. These arrhythmias may further compromise the prognosis of the CNS disease: 4–5% of sudden deaths in patients with subarachonid hemorrhage are attributed to this complication. Arrhythmias occur because of an imbalance between sympathetic and parasympathetic influences on the heart, presumably from an enhanced release of peripheral catecholamines triggered by the central lesion.

32. What is the nature of the myocardial injury associated with CNS disease?
CNS lesions, particularly intracerebral and subarachnoid hemorrhage, may cause a number of EKG abnormalities suggestive of myocardial ischemia. These changes may closely resemble myocardial infarction and include prolongation of the QT interval, ST segment depression, flattening or inversion of T waves, and the appearance of U waves. With the exception of QT interval prolongation and the U waves, these changes usually revert to normal within 2 weeks after the CNS event. Other less frequently observed EKG changes are increased amplitude of the P wave, development of Q waves, ST segment elevation, and T wave elevation, notching, or peaking. Differentiation between a centrally induced EKG abnormality and a true myocardial infarction may be difficult, but the patient must be cared for in a monitored setting until a "true" myocardial infarction is excluded. The EKG changes are thought to be due to a neurogenically mediated excessive release of catecholamines upon cardiac myocytes, resulting in myonecrotic changes. In fact, a higher level of serum catecholamines correlates with a poor outcome in patients with subarachnoid hemorrhage.

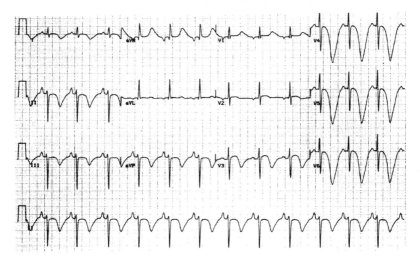

Electrocardiogram of a 41-year-old woman showing typical CNS changes of prolonged QT interval and deep, inverted, peaked T waves. These EKG changes were secondary to the traumatic basal ganglion hemorrhage shown on her CT scan (*see figure on following page*).

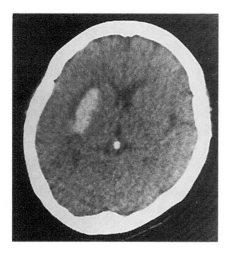

CT scan showing traumatic basal ganglion hemorrhage.

33. What is the relationship of changes in blood pressure to CNS disease?

Lesions of the hypothalamus and medulla oblongata or tumors of the posterior fossa may cause arterial hypertension. Ischemic, degenerative, or destructive lesions of the nucleus tractus solitarius in the medulla may result in chronic lability of blood pressure. Cushing's response of hypertension, bradycardia, and apnea, an important sign of increased intracranial pressure and potential herniation, also may develop after ischemic lesions of the dorsal medullary reticular formation along the floor of the fourth ventricle. Hypertension caused by posterior fossa tumors is due to the local distortion of the brainstem. Such an increase in blood pressure may be episodic and indistinguishable from a pheochromocytoma. Patients with normal-pressure hydrocephalus also may have chronic hypertension. Decreased blood pressure is rare with CNS disease, but orthostatic hypotension may accompany brainstem tumors, although the exact mechanism and the specific nuclei involved are not clear.

34. What autonomic dysfunctions occur following heart transplantation?

Heart or heart-lung transplantation results in afferent and efferent denervation (i.e., loss of autonomic control) of the transplanted organ with a relative resting tachycardia, little or no rise in heart rate after standing, and a delayed increase in heart rate in response to exercise. Also, there are no changes in heart rate with the Valsalva maneuver or carotid sinus massage. In general, the heart rate response in such patients depends on the circulating catecholamines. The resting tachycardia seen in severe autonomic neuropathies (e.g., diabetes) resembles that seen in a denervated transplanted heart.

35. Which neurologic conditions cause hypothermia?

Experimental studies suggest that lesions of the anterior hypothalamus cause hyperthermia, lesions of the posterior hypothalamus hypothermia, and lesions of the suprachiasmatic nucleus alteration in the circadian rhythm of temperature. Tumors and degenerative or inflammatory processes involving the hypothalamus may produce hypothermia (core body temperature below 35°C).

Wernicke's encephalopathy, by damaging the posterolateral hypothalamus and the floor of the fourth ventricle, may present with continuous hypothermia. Prompt treatment with thiamine results in normalization of temperature.

Shapiro's syndrome (agenesis of the corpus callosum) may be associated with episodic hypothermia and hyperhidrosis. Lesions of the posterior or anterior hypothalamus, infundibular nuclei, septal region, and cingulate gyrus may be seen on postmortem examination. Anticonvulsants, cyproheptadine, clonidine, or oxybutynin may control the hypothermia and diaphoresis.

36. What are the major differences between the syndrome of pure autonomic failure (PAF) and multiple-system atrophy (MSA)?

MSA, also called Shy-Drager syndrome, is associated with autonomic dysfunction, particularly orthostatic hypotension, and parkinsonian symptoms of akinesia and ridigity, leading to incapacity in a few years. Clinical variants of striatonigral degeneration (predominant symptoms = rigidity and dysarthria) and olivopontocerebellar atrophy (predominant symptoms = ataxia, incoordination, or bradykinesia) have been identified. PAF, also called idiopathic orthostatic hypotension and Bradbury-Eggleston syndrome, is an idiopathic sporadic disorder characterized by orthostatic hypotension, usually accompanied by evidence of more widespread autonomic failure. There are no other neurologic signs, and the natural history is slow progression over 10–15 years. Symptoms of autonomic dysfunction in MSA may precede the appearance of neurologic symptoms by up to 5 years. Accordingly, the diagnosis of PAF cannot be made with certainty until prolonged follow-up has been established.

37. Which autonomic dysfunctions occur in Parkinson's disease (PD)?

In the classic forms of PD, disturbances in salivation, sweating, and bladder and bowel functions may be seen. Some patients may have orthostatic dizziness, but a significantly lower resting or orthostatic blood pressure is usually not present. One should not overlook the possibility that orthostatic symptoms may result from dopaminergic agents used in treatment. The cardiovascular reflexes are generally preserved, although responses may be somewhat reduced. The resting recumbent levels of plasma NE are slightly lower than in healthy subjects. These subtle autonomic disturbances in PD are thought to be due to a central rather than a peripheral lesion. Of interest, however, Lewy bodies may be present in the sympathetic ganglia of patients with PD.

38. What are the most important genetic causes of autonomic failure?

1. Dopamine/beta-hydroxylase deficiency
2. Familial dysautonomia
3. Fabry's disease
4. Familial amyloidosis
5. Multiple endocrine neoplasia, type 2b
6. Porphyria

39. What is familial dysautonomia?

Familial dysautonomia (Riley-Day syndrome, hereditary sensory-autonomic neuropathy type III [HSAN-III]) is an autosomal recessive disorder affecting primarily people of Ashkenazi Jewish extraction. It is classified as one of the hereditary sensory autonomic neuropathies (HSAN), of which at least seven clinically and genetically distinct entitites have been identified. It affects the development and survival of sensory, sympathetic, and some parasympathetic neurons. The frequency of occurrence is 1 in 3,600 live briths among Ashkenazi Jews. The parents are usually unaffected, but less pronounced autonomic dysfunction has been reported in the parent of a son with familial dysautonomia. The location of the candidate gene has been narrowed to a small region on the long arm of chromosome 9. The identification of close flanking markers allows accurate genetic testing, prenatal diagnosis, and carrier identification.

40. What are the five cardinal clinical criteria for Riley-Day syndrome?

1. Alacrima
2. Absent fungiform papillae of tongue
3. Depressed patellar reflexes
4. Absent skin response to scratch and histamine injection
5. Pupillary hypersensitivity to parasympathomimetic agents

Supportive evidence includes relative insensitivity to pain and temperature, transient and emotionally induced erythematous skin blotching, orthostatic hypotension, hyperhidrosis or erratic sweating, and esophageal and GI transit dysfunction. Sural nerve biopsy reveals a markedly diminished number of unmyelinated and small-diameter myelinated axons.

41. What is Fabry's disease?

This X-linked recessive metabolic disease, also known as angiokeratoma corporis diffusum, is due to a deficiency of the lysosomal enzyme alpha-galactosidase, with resulting cell storage of the glycolipid ceramide trihexoside in several organs, including the skin (corpora angiokeratomas), kidneys, cardiovascular and pulmonary systems, blood vessels, and central and peripheral nervous systems. Because the neuropathy is prominent, the disease should be suspected in any boy or young man who presents with episodes of tender feet and painful burning sensation of the lower legs. Vascular disease develops at a young age, and many patients have a stroke or myocardial infarction before the age of 50. The posterior cerebral circulation appears more vulnerable, as suggested by the disproportionately high number of brainstem strokes in this population. The disease displays a remarkable genetic heterogeneity; more than 50 mutations in the alpha-galactosidase A gene have been identified.

Pathologically, there is a prominent lipid deposition in the dorsal root and peripheral autonomic ganglia, which are known to have fenestrated blood vessels and a permeable blood-nerve barrier. It appears that much of the stored ceramide trihexoside originates systemically and enters brain and nerve through permeable sites. Storage of lipids within central autonomic nuclei of the brainstem and spinal cord, areas protected by the blood-brain barrier, cannot be readily explained.

The clinical presentation of autonomic dysfunction includes diminished sweating (which may be due to lipid accumulation in sweat glands rather than neuropathy), absent skin wrinkling after immersion in warm water, reduced cutaneous flare response, reduced tear and saliva production, disturbed intestinal motility, abnormal cardiovascular responses, and abnormal pupillary response to pilocarpine. Responses to postural change and plasma NE levels are normal. Peripheral nerve pathology consists of degenerative changes of unmyelinated and small myelinated fibers. Successful renal transplantation corrects many of the abnormalities and increases survival. Intravenous infusion of alpha galactosidase appears to improve neuropathic pain, renal function, and glomerular pathology.

42. What is familial amyloidosis?

Hereditary amyloidosis is a heterogeneous group of familial diseases that have in common the systemic or localized accumulation of polypeptide amyloid fibrils arranged in beta-pleated sheets. Extracellular amyloid deposits result in disruption of normal tissue structure and function. Different subunits of proteins of 10–15 kda form the fibril structure, which has a beta configuration, giving the substance the property of birefringence. The chemical properties of different amyloid protein subunits, as determined by varied amino acid sequences, define the different amyloid diseases. In hereditary amyloidosis, the major component of subunit protein is a prealbumin (transthyretin), a normal constituent of plasma synthesized in the liver and choroid plexus. It is a tetramer composed of four identical subunits, each being a single polypeptide chain of 127 amino acid residues encoded by a single gene on human chromosome 18. It has no structural relationship to albumin and on electrophoresis migrates faster than albumin (hence, prealbumin). Unlike primary amyloidosis, the amyloid of hereditary amyloidosis is without light chains. Different mutants of the prealbumin protein with single amino acid substitutions are associated with most of the clinical varieties of systemic autosomal dominant amyloidosis. Although some of the mutations correlate with the clinical classification of amyloidosis, clinical pictures may overlap considerably. Future classification of hereditary amyloidosis will take into account the biochemical analysis of the condition.

Of more than 50 disease-causing mutations in the transthyretin gene, at least 20 are associated with autonomic dysfunction of differing severity. The autonomic dysfunction involves both sympathetic and parasympathetic systems. Late onset, predominant sensory symptoms, prominent early autonomic involvement, and frequent association with carpal tunnel syndrome should strongly favor the diagnosis of familial amyloidosis. Genetic testing for detection of Met 30 transthyretin mutation, the most common mutation, is now commercially available. The only treatment for familial amyloidosis is liver transplantation. When performed early in the course of the disease, it may stop clinical progression and modestly improve symptoms.

43. What is multiple endocrine neoplasia type 2b (MEN 2b)?

MEN 2b, an autosomal dominant inherited disorder, is characterized by multiple mucosal neuromas (conjunctivae, oral cavity, tongue, pharynx, and larynx), medullary thyroid carcinoma, pheochromocytoma, ganglioneuromatosis, bony deformities, marfanoid appearance, muscle underdevelopment, and hypotonia. Gross and microscopic abnormalities of the peripheral autonomic nervous system affect both sympathetic and parasympathetic systems. Patients have disorganized hypertrophy and proliferation of autonomic nerves and ganglia (ganglioneuromatosis). Neural proliferation of the alimentary tract (Auerbach and Meissner's plexi), upper respiratory tract, bladder, prostate, and skin also may be seen. The clinical autonomic manifestations include impaired lacrimation, orthostatic hypotension, impaired reflex vasodilation of the skin, and parasympathetic denervation supersensitivity of pupils, with intact sweating and salivary gland function. Nerve biopsy shows degeneration and regeneration of unmyelinated fibers. A few point mutations in the RET proto-oncogene located on chromosome 10 have been associated with the disease. Genetic testing is critical for detection of young carriers, who can undergo prophylactic thyroidectomy to prevent the development of medullary thyroid carcinoma

44. What is porphyria?

Acute hepatic porphyrias (acute intermittent porphyria, variegate porphyria, and hereditary coproporphyria) are autosomal dominant hereditary disorders that manifest as acute or subacute, severe, life-threatening neuropathy. The basic genetic defect is a 50% reduction in porphobilinogen deaminase activity (acute intermittent porphyria), protoporphyrinogen-IX oxidase (variegate porphyria), and coproporphyrinogen oxidase (coproporphyria), resulting in abnormalities of heme biosynthesis. In the presence of sufficient endogenous or exogenous stimuli (e.g., drugs, hormones, menstruation, starvation), this partial deficiency may lead to clinical manifestations, including peripheral neuropathy, autonomic dysfunction, skin symptoms, and CNS abnormalities.

Pathologic involvement of the autonomic nervous system (degeneration of the vagus nerve and sympathetic trunk) may explain certain features of acute attacks, including abdominal pain, severe vomiting, constipation, intestinal dilatation and stasis, persistent sinus tachycardia (100–160 minute), labile hypertension, postural hypotension, hyperhidrosis, and sphincteric bladder problems. Persistent tachycardia invariably precedes the development of peripheral neuropathy and respiratory paralysis and, along with labile hypertension, may be explained by vagus nerve damage. Tachycardia and hypertension may be associated with increased catecholamine release. It has been suggested that autonomic neurons may be more sensitive to the biochemical derangement of porphyria than are somatic neurons. Employment of a battery of baroreflex tests during the acute attack reveals mostly reversible parasympathetic and sympathetic dysfunction. The parasympathetic tests, however, become abnormal earlier and more frequently than the sympathetic tests. The heart rate variation with the Valsalva maneuver may be abnormal in asymptomatic subjects with acute intermittent porphyria.

Detailed studies of proximal GI tract motility and circulating gut peptide levels in acute intermittent porphyria suggest that the characteristic but rarely reversible disturbances of gut motor activity are due to autonomic and/or enteric nerve damage.

45. What are the most important factors in the maintenance of normal blood pressure?

1. Blood volume
2. Vascular reflexes (e.g., reflex arteriolar-venous constriction, baroreflex-induced tachycardia, and cerebellar reflexes)
3. Hormonal mechanisms (e.g., increased plasma catecholamines, renin-angiotensin-aldosterone system, arginine-vasopressin, atrial natriuretic factor)

46. What age-related physiologic changes predispose to hypotension?

Decreased baroreflex sensitivity, impaired neuroendocrine response to changes of intravascular volume (e.g., reduced secretion of renin, angiotensin, and aldosterone) and impaired early cardiac ventricular filling (diastolic dysfunction).

47. What are the baroreceptors? What is their significance?

Baroreceptors are spray-type nerve endings in the walls of blood vessels and the heart that are stimulated by the absolute level of, and changes in, arterial pressure. They are extremely abundant in the wall of the bifurcation of the internal carotid arteries (carotid sinus) and in the wall of the aortic arch. The primary site of termination of baroreceptor afferent fibers is the NTS, but the afferent fibers of the carotid sinus, carried by the glossopharyngeal nerve, terminate more caudally near the obex.

The function of the baroreceptors is to maintain systemic blood pressure at a relatively constant level, especially during a change in body position. The system, in general, reduces daily variation in arterial pressure by approximately one-half to one-third of that which would occur if the baroreceptor systems were absent. The relative influence of the carotid sinus and aortic arch baroreceptors on the control of blood pressure is debatable, but data obtained from direct sympathetic nerve recordings in humans indicate that the aortic baroreflex is a more important regulator of efferent sympathetic responses during acute hypotension in healthy subjects than are carotid sinus baroreflexes. Intact baroreceptors are extremely effective in preventing rapid changes in blood pressure from moment to moment or hour to hour, but because of their adaptability to prolonged changes of blood pressure (> 2 or 3 days), the system is incapable of long-term regulation of arterial pressure.

Baroreceptors are activated with each arterial pulse wave, and their rate of firing increases with raised arterial pressure and decreases when arterial pressure falls. Stretching of baroreceptors causes them to transmit signals to the NTS, resulting in efferent discharges via sympathetic (decreased signal) and parasympathetic (increased signal) systems to the decreased cardiac output. In executing such a complex reflex function, several groups of excitatory and inhibitory chemical messengers play major roles, including amino acids (L-glutamate, gamma-aminobutyric acid [GABA], and glycine), monoamines (norepinephrine, epinephrine, dopamine, serotonin, histamine, and acetylcholine), and neuropeptides. Information obtained largely from experimental animals indicates that inhibition of sympathoexcitatory neurons in the rostral NTS is mediated by GABAergic or noradrenergic mechanisms, whereas L-glutamate is a likely candidate as a primary neurotransmitter for excitatory inputs from these neurons. The monoamines and neuropeptides act mostly as modulators via the descending pathways, setting the level of excitability of sympathetic preganglionic neurons. Interruption of these pathways (e.g., cervical cord transection) results in release of these neurons from suprasegmental control of baroreflexes (autonomic hyperreflexia of chronic tetraplegics).

48. How is baroreceptor function evaluated?

The evaluation of arterial and cardiopulmonary baroreflex function in the clinical setting is indirect and therefore imprecise. Interpretation of overall baroreflex function based on any single test should be cautious unless an abnormality is gross. When different techniques are compared, the correlation is often poor. Apart from disease states, baroreflexes also may be depressed in old age due to both decreased arterial wall distensibility and degenerative changes of the baroreflex arc nerves. During sleep, the baroreflex activity is increased so that arterial blood pressure tends to fall. Four noninvasive tests of baroreflex function have emerged as most popular and fairly reliable. There is agreement that these tests and other noninvasive cardiovascular reflex tests can provide objective evidence of autonomic involvement:

1. Beat-to-beat heart rate variation
2. Heart rate response to the Valsalva maneuver
3. Heart rate and blood pressure response to standing
4. Blood pressure response to sustained hand grip

49. What is the basis for the beat-to-beat heart rate test?

Normally inspiration increases heart rate and expiration decreases it (sinus arrhythmia). This phenomenon is mediated primarily by the vagus nerve; pulmonary stretch receptors and cardiac mechanoreceptors as well as baroreceptors contribute to its generation. The variation of heart rate in inspiration and expiration is age-dependent and is reduced in elderly people (e.g., normal maximal-to-minimal variation in people 10–40 years old is > 18 beats per minute, but in people 61–70 years old it declines to > 8 beats per minute). The test is easy to perform with a commercial EKG machine or appropriately set EMG equipment. While supine (head elevated to 30°), the patient breathes deeply at 6 respirations per minute, and minimal and maximal heart rate within each respiratory cycle (5 seconds inspiration followed by 5 seconds expiration) is measured. The longest R-R interval on EKG (slow heart rate) is divided by the shortest R-R interval (fast heart rate), and the expiration-to-inspiration (E:I) ratio is determined. Normal values for 16–20 year olds are more than 1.23; for 76–80 year olds, more than 1.05. An abnormal test indicates parasympathetic dysfunction.

50. What is the difference in orthostatic hypotension caused by autonomic dysfunction and that caused by hypovolemia?
   In most autonomic neuropathies associated with orthostatic hypotension, failure of vascular reflexes to increase sympathetic outflow to splanchnic and muscular vasculature results in a drop in both systolic and diastolic pressures. However, there is no increase in plasma norepinephrine (hypoadrenergic response). Conversely, in orthostatic hypotension secondary to hypovolemia, plasma norepinephrine increases excessively in response to standing (hyperadrenergic response).
   In orthostatic hypotension secondary to generalized sympathetic failure, a drop in systolic blood pressure is not associated with reflex tachycardia, whereas in orthostatic hypotension secondary to hypovolemia or deconditioning, with intact sympathetic nerves, reflex tachycardia is prominent. A fall in systolic pressure alone is most likely caused by a nonneurologic disturbance (e.g., hypovolemia).

51. What are the three main mechanisms of syncope?
   1. **Orthostatic hypotension** may be due to a reduction in vascular resistance, hypovolemia (or both), drugs, chronic baroreflex failure, or a neurally mediated mechanism (vasovagal syncope triggered by pain or fear). Reflex syncope and vasodepressor syncope are synonymous with vasovagal syncope.
   2. **Fall in cardiac output** may be due to cardiac arrhythmias, obstructions to flow, or myocardial infarction.
   3. **Increased cerebrovascular resistance** may be due to hyperventilation or increased intracranial pressure.

52. What general advice should you give to a patient with orthostatic hypotension secondary to dysautonomia?
   1. Avoid straining, which results in the Valsalva maneuvers, by treating and preventing constipation with a high-fiber diet.
   2. Avoid severe diurnal variation, particularly morning postural hypotension, by head-up tilt or sleeping in a sitting position at night, sitting for several minutes at the edge of the bed before standing, shaving while sitting, or immediately assuming a squatting position, crossing the legs, bending forward and placing the head between the knees, or placing one foot on a chair when presyncopal symptoms occur.
   3. Avoid exposure to a warm environment to prevent uncompensated vasodilation (e.g., travel to warm countries, hot baths).
   4. Avoid postprandial aggravation of orthostatic hypotension by eating smaller and more frequent meals with a reduced carbohydrate content.
   5. Avoid a low-sodium diet by increasing the food sodium content to at least 150 mEq.
   6. Avoid dehydration by increasing fluid intake to 2.0–2.5 L/day.
   7. Avoid vigorous exercise; moderate isotonic exercises are preferable to isometrics.
   8. Avoid prolonged recumbency.
   9. Avoid vasodilators such as alcohol.
   10. Avoid drugs known to cause vasodilation and/or bradycardia (nitroglycerin or beta blockers).

53. What are the most important nonneurogenic causes of orthostatic hypotension?

1. Volume loss (e.g., bleeding, burns)
2. Dehydration and electrolyte disturbances (e.g., vomiting, diarrhea, adrenal insufficiency, diuretic use)
3. Vasodilation (e.g., vasodilator drugs, heat, alcohol, varicose veins, hyperbradykininism)
4. Cardiac diseases (aortic stenosis, atrial myxoma, pericarditis, myocarditis)

54. What is postural tachycardia syndrome (POTS)? How is it treated?

This increasingly recognized condition, often observed in females aged 15–50, is defined as a syndrome of consistent orthostatic symptoms associated with an excessive heart rate increase of 30 beats/minute or greater within 5 minutes of standing or tilt-up. The heart rate is usually equal to or greater than 120 beats/minute after 5 minutes of standing. There is only a minimal or no drop in blood pressure after standing, but the patient feels many of the orthostatic symptoms, including dizziness, fatigue, tremulousness, palpitations, nausea, vasomotor skin changes, hyperhidrosis, or chest wall pain. Some patients have a history of an antecedent viral infection. Standing plasma norepinephrine levels may be increased. Some patients with the diagnosis of chronic fatigue syndrome or anxiety or panic disorder may instead have POTS, especially if their symptoms are consistently reproduced after standing and cease after assuming a recumbent position.

The exact etiology of POTS has remained elusive, but a partial autonomic dysfunction, resulting from sympathetic denervation limited to the lower limbs, is suspected. Treatment options include increased intake of fluids and salt (to increase blood volume), fludrocortisone, midodrine, α_1-adrenergic agonists (which induce vasoconstriction), and measures to reduce blood pooling in the legs.

Jacob J, Costa F, Shannon JR, et al: The neuropathic postural tachycardia syndrome. N Engl J Med 343:1008–1014, 2000.

55. What cardiovascular autonomic changes are seen during rapid eye movement (REM) sleep?

During REM sleep sympathetic activity of the splanchnic and renal circulation is decreased, but activity by skeletal muscles is increased. Whereas the slow phases of sleep are accompanied by hypotension and bradycardia, which become increasingly more pronounced with the progression of sleep from stage 1 to stage 4, REM sleep is associated with large, transient increases in blood pressure, reversing the hypotension of slow-wave sleep. Direct recording of sympathetic nerve traffic to the skeletal-muscle vascular bed by microneurography shows more than a 50% reduction in sympathetic activity during the slow phases of sleep but a significant increase to the level of wakefulness during REM. This finding may suggest that slow-wave sleep provides a protective effect on the cardiovascular and cerebrovascular systems; during REM sleep or immediately afterward, such protective effects may disappear. This phenomenon may explain why cardiovascular and cerebrovascular events occur more frequently in the early morning hours after awakening.

Somers VK, Dyken ME, Mark AL, Abboud FM: Sympathetic-nerve activity during sleep in normal subjects. N Engl J Med 328:303, 1993.

56. Why does skin turn red (flare) after it is scratched?

The normal skin axon-reflex vasodilation (flare) follows skin stimulation from a simple scratch. The scratch causes activation of unmyelinated sensory nerve terminals (C fibers). The impulse generated by this stimulus travels antidromically, reaches a branch point, then orthodromically arrives at a skin blood vessel, releasing one or more vasodilating peptides or adenosine triphosphate (ATP). The released substance leads to further histamine release, activating other sensory terminals, creating a cascade of spreading flare response. Released histamine also causes itching. Both the flare response and the itching may be reduced by antihistamines. The absence of a flare response provides evidence of dysfunction of unmyelinated sensory fibers in peripheral neuropathies.

57. What is a sudomotor axon reflex?

The sudomotor axon reflex employs the same mechanism as the skin axon-reflex flare, but the neural pathway consists of an axon reflex mediated by the postganglionic sympathetic axon (C fibers) that innervates sweat glands. The axon terminals of these fibers are activated by the local injection of acetylcholine: the generated impulse travels to a branch point where it is deflected and then travels orthodromically to activate a different sweat gland, releasing acetylcholine, which binds to M3 muscarinic receptors. In other words, in the sudomotor axon reflex the activation of sweat glands results in the reflex activation of another population of nearby glands, the sweat output of which can be quantitatively measured. The quantitative sudomotor axon-reflex test (Q-SART) is, therefore, a sensitive and reproducible test of the integrity of the postganglionic sympathetic sudomotor axon.

58. There is a higher incidence of sudomotor and vasomotor disturbances of the arm with injuries to the lower trunk of the brachial plexus than with injuries to the upper trunk. Why?

There is a higher density of postganglionic sympathetic fibers in the medial cord of the brachial plexus and the median and ulnar nerves.

59. During examination of the external ear canal with an otoscope, the patient developed dry cough and became dizzy. Why?

There is an anatomic explanation. The second branch of the vagus nerve, the auricular nerve, which originates after the vagus nerve has exited from the jugular foramen, is a somatic afferent nerve that provides the sensory fibers for the posterior wall and floor of the external acoustic meatus and the outer surface of the tympanic membrane. Irritation of the external auditory canal and the tympanic membrane by instruments, cerumen, or syringing may therefore cause abnormal vagal reflexes, resulting in coughing, vomiting, slow heart rate, or even cardiac inhibition.

60. What is the syndrome of autonomic dysreflexia observed in tetraplegics?

Traumatic spinal cord lesions result in markedly abnormal cardiovascular, thermoregulatory, bladder, bowel, and sexual function. In a recently injured tetraplegic in spinal shock, tactile or painful stimuli originating below the level of the lesion induce no change in blood pressure or heart rate. In the chronic stages of spinal cord injury at a level above T5, however, there is an exaggerated rise in the systolic and diastolic blood pressure, accompanied by bradycardia. Transient tachycardia may precede the drop in heart rate. The plasma norepinephrine levels are only marginally elevated. The marked hypertension may lead to neurologic complications, including seizures, visual defects, and cerebral hemorrhage. This phenomenon, called autonomic dysreflexia, is caused by the increased activity of target organs below the lesion supplied by sympathetic and parasympathetic nerves lacking supraspinal modulation. Other clinical manifestations of autonomic dysreflexia include headache, chest tightness and dyspnea, pupillary dilation, cold limbs, flushing of face and neck, excessive sweating of the head, penile erection and discharge of seminal fluid, and contraction of bladder and bowel.

61. What is the best management of autonomic dysreflexia?

The prolonged episodes of this syndrome may be prevented if the precipitating cause (e.g., painful tactile or visceral urinary and rectal stimuli) are corrected. It is important that the bladder be emptied before performing any procedure on tetraplegics. Blood pressure can often be decreased by elevating the head of the bed. Clonidine, an alpha$_2$ and imidazoline receptor agonist, acting at the level of the medulla, is useful in prophylaxis of autonomic dysreflexia.

62. What are the pathologic causes of hyperhidrosis? How is it treated?

Spinal cord damage or lesions of the peripheral sympathetic nerves may cause localized hyperhidrosis. **Generalized and episodic hyperhidrosis** may occur in patients with infectious diseases (night sweats), malignancies, hypoglycemia, thyrotoxicosis, pheochromocytomas, carcinoid syndrome, acromegaly, or diencephalic epilepsy and in patients receiving cholinergic agents.

Primary or essential hyperhidrosis usually involves limited areas of the body, particularly the axilla, palms, and plantar regions. Axillary hyperhidrosis predominantly affects younger people and may cause social embarrassment. Essential hyperhidrosis is, however, usually self-limiting by the fourth or fifth decade of life. There is no known cause for essential hyperhidrosis, but up to one-half of patients have a family history of a similar condition. Several studies have demonstrated no abnormalities of the sweat glands and have implicated central and preganglionic sympathetic pathway hyperactivity.

The treatment of essential generalized hyperhidrosis is difficult and requires systemic pharmacotherapy (anticholinergics and diltiazem), topical agents (aluminum chloride), excision of axillary sweat glands, and sympathectomy as the last resort. Recent experience suggests that botulinum toxin injections are a safe and effective treatment for focal or localized hyperhidrosis.

63. How may mastocytosis be confused with autonomic dysfunction?

Mastocytosis, i.e., abnormal proliferation of tissue mast cells, may be confused with autonomic dysfunction because of symptoms of flushing, palpitation, dyspnea, chest discomfort, headache, light-headedness and dizziness, fall in blood pressure, nausea, abdominal cramps, and diarrhea, which occur episodically. Some patients may have an elevation of blood pressure. Each attack is followed by profound lethargy and fatigue. Episodes may be brief, lasting several minutes, or protracted, lasting 2–3 hours. Exposure to heat or emotional or physical stress may precipitate an attack. Flushing and warm sensations are the most important clues differentiating this syndrome from syndromes of orthostatic intolerance.

In adults there are two main forms of abnormal proliferation of mast cells: cutaneous mastocytosis and systemic mastocytosis. Some patients may experience episodes of systemic mast cell activation but show no evidence of mast cell proliferation in the skin or bone marrow. During an attack, increased serum histamine and prostaglandin D_2 may be demonstrated. Pigmented cutaneous lesions (urticaria pigmentosa) that characteristically urticate when stroked (Darier's sign) are frequently observed. Some patients with systemic mast cell activation are hypersensitive to aspirin, and any prostaglandin inhibitor may provoke severe mast cell activation.

64. When your attending pimps you on rounds, why do you get sweaty palms but not sweaty armpits?

Anxiety and emotional stress primarily aggravate the hyperhidrosis of the palms and soles, but not of the axilla. The eccrine sweat glands of the palms and soles, as well as those of the forehead, respond to emotional, mental, or sensory stimuli, whereas the axillary glands respond primarily to thermal stimuli.

BIBLIOGRAPHY

1. Appenzeller O, Oribe E: The Autonomic Nervous System. Amsterdam, Elsevier, 1997.
2. Bannister R, Mathias C: Autonomic Failure, 3rd ed. Oxford, Oxford University Press, 1992.
3. Harati Y: Diabetes and the autonomic nervous system. In Appenzeller O (ed): The Autonomic Nervous System, Part II, Revised series 31. Amsterdam, Elsevier, 2000.
4. Low PA: Clinical Autonomic Disorders, 2nd ed. Philadelphia, Lippincott-Raven, 1997.
5. Robertson D, Low PA, Polinsky RJ: Primer on the Autonomic Nervous System. San Diego, Academic Press, 1996.
Websites
www.ninds.nih.gov/health_and_medical/disorders/syncope
www.mdausa.org/disease/les.html

13. DEMYELINATING DISEASE

Loren A. Rolak, M.D.

1. What is myelin?

Myelin is the proteolipid membrane that ensheathes and surrounds nerve axons to improve their ability to conduct electrical action potentials. Oligodendrocytes make myelin and wrap it around axons, leaving gaps called nodes of Ranvier, where membrane ionic channels are heavily concentrated and powerful action potentials can thus be generated.

2. How does demyelination cause symptoms?

When myelin is stripped away from the axon, the underlying membrane does not contain a high enough concentration of sodium, potassium, and other ionic channels to permit a sufficient flow of ions to cause depolarization. The membrane thus becomes inert. The loss of myelin makes it impossible to depolarize the membrane to conduct an action potential, so the nerve is rendered useless.

3. What is multiple sclerosis? What is its incidence?

Multiple sclerosis (MS) is the most common condition that destroys myelin in the central nervous system. It affects approximately 250,000 Americans, mostly between the ages of 20 and 40, making it the leading disabling neurologic disease of young people.

4. How does MS cause demyelination?

MS is an inflammatory disease. Lymphocytes, macrophages, and other immunocompetent cells accumulate around venules in the central nervous system and exit into the brain, attacking and destroying the myelin.

5. Are there other demyelinating diseases?

Yes, but they are rare. MS is the only common demyelinating disease in adults. Other rare conditions include:

1. **Central pontine myelinolysis**, a syndrome of myelin destruction in the pons, associated with rapid correction of hyponatremia.

2. **Progressive multifocal leukoencephalopathy**, an opportunistic viral infection of oligodendrocytes, seen most often in patients with acquired immunodeficiency syndrome (AIDS).

3. **Acute disseminated encephalomyelitis**, a postinfectious, acute, autoimmune demyelination.

4. **Inborn errors of myelin metabolism**, usually presenting in childhood:
   • Metachromatic leukodystrophy, a deficiency of the enzyme aryl sulfatase
   • Adrenoleukodystrophy, a defect in metabolism of very long chain fatty acids
   • Krabbe's globoid leukodystrophy, a deficiency of the enzyme galactosylceramidase

O'Riordan JI: Central nervous system white matter diseases other than multiple sclerosis. Curr Opin Neurol 10:211–214, 1997.

CLINICAL FEATURES OF MULTIPLE SCLEROSIS

6. What are the most common symptoms of MS?

1. Pyramidal weakness	45%
2. Visual loss	40%
3. Sensory loss	35%
4. Brainstem dysfunction	30%

5. Cerebellar ataxia and tremor   25%
6. Sphincter disturbances   20%

7. What is the relationship of optic neuritis to MS?

A patient presenting with acute inflammatory demyelination of the optic nerve (optic neuritis) has approximately a 30–60% chance of suffering further demyelinating episodes in the CNS—i.e., of developing clinical MS. The strongest predictive factor for subsequent development of MS is an abnormal magnetic resonance imaging (MRI) study of the brain at initial presentation. An analogous argument applies to monophasic demyelination of the spinal cord—transverse myelitis.

8. Are there any symptoms that MS does not cause?

Not many. Virtually every neurologic problem has been described in MS, at least as a case report. However, because MS is a disease of myelin (white matter), it rarely causes neuronal (gray matter) symptoms. Uncommon symptoms include dementia, aphasia, seizures, pain, and movement disorders.

9. What is the clinical course of MS?

MRI studies show that inflammatory demyelinating lesions appear and disappear almost constantly in patients with MS, but very few of these lesions (in some patients only 1–2%) ever cause symptoms. The clinical course of MS is highly variable and can follow almost any pattern, but most patients are pigeon-holed into one of four types:

1. **Relapsing–remitting.** Patients have the sudden onset (over hours or days) of neurologic symptoms that usually last several weeks and then resolve, often leaving few or no deficits. The frequency of clinical attacks is highly variable but averages about one per year.

2. **Secondary progressive.** After an initial relapsing–remitting course, most patients gradually develop progressive disability without further acute relapses. The transition from a relapsing–remitting course to a secondary progressive course takes about 10 years.

3. **Primary progressive.** Approximately 15% of patients have progressive symptoms from the onset, which are not preceded by acute relapses. Such patients are often older and have spinal cord symptoms.

4. **Progressive relapsing.** Rare patients have progressive disease punctuated by acute relapses.

Confaureux C, Vukusic S, Moreau T, Adeleine P: Relapses and progression of disability in multiple sclerosis. N Engl J Med 343:1430–1433, 2000.

10. What is the prognosis of MS?

MS varies greatly, not only in its symptoms and clinical course, but also in its prognosis. Although not a fatal disease, MS is associated with a slight statistical shortening of lifespan as a result of secondary complications that may afflict severe cases, such as aspiration pneumonia, decubitus ulcers, urinary tract infections, and falls. As a general rule, approximately one-third of patients with MS do well throughout their life, without accumulating significant disability. Another one-third accumulate neurologic deficits sufficient to impair activities but not serious enough to prevent them from leading a normal life—holding a job, raising a family. The final third of people with MS become disabled, requiring a walker, wheelchair, or even total care.

11. What factors help to predict the course of MS?

The variability of MS makes accurate prediction fallible, but a few factors portend a good prognosis:

1. Early age of onset (first symptoms before age 40)
2. Sensory symptoms at onset (as opposed to weakness, ataxia, or other motor abnormalities)
3. Pattern of exacerbations and remissions (vs. a primary progressive symptom at onset)
4. Female gender. Women do better than men.

Rolak LA: Multiple sclerosis. In Evans R (ed): Prognosis of Neurological Disorders. New York, Oxford University Press, 1992, pp 295–300.

DIAGNOSIS

12. Given the great variability in the signs, symptoms, and clinical course of MS, how can it be accurately diagnosed?

The diagnosis of MS is one of the most difficult in neurology. Nevertheless, careful analysis has shown that certain clinical criteria can accurately diagnose MS.

Clinical Criteria for Definite Multiple Sclerosis

1. Two separate central nervous system symptoms.
2. Two separate attacks—onset of symptoms is separated by at least 1 month.
3. Symptoms must involve the white matter.
4. Age 10–50 (although usually 20–40)
5. Objective deficits are present on the neurologic examination.
6. No other medical problem can be found to explain the patient's condition.

The key to the clinical criteria for the diagnosis of MS is two separate symptoms at two separate times, or lesions disseminated in space and in time.

13. Are laboratory tests useful for diagnosing MS?

Yes—in the proper setting and with proper caution. The diagnosis of MS is seldom made without some laboratory support, especially in patients who do not quite meet all of the clinical criteria. However, no one test proves the diagnosis, and all laboratory data have sufficient problems with sensitivity and specificity to impair their usefulness.

Rolak L: The diagnosis of multiple sclerosis. Neurol Clin 14:27–43, 1996.

14. How can the cerebrospinal fluid (CSF) be used to diagnose MS?

Immunoglobulins are increased in the central nervous system in patients with MS, and the CSF often reflects elevations of both total IgG and IgG synthesis rates. Also, when the IgG is examined by electrophoresis, it may clump together in specific bands. The finding of several of these bands in the IgG region, called oligoclonal bands, is reasonably sensitive and specific for MS. However, it remains unclear how or why oligoclonal bands are produced or exactly what they represent.

15. Do other diseases have oligoclonal bands?

Yes, especially inflammatory conditions, such as syphilis, meningoencephalitis, and subacute sclerosing panencephalitis (SSPE, a latent measles infection), and autoimmune processes such as Guillain-Barré syndrome.

16. How are evoked potentials used to assist in the diagnosis of MS?

Because evoked potentials measure conduction through the central nervous system, they reveal areas of demyelination by showing slowed conduction through pathways where the myelin has been damaged. MS is the most common cause of a slowing detected by evoked potentials.

17. What are the evoked potentials usually used to diagnose MS?

1. **Visual evoked potentials** (VEPs) are performed by flashing a checkered pattern in the patient's eyes while recording the electrical response from the visual cortex in the occipital lobe. Normally, a response appears approximately 100 ms after the stimulus is presented to the eye, and a delay implies demyelination in the visual pathways.

2. **Brainstem auditory evoked potentials** (BAEPs) are performed by giving an auditory stimulus in the ear, such as a clicking sound, while recording from the auditory cortex in the temporal lobe. The sound generates a series of waves as it travels through the brainstem and hemispheres, and a delay in these waves is presumptive evidence of a demyelinating slowing.

3. **Somatosensory evoked potentials** (SSEPs) are performed by applying an electrical stimulus to the wrist or ankle while recording from the sensory area of the cortex. Slowing can often be detected in the spinal cord, brainstem, or hemispheres.

18. How valuable are evoked potentials for diagnosing MS?

Studies disagree considerably, but probably about 75% of people with definite MS have an abnormal VEP; about 50% have abnormal SSEPs. BAEPs are abnormal in about 25%. Most of these patients also have an abnormal MRI scan, however, so evoked potentials seldom add much to the diagnosis.

Gronseth GS, Ashman EJ: Practice parameter: The usefulness of evoked potentials in identifying clinically silent lesions in patients with suspected multiple sclerosis. Neurology 54:1720–1725, 2000.

19. How is MRI used to diagnose MS?

MRI shows abnormalities in at least 80% of patients with MS. Because of its sensitivity and noninvasive nature, MRI has become the most common procedure to confirm the diagnosis of MS. The drawback to MRI is its lack of specificity. Unfortunately, the scattered subcortical periventricular white matter abnormalities that characterize MS may occur in various other settings, including cerebrovascular disease, vasculitis, migraine, hypertension, and some subjects who appear to be normal. For this reason, reliance strictly on MRI may lead to overdiagnosis of MS.

Pirtilla T, Nurmikko T: CSF oligoclonal bands, MRI, and the diagnosis of multiple sclerosis. Acta Neurol Scand 92:468–471, 1995.

Wallace CJ, Sevick RJ: Multifocal white matter lesions. Semin Ultrasound CT MRI 17:251–264, 1996.

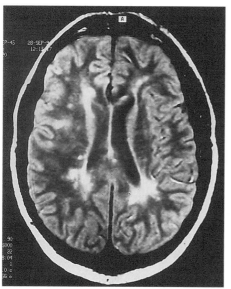

Axial flair MRI of the brain shows typical confluent, deep white matter signal intensities characteristic of MS.

ETIOLOGY

20. How does the epidemiology of MS provide clues to its cause?

Some unusual features characterize the epidemiology of MS. MS is more common the farther one moves away from the equator. Although MS is virtually unheard of in the tropics, its incidence is approximately 1 per 1,000 in in Northern Scotland, Scandinavia, and Iceland.

It most frequently afflicts high socioeconomic classes, such as literate, educated professionals. It is more common in women than men by a ratio of at least 3:2. It primarily strikes people of northern European ancestry and is almost unknown in other racial groups such as Eskimos and gypsies. This finding may be related to specific human leukocyte anigen (HLA) type (i.e., immune functions).

The chance of developing MS seems to be set by approximately age 15. A person born in a high-risk area (such as Scandinavia) who leaves for a low-risk area (in the tropics) after age 15 will carry the high risk for developing MS. A person who emigrates before age 15 acquires the low risk of the new home. In short, the risk of MS is determined before age 15, even though the disease itself does not appear, on average, until age 30. Unfortunately, none of these tantalizing epidemiologic findings has yet led to a coherent hypothesis for the etiology of MS.

Hogancamp WE, Rodriguez M, Weinshenker BG: The epidemiology of multiple sclerosis. Mayo Clin Proc 72:871–878, 1997.

21. What evidence suggests that MS is an autoimmune disease?

1. Pathologically, MS is an inflammatory disease involving lymphocytes and other immuno-competent cells.

2. MS is most common in patients with certain HLA types, implying that genes that control the immune system are related to the development of MS.

3. Oligoclonal bands in the CSF imply an abnormality in the immune system.

4. T-cell subsets are abnormal in MS. Most researchers report decreased numbers of suppressor T-lymphocytes.

5. The animal model of MS, experimental autoimmune encephalomyelitis (EAE), is an immune-mediated disease. Animals injected with myelin basic protein and immune adjuvants can be induced to mount an immune response against the myelin antigens, which cross-reacts and damages their own myelin.

Rolak LA: Multiple sclerosis. In Rolak L, Harati Y (eds): Neuro-immunology for the Clinician. Boston, Butterworth-Heinemann, 1997, pp 107–132.

22. What evidence suggests that MS is a viral disease?

1. MS is more common in certain parts of the world than others, suggesting an environmental factor. A virus could be this environmental factor.

2. Viral demyelinating diseases are known in animals, some of which serve as a model for MS. Canine distemper virus and Theiler's virus are examples of viral models of MS.

3. Latent viruses and slow viruses are well known in the human central nervous system, fitting the epidemiologic data that suggest latent and relapsing disease as a feature of MS.

4. The immune system in patients with MS reacts abnormally to viral antigens. This is true of both humoral (antibodies) and cell-mediated immunity.

23. Is MS all one disease?

That is not clear. Clinically, it is quite heterogeneous, and, pathologically, it may be also. New immunopathologic techniques suggest that there may be different patterns of demyelination and immune activation among different patients.

Luchinetti C, Bruck W, Parisi J, et al: Heterogeneity of multiple sclerosis lesions: Implications for the pathogenesis of demyelination. Ann Neurol 47:707–717, 2000.

TREATMENT

24. What is the role of steroids in MS?

A number of studies have indicated that steroids are superior to placebo for alleviating attacks of MS. Symptoms resolve more quickly, although it is not clear if treatment of attacks will ultimately prevent disability or mitigate the final outcome of the disease. There remains much controversy about the most appropriate steroid preparation, dosage, route of administration, and duration of treatment.

25. What is the usual steroid regimen in MS?

The most popular therapy now employs intravenous methylprednisolone (Solu–Medrol) in a dose of 500–1000 mg daily for 3–7 days. This "pulse" of steroids is effective, at least in the short term, for improving MS symptoms.

26. What is the role of immunosuppressants in MS?

Many immune-altering regimens have been used in MS, but prospective, randomized, blinded, controlled, multicentered trials have been few and disappointing. Nevertheless, drugs such as cyclophosphamide, azathioprine, methotrexate, and intravenous immunoglobulin are still occasionally used because of their theoretical benefits for immune-mediated diseases and because of the desperate disabilities in some young people with MS.

Mitoxantrone (Novantrone), a broad-spectrum immunosuppressant, can slow the accumulation of disability in secondary progressive MS and is the best available treatment for that form of the disease. However, its benefits are modest, and its cardiotoxicity is considerable. Thus, its therapeutic role is limited.

Rudick RA, Cohen JA, Weinstock-Guttman B, et al: Management of multiple sclerosis. N Engl J Med 337:1604–1611, 1997.

27. What prophylactic drugs are available to decrease attacks of MS?

There is no cure for MS, but three drugs have been approved in the United States to reduce the rate of attacks in relapsing–remitting MS. They seem about equally effective, decreasing attacks by approximately 30%:

1. **Beta-interferon-1b** (Betaseron)—differs from natural human interferon by a single amino acid. It is given in a dose of 8 million units subcutaneously every other day but produces flulike side effects in a substantial number of patients.

2. **Beta-interferon-1a** (Avonex)—identical to Betaseron except for one amino acid and added glycosylation. It is unclear to what extent Avonex is really a different drug from Betaseron, but the dosage is different (6 million units/week intramuscularly). It causes the same flulike symptoms.

3. **Glatiramer acetate** (Copaxone)—a synthetic polypeptide resembling a fragment of myelin basic protein. The dose is 20 mg/day subcutaneously, which causes no systemic side effects.

Rolak LA: New prophylactic treatments for multiple sclerosis. Drugs Today 33:175–182, 1997.

28. What is the best drug to prevent attacks of MS?

There is no consensus about which of the three drugs is superior or even which patients with MS should be treated at all, although most patients with relapsing–remitting disease are started on therapy. The mechanism of action is not definitely known for any of the drugs, and none has yet been proved to reduce long-term disability significantly. The choice of therapy thus depends largely on convenience, toxicity, and personal preferences of doctors and patients.

Rolak LA: Multiple sclerosis. Neurol Clin North Am 19:107–118, 2001.

SYMPTOMATIC TREATMENT

29. What is the role of symptomatic treatments for MS?

If MS were cured today, the many sufferers from the disease would still have neurologic deficits. Management of these deficits is an important part of the treatment of MS. The most disabling symptoms reported by patients are fatigue, motor deficits, cerebellar problems, and sphincter disturbance.

30. What is the best treatment for fatigue in MS?

Although fatigue seems to be a vague and subjective symptom, it is one of the leading reasons for inability to work among MS victims. Amantadine has been shown in careful studies to reduce fatigue, usually in doses of 100 mg twice daily, and is the mainstay of treatment. Modafinil and selective serotonin reuptake inhibitors such as fluoxetine are also prescribed, but without much scientific basis. Pemoline (Cylert), a mild stimulant, is often used but has not been proved effective. Of course, simple commonsense measures are also useful, such as resting during the day and reorganizing the home and workplace for better efficiency.

Rolak LA: Fatigue and multiple sclerosis. In Dawson DM, Stabin TD (eds): Chronic Fatigue Syndrome. Boston, Little, Brown, 1993, pp 153–161.

31. What is the best treatment for motor deficits in MS?

Unfortunately, little can be done to restore muscle strength. However, spasticity often improves with the use of baclofen (Lioresal) in doses of 60 mg/day or more. Tizanidine (Zanaflex), given up to 8 mg four times/day, produces similarly potent muscle relaxation. Dantrolene (Dantrium) and diazepam (Valium) are also useful oral antispasticity agents, although their side effects make them less attractive as first-line drugs. Physical therapy can also minimize spasticity.

Nance PW: Tizanidine: An alpha-agonist imidazole with antispasticity effects. Ther Trends 15:11–25, 1997.

32. What is the best treatment for cerebellar tremor and ataxia in MS?

Therapy for cerebellar deficits is frustrating—these are among the most difficult symptoms to alleviate. Sometimes simple mechanical measures are helpful, such as attaching weights to the ankles or wrists. Drug treatment usually focuses on agents that increase levels of gamma-aminobutyric acid (GABA), which is the primary neurotransmitter of the cerebellum. Benzodiazepines such as clonazepam (Klonopin) may help in a dose of 0.5 mg or more twice daily. Other agents that increase GABA include valproic acid (Depakote) in the usual anticonvulsant doses and isoniazid, which must be used in high doses of 900–1200 mg/day. A novel but risky surgical approach uses deep brain stimulation of the thalamus to reduce contralateral tremors.

Whittle IR, Haddow LJ: CT guided thalamotomy for movement disorders in multiple sclerosis. Acta Neurochir 64:13–16, 1995.

33. What is the best treatment for urologic problems in MS?

Urologic consultation is often useful to manage the neurogenic bladder. The most common problem is a hyperreflexic bladder with a small capacity, early detrusor contraction, urinary frequency, and urgency. It can be managed with medications such as oxybutinin (Ditropan), toprolidine (Detrol), or hyoscyamine (Levsinex). A flaccid bladder (more rare) may require self-catheterization. When sphincter-detrusor dyssynergia appears, medications to relax the sphincter, such as the alpha-adrenergic blocking agent prazosin (Minipress), may be useful.

BIBLIOGRAPHY

1. Burks JS, Johnson KP: Multiple Sclerosis: Diagnosis, Medical Management, and Rehabilitation. New York, Demos, 2000.
2. Compston A, Ebers G, Lassmann H, et al: McAlpine's Multiple Sclerosis, 3rd ed. London, Churchill Livingstone, 1998.
3. Paty DW, Ebers GC: Multiple Sclerosis. Philadelphia, F.A. Davis, 1998.
4. Raine CS, McFarland HF, Tourtellotte WW (eds): Multiple Sclerosis: Clinical and Pathogenetic Basis. London, Chapman & Hall, 1997.
5. Rolak LA, Harati Y (eds): Neuro-immunology for the Clinician. Boston, Butterworth-Heinemann, 1997.
Website
www.nmss.org

14. DEMENTIA

Rachelle S. Doody, M.D., Ph.D.

GENERAL CONSIDERATIONS

1. How is dementia defined? How do definitions vary?

Dementia is generally regarded as an acquired loss of cognitive function due to an abnormal brain condition. The National Institutes of Health criteria (formerly NINCDS-ADRDA criteria) for the diagnosis of Alzheimer's disease (AD) stress that there must be **progressive** loss of cognitive function, including but not limited to memory loss. The DSM-IV general criteria for dementia include the requirement of **functional decline** that interferes with work or usual social activities in addition to cognitive decline.

American Psychiatric Association: Diagnostic and Statistical Manual of Mental Disorders, 4th ed. Washington, D.C., American Psychiatric Association, 1994.

McKhann G, et al: Clinical diagnosis of Alzheimer's disease. Report of the NINCDS-ADRDA Work Group under the auspices of Department of Health and Human Services Task Force on Alzheimer's Disease. Neurology 34:939–944, 1984.

2. What is senility? Is it normal?

Senility is an outdated term. It used to mean cognitive impairment due to aging, which was assumed to be normal. Although memory, learning, and thinking change with age in subtle ways, memory loss and cognitive impairment are not features of normal aging.

3. What is pseudodementia?

Pseudodementia has many meanings. It refers to depressed patients who are cognitively impaired and often have motor slowing but do not have one of the well-defined dementia syndromes. The term does not mean that the patient is consciously simulating dementia (malingering) or is cognitively intact but believes himself or herself to be demented (Ganser's syndrome). Some researchers believe that pseudodementia may be a precursor to dementia.

Folstein M, Rabins P: Replacing pseudodementia. Neuropsychiatry Neuropsychol Behav Neurol 4:36–40, 1991.

4. What features are characteristic of pseudodementia associated with depression?

Patients with pseudodementia may or may not have a history of depressive or vegetative symptoms. They tend to have flat affect, to give up easily when mental status is examined, or to say that they cannot perform a task without even trying it. They often respond surprisingly well when given extra time and encouragement, but they may deny their success. Results of mental examination are inconsistent; for example, they may fail a simple task but perform a similar, more difficult one correctly. Or they may have variable strengths and weaknesses over repeated testing sessions.

5. What is Ganser's syndrome?

It is an involuntary and unconscious simulation of altered mental status (confusion or dementia) in a patient who is not malingering and believes in the validity of his or her symptoms.

6. What is delirium?

Delirium is an acute confusional state.

7. What features distinguish delirium from dementia?

Although this distinction cannot always be made with certainty, several features are helpful. Sudden onset suggests delirium, as do findings of altered consciousness, marked problems with attention and concentration out of proportion to other deficits, cognitive fluctuations (e.g., lucid intervals), psychomotor and/or autonomic overactivity, fragmented speech, and marked hallucinations (especially auditory or tactile). Chronically demented patients may develop delirium in addition to dementia, which will change the clinical picture.

8. Do all patients with dementia develop psychotic features?

No. Psychosis is a variable finding in all types of dementia and is not even clearly related to the stage or severity of dementia.

Doody RS, et al: Positive and negative neuropsychiatric features in Alzheimer's disease. J Neuropsychol Clin Neurosci 7(1):54–60, 1995.

9. Which screening instruments are commonly used in diagnosing dementia?

The Folstein Mini-Mental Status Examination (MMSE), Short Blessed, and Mattis Dementia Rating Scale are commonly used clinically and in experimental studies to screen for dementia and to rate severity of dementia.

10. What are the limitations of the MMSE in the assessment of dementia?

Besides the fact that it has both false-positive (usually depression) and false-negative results (usually early dementia in highly functioning patients), the MMSE also has limitations based on its lack of comprehensiveness.

Feher E, et al: Establishing the limits of the mini-mental state. Arch Neurol 49:87–92, 1992.

11. At what point is a patient too demented to require an evaluation?

No patient is too demented to be evaluated. The need to rule out reversible causes and structural lesions always remains. Neurologic and psychometric examinations can be tailored to the level of even the most profoundly demented patients.

12. What are the most common causes of dementia or conditions resembling dementia?

Alzheimer's disease is the most common form of dementia in adults (> 50% in most series). Depression with pseudodementia is a frequent cause of cognitive loss and must be ruled out in all patients. Other important causes include multi-infarct or vascular dementia, Lewy body dementia, and dementia-like syndromes due to alcohol or chronic use of certain prescription drugs.

13. What uncommon causes of dementia must be considered in the differential diagnosis of every patient with dementia?

1. Toxins (lead, organic mercury)
2. Vitamin deficiencies (B_{12}, B_1, and B_6, in particular)
3. Endocrine disturbances (hypothyroidism or hyperthyroidism, hyperparathyroidism, Cushing's disease, Addison's disease
4. Chronic metabolic conditions (hyponatremia, hypercalcemia, chronic hepatic failure, renal failure)
5. Vasculopathies affecting the brain
6. Structural abnormalities (chronic subdural hematomas, normal-pressure hydrocephalus, slow-growing tumors)
7. CNS infections (including AIDS, Creutzfeldt-Jakob disease, cryptococcal or tuberculous meningitis)

14. Which dementia syndromes are associated with alcohol?

The DSM-IV includes alcohol amnestic syndrome (Korsakoff's syndrome), in which the amnestic disorder predominates, as well as a more generalized dementia associated with alcoholism. Both are associated with some degree of visuospatial impairment; neither includes aphasia.

ALZHEIMER'S DISEASE

15. How is Alzheimer's disease (AD) diagnosed?
First, the presence of dementia must be established clearly by clinical criteria and confirmed by neuropsychological testing. The clinical manifestations must include impairment of memory and at least one other area of cognition. There must be no evidence of other systemic or brain disease sufficient to cause the dementia, and the NIH criteria suggest basic laboratory studies (which are not all-inclusive) to exclude other disease. The diagnosis is both a diagnosis of exclusion and a diagnosis based on the establishment of certain characteristic features.
McKhann G, et al: Clinical diagnosis of Alzheimer's disease: Report of the NINCDS-ADRDA Work Group under the auspices of Department of Health and Human Services Task Force on Alzheimer's Disease. Neurology 34:939–944, 1984.

16. When should the designations of probable, possible, and definite AD be used?
Probable AD refers to a clinical diagnosis based on the NIH criteria. Most patients have this diagnosis.
Possible AD refers to patients with atypical features (progressive isolated memory or language dysfunction, for example) or patients with a concurrent disorder that may cause cognitive impairment, but it is not believed to be the only factor (concomitant cerebrovascular accident, for example).
Definite AD is reserved for patients with biopsy- or autopsy-proved AD.
McKhann G, et al: Clinical diagnosis of Alzheimer's disease: Report of the NINCDS-ADRDA Work Group under the auspices of Department of Health and Human Services Task Force on Alzheimer's Disease. Neurology 34:939–944, 1984.

17. How are the alcohol-related dementias differentiated from AD?
No absolute features distinguish these conditions. If the patient has a systemic disorder (such as alcoholism) that, in the clinician's opinion, is sufficient to cause dementia, the diagnosis should **not** be probable AD. Possible AD may be used if underlying AD is suspected in an actively drinking patient. The patient should stop drinking with the help of appropriate rehabilitative services. If the dementia improves and the improvement continues or persists for 1 year or more, the diagnosis is not likely to be AD.

18. Which blood tests are typically ordered in a patient with suspected AD to rule out other causes of dementia?

1. Chemistry analysis (including sodium, blood sugar, calcium, liver enzymes, renal function)
2. Complete blood count with differential
3. Thyroid function tests
4. Venereal Disease Research Laboratory or equivalent test for syphilis
5. Vitamin B_{12}
6. Antinuclear antibody (extractable nuclear antigen panel, if positive)
7. Serum protein electrophoresis
8. HIV
9. Sedimentation rate
10. Serum cholesterol and triglycerides

Additional tests:

Prothrombin time/partial thromboplastin time
Folate
Serum arterial ammonia
Parathyroid hormone
Serum protein electrophoresis
Sedimentation rate

Cortisol levels
Rheumatoid factor
Serum (and urine) drug screens
Hexosaminidase levels
HIV
Serum cholesterol and triglycerides

19. Which ancillary studies (in addition to blood tests) are useful to evaluate patients with suspected AD?
An imaging study (MRI or CT with contrast) and neuropsychological testing to confirm dementia are necessary. Electroencephalography (EEG), single-photon emission CT (SPECT), or

positron emission tomography (PET) studies and lumbar puncture may be useful or even necessary. Also consider an EKG (to look for evidence of cardiovascular disease) and chest radiograph.

20. When is lumbar puncture (LP) necessary in the diagnostic work-up?

When symptoms are of short duration (< 6 months) or have atypical features, such as rapid progression or severe confusion, an LP should be performed early. It also should be done if clinical or laboratory features suggest a specific etiology that is an indication for LP, such as CNS meningitis or CNS vasculitis.

21. What are typical symptoms of early AD?

Early symptoms of AD include forgetfulness for recent events or newly acquired information, often causing the patient to repeat himself or herself. Other early features are disorientation, especially to time, and difficulty with complex cognitive functions such as mathematical calculations or organization of activities that require several steps.

22. What are typical symptoms of moderately advanced AD?

Advanced AD includes a history of progression of pervasive memory loss sufficient to impair everyday activities, disorientation to place and/or aspects of person (e.g., age), inability to keep track of time, and problems with personal care (such as forgetting to change clothes). Behavioral changes, such as depression, paranoia, or aggressiveness, are more likely in these stages.

23. Does progression of AD follow a consistent pattern?

Definitely not. Salient symptoms and rates of progression vary tremendously.

24. What language disturbances do patients with AD experience?

Early in the disease, most patients have word-finding difficulties that may cause pauses in spontaneous speech or may be detected by asking the patient to name objects (particularly objects with low frequency in the language). As AD progresses, most patients develop problems with comprehension with intact repetition (similar to transcortical sensory aphasia); then repetition becomes affected while speech remains fluent (similar to Wernicke's aphasia). Ultimately, some patients develop expressive speech problems in addition to the above symptoms, or they may just stop talking secondary to inanition and apparent lack of anything to say.

25. Does the presence or absence of insight differentiate AD from other dementias?

Lack of insight into their memory disorder (or anosognosia) occurs in some patients with AD as well as in patients with other dementing disorders. It does not appear to correlate with disease severity and is not useful in differential diagnosis.

Feher E, et al: Mental status assessment of insight and judgment. Clin Geriatr Med 5:477–498, 1989.

26. What motor features may be associated with AD? What is their significance?

Rigidity, bradykinesia, and parkinsonian gait may be associated with more rapid progression of disease (both cognitive decline and activities of daily living). Tremor is rare, differentiating patients with AD from patients with Parkinson's disease to some extent. Myoclonus may occur, and recent evidence suggests its association with a younger age of onset of AD.

27. Are there specific clinical subtypes of AD?

Clinical subtypes are unclear, but possibilities include early-onset AD (< 65 yr), AD with extrapyramidal features, and AD with psychosis. Familial AD is well recognized (about 10% of cases) and characterized by early onset and autosomal dominant transmission.

28. What is the genetic defect in early-onset familial AD?

Some families show a mutation in the gene that encodes amyloid precursor protein on chromosome 21. Other families show mutations on chromosome 14 (in the gene for presenilin 1) or chromosome 1 (in the gene for presenilin 2). It is likely that other genes will be linked to the early-onset familial form of AD.

29. What is the genetic defect in late-onset familial AD?

Late-onset familial AD is linked to chromosome 19. It also has been demonstrated that the particular inherited form of apolipoprotein E (coded by a gene on chromosome 19) determines the age-dependent risk and age of onset of AD in some patients. Patients who inherit one or more E_4 alleles are at greater risk. Other families have been linked to variant forms of alpha 2 macroglobulin on chromosome 12. These gene associations likely represent inherited risk factors rather than genetic forms of AD.

30. Is there a genetic component to all cases of AD?

The answer is not clear. Patients with a family history of AD in even one primary relative appear to be at increased risk, and the risk is higher if both parents have AD. Cases that seem to be sporadic are common, although the apolipoprotein E (ApoE) genotype is a clear risk factor for both sporadic and late-onset familial cases. Multiple genetic factors probably account for a predisposition for AD.

31. What is apolipoprotein E? What is its importance?

ApoE is a cholesterol-carrying blood protein that comes in three forms: $ApoE_2$, E_3, and E_4. We inherit one ApoE allele from each parent, and people with one or more E_4 alleles have an increased risk for developing AD.

32. What other disorders have been associated with AD in epidemiologic surveys?

Patients with Down syndrome are at high risk for AD. Whether families of patients with AD have a higher incidence of Down syndrome remains controversial. Parkinson's disease and a history of head trauma have been associated with AD in some large studies but not in others.

33. What are the risk factors for AD?

The presence of $ApoE_4$ and serious head injury in $ApoE_4$-positive people, aging, postmenopausal estrogen deficiency, positive family history (independent of ApoE genotype), and low education level (especially early in development) may be risk factors. Aluminum exposure is frequently cited, but no sound evidence supports the association.

34. What factors reduce the risk for AD?

Although definite proof is lacking, estrogen replacement, anti-inflammatory drugs (including nonsteroidal agents), and antioxidants have been proposed and are under study.

35. What are the classic neuropathologic changes in AD?

Senile plaques, neurofibrillary tangles, granulovacuolar degeneration, and amyloid in blood vessels and plaques are classic changes. Plaques and tangles also may be seen in normal brains but are far less numerous; tangles outside the hippocampus are rare.

36. Which neuropathologic changes correlate best with the severity of dementia?

In most studies, neurofibrillary tangles correlate best with the severity of dementia. Synaptic density has been shown to have an inverse correlation with severity of dementia, at least in some brain regions. Because education seems to increase synaptic density, some have suggested that education may have a protective effect against the manifestation of AD cognitive changes.

Terry R, et al: Physical basis of cognitive alterations in Alzheimer's disease: Synapse loss is the major correlate of cognitive impairment. Ann Neurol 30:572–580, 1991.

37. Which neuropathologic entities overlap with AD?

Besides normal aging, dementia with Lewy bodies, Parkinson's dementia, progressive supranuclear palsy, and vascular dementias are sometimes difficult to distinguish from AD, because plaques and tangles may occur with other pathologic changes. Clinical correlations are extremely important in such cases.

38. Which neuropathologically distinct entities may be clinically indistinguishable from AD?

Vascular dementias (without plaques and tangles), dementia with Lewy bodies, Pick's disease, dementia lacking distinctive histology, and other frontal lobe dementia syndromes may be impossible to distinguish from AD on clinical grounds alone.

39. What is the clinical picture of frontotemporal dementia?

This designation includes a group of entities with variable neuropathologic findings and similar clinical features. Patients have early personality changes, particularly impulsivity and Klüver-Bucy type symptoms or withdrawal and depression. Psychiatric symptoms may precede dementia by several years. Memory and frontal executive tasks (e.g., planning, set-shifting, set maintenance) are much more impaired than attention, language, and visuospatial skills. SPECT studies may show hypofrontality. Neuropathology includes Pick's disease or primary degeneration at multiple brain sites (dementia lacking distinctive histology), usually with gliosis. Many of these cases have been linked to genetic mutations in the tau protein on chromosome 17.

The Lund and Manchester Groups: Clinical and neuropsychological criteria for frontotemporal dementia. J Neurol Neurosurg Psychiatry 57:416–418, 1994.

40. What is the cholinergic hypothesis?

This hypothesis attempts to explain many of the cognitive deficits in AD (particularly memory disturbance) by a deficiency of cholinergic neurotransmission. Evidence includes the fact that poor memory can be induced in normal people by anticholinergic drugs. Loss of cholinergic projection neurons in the nucleus basalis of Meynert and loss of choline acetyltransferase activity throughout the cortex of patients with AD correlate with the severity of memory loss.

41. Besides acetylcholine, which transmitters are affected by AD?

Norepinephrine, somatostatin, dopamine, serotonin, and neuropeptide Y are decreased. Glutamate dysfunction also may play a role in AD.

42. What is the role of amyloid in AD?

Clearly AD is associated with abnormal accumulation of a breakdown product of the amyloid precursor protein known as beta-amyloid or $A\beta$ amyloid, especially in the insoluble form. Amyloid appears to be toxic to cells in vitro, and abnormal accumulation may actually cause cell loss. No one knows why the $A\beta$ amyloid accumulates, but accumulation may be secondary to abnormal processing within neurons.

43. What is the role of tau protein in AD?

Tau protein is expressed in association with the cytoskeleton of neuronal cells. In damaged cells (e.g., after heat shock), its expression is increased. Tau appears to be hyperphosphylated in cells destined to develop neurofibrillary tangles. It may be an early marker of cells with abnormal cytoskeletal function and abnormal metabolism.

44. Discuss the possible role of nerve growth factor (NGF) in AD.

NGF is a trophic hormone that maintains the integrity of cholinergic neurons. Loss of NGF may contribute to the loss of such neurons in AD, and increases in NGF (and other growth factor production) may improve the course or symptoms of the disease by preserving and enhancing the function of remaining cholinergic neurons.

45. What is the treatment for the noncognitive secondary behavioral effects of AD?

Behavioral symptoms, such as disturbed sleep, depression, anxiety, psychotic features, agitation, and aggressiveness, are amenable to treatment. Behavioral modification, such as entraining sleep-wake cycles and increasing daytime activity, should be tried first for **sleep disorders**, but mild hypnotics may be useful. Clinical trials of melatonin are under way.

Depression, particularly early in the disease, may respond to low doses of antidepressants, but drugs with anitcholinergic side effects should be avoided. Drugs that act on the serotonergic system may be better tolerated (fluoxetine, paroxetine, citalopram, trazodone), although controlled studies are lacking for patients with AD.

Anxiety and agitation frequently respond to behavioral interventions, such as day center participation, that engage the patient and reduce caregiver stress. Other respite interventions for caregivers may help to reduce patient stress. If symptoms are infrequent, anxiety or agitation may be treated with low doses of anxiolytics as needed, such as chloral hydrate or lorazepam (avoid long-acting drugs). Chronic anxiolytics are not indicated for AD, but short-term therapy with buspirone or lorazepam may be justified during periods of transition or change.

Severe agitation, aggressiveness, and psychotic features that disturb the patient should be treated with antipsychotics such as olanzepine, respiridone, and quetiapine, in the lowest doses possible, because these drugs further impair cognition (and sometimes motor performance). Psychotic features that do not disturb the patient or disrupt the household need not be treated.

Doody RS: Treatment strategies in Alzheimer's disease. In Clark C, Trojanowski J (eds): Neurodegenerative Dementias. New York, McGraw-Hill, 1998.

46. What treatments exist for the primary process of AD?

The Food and Drug Administration has approved four treatments specifically for AD—tacrine, donepezil, rivastigmine, and galantamine. All are cholinesterase inhibitors. Experimental studies are under way with additional cholinesterase inhibitors, muscarinic and nicotinic agonists, antioxidants, anti-inflammatory agents, substances that act as or upregulate growth factors, and strategies designed to interfere with amyloid metabolism. Studies of estrogen as a treatment for AD have been negative. Many patients can qualify for these studies and should be referred to AD research centers that test medications if they are interested. Available drugs and sites can be identified by calling the National Alzheimer's Disease Association in Chicago.

Corey-Bloom, et al: A randomized trial evaluating the efficacy and safety of ENA 713 (rivastigmine tartrate), a new acetycholinesterase inhibitor, in patients with mild to moderately severe Alzheimer's disease. J Geriatr Psychopharmacol 1:55–65, 1998.

Schneider LS, Tariot PN: Emerging drugs for Alzheimer's disease. Med Clin North Am 78:911–917, 1994.

Raskind, et al: Galantamine in Alzheimer's disease: A 6-month randomized, placebo-controlled trial with a 6-month extension. Neurology 54:2261–2268, 2001.

Rogers, et al: A 24-week double-blind, placebo-controlled trial of Donepezil in patients with Alzheimer's disease. Neurology 50:136–145, 1998.

47. Are there any agents besides cholinesterase inhibitors that improve cognition or slow functional loss in AD?

One large-scale double-blind study supports the benefits of vitamin E (1000 IU twice daily) or selegiline, an MAO-B inhibitor (5 mg twice daily) for slowing the time to significant worsening. Vitamin E is better tolerated, and the two should not be used together, because combination therapy reduces the benefits.

Sano, et al: A controlled trial of selegiline, alpha-tocopherol or both as treatment for Alzheimer's disease. N Engl J Med 336:1216–1222, 1997.

48. What is respite care?

Respite care is any caretaking arrangement for the patient that temporarily relieves the primary caregiver. It may be as informal as a friend or relative who comes to the home to care for the patient, part-time in-home aid, or a few days per week at a day center. It also may apply to short-term stays in residential facilities.

49. What are the responsibilities of physicians and health-care workers with respect to respite care?

The physician or health-care worker must introduce the concept of respite care and assure every primary caregiver that he or she will need it sooner or later. Even early in the disease process, activities that are directed toward patients (such as day centers) help promote their autonomy and provide supervision while providing respite to caregivers. Many caregivers feel guilty about not being able to care for the patient alone every day and night. They need to know that all affected families require help in caregiving.

VASCULAR DEMENTIAS

50. What entities constitute the vascular dementias?
1. Multiple large infarctions, which usually involve cortical and subcortical tissue
2. Multiple smaller infarctions that involve critical brain regions
It is less clear whether diffuse, chronic vascular processes such as Binswanger's disease, leukoaraiosis, or diffuse changes in white matter due to microinfarcts also cause dementia.

51. Can vascular dementia be diagnosed by CT or MRI alone?
No. Patients who have changes in white matter on scans or even multiple, definite infarctions may be clinically normal. It is not known how many infarcts or how much change in white matter on a scan translates into dementia for patients who suffer cognitive impairments. Many white matter signal changes, especially on MRI, do not represent strokes
Román GC, et al: Vascular dementia: Diagnostic criteria for research studies. Neurology 43:250–260, 1993.

52. Can dementia occur after a single stroke?
One prospective study of patients after acute stroke showed that the risk of dementia was 9–10 times greater than for matched controls without a stroke. A single stroke also can lead to dementia by "unmasking" underlying Alzheimer's disease that has not yet become symptomatic.
Tatemichi TK, et al: Dementia after stroke: Baseline frequency, risks, and clinical features in a hospitalized cohort. Neurology 42:1185–1193, 1992.

53. Can neuropsychological testing differentiate vascular dementia from AD?
Not absolutely. Patchy performances across tests, unilateral motor impairments (e.g., reaction times or finger tapping), and improvements in some but not all areas of cognition over time are typically seen in vascular dementias. Asymmetric finger tapping, however, is also common in AD.
Massman P, Doody R: Hemisphere asymmetry in Alzheimer's disease is apparent in motor functioning. J Clin Exp Neuropsychol 18:110–121, 1996.

54. What basic work-up should be done when vascular dementia is suspected?
The work-up should begin with imaging studies and psychometric testing in addition to the history and physical exam. In most cases, all tests recommended for the diagnosis of AD should be pursued to rule out additional conditions that may cause or contribute to the dementia, including a lipid profile. Some patients, especially those with clear-cut strokes, may benefit from imaging of the carotid arteries, especially when high-grade stenosis or ulcerated plaques are suspected. An echocardiogram is indicated in patients who have a cardiac history or appear to have had embolic strokes.

55. What ancillary tests may be useful in diagnosing vascular dementia?
The EEG may show multiple slow-wave foci, and SPECT or PET scans may show multiple areas of decreased flow or altered metabolism. These tests have not been adequately studied to assess their utility for differentiating the various forms of vascular dementia.

56. Can vascular dementia be diagnosed in patients with aphasia due to a left hemisphere infarct?
Patients should not be tested for dementia in the acute phase of stroke, whether aphasic or otherwise. Although most tests for cognitive functioning rely heavily on language abilities, tests of nonverbal memory and reasoning help to support the diagnosis of dementia in an aphasic patient. A history of functional decline not related to language-based tasks is also helpful.

57. What is the treatment of vascular dementia?
As for AD, noncognitive behavioral effects of dementia are amenable to therapy, and respite care should be introduced early. In addition, it is advisable to control vascular risk factors as much as possible (blood pressure, cholesterol, hypertension). Prophylactic antiplatelet therapy (aspirin, clopidogrel, or ticlopidine), although not of proven benefit for dementia, may be helpful by reducing the risk of future strokes.

SUBCORTICAL DEMENTIAS

58. What are the characteristics of subcortical dementias?

Subcortical dementias lack cortical features, such as aphasia, apraxia, and acalculia. Recall memory is impaired worse than recognition memory. Visuospatial skills are often impaired. Frontal executive deficits, bradyphrenia, anomia, personality changes, and psychomotor slowing are prominent. Dysarthria, abnormal posture and coordination, and adventitious movements may be present.

Cummings JL: Subcortical Dementia. New York, Oxford Press, 1990.

59. How do the general features of subcortical dementias differ from cortical dementias?

The cortical dementias, such as AD, usually involve language and calculations and may involve apraxia and cortical sensory disturbances (e.g., astereognosis, graphesthesia), whereas subcortical dementias do not. Both recall and recognition memory are usually impaired in cortical dementia, whereas recognition memory is relatively preserved in subcortical dementia. Frontal executive functions are lost in proportion to the overall dementia in cortical processes but are especially prominently affected in subcortical dementia. Bradykinesia and bradyphrenia, as well as other motor features, are usually absent or late findings in cortical dementias but occur early in subcortical dementias. Personality changes are variable in both types but are said to be more prominent early in the course of subcortical dementia.

Cummings JL: Subcortical Dementia. New York, Oxford Press, 1990.

60. In what ways do the specific memory disturbances of subcortical dementias differ from those of cortical dementias?

Problems with short-term spontaneous recall occur in both types, but strategies to enhance encoding and recognition cuing are mainly helpful in subcortical dementias. Incidental memory (details not related to the task at hand, such as what the examiner was wearing) is better in subcortical dementias. Procedural memory (memory involved in learning tasks) is better preserved in cortical dementias. Remote memory usually shows a temporal gradient in cortical dementias but not in subcortical dementias.

61. Is there a rigid anatomic or functional distinction between cortical and subcortical dementia?

No. So-called subcortical dementias may give rise to or be associated with cortical changes and vice versa. Huntington's dementia, like most subcortical dementias, causes disturbances of cortical frontal lobe functioning. Patients with Parkinson's disease may show atrophy of cortical cells. Patients with AD have subcortical changes in deep nuclei, such as the nucleus basalis of Meynert and locus ceruleus.

62. What disorders or clinical syndromes are associated with subcortical dementia?

1. Parkinson's disease
2. Huntington's disease
3. Progressive supranuclear palsy
4. Spinocerebellar degeneration
5. Idiopathic basal ganglia calcification
6. Multiple sclerosis
7. Inflammatory conditions involving the basal ganglia and/or thalamus
8. AIDS
9. Corticobasal degeneration

63. What are the clinical features of Parkinson's dementia?

Parkinsonian features sufficient to make a diagnosis of Parkinson's disease usually predate the dementia by at least 1 year. Typically bradyphrenia, dysnomia, and frontal executive dysfunction are present, and depression is common. There may be visuospatial abnormalities, especially on formal testing.

64. What are the clinical features of Huntington's dementia?

Psychiatric symptoms or dementia may occur before or after the features of Huntington's disease (e.g., chorea) are well established. Psychiatric features include personality changes, depression, and psychosis. The memory disorder is typical of the subcortical pattern. Language and speech disorders, including dysarthria, reduced spontaneous speech, impaired syntactic complexity, and impaired comprehension, are common, as are visuospatial abnormalities.

65. What are the clinical features of the dementia associated with progressive supranuclear palsy (PSP)?

PSP is a syndrome characterized by supranuclear gaze palsy, dystonic rigidity of axial musculature, dysarthria, and pseudobulbar palsy. The dementia is not clearly present in all patients and is difficult to characterize because the associated visual scanning disorder interferes with testing. Memory impairments tend to be mild relative to frontal executive functions.

66. What is dementia with Lewy bodies?

A spectrum of disorders probably makes up Lewy body disease, ranging from Parkinson's disease (with Lewy bodies primarily in the subcortical and brainstem regions) to diffuse Lewy body disease, in which Lewy bodies are present throughout the cortex, subcortex, and brainstem. Some authorities describe an intermediate form of Lewy body dementia (senile dementia of the Lewy body type), which is associated with many Lewy bodies in the brainstem and subcortical regions, fewer in the hippocampus, and fewer still in the neocortical region.

Doody R, Massman P: Other extrapyramidal dementias. In Morris JC (ed): Handbook of Dementing Illnesses. New York, Marcel Dekker, 1994, pp 319–334.

67. What are the clinical characteristics of dementia with Lewy bodies?

Patients typically exhibit fluctuating confusion and dementia, usually with vivid visual hallucinations and mild extrapyramidal features. The neuropsychological deficits are not well characterized, and little is known about the natural history of the disorder.

McKeith IG, et al: Consensus guidelines for the clinical and pathologic diagnosis of dementia with Lewy bodies (DLB). Neurology 47:1113–1124, 1996.

68. What other disorders are in the differential diagnosis of dementia (not necessarily subcortical) with extrapyramidal features?

1. Alzheimer's disease
2. Parkinson's disease plus dementia
3. Creutzfeldt-Jakob disease
4. Binswanger's disease
5. Multiinfarct or vascular dementia
6. Normal pressure hydrocephalus
7. Dementia lacking distinctive histology
8. Corticobasal ganglionic degeneration
9. AIDS dementia
10. Hallervorden-Spatz disease
11. Neuronal intranuclear inclusion disease
12. GM_1 gangliosidosis type III
13. Striatonigral degeneration

69. How do patients with corticobasal ganglionic degeneration (CBGD) present?

Patients tend to present either with an alien limb phenomenon and associated motor features (tremor, rigidity, grasp reflex, apraxia, myoclonus) or with an akinetic-rigid syndrome similar to Parkinson's disease. Dementia frequently develops over time and affects cognitive function pervasively. The neuropsychological deficits are typical of subcortical dementia.

Doody RS, Jankovic JJ: The alien hand and related signs. J Neurol Neurosurg Psychiatry 55:806–810, 1992.

Massman PJ, et al: Neuropsychological functioning in cortical-basal ganglionic degeneration: Differentiation from Alzheimer's disease. Neurology 46:720–726, 1995.

BIBLIOGRAPHY

1. Adams RD, Victor M, Ropper AH: Principles of Neurology, 6th ed. New York, McGraw-Hill, 1997.
2. Cummings JL: Subcortical Dementia. New York, Oxford Press, 1990.
3. Morris J (ed): Handbook of Dementing Illnesses. New York, Marcel Dekker, 1994.
4. Trimble MR, Cummings JL: Contemporary Behavioral Neurology. Boston, Butterworth-Heinemann, 1997.
5. Trojanowski J, Clark C (ed): Neurodegenerative Dementias. New York, McGraw-Hill, 1998.
Websites
www.alzforum.org
www.alz.org
www.nlm.nih.gov/medlineplus/dementia.html

15. APHASIA AND BEHAVIORAL NEUROLOGY

David B. Rosenfield, M.D.

LANGUAGE DISTURBANCES

1. What is the definition of aphasia?

Aphasia is an acquired disturbance of language. Someone who has been mentally retarded from birth and never developed normal language is not considered to be aphasic.

2. What is the most common cause of aphasia in adults?

Vascular disease or trauma.

3. What is the difference between language, speech, and phonation?

Language is a set of symbols that are constrained in their interrelationship by perception, production, and central processing rules. Language consists of semantics (meaning of words), phonology (sound of words), and syntax (rules of grammar).

Speech is the neuromechanical process of the actual production of the sound and depends on respiratory input, articulatory input, and phonation.

Phonation refers to sounds produced from the larynx.

4. What percentage of people are right-handed?

Over 90% of humans state that they are right-handed. However, if one provides them a list of tasks, ranging from how one strikes a match to what hand is on top of a broom, 60% are strongly right-handed, and 35% have a mixed hand preference.

5. What percentage of people are left-handed?

Less than 5% of people use their left hands for all skilled tasks.

6. What is the effect on aphasia of knowing more than one language?

If one is aphasic in one language, one is aphasic in all others. There might be some differences in the degree of aphasia, depending on the language; variations have been found in tonal languages such as Thai and Japanese and in other languages such as Hebrew. Factors such as the age at which one acquired a language, whether more than one language was simultaneously vs. sequentially acquired, skill at both languages, and context of the acquisition (such as home, work, or school) influence the degree of aphasia.

7. What is the rule of Ribot?

Ribot contended that the language that one learns first is the most "automatic" or "overlearned" and, consequently, the best preserved if one is rendered aphasic.

8. What is Pitres' law?

Pitres contended that the language most recently learned and used is best preserved in aphasia. The discrepancy between Ribot's rule and Pitres' law has not been completely resolved.

9. What is the difference between nonfluent aphasia and fluent aphasia?

Aphasics who use short phrases (less than five words) and have a reduced grammatical form are considered to be nonfluent. Those who produce phrases longer than five words and have fairly normal grammatical output are considered to be fluent, although their language may be impaired in other ways. Thus, a nonfluent aphasic may say, "Where is book?" and a fluent aphasic may say, "Where is the paper of the cover?"

10. What are the clinical characteristics of nonfluent aphasia?
1. Impaired articulation
2. Impaired melodic production
3. Reduced phrase length (five or less words per phrase)
4. Decreased grammatical complexity

Some patients do not have all of the elements of nonfluency. Thus, some may be nonfluent, partially fluent, or dysarthric.

11. What are the features of Broca's aphasia?
1. Nonfluency
2. Effortful initiation of speech production
3. Poor repetition
4. Poor ability to name
5. Paraphasic errors (semantic and phonemic)
6. Moderately good comprehension but difficulty with understanding syntactically complex sentences

Broca's aphasia is usually associated with right hemiparesis, hemisensory loss, buccofacial apraxia, and left limb ideomotor apraxia.

12. Where is the lesion that causes Broca's aphasia?

The lesion that causes Broca's aphasia usually involves the frontal operculum (Brodmann areas 45 and 44) and the deep frontal white matter, sparing the lower motor cortex and the middle paraventricular white matter. Some patients have compromise of the periolandic cortex, especially in Brodmann's area 4. Still others have compromise in the periolandic region with extensive subcortical white matter damage. Some contend that damage *only* to Broca's area in the cortex, without compromising surrounding tissue, does not cause a true aphasia.

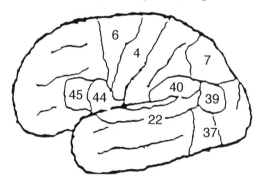

Diagram of the left cerebral cortex, showing the Brodmann's areas important for language function. (From Alexander MP, Benson DF: The aphasias and related disturbances. In Joynt RJ (ed): Clinical neurology. Philadelphia, J.B. Lippincott, 1992, with permission.)

13. What are paraphasias? Describe the two types.
Paraphasias are substitutions for and within words.
1. **Semantic (verbal) paraphasia** is a substitution of one word for another ("cat" for "dog"). Often pronouns or prepositions are changed.
2. **Phonemic (literal) paraphasia** is a substitution of one sound for another (e.g., "breen" for "green").

14. What is jargon aphasia?
Jargon aphasia is a fluent, paraphasic output with many phonemic substitutions in a sentence.

15. What are neologisms?
Neologisms are new words ("I am going to the tramechon"). Their use may be considered a type of paraphasia or word substitution.

16. What is logorrhea?

Logorrhea ("press of speech") refers to fluent speech with far too many unnecessary words and frequent neologisms (new words that make no sense). This type of deficit is often seen in Wernicke's aphasia.

17. What are the features of Wernicke's aphasia?

1. Fluent aphasic output
2. Normal sentence length
3. Good articulation
4. Good (sometimes exaggerated) prosody
5. Anomia
6. Phonemic and semantic paraphasias
7. Poor auditory and reading comprehension
8. Impaired repetition
9. Fluent but empty writing

18. Where is the lesion that causes Wernicke's aphasia?

Classic Wernicke's aphasia usually indicates an extensive lesion of the posterosuperior temporal region, including the superior and middle temporal gyrus, supramarginal-angular regions, and sometimes part of the laterotemporal-occipital junction. It also may be seen in subcortical lesions that block the inferior afferent signals to the temporal cortex by damaging the temporal isthmus.

19. What are the characteristics of conduction aphasia?

1. Fluent aphasia
2. Good comprehension
3. Poor repetition
4. Paragrammatic
5. Anomia
6. Paraphasic errors
7. Good recitation
8. Good reading aloud

Most paraphasic distortions are phonemic. Repetition and oral reading frequently exaggerate these errors. Conduction aphasia is usually associated with agraphia and some degree of limited reading comprehension.

20. Where is the lesion responsible for conduction aphasia?

The lesion usually involves the left inferior parietal lobule, especially the anterior supramarginal gyrus. Often the lesion is in the subcortical white matter, deep to the inferior parietal cortex, affecting the arcuate fasciculus or the extreme capsule immediately below the arcuate fasciculus, both of which are connected to the temporal and frontal cortex.

21. What is word deafness?

Pure word deafness is a disturbance in which auditory comprehension is compromised, but there are no other disturbances of hearing. Patients are "deaf" only for words.

22. Describe the three types of pure word deafness.

1. Language is fluent, grammar may be normal or slightly abnormal, and speech is rather empty. Reading comprehension is normal or near normal. Writing is similar to speech. Many patients present initially with Wernicke's aphasia.

2. As above, but greater deficits in auditory perception. Patients fail to recognize many sounds (e.g., guitar, piano, bells, chimes, buzz saw) and thus have auditory agnosia.

3. Patients have impairment in sequencing a rapid array of sounds.

All three groups behave as though they were deaf. All have better comprehension when the rate of speech is slowed, but all still have difficulty. Many have a questioning type of echolalia, repeating what the examiner says but adding a pitch intonation that implies a question.

23. Where are the lesions for the three types of pure word deafness?

1. In the first group (see above), the lesion involves the left superior temporal gyrus, usually the anterior portion of the classic Wernicke's aphasia lesion. Often patients have damage to the left auditory cortex and partial damage to connections with the posterosuperior temporal gyrus, presumably underlying the disordered auditory processing, mild anomia, and paraphasia. Sparing

of the posterior temporal and parietal regions accounts for the generally spared reading comprehension. Injuries are unilateral. Prognosis is good.

2. The second type occurs with bilateral superior temporal gyrus damage, at least in part, involving both auditory association cortices. If the lesions are extensive, the patient has cortical
deafness. If the lesions are partial, the patient has reduced auditory comprehension.

3. The third type is associated with bilateral lesions, but the left lesion is usually restricted
to the auditory cortex and auditory pathways with little, if any, involvement of the posterosuperior temporal gyrus.

24. What are the characteristics of aphemia?

Patients who are aphemic have a slow and halting articulation, altered prosody, and an almost
dystonic quality of articulatory movements. Writing is usually normal. Their compromise is fairly
modality-limited—the deficit is mainly in speech output, sparing comprehension and writing.
When writing is compromised, it resembles speech in that the syntax is normal, although there
may be mild anomia. Such patients have a right facial paresis and sometimes have mild apraxia.

25. Where is the lesion that causes aphemia?

The location of the classic lesion causing aphemia is not known. When described as cortical
dysarthria or cortical dysprosody, involvement has been noted in the white matter, deep to the
lower motor cortex. Indeed, some contend that aphemias are a mild form of Broca's aphasia.
Aphemia has been described with lesions of the lower motor cortex (cortical dysarthria, cortical
dysprosody), subcortical white matter deep to the lower motor cortex (subcortical dysarthria),
middle superior paraventricular white matter, and genu of the internal capsule (capsular dysarthria, dysarthria-clumsy hand syndrome).

26. What are the characteristics of global aphasia?

1. Poor fluency
2. Poor comprehension
3. Poor repetition

The output is often restricted to meaningless speech sounds or stereotypes. Comprehension
and repetition are severely compromised.

27. Where are the lesions that cause global aphasia?

Such lesions concurrently involve Broca's area and Wernicke's area. They may be cortical-
subcortical or purely subcortical.

28. What are the features of transcortical sensory aphasia?

1. Fluent output
2. Poor comprehension
3. Good repetition
4. Many phasic disturbances
5. Echolalia
6. Impaired auditory and reading comprehension
7. Motor and sensory deficits are seldom seen
8. Right visual field deficits

29. Where is the lesion that causes transcortical sensory aphasia?

Such lesions usually involve the temporal parietal-occipital junction posterior to the superior
temporal gyrus and overlapping with the posterior portions of Wernicke's area. Some investigators believe that compromise to Brodmann's area 37, the posteroinferior temporal gyrus, is the
critical lesion.

30. What are the features of transcortical motor aphasia?

1. Nonfluent
2. Good comprehension
3. Good repetition
4. Delayed initiation of output
5. Brief utterances
6. Semantic paraphasia
7. Echolalia

Patients usually do not have impaired articulation or dysprosody of the classic nonfluent (e.g, Broca's aphasia), nor do they have agrammatical speech output.

31. Where is the lesion responsible for transcortical motor aphasia?
Such lesions have been associated with just about any site in the left frontal lobe, from the operculum to the supplementary motor area.

32. What are the features of of mixed transcortical aphasia?
1. Nonfluency
2. Poor comprehension
3. Good repetition
4. Stock phrases (e.g., "you know," "the thing is") and echolalia are pronounced

33. Where is the lesion responsible for mixed transcortical aphasia?
The lesion responsible for mixed transcortical aphasia overlaps lesions that cause transcortical motor aphasia and transcortical sensory aphasia: the dorsolateral frontal region anterior to the motor cortex and the temporal-parietal-occipital junction. This syndrome frequently follows anoxia.

34. What are the characteristics of anomic aphasia?
1. Fluent output
2. Good comprehension
3. Good repetition
4. Word-finding deficits
The term *anomic aphasia* indicates that the word-finding deficit is the only significant impairment in spoken language. Output is fluent and grammar is good, although grammar may be better in some parts of the sentence than in others.

35. Where is the lesion responsible for anomic aphasia?
Such lesions usually involve the temporal-parietal-occipital junction association cortex, Brodmann's area 37, 39, 40, 19, or 7.

36. What is a useful algorithm for classifying the cortical aphasias?

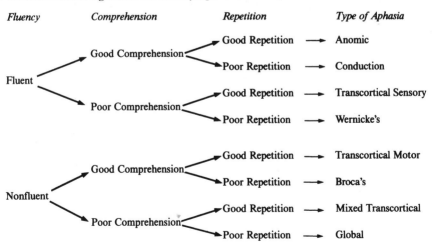

37. What are the characteristics of subcortical aphasia? When should one suspect subcortical aphasia?
Subcortical aphasias are a set of syndromes that have been defined in patients whose lesions are primarily restricted to the subcortical regions, such as the thalamus, basal ganglia, and deep

white matter pathways. Heretofore neurologists assumed that only cortical lesions were responsible for aphasic syndromes. Subcortical lesions produce aphasia but not as frequently as cortical lesions. The language characteristics of subcortical aphasias are often atypical, whereas language dysfunction associated with cortical compromise is fairly well characterized. Aphasia that is difficult to classify, in the presence of dysarthria and right hemiparesis, should cause one to suspect a subcortical lesion.

There are two main types of subcortical aphasia: one due to nonthalamic subcortical lesions and the other due to thalamic lesions.

38. What types of aphasia are associated with damage to the left basal ganglia?

Strokes in the vicinity of the left basal ganglia, particularly the putamen, sometimes produce aphasia. The types of aphasic syndromes are variable, depending on the size of the hemorrhage, but often global aphasia or Wernicke's aphasia is produced. The most common left basal ganglia infarctions causing aphasia include the anterior putamen, caudate nucleus, and anterior limb of the internal capsule, which produce the anterior subcortical syndrome, including dysarthria, decreased fluency, mildly impaired repetition (less impairment than Broca's aphasia), and mild comprehension compromise. Evidence from positron emission tomography (PET) suggests that basal ganglia lesions affect language directly as well as indirectly via decreased activation of cortical language areas.

39. What are the thalamic subcortical aphasias?

There are different types of thalamic aphasia. Lesions in the posterior left thalamus produce no definite language impairment. Lesions in the left paramedial thalamic area, including the dorsum medial and centromedian nuclei as well as the medial intramedullary laminar, produce deficits in attention and memory. When language is compromised, the compromise is limited to anomia; the impairments are probably due to lack of attention. Patients with bilateral paramedian lesions have amnesia and a broader cognitive deficit, mainly due to inattention. Such patients may appear grossly normal.

Lesions involving the anterior, ventroanterior, dorsal lateral, ventral lateral, and anterior dorsal medial nuclei or the anterior medial intramedullary region produce an aphasia similar to mixed transcortical or transcortical sensory output. Output is grammatic but terse, with some elements of echolalia. Comprehension is impaired, and repetition is fairly good. Severe anomia, agraphia, and impaired reading are usually present. Most patients are apathetic, and some are demented.

40. Does the concept of cerebral laterality for language also apply to the thalamus?

Right thalamic lesions have been associated with aphasia in left-handed patients. This suggests that hemispheric language dominance extends to the thalamic level.

41. What is primary progressive aphasia?

Progressive aphasia is a progressive deterioration of language with an insidious onset and relative absence of decline in other aspects of cognition. Careful neuropsychological testing in the majority of patients with progressive aphasia reveals cognitive impairment in nonlanguage domains. However, such patients manifest a disturbance in speech and language considerably out of proportion to other cognitive deficits. Pathologic changes are found primarily in the left temporal lobe.

42. Name, in decreasing order of frequency, the neuropathologic substrates associated with progressive aphasia.

1. Pick's disease
2. Focal spongiform degeneration
3. Alzheimer's disease

43. What is prosody?

Prosody is a suprasegmental feature of language that conveys information beyond that transmitted by word choice and word order alone. Acoustic features associated with prosody include pitch, intonation, melody, cadence, loudness, timbre, tempo, stress, accent, and timing of pauses.

44. What are the functional-anatomic correlates of prosody?

Right frontal opercular lesions impair spontaneous production of prosody, whereas posterior temporal parietal lesions usually impair comprehension of prosody.

45. How is aphasia in childhood different from aphasia in adulthood?

Most childhood aphasics are nonfluent. Until the age of 6 or 7 years, the main fundamentals of phonology, phonemics, lexicon (dictionary of words in our brain), semantics, grammar, syntax, writing, and reading are in the process of being acquired. Brain damage at this time disrupts acquisition and decreases capacity. Brain injury during early infancy usually does not cause major compromise in language. Injury after the age of 1 year causes aphasia if the injury is in the dominant hemisphere. Between the ages of 2 and 9 years, an atypical aphasia profile occurs. Fluent aphasia is rare, even with posterior left hemisphere compromise. After the age of 10, the aphasia profiles are increasingly adultlike. Recovery is more complete in children than in adults, especially up to the ages of 8–10 years.

46. What is the most common cause of childhood aphasia?

Vascular disease or trauma.

47. What is alexia?

Alexia is the disordered comprehension of written language, i.e., difficulty in reading.

48. What is dyslexia?

Alexia is the term commonly used in the United States to describe altered reading comprehension. However, in some countries, the term dyslexia is preferred. In the U.S., however, the term dyslexia generally denotes identified developmental inability to learn to read, due either to inborn deficits or perinatal injury. Alexia refers only to an acquired loss.

49. What are the three different types of alexia?

1. **Posterior alexia**, also known as pure alexia and alexia without agraphia, is characterized by inability to read but intact ability to write. Patients cannot read what they have written. Approximately 60% have an associated color anomia. If one spells a word, they can usually understand what the word is. They can spell aloud themselves. Usually, a right homonymous visual field deficit is present.

2. **Central alexia** is alexia with agraphia. Patients can neither read nor write. They can comprehend spoken language much better than written language but cannot recognize words that are spelled aloud. They can neither spell aloud nor produce written language.

3. **Anterior alexia** usually accompanies classic Broca's aphasia. Patients cannot comprehend grammatically significant relational words, such as prepositions or articles. They may comprehend written substantive words. They often fail to read aloud individual letters (literal alexia), but they may read a word that is a homophone for the latter (e.g., "see" for "sea"). Anterior alexia is associated with anterior language compromise, usually Boca's aphasia.

50. Where are the lesions that produce the different types of alexia?

1. **Posterior alexia.** The lesion usually involves the medial aspect of the dominant occipital lobe as well as to the splenium of the corpus callosum.

2. **Central alexia.** The lesion involves the dominant angular gyrus.

3. **Anterior alexia.** The lesion is similar in location to that causing Broca's aphasia.

51. What is agraphia?

Agraphia is compromised production of written language (i.e., difficulty in writing).

52. What are the clinical features of Gerstmann's syndrome?
- Acalculia
- Agraphia
- Right/left discrimination
- Finger agnosia

53. Where is the lesion responsible for Gerstmann's syndrome?
The dominant angular gyrus.

AGNOSIAS

54. What is agnosia?
Agnosia is the inability to recognize objects despite adequate perception in the modality (i.e., visual, tactile, auditory) in which the object is presented.

55. What are two types of visual agnosia?
1. **Apperceptive agnosia** is characterized by good acuity, good perception of movement, and good ability to perceive color. Yet the perception of form is poor, and patients complain of poor vision. They are unable to draw objects or copy pictures. They cannot distinguish different shapes. Although they cannot name objects, they can name colors.
2. **Associative visual agnosia** is not accompanied by complaints of poor vision. Patients can draw, copy, and distinguish shapes. They do not describe the object, circumlocute, gesture, or mimic the use and can neither recognize nor name the object. Patients with associative visual agnosia cannot recognize objects through vision alone.

56. Pinpoint the location of the lesions responsible for visual agnosia.
Apperceptive visual agnosia usually results from compromise in the calcarine cortex. Patients with associative visual agnosia usually have bilateral, inferior, temporal-occipital lesions that involve the inferior visual association cortex and the white matter pathways into the parahippocampal gyrus. Patients usually have bilateral upper visual field compromise, mild general anomia, severe alexia, and memory impairment.

57. What is prosopagnosia?
Prosopagnosia is the inability to recognize familiar faces. It is frequently associated with achromatopsia or agraphia and is always associated with unilateral or bilateral visual field deficits.

58. Where is the lesion responsible for prosopagnosia?
Prosopagnosia is associated with bilateral occipital-temporal lesions.

59. What is anosognosia?
Anosognosia refers to denial of illness. There are two types: verbal, explicit denial of illness and lack of concern about the deficit.

60. In which four different behavioral syndromes can anosognosia occur?
Wernicke's aphasia   Left hemianopsia
Anton's syndrome   Left hemiplegia
It also may occur in patients with Korsakoff's syndrome or frontal lobe dysfunction.

61 What is Anton's syndrome?
It is a syndrome of cortical blindness in which patients deny being blind and confabulate responses when confronted with their errors, making excuses. They may have simple or complex visual hallucinations. The syndrome is usually associated with bilateral cerebral infarcts in the distributions of the posterior cerebral arteries that involve the primary visual areas of the

calcarine cortex (Brodmann's area 17) and visual association areas. Parietal and temporal lobes are sometimes injured.

APRAXIAS

62. What is apraxia?

Apraxia is the inability to perform a skilled, learned, purposeful motor act in the absence of a primary disturbance in attention, comprehension, motivation, power, tone, coordination, or sensation that would preclude that act. Individuals must be able to perform the act spontaneously. Thus, an individual may not be able to wave goodbye when so instructed but can wave goodbye when he or she spontaneously chooses to do so.

63. What are the three major types of apraxia?

1. **Motor ataxia** represents a breakdown in the smooth execution of a movement despite perseveration of the intended motor pattern. The performance is not affected by the modality of request (e.g., spoken or written). The disturbance is purely one of output.

2. **Ideomotor apraxia** is the inability to carry out a learned motor pattern to a stimulus that should elicit it (verbal command or gesture for initiation). The errors are usually perseverations or crude undifferentiated movements.

3. **Ideational apraxia** is due to consternation about how to carry out a movement, but once the patient has been cued, he or she produces the correct response. Such patients fail to use everyday objects correctly.

64. Where are the lesions responsible for apraxias?

1. **Motor apraxia** usually results from damage to the motor association cortex, contralateral to the affected limb.

2. **Ideomotor apraxia** is often associated with large parietal lesions, especially involving the inferior part of the parietal lobe. Large lesions may be deep in the periolandic region, compromising the deep parietal-frontal connections and/or input to the callosal pathways.

3. **Ideational apraxia** often involves compromise in the dominant parietal lobe, but this has not been well delineated.

65. What is dressing apraxia?

Dressing apraxia is not a true apraxia. It is an inability to dress that is often associated with left visual field deficits and topographic disorientation. Lesions in the right parietal-occipital-temporal region cause problems with complex perceptual-spatial actions, including dressing. Another problem arising from this region is hemineglect, in which one-half of the body is neither clothed nor groomed.

66. What is constructional apraxia?

Constructional apraxia is also a misnomer. Patients have difficulty in copying figures, but this difficulty does not imply apraxia. It is also associated with right parietal lobe lesions.

67. What is apraxia of speech?

Apraxia of speech is a controversial term. In its classic concept, it is characterized by articulatory imprecision that worsens with increased phonetic complexity. However, it is not a true apraxia. All patients have some deficit in comprehension. The disturbance is thought to represent an interaction of the phonologic errors due to paresis and ataxia of the articulatory system and of phonemic errors due to damage anywhere in the functional system for phonemic production (upper temporal gyrus to the lower motor cortex).

BIBLIOGRAPHY

1. Damasio AR, Damasio AH: Aphasia and the neural basis of language. In Marsel Mesulam M (ed): Principles of Behavioral and Cognitive Neurology, 2nd ed. Oxford, Oxford University Press, 2000, pp 294–315.
2. Galaburda AM: Anatomy of developmental disorders: Geschwind's last legacy. In Schachter SC, Davinsky O (eds): Behavioral Neurology and the Legacy of Norman Geschwind. Philadelphia, Lippincott-Raven, 1997, pp 89–100.
3. Kirshner KS: Aphasia. In Bradley WG, et al (eds): Neurology and Clinical Practice, 3rd ed. Boston, Butterworth-Heinemann, 2000, pp 141–160.
4. Mega MS, Alexander MP, Cummings JL, Benson DF: The aphasias and related disturbances. In Joint RJ, Griggs RC (eds): Baker's Clinical Neurology on CD-ROM. Philadelphia, Lippincott Williams & Wilkins, 2000.
5. Rosenfield DB, Barroso AO: Difficulties with speech and swallowing. In Bradley WG, et al (eds): Neurology and Clinical Practice, 3rd ed. Boston, Butterworth-Heinemann, 2000, pp 171–186.
6. Ross ED: Affective prosody in the aprosodias. In Marsel Mesulam M (ed): Principles of Behavioral and Cognitive Neurology, 2nd ed. Oxford, Oxford University Press, 2000, pp 316–331.

Website
www.bcm.tmc.edu/neurol/challeng/pat 23/summary.html

16. DYSARTHRIA, DYSFLUENCY, AND DYSPHAGIA

David B. Rosenfield, M.D.

DYSARTHRIA

1. Which parts of the brain are involved in speech motor output?

Human speech production involves coordination among respiration, laryngeal activity, and supralaryngeal articulatory movement. The lower motoneurons that control the respiratory movements reside in the anterior portion of the cervical, thoracic, and upper lumbar spinal cord. Motoneurons controlling laryngeal closure reside in the nucleus ambiguus. Neurons directly responsible for the supralaryngeal musculature are the trigeminal motor nucleus, facial nucleus, rostral portion of the nucleus ambiguus, hypoglossal nucleus, and anterior horn cells at the rostral portion of the cervical spinal cord. These lower motor neurons and the bilateral inputs from multiple realms (including motor cortex) of both hemispheres constitute the underlying neural input of speech motor production.

2. What is dysphonia?

Dysphonia is an abnormality in phonation (sound output from the larynx).

3. What is the difference between speech compromise and language compromise?

Speech is motor output. **Speech compromise** is a deficiency in the way speech sounds. It refers to the underlying motor component. **Language compromise** involves errors in syntax, word choice, or how sounds are put together. Talking with food in one's mouth causes speech compromise. An aphasic patient has acquired language compromise.

4. What is the primary difference between communication among animals and humans?

Animals have a system of communication, whereas humans have a system of language. Animals do not have a generative grammar, whereas humans do. However, the brain of an animal must learn to control the sound output, just as a human does.

5. What is dysarthria?

Dysarthria, although implying a problem of articulation only, is a defect in phonation as well as resonance. Phonation is sound production (from larynx). Resonance is how the sounds are altered in the cavity between the larynx and vocal fold and the lips/nares (e.g., hyponasal, hypernasal).

6. What are the causes of dysarthria?

Dysarthria may be due to compromise of the brain, brainstem, cerebellum, nerve, neuromuscular junction, or muscle. All diseases that affect these regions, considerable in number, may cause dysarthria, particularly myopathy, myositis, myasthenia gravis, neuropathies, motor neuron disease, cerebellar disease, tumors of the brain and brainstem, Parkinson's disease, and various other movement disorders.

7. What determines prognosis in dysarthria when it is caused by damage to the cerebral hemispheres?

Patients with damage in only one hemisphere have a much better prognosis for dysarthria than patients with damage in both hemispheres.

8. Where can the brain be stimulated during ongoing speech to cause speech arrest?

In right-handed people, just about anywhere in the left hemisphere and in the area of the motor strip on the right. Stimulation of the supplementary motor area, bilaterally, induces speech arrest.

9. What happens when Broca's area is electrically stimulated?

If Broca's area is stimulated while someone is talking, the persons stops talking. If it is stimulated while a person is not talking, a grunted sound is elicited.

10. What happens when Wernicke's area is electrically stimulated?

If Wernicke's area is electrically stimulated while someone is talking, the person stops talking. If it is stimulated during silence, a sound may be elicited but not a sentence of word output.

11. What is the Wada test?

The Wada test involves injection of a short-acting barbiturate into the carotid artery of one hemisphere to render the patient plegic, numb, and blind on the side opposite the injection. If language "resides" on the injected side, the patient also becomes aphasic. The test is named after Dr. Jun Wada.

12. How does the Wada test relate to handedness?

The correlation is excellent. Over 95% of persons who become aphasic when only one particular hemisphere is injected during the Wada test have handedness pertaining to dominance of the injected hemisphere.

13. List common brain/brainstem causes of dysarthria.

Structural compromise of the corticobulbar tracts (unilaterally or bilaterally) or cranial nerve nuclei V, VII, X, or XII may cause dysarthria. Common diseases that cause such compromise are stroke, tumor, demyelinating disease, motor neuron disease, and collagen disease.

14. What are the speech signs in Parkinson's disease?

Phonation is weak, pitch varies little, volume is low, and the patient is hoarse. Accelerated rate, repetitive dysfluencies, and imprecise consonants may occur. Reduced vocal intensity and abnormal articulation contribute to the impaired intelligibility of many patients with Parkinson's disease. Speech treatment usually focuses on improving articulation and rate but has met with limited success.

15. What are the speech signs in hyperkinetic dysarthria-chorea?

Sudden alterations in pitch and loudness, phonatory arrest, strained hoarseness, and sudden alterations in precision of vowels and consonants.

16. What are the speech signs in hyperkinetic dysarthria-phonatory tremor?

Rhythmic alterations in pitch and loudness, adductor phonatory arrests, and compensatory strain or strangle.

17. What are the speech signs in Gilles de la Tourette syndrome?

Grunts, barks, squeaks, throat clearing, gurgling, moaning, snorting, sniffing, whistling, clicking, lip smacking, spitting, unintelligible sounds, echolalia, coprolalia, and dysfluencies.

18. What are the speech signs in cerebellar disease?

Phonation may be associated with tremor and variations in loudness. Irregular articulatory breakdown, imprecise consonants, and sometimes excessive and equal stress in all syllables of words are present.

19. List the nerve-damage causes of dysarthria.

Collagen disease, viral infection, diabetes, and alcohol.

20. What are the speech signs in motor neuron disease?

Phonation is strained, harsh, wet, and sometimes fluttering during vowel prolongation. Speech is hypernasal. Articulation is slow, consonants are imprecise, phrases are short, and vowels are distorted.

21. What is the effect of a fifth cranial nerve (trigeminal) lesion on speech output?

Phonation and velopharyngeal function are normal, mandibular muscles are weak, and vowels and consonants are imprecise.

22. How does a lesion of the seventh cranial nerve (facial) affect speech?

Phonation and velopharyngeal function are normal, the orbicularis orbis is weak (causing difficulty in producing /p/ sounds), vowels are imprecise, and labial consonants are imprecise.

23. How does the tenth cranial nerve (vagus) lesion affect speech?

Phonation is hoarse and breathy, and volume is low. Speech is hypernasal if the lesion is above the pharyngeal branch.

24. What is the effect of a twelfth cranial nerve (hypoglossal) lesion on speech?

Phonation and velopharyngeal function are normal. The tongue is weak, demonstrating atrophy and fasciculation. The patient may have drooling, imprecise vowels, and imprecise lingual consonants.

25. Which muscles adduct the vocal folds?

Thyroarytenoid, interarytenoid, lateral cricothyroid, and lateral cricoarytenoid.

26. Which muscles abduct the vocal folds?

Posterior cricoarytenoid.

27. Which nerves innervate which muscles in the larynx?

All of the muscles in the larynx are innervated by branches from the recurrent laryngeal nerve.

28. What are the causes of recurrent laryngeal nerve paralysis?

1. Inflammation (viral disease, collagen disease, pulmonary tuberculosis, coccidioidomycosis)
2. Polyneuropathy (especially diabetes and alcohol)
3. Trauma (intubation, neck trauma, head trauma, mediastinoscopy, radical neck dissection, carotid endarterectomy, cardiovascular surgery, thyroidectomy, esophageal resection for carcinoma)
4. Neoplasm
5. Syringomyelia
6. Idiopathic

29. List the causes of bilateral abductor vocal cord paralysis in adults.

1. Thyroidectomy
2. Neck malignancy
3. Poliomyelitis
4. Brainstem stroke
5. Guillain-Barré syndrome
6. Demyelinating disease
7. Central nervous system neoplasm
8. Central nervous system infection
9. Charcot-Marie-Tooth disease

Rare causes: foreign bodies near the larynx, bilateral carotid dissection, neck infection, head or neck trauma, substernal thyroid, idiopathic.

30. How does myasthenia affect speech?

Its effects are similar to those of a myopathy, but speech improves with rest.

31. What is the effect of myopathy/myositis on speech output?

Phonatory output is hoarse, breathy, and diplophonic and has low volume. The speech is hypernasal, and vowels and consonants may be compromised, depending on the muscles involved.

32. Name four muscle disturbances that can cause dysarthria.

Collagen disease, polymyositis, dermatomyositis, hypothyroidism.

33. Define spasmodic dysphonia.

Spasmodic dysphonia is effortful, strained speech associated with a sensation of strain and strangle.

34. What is the most common presentation of spasmodic dysphonia?

Strain in the throat, interruption of sound while talking, and difficulty in getting words out, but with no evidence of associated aphasia.

35. What are the neurologic causes of spasmodic dysphonia?

Laryngeal tremor, laryngeal dystonia, and other movement disorders involving the laryngeal neuromotor system. It also may be a symptom of psychiatric disease.

36. What is the prognosis in spasmodic dysphonia?

When the condition is associated with tremor, the prognosis is fairly good with therapy. Many experts contend that patients do fairly well with speech therapy; others opt more strongly for various medications, including botulinum toxin injections.

37. What are the speech characteristics of corticobasal degeneration?

Speech characteristics of corticobasal degeneration (CBD) include dysfluency, nonfluentlike aphasia, phonologic errors incorporating what some term *speech apraxia*, and elements of oral (buccofacial) apraxia. Be careful about diagnosing CBD as the culprit of speech compromise unless oral apraxia is also present.

DYSFLUENCY

38. What are the prevalence and characteristics of developmental stuttering?

Developmental stuttering is much more common among males than females (ratio of 4:1). Some argue that everyone stutters, some for just a few minutes or few hours. The prevalence of stuttering in childhood is 4% and in adulthood slightly over 1%. Developmental stutterers stutter at the beginning of sentences and phrases, are more fluent when their speech is markedly slowed and drawn out, and do not stutter when they sing. Other fluency-evoking maneuvers include repetitive reading, choral reading, and interference by loud, broad-band noise with hearing of one's own speech. Development stutterers are emotionally bothered by their dysfluent output.

39. Can a previously fluent person become a stutterer after brain injury?

Yes. Acquired stutterers stutter throughout the sentence, whereas developmental stutterers usually stutter at the beginning of sentences and phrases. In addition, fluency-evoking maneuvers, such as singing, do not help acquired stutterers but render developmental stutterers almost totally fluent. As opposed to developmental stutterers, acquired stutterers are only minimally distraught at their compromised output.

40. What are the causes of acquired stuttering?

The causes of acquired stuttering include compromise to either hemisphere, anterior or posterior. The damage is usually mild. The damage may be due to stroke, vasculitis, infection, tumor, trauma, or metabolic compromise. Psychogenic causes also exist.

41. Describe the characteristics of cluttering.

The clutterer's speech is characterized by excessive speed, repetitions, interjections, disturbed prosody, and sometimes inconsistent articulatory disturbances. Some contend that such patients have errors in grammar, are hyperactive, and have poor concentration. Although their rate of speech may not always be markedly increased, the listener usually has the sensation that it is. As opposed to developmental stutterers, clutterers frequently are unconcerned about their speech deficit.

42. What are the characteristics of palilalia?

Palilalics compulsively repeat phrases or words with reiteration at increasing speed and with a decrescendo volume.

43. Which diseases are associated with palilalia?

Postencephalitic Parkinson's disease, idiopathic Parkinson's disease, and pseudobulbar palsy.

DYSPHAGIA

44. What is dysphagia?
Dysphagia (difficulty in swallowing) is a subjective symptom as opposed to an objective sign until delay or disruption in the swallowing mechanism can be documented. If no objective evidence of dysphagia can be documented, globus hystericus should be considered. Dysphagia may be due to mechanical factors that physically narrow the oropharyngeal lumen and obstruct food passage or to neuromotor diseases that cause inadequate food bolus propulsion into the stomach.

45. List the three stages of swallowing.
1. Oropreparatory stage (food passes from mouth into pharynx).
2. Pharyngeal transfer stage (food passes through the pharynx, over the larynx, and into the esophagus).
3. Esophageal stage (food is transported from proximal esophagus, the upper one-third of which contains striated muscle, to the lower two-thirds, which consists of smooth muscle, across the lower esophageal sphincter, and into the stomach).

46. What is the swallow reflex?
The swallow reflex mediates the first stage of swallowing into the second. It consists of several movements. The soft palate moves upward (velar elevation), closing the passageway between the oral and nasal cavity; the pharyngeal muscles contract (pharyngeal peristalsis), the larynx elevates, and posterior flexion of the epiglottis closes the airway to the trachea. Vocal cord closure occurs, followed by relaxation of the cricopharyngeus muscle, the upper esophageal sphincter.

47. What is the role of the vagus nerve in swallowing?
The vagus nerve supplies motor fibers to the striated muscle of the esophagus. Thus, a serious consequence of damaging the vagus at the origin of the esophageal branch is dysphagia. A high vagotomy permanently paralyzes the striated muscle at the upper one-third of the esophagus. Peristalsis in the lower two-thirds of the esophagus is an automatic function, mediated by the intrinsic myoenteric plexuses and smooth muscle.

48. Are there different types of dysphagia?
Dysphagia may be due to mechanical problems or neuromotor problems. Each of these realms has an oropharyngeal and an esophageal component.

49. What are the symptoms of oropharyngeal dysphagia?
The symptoms typically occur immediately upon swallowing and include the sensation of food sticking in the neck, pain while swallowing, nasal regurgitation of food or fluids, and coughing and choking due to aspiration. Discomfort in the midneck area may be present.

50. List the cause of oropharyngeal neuromotor dysphagia.
1. Motor neuron disease
2. Brain tumor
3. Stroke
4. Neuropathy (includes mechanical nerve injury)
5. Demyelinating disease
6. Degenerative disease (especially spinocerebellar)
7. Syringobulbia
8. Myasthenia gravis
9. Myopathy (including oculopharyngeal muscular dystrophy, hypothyroidism, polymyositis, dermatomyositis)

10. Parkinson's disease
11. Cerebral palsy
12. Tardive dyskinesia
13. Cricopharyngeal achalasia
14. Xerostomia (dry mouth)
15. Sjögren's syndrome
16. Scleroderma

51. What are the causes of oropharyngeal mechanical dysphagia?
1. Oropharyngeal tumor
2. Zenker's diverticulum
3. Cervical osteophytes
4. Dislocation of temporomandibular joint
5. Macroglossia
6. Congenital abnormalities
7. Tight circumoral tissue due to scleroderma/burns
8. Neck surgery
9. Retropharyngeal mass
10. Large goiter

52. What are the symptoms of mechanical dysphagia?
Symptoms related to mechanical (oropharyngeal, oroesophageal) dysphagia are usually caused by difficulty in swallowing solid foods, progressing to difficulty in swallowing liquids. When the disorder is advanced, patients cannot swallow their own salivary secretions. Symptoms may occur immediately, seconds, or minutes after swallowing, depending on the level and chronicity of the underlying process. More rostral levels of dysfunction cause earlier symptoms.

53. What causes esophageal neuromotor dysphagia?
1. Scleroderma
2. Achalasia
3. Diffuse esophageal spasm
4. Polymyositis and dermatomyositis (usually oropharyngeal)
5. Idiopathic autonomic dysfunction
6. Postvagotomy dysphagia
7. Neuropathy (vagal disease, especially diabetes)
8. Amyloidoses (primary or secondary)
9. Symptomatic esophageal peristalsis (nutcracker esophagus)

54. List the causes of esophageal mechanical dysphagia.
1. Esophageal carcinoma
2. Metastases to esophagus
3. Benign esophageal tumor
4. Inflammation
5. Strictures of the esophagus
6. Pancreatitis with pseudocysts
7. Pancreatic tumors
8. Postvagotomy hematoma/fibrosis
9. Thoracic aorta aneurysm
10. Posterior mediastinal mass
11. Large hiatal hernia
12. Dysphagia lusoria (abnormal origin of the right subclavian artery)

BIBLIOGRAPHY

1. Damasio AR, Damasio AH: Aphasia and the neural basis of language. In Marsel Mesulam M (ed): Principles of Behavioral and Cognitive Neurology, 2nd ed. Oxford, Oxford University Press, 2000, pp 294–315.
2. Mega MS, Alexander NP, Cummings JL, Benson DF: The aphasias and related disturbances. In Joint RJ, Griggs RC (eds): Baker's Clinical Neurology on CD-ROM. Philadelphia, Lippincott William & Wilkins, 2000.
3. Rosenfield DB, Barroso AO: Difficulties with speech and swallowing. In Bradley WG, et al (eds): Neurology and Clinical Practice, 3rd ed. Boston, Butterworth-Heinemann, 2000, pp 171–186.
4. Rosenfield DB: Stuttering. In Schachter SC, Davinsky O (eds): Behavioral Neurology and the Legacy of Norman Geschwind. Philadelphia, Lippincott-Raven, 1997, pp 101–114.
5. Rosenfield DB, Viswanath NS, Helekar SA: An animal model of stuttering. In Peters HSM (ed): Proceedings of the Third World Congress on Fluency Disorders, Elsevier [in press].

Website
www.voice-center.com/dystonia.html

17. VASCULAR DISEASE

David Chiu, M.D., and John P. Winikates, M.D.

CLINICAL FEATURES

1. What is stroke?

Stroke is a clinical syndrome defined by acute neurologic deficits in the setting of focal disruption of the cerebral circulation. There are a number of subtypes, including atherothrombotic, cardioembolic, lacunar, and hemorrhagic strokes. Rather than representing diagnostic closure, a stroke should prompt the search for an etiologic explanation.

2. How common is stroke?

Stroke is the most common disabling neurologic disease. It is the third leading cause of death in the industrialized world after heart disease and cancer. In the United States, about 750,000 strokes and 150,000 resultant deaths occur annually. Stroke is also the leading cause of serious disability in adults.

3. What is the most common presenting symptom of stroke?

About 70% of strokes present with hemiparesis. The second most common disabling symptom is aphasia.

4. Describe the clinical profile of a thrombotic stroke.

An atherothrombotic stroke may be sudden, stuttering, or stepwise in onset. The classic history is a patient who awakens from sleep with the deficit. This stroke subtype results from thrombosis associated with atherosclerotic lesions of the large and medium-sized arteries in the neck or brain. Strokes caused by carotid disease are included in this category. The mechanism of cerebral infarction in this setting is often artery-to-artery embolism of platelet-fibrin thrombi or atherosclerotic material rather than purely hemodynamic.

5. Describe the clinical profile of a cardioembolic stroke.

The typical cardioembolic stroke has an abrupt temporal profile, with deficits that are maximal at onset. Deficits may improve shortly afterward if the embolus breaks up and travels to more distal branches of the affected artery. The classic history is an onset of symptoms during activity or in association with palpitations or a Valsalva maneuver. The heart and aortic arch are sources of such emboli.

6. Describe the clinical profile of a lacunar stroke.

There are four classic lacunar stroke syndromes: (1) pure motor hemiparesis, with face, arm, and leg equally affected; (2) pure hemisensory stroke; (3) clumsy hand–dysarthria; and (4) ataxia hemiparesis, characterized by ipsilateral incoordination out of proportion to the degree of weakness. Other lacunar stroke syndromes have been described, but these four are the most widely recognized. Lacunar strokes are associated with hypertension and/or diabetes and are related to occlusion of small perforating arterioles by lipohyalinosis or microatheroma

7. Describe the clinical profile of a hemorrhagic stroke.

Hemorrhagic strokes have a clinical profile that may not be clearly distinguishable from ischemic strokes. A prominent decrease in level of consciousness can be a clue. Headache, nausea, vomiting, severe hypertension, or other signs of raised intracranial pressure also suggest a hemorrhagic stroke. Common sites for hypertensive intracerebral hemorrhage are the putamen, thalamus, pons, cerebellum, and hemispheric lobes. Hemorrhagic strokes can result from ruptured cerebral aneurysms with subarachnoid hemorrhage, ruptured arterial venous malformations, or amyloid angiopathy.

8. What percentage of strokes can be attributed to each type? Describe onset, imaging findings, and other salient features of each type.

Types of Strokes

TYPE	% OF STROKES	ONSET	MRI OR CT SCAN	OTHER FEATURES
Atherothrombotic	20	May be gradual	Infarction	Carotid bruit
Cardioembolic	30	Sudden	Cortical infarction, may undergo spontaneous hemorrhagic transformation	Underlying heart disease, peripheral emboli, strokes in different vascular territories
Lacunar	20	May be gradual	Small, deep infarction	Pure motor or sensory
Other ischemic/ cryptogenic	20	Varied	Varied	Young patient, risk factors absent
Hemorrhagic	10	Sudden	Hyperdensity on CT	Depressed level of consciousness, nausea and vomiting, headache

9. What are the main anatomic syndromes in cerebrovascular disease?
The first anatomic challenge is to localize the lesion to the anterior or posterior circulation. The anterior or carotid artery territory encompasses the frontal lobes, parietal lobes, basal ganglia, internal capsule, and a major portion of the temporal lobes. The posterior or vertebrobasilar territory includes the brainstem, cerebellum, thalamus, occipital lobes, and mesial and inferior temporal lobes.

10. What are the major symptoms of a vascular event affecting the anterior circulation?
Hemiparesis with or without ipsilateral hemisensory loss is the most common symptom of a stroke in the carotid circulation, although lesions in the brainstem also can produce hemiplegia. A specific pattern of hemiparesis can be a helpful clue. Weakness affecting the face and arm more than the leg suggests a stroke in the middle cerebral artery territory, whereas a deficit mainly involving the leg is characteristic of an anterior cerebral artery stroke.

Aphasia, neglect, apraxia, and seizures are other signs of involvement of the internal carotid artery territory. Gaze deviation to the side opposite the hemiparesis is highly suggestive as well.

Amaurosis fugax or transient monocular visual loss implies ischemia in the territory of the ophthalmic artery, the first branch of the internal carotid artery. Homonymous hemianopia, if associated with some of the deficits discussed above, usually represents subcortical involvement of the optic radiations.

11. What signs suggest posterior circulation localization?
Brainstem findings suggest disease involving the vertebrobasilar system and its branches. Diplopia, dysarthria, dysphagia, dizziness/vertigo, and ataxia are among the classic symptoms of vertebrobasilar disease. Dizziness is the least specific symptom of vertebrobasilar disease but the most common. Crossed findings (e.g., loss of pinprick and temperature sensation on one one side of the face and the contralateral extremities) is a brainstem pattern that stems from the decussation of various long tracts at different levels of the brainstem.

Vertebrobasilar insufficiency is in the differential diagnosis of syncope, although other focal findings are typically present. A major stroke in the territory of the basilar artery can produce coma, quadriparesis, and decerebrate posturing.

12. What are the most important causes of stroke in the anterior circulation?

The most important causes of stroke in the anterior circulation are internal carotid artery stenosis, cardiac embolism, atherothrombotic disease of the major intracranial branches (especially the middle cerebral artery), and small vessel disease of the penetrating arteries.

13. What are the most important causes of stroke in the posterior circulation?

Posterior circulation symptoms often relate to atherosclerosis of the vertebrobasilar arteries or aortic arch or to small vessel disease in the penetrating branches. Cardiac embolism to the vertebrobasilar circulation has a predilection for the distal basilar territory, especially the terminal branches of the basilar artery (posterior cerebral arteries).

14. Describe the basic evaluation of a suspected stroke.

The first stage in evaluation is the **history**. The described symptoms suggest the initial localization. The time course of stroke is relatively acute, but some details may be clues to the pathogenesis of the individual event. Onset during sleep or a stuttering progression suggests an atherothrombotic mechanism or a lacunar stroke, whereas sudden onset with maximal deficit at the beginning suggests a cardiac embolism. The **physical examination** includes assessment of the cardiovascular system for the presence of heart murmurs, congestive heart failure, cardiac arrhythmias, carotid bruits, and signs of peripheral vascular disease. The **neurologic exam** focuses on the major deficit and a search for important associated signs that aid in localization.

15. Which initial laboratory studies should be obtained for patients with a stroke?

Laboratory studies indicated during the initial evaluation include complete blood count (CBC), platelet count, prothrombin time (PT) and partial thromboplastin time (PTT), electrolytes, glucose, blood urea nitrogen (BUN), creatinine, chest radiograph, and electrocardiogram (EKG). These provide both general medical assessment and evaluation for some of the complications and underlying risk factors. Subsequent laboratory analysis should include a fasting lipid profile.

In selected cases, antithrombin III, protein C and protein S, activated protein C resistance, and prothrombin gene mutation studies may indicate an inherited hypercoagulable state. Anticardiolipin antibody and lupus anticoagulant can point to antiphospholipid antibody syndromes a cause of stroke. Hyperhomocysteinemia is a risk factor for atherosclerosis and thrombosis. Blood cultures should be obtained in any patient with suspected endocarditis.

If vasculitis is suspected as the underlying cause, screening is done by measurement of erythrocyte sedimentation rate (ESR), rapid plasma reagin (RPR), antinuclear antibody (ANA), rheumatoid factor, serum protein electrophoresis (SPEP), and complement levels C3, C4, and CH50.

16. What initial imaging should be performed in acute stroke?

Noncontrast CT scanning of the brain is the initial imaging study of choice. The distinction between ischemic and hemorrhagic stroke is readily made by CT. Routine MR imaging can miss the diagnosis of subarachnoid hemorrhage. Other practical advantages of CT over MRI are its more rapid availability, less need for patient cooperation, and greater suitability for critically ill or potentially unstable patients.

MRI is often the favored imaging modality for patients with nonacute stroke, in whom its greater sensitivity for ischemic stroke, especially in the posterior fossa, becomes an important advantage. Special MR sequences add to the range of information provided. Diffusion-weighted imaging, for example, allows determination of the acuity of ischemic lesions. MR angiography is a valuable screening study for arterial stenosis or aneurysms.

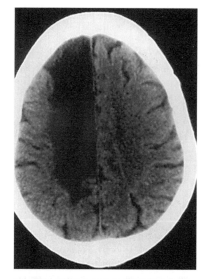

Noncontrast CT scan of the brain showing a well-established ischemic stroke in the territory of the anterior
cerebral artery.

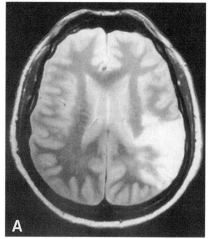 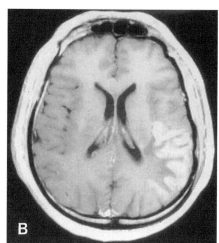

MR of an acute ischemic stroke in the posterior area of the middle cerebral artery territory. The stroke is
shown on a proton density technique *(A)* and a gadolinium-enhanced T1 image *(B)*, which demonstrates the
gyral enhancement characteristic of many infarcts.

17. What cardiac work-up may be useful in stroke?

A cardiac exam, EKG, and chest radiograph may be all that is necessary in some cases of
stroke. Transthoracic echocardiography is frequently performed and is useful in assessing ventricular and valvular function. Transesophageal echocardiography (TEE) is more sensitive than
transthoracic echo for the detection of atrial and aortic abnormalities, especially patent foramen ovale, atrial septal aneurysm, left atrial appendage thrombus, and aortic arch atheroma.

Cardiac and/or Holter monitoring is frequently performed and occasionally reveals unsuspected
cardiac arrhythmias such as intermittent atrial fibrillation. Myocardial infarction is a common cause
of death after stroke, especially in patients with cardiac risk factors. Evaluation for coronary artery
disease can be performed with stress thallium cardiac scans. Although this technique may be
useful in identifying occult coronary artery disease, its routine use has not yet been established.

18. What other imaging methods may be useful in evaluating stroke?

Carotid Doppler ultrasound may be useful in screening the extracranial internal carotid arteries for atherosclerotic disease. Its accuracy depends on the experience of the laboratory performing the test. Magnetic resonance angiography (MRA) also may be used to evaluate the carotid circulation, the vertebrobasilar system, the circle of Willis, and the anterior, middle, and posterior cerebral arteries and their major branches. MRA can provide valuable information about the intracerebral circulation not otherwise available without cerebral angiography. Because of turbulence at a site of stenosis, MRA overestimates the degree of stenosis compared with contrast angiography.

Contrast cerebral angiography provides the most detailed and reliable information about carotid and intracranial disease. In experienced hands, the complication rate should be < 1%.

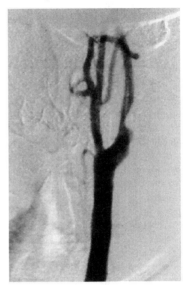

Contrast angiography showing atherosclerotic stenosis of the left internal carotid artery.

19. What is the role of transcranial Doppler imaging in assessment of strokes?

Transcranial Doppler can provide information about blood flow in intracranial arteries. Blood flow velocities can be measured in the middle cerebral, anterior cerebral, posterior cerebral, vertebral, and basilar arteries by using different ultrasound "windows" in the skull. Decreased flow in the middle cerebral artery may be evidence of stenosis more proximally in the internal carotid; increased flow velocity may be evidence of stenosis or vasospasm in the middle cerebral artery. The technique also may be used to confirm cross-filling of the middle cerebral artery on one side from the contralateral internal carotid artery via the circle of Willis.

RISK FACTORS

20. What are the major risk factors for stroke?

The most important established risk factor for stroke is age, and second is probably hypertension. Additional well-established risk factors are:

1. Gender (male > female)
2. Family history
3. Diabetes mellitus
4. Cardiac disease
5. Prior stroke
6. Transient ischemic attacks
7. Carotid bruits
8. Smoking
9. Increased hematocrit
10. Elevated fibrinogen level
11. Hemoglobinopathy
12. Drug abuse, such as cocaine

Wolf PA: Epidemiology and stroke risk factors. In Samuels MA, Feske S (eds): Office Practice of Neurology. New York, Churchill-Livingstone, 1996, pp 224–237.

21. What other risk factors have been described?
1. Hyperlipidemia
2. Diet
3. Oral contraceptives
4. Sedentary lifestyle
5. Obesity
6. Peripheral vascular disease
7. Hyperuricemia
8. Infection
9. Hyperhomocysteinemia
10. Migraine
11. African-American race
12. Geography ("the Stroke Belt")
13. Alcohol consumption

22. What is the significance of hypertension as a risk factor for stroke?
From a public health standpoint, hypertension is the most important modifiable risk factor for stroke. The risk of all stroke subtypes is increased 3- to 4-fold by hypertension. Included is the isolated systolic hypertension of the elderly, once thought to be relatively benign. Treatment significantly lowers stroke incidence.

23. What forms of cardiac disease are risk factors for stroke?
People with heart disease of almost any type have more than twice the risk of stroke compared with people with normal cardiac function. Coronary artery disease is a major association, both as an indicator of the presence of systemic atherosclerosis and as a potential source of emboli from mural thrombi due to myocardial infarction. Congestive heart failure of any etiology is associated with an increased incidence of stroke. Hypertensive heart disease, whether detected clinically, by left ventricular hypertrophy (LVH) on EKG, or by echocardiogram, is associated with an increased risk of both thromboembolic and hemorrhagic strokes.

Another major stroke risk factor is atrial fibrillation, which is strongly associated with cerebral embolism. Atrial fibrillation due to rheumatic valvular disease has the strongest association, increasing stroke risk by 17 times. Nonvalvular and lone atrial fibrillation also have been shown to increase stroke risk, especially with advancing age.

Various other cardiac lesions have been associated with stroke, such as patent foramen ovale, atrial septal aneurysm, aortic arch atheroma, left atrial appendage thrombus, spontaneous echo contrast, and mitral valve prolapse. Many of these are poorly seen with transthoracic echo but readily detected on transesophageal echo. The clinical significance and appropriate therapy of many of these lesions with respect to stroke remain to be clarified.

24. Is smoking an established risk factor for stroke?
Meta-analysis of epidemiologic studies has shown that cigarette smoking confers an increased risk for stroke, that the degree of risk correlates with the number of cigarettes smoked, and that smoking cessation decreases risk, with the incidence reverting to that of nonsmokers by 5 years after smoking cessation. Smoking confers increased risk in all age groups and both sexes. The association applies not only to ischemic stroke but also to subarachnoid hemorrhage due to cerebral aneurysms.

25. What is the single strongest risk factor for stroke?
Age is the strongest single stroke risk factor. About 30% of strokes occur before the age of 65; 70% occur in those 65 and over. Stroke risk roughly doubles for every decade of age after 55 years.

26. What is the role of abnormal lipids in stroke? What is the role of drugs abuse?
Although elevated cholesterol clearly has been related to ischemic heart disease, its relation to stroke was less clear until recently. Elevated cholesterol is a risk factor for carotid atherosclerosis. Lipid-lowering therapy with statins in patients with ischemic heart disease reduces the incidence of stroke by approximately 30%. Very low cholesterol, on the other hand, may be a risk factor for hemorrhagic stroke.

Drugs of abuse also increase stroke risk. Cocaine and amphetamines are associated with intracerebral and subarachnoid hemorrhage. Intravenous drug use increases the risk of endocarditis and ischemic stroke.

27. Do oral contraceptives increase stroke risk in women?

The early, high-estrogen oral contraceptives were reported to increase the risk of stroke in young women. Lowering the estrogen content has decreased this problem but not eliminated it altogether. The risk factor is strongest in women over 35 years who are also smokers. The presumed mechanism is an increased coagulation tendency mediated by estrogen stimulation of liver protein production, including clotting factors. An autoimmune mechanism has also been suggested in rare cases.

Recent randomized clinical trials showed that postmenopausal hormone replacement therapy has no effect on stroke incidence.

28. Which clotting system abnormalities are associated with stroke?

Rare inherited abnormalities of the blood clotting system include antithrombin III deficiency, protein C and protein S deficiency,activated protein C resistance (factor V Leiden mutation), and prothrombin gene mutation. Antiphospholipid antibodies and hyperhomocysteinemia also promote thrombosis.

29. Summarize the most important treatable stroke risk factors.

The most important modifiable risk factors for stroke are hypertension, smoking, heart disease, hyperlipidemia, and hyperhomocysteinemia. The presence of prior stroke or TIA is also an important treatable risk factor. Other modifiable risks include diabetes, alcohol consumption, drugs of abuse, oral contraceptives, and obesity.

Rokey R, Rolak LA: Epidemiology and risk factors for stroke and myocardial infarction. In Rolak LA, Rokey R: Coronary and Cerebral Vascular Disease. Mt. Kisco, NY, Futura, 1990, pp 83–117.

THERAPY

30. What are the most common causes of death in patients admitted to the hospital with a stroke?

The leading causes of death in the first month after a stroke are (1) the neurologic sequelae of the stroke, (2) pneumonia, (3) pulmonary embolism, and (4) cardiac disease. An essential part of stroke treatment, therefore, is the treatment and prevention of medical complications.

31. What is the treatment for a completed stroke?

Intravenous tissue plasminogen activator (t-PA) given within the first 3 hours of an acute ischemic stroke significantly improves the likelihood of a good neurologic outcome. Candidates for thrombolytic treatment should have a potentially disabling deficit that is not rapidly resolving. Important contraindications include the presence of hemorrhage or extensive acute hypodensity on the CT scan, a stroke or severe head injury in the previous 3 months, history of intracranial hemorrhage, major surgery in the previous 2 weeks, active or recent bleeding, severe uncontrolled hypertension (SBP > 185 mmHg or DBP > 110 mmHg), thrombocytopenia, abnormal prothrombin or partial thromboplastin time, pregnancy, and myocardial infarction-related pericarditis.

A 0.9 mg/kg dose of t-PA is given as an intravenous infusion, 10% as a bolus and the remainder over 1 hour to a maximal dose of 90 mg. Other antithrombotic drugs, such as aspirin and heparin, should be withheld in the first 24 hours, and blood pressure should be maintained under 185/110 mmHg.

32. What are the risks of thrombolytic therapy?

Under strict adherence to the above guidelines, the risk of symptomatic intracerebral hemorrhage is 6%. One-half are fatal. The risk of intracranial hemorrhage increases significantly if the guidelines are violated. Thrombolysis may be associated with a higher risk of hemorrhage if treatment is administered after 3 hours, a higher dose or different thrombolytic agent is used, aspirin or heparin is given in the first 24 hours, or blood pressure is not maintained under 185/100 mmHg. Despite the recognized risks of thrombolysis, the treatment increases by 50% the likelihood of an excellent recovery and reduces the number of patients who die or are left severely disabled.

33. What is the role of intra-arterial thrombolysis?

Intra-arterial thrombolytic therapy has been shown to be beneficial in patients with strokes due to middle cerebral artery occlusion up to 6 hours after onset of symptoms. The potential advantages of intra-arterial administration (confirmation of the arterial occlusion, lower doses of thrombolytic agent, higher patency rates) need to be balanced against the disadvantages (time delay to treatment, less readily available resources).

34. What advances in acute stroke treatment may be anticipated?

Several putative neuroprotective drugs are currently in clinical trial testing. By targeting one or more steps of the ischemic cascade, these drugs reduce neuronal injury and neurologic disability in experimental models of stroke.

35. What is the role of warfarin (Coumadin) therapy in cerebrovascular disease?

Warfarin is the stroke preventive treatment of choice in patients at high risk for cardiogenic emboli. Therapy ideally is initiated while the patient is receiving standard or low-molecular-weight heparin. Warfarin is effective in long-term use for the reduction of stroke risk in non-valvular atrial fibrillation as well as in rheumatic valvular-related atrial fibrillation and intracardiac thrombus. The benefit of warfarin depends on the risk of stroke versus the risk of a major bleeding event. Although the target international normalized ratio (INR) is 2–3 in most cases, it is higher for patients with mechanical cardiac valves and may be lower for very elderly patients or patients at higher risk for hemorrhagic complications. The bleeding risk to related to the intensity of anticoagulation. The risk of embolic stroke with different cardiac lesions can be stratified as follows:

Risk Stratification for Patients in Atrial Fibrillation

High risk (≥ 5% per year)
  Valvular heart disease (e.g., mitral stenosis, prosthetic mechanical valve)
  Recent-onset congestive heart failure (within 3 months)
  Prior thromboembolism
  Thyrotoxicosis
  Systolic hypertension
  Severe left ventricular dysfunction by echocardiogram
  Demonstration of intracardial thrombus

Moderate risk (3–5% per year)
  Age ≥ 60 years
  Mitral anulus calcification
  Diuretic therapy
  Silent cerebral infarction by CT

Low risk (< 3% per year)
  Lone atrial fibrillation, chronic or paroxysmal, age < 60 years

Uncertain risk
  Diabetes mellitus
  Left atrial enlargement
  Coexistent carotid artery disease
  Recent-onset vs. chronic atrial fibrillation
  Reduced cerebral blood flow

From Halperin JL, Hart RG: Atrial fibrillation and stroke: New ideas, persisting dilemmas. Stroke 19:937, 1988, with permission.

36. Describe the approach to primary stroke prevention.

The mainstay of primary stroke prevention is risk factor management. Although aspirin lowers the incidence of first-time myocardial infarction, it has not been shown to be useful for primary prevention of stroke.

37. What treatment is used to prevent a stroke in patients with TIA or prior stroke?

Aspirin remains the most popular drug for secondary stroke prevention. The standard dose is 325 or 81 mg/day. There are proponents of higher doses of aspirin, but higher doses are associated with greater gastrointestinal side effects without proof of greater benefit.

38. Which antiplatelet agents other than aspirin are used for the prevention of stroke?

Clopidogrel, 75 mg/day, is more effective than aspirin in preventing secondary ischemic events (stroke, myocardial infarction, and vascular death). The relative risk reduction is 8–9%. Clopidogrel is indicated in patients who are aspirin-intolerant and should be considered in high-risk patients (e.g., those who fail aspirin monotherapy).

Aspirin combined with extended-release dipyridamole is another effective secondary stroke prevention regimen. The benefits of the two agents are additive. Headache, the most common side effect, is attributable to the dipyridamole component.

Ticlopidine is a platelet ADP receptor antagonist chemically related to clopidogrel. It has superior efficacy compared with aspirin, but side effects include rash, diarrhea, and neutropenia, which necessitates CBC monitoring. For these reasons, ticlopidine is rarely used as a first-line agent.

39. What is the role of carotid endarterectomy in cerebrovascular disease?

Carotid endarterectomy has been proved to prevent recurrent ischemic stroke in patients with high-grade carotid stenosis. In symptomatic patients with an internal carotid artery stenosis of 70% or greater, surgery significantly reduces the risk of subsequent stroke. There is a smaller benefit in symptomatic patients with 50–70% stenosis. Lesions less than 50% are better treated medically. An advantage for carotid endarterectomy also has been demonstrated for asymptomatic lesions of 60% or greater, but the absolute reduction in stroke risk is much smaller.

40. Which factors affect the benefit of carotid endarterectomy?

Surgical morbidity and mortality are the key factors determining benefit in carotid surgery. The efficacy of endarterectomy assumes a surgical morbidity and mortality rate of 6% or less for symptomatic carotid disease and 3% or less for asymptomatic disease. The benefit of surgery may be lost when surgical morbidity and mortality exceed these rates.

41. What other interventions are available for severe cerebrovascular disease?

- Angioplasty and/or stenting is currently performed as an investigational technique, particularly for severe symptomatic lesions of the carotid, vertebral, basilar, or middle cerebral arteries not amenable to surgical treatment.
- Extracranial-intracranial bypass surgery may be considered in selected patients with ischemic symptoms secondary to carotid occlusion and demonstrated hemodynamic insufficiency.
- Hemicraniectomy is a life-saving decompressive procedure that may be appropriate in younger patients with malignant nondominant hemispheric brain infarction with resulting cerebral edema and incipient brain herniation.
- Surgical evacuation of intracerebral hematomas is sometimes indicated as a life-saving procedure. As a routine treatment for intracerebral hemorrhages, surgery has not been shown to improve neurologic outcome.

SUBARACHNOID HEMORRHAGE

42. What percentage of strokes are due to hemorrhage?

About 15–20% of strokes are due to hemorrhage; roughly one-half of these are due to subarachnoid hemorrhage (SAH). SAH is a relatively more common cause of stroke in the young. The actual incidence of SAH increases with age, but SAH becomes a less important cause of stroke overall as the incidence of atherothrombotic stroke rises.

43. What predisposes to SAH?

SAH is common after trauma. SAH due to ruptured arterial aneurysm is the most serious type with the greatest morbidity and mortality. SAH also may be a consequence of rupture of an arteriovenous malformation (AVM). Ingestion of cocaine or amphetamines may be associated with SAH. Hypertension, cigarette smoking, and alcohol consumption are also risk factors.

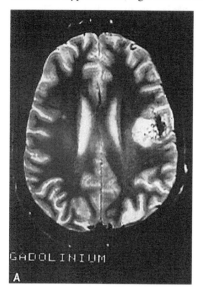
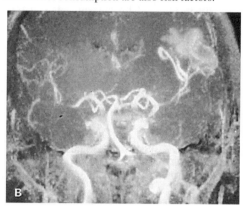

A, MR appearance of a left frontoparietal arteriovenous malformation. *B*, The characteristic appearance on an MR angiogram.

44. Where are most intracerebral aneurysms located?

Eighty percent of aneurysms occur in the anterior circulation and 20% in the posterior circulation. The most common locations are (1) the anterior communicating artery (30%); (2) the junction of the posterior communicating artery with the internal carotid artery (25%); and (3) the bifurcation of the internal carotid and middle cerebral artery (20–25%). Aneurysms are multiple in about 25% of patients. About 3% of intracerebral aneurysms are associated with polycystic kidney disease. Fibromuscular dysplasia of the internal carotid artery is accompanied by intracranial aneurysms in about 25% of cases.

45. What is the clinical profile of SAH?

SAH is characterized by sudden severe headache, often described as "the worst headache of my life," with or without focal neurologic deficit, and often with altered mental status. Aneurysmal SAH may be preceded by a moderately severe headache caused by an initial "sentinel bleed." Clinical deterioration can result from rebleeding from untreated aneurysms. SAH may not be suspected from the initial headache, causing delay in diagnosis and treatment.

46. What is the work-up of SAH?

The initial test in suspected SAH is a noncontrast CT scan of the brain, which may reveal blood in the cisterns, sylvian fissure, or sulci around the convexities. There also may be intraparenchymal blood, suggesting the location of the ruptured aneurysm responsible for the hemorrhage. The aneurysm itself may be visible. The amount of subarachnoid blood visible on CT scanning correlates with extent of bleeding and prognosis. The CT scan may be negative in 10% of SAHs. When SAH is strongly suspected clinically and the initial CT scan is negative, a lumbar puncture is necessary.

Once SAH is confirmed, neurosurgical consultation should be obtained to plan possible surgical management. Cerebral angiography is necessary for identification of the site of bleeding. Angiography should be obtained emergently if early surgical management is a consideration. Angiography may fail to identify the underlying lesion because vasospasm or thrombosis may prevent visualization of the responsible aneurysm. Repeat angiography may be necessary if initial angiography fails to identify the bleeding source.

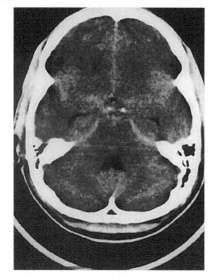

Noncontrast CT scan showing an acute subarachnoid hemorrhage, with blood diffusely filling CSF spaces.

47. What are the treatment options for SAH due to ruptured aneurysm?

Early surgical repair of a ruptured aneurysm is indicated in patients with a favorable clinical grade to prevent rebleeding. The definitive treatments are surgical clipping of the aneurysm or endovascular obliteration by catheter-directed placement of thrombogenic coils. In patients undergoing aneurysm clipping, surgery should be performed within the first 48 hours from onset of symptoms or be postponed 10–14 days because of the risk of vasospasm. Careful blood pressure control is necessary to prevent rebleeding in patients with unclipped aneurysms, and blood pressure must be monitored continuously during this phase.

48. Describe the basic medical management of SAH.

The general nonsurgical management centers on treatment and prevention of vasospasm and medical complications. Hypertensive hypovolemic therapy is often used to ameliorate the ischemic complications of vasospasm. Nimodipine is administered at a dosage of 60 mg every 4 hours for 3 weeks. If the patient cannot take the medication by mouth, it is administered by nasogastric tube. Because nimodipine lowers blood pressure and may cause bradycardia or atrioventricular (AV) block, the patient's blood pressure and EKG must be monitored during initial therapy.

49. What clinical grading system is used to characterize patients with SAH?

Patients with SAH are graded on a clinical scale of I to V, based primarily on level of consciousness and presence of focal neurologic signs.

Grade I	Awake, with no symptoms or mild headache and/or nuchal rigidity
Grade II	Awake, with moderate-to-severe headache and nuchal rigidity
Grade III	Drowsy or confused, with or without focal deficits
Grade IV	Stuporous, with moderate-to-severe hemiparesis and signs of increased intracranial pressure
Grade V	Comatose with signs of severe increased intracranial pressure

This clinical grading scale has prognostic significance. Grade I or II patients have the best prognosis and should undergo early cerebral angiography and definitive intervention, particularly if evaluation is within the first 48 hours of onset. Grade IV and V patients have a poor prognosis and warrant medical management until their clinical state improves. Angiography may be performed later if patients improve sufficiently to warrant more definitive care.

50. Which focal neurologic signs commonly accompany SAH? What is their mechanism?

Focal neurologic signs associated with an aneurysm of the posterior communicating artery are ptosis, pupillary dilatation, and impaired extraocular movements due to compression of the third nerve. Pupillary dilatation suggests external compression of the third nerve because the fibers for pupillary constriction are superficial, whereas those for the extraocular muscles are deeper in the nerve. Development of focal neurologic signs may be a consequence of intra-parenchymal bleeding or ischemia due to vasospasm.

51. What systemic complications are common in SAH?

Fever may occur in SAH due to infection, especially pneumonia or urinary tract infection. An inflammatory response to the blood in the CSF also may lead to fever, and the clinical picture may mimic acute meningitis. Hyponatremia may result from cerebral salt-wasting syndrome or syndrome of inappropriate secretion of antidiuretic hormone; the proper treatment (fluid and electrolyte resuscitation vs. free water restriction) requires an assessment of the patient's volume status. SAH may cause acute EKG changes, especially prolongation of the QT interval, T-wave inversion, and arrhythmia. An EKG should be obtained during the initial evaluation, and the cardiac rhythm should be monitored continuously in the ICU, with treatment of rhythm disturbances as necessary. A rare complication of SAH is neurogenic pulmonary edema. Development of congestive heart failure due to underlying heart disease or respiratory failure due to acute respiratory distress syndrome also may occur.

52. What CNS complications occur in SAH?

Rebleeding can cause worsening headache or declining level of consciousness. **Intraparen-chymal extension** can cause focal deficits due to mass effect, including development of cerebral edema and herniation. **Seizures** are another complication of SAH related to the irritant effect of blood.

Vasospasm occurs with aneurysmal SAH but usually not with other causes of SAH. It can lead to local ischemic injury and infarction. Transcranial Doppler can be used to monitor the flow velocity of the middle cerebral artery; vasospasm leads to a characteristic increase in the measured flow velocity.

Acute hydrocephalus may develop, usually communicating hydrocephalus due to obstruction of the pacchionian granulations in the venous sinuses by subarachnoid blood. It may be treated in the short term by ventriculostomy or permanently by ventriculoperitoneal shunt, if necessary. Patients in higher clinical grades are more likely to experience further deterioration.

53. What is the prognosis in patients with SAH?

The prognosis of SAH correlates with the clinical grade. Prognosis is best in grade I or II.

Grade	Deterioration (%)	Rebleed (%)	Death (%)
I	5	10–15	3–5
II	20	10–15	6–10
III	25	10–20	10–15
IV	50	20–25	40–50
V	80	25–30	50–70

BIBLIOGRAPHY

1. Caplan LR: Brain Ischemia: Basic Concepts and Clinical Relevance. London, Springer, 1995.
2. Daniel WG, Kronzon I, Mugge A (eds): Cardiogenic Embolism. Baltimore, Williams & Wilkins, 1996.
3. Kase CS, Caplan LR: Intracerebral Hemorrhage. Boston, Butterworth-Heinemann, 1994.
4. NASCET Collaborators: Beneficial effect of carotid endarterectomy in symptomatic patients with high-grade carotid stenosis. N Engl J Med 325:445–453, 1991.
5. National Institute of Neurological Disorders and Stroke t-PA Study Group: Tissue plasminogen activator for acute ischemic stroke. N Engl J Med 333:1581–1587, 1995.
6. Vermeulen M, Lindsay KW, Van Gihn J: Subarachnoid Hemorrhage. London, W.B. Saunders, 1992.
Websites
www.neuro.wustl.edu/stroke/stroke-trials.htm
stroke.ahajournals.org

18. NEURO-ONCOLOGY

Everton A. Edmondson, M.D.

NEUROLOGIC COMPLICATIONS RELATED TO CANCER

1. How often are neurologic problems encountered in patients with cancer? Name several common and uncommon examples.

Neurologic complications are seen in approximately 30% of patients with cancer. The most common problem is metabolic encephalopathy, followed by metastatic disease to the CNS. Unique neurologic complications of cancer include paraneoplastic syndromes and complications related to cancer therapy (e.g,. radiation encephalopathy, radionecrosis, chemotherapy-induced neuropathies, psychosis, cerebellar dysfunction, leukoencephalopathy). It is not uncommon to find multiple neurologic problems in the same patient. Multifocal structural disease may coexist with metabolic or infectious complications, creating a major diagnostic challenge.

2. What are the most important paraneoplastic syndromes affecting the nervous system?

1. Lambert-Eaton syndrome
2. Dermatomyositis
3. Carcinomatous neuromyopathy
4. Acute necrotizing myopathy
5. Subacute/chronic sensorimotor polyneuropathy
6. Sensory neuropathy
7. Autonomic neuronopathy
8. Polyradiculopathy
9. Subacute motor neuronopathy
10. Retinal degeneration
11. Opsoclonus-myoclonus
12. Myelitis
13. Necrotizing myelopathy
14. Limbic encephalitis/encephalomyelitis
15. Cerebellar degeneration

3. How common are paraneoplastic syndromes?

If one excludes coexisting problems such as nutritional deficiencies and complications related to cancer treatment, the incidence of a true remote effect of cancer on the nervous system is less than 1%.

Dropcho EJ: Pananeoplastic diseases of the nervous system. Curr Treatment Options Neurol 1:417–427, 1999.

4. What are the characteristic features of Lambert-Eaton syndrome?

This disorder of the neuromuscular junction is characterized by fatigability, limb-girdle weakness (usually more in the legs than arms but not invariably), marked incremental response to 20–50 Hz of repetitive electrical stimulation, and, in roughly half of cases, dryness of the mouth and impotence due to cholinergic interference. **Ptosis and extraocular dysmotility are not features of this syndrome.**

5. How frequently is dermatomyositis seen as a paraneoplastic problem in adults?

Roughly 10% of cases are associated with underlying malignancy. The most common sources are lung, breast, ovaries, and GI tract. The index of suspicion should be higher in patients over 40 years of age.

6. What is carcinomatous neuromyopathy?

This is not a discrete entity. Commonly weakness and reduced reflexes are accompanied by muscle atrophy, but the problem could be primarily a neuropathy or neuronopathy or a combination of myopathy and neuropathy. Findings on neurodiagnostic studies vary significantly.

7. Which neoplasms are associated with cerebellar degeneration?

Oat-cell carcinoma and other lung cancers, breast cancer, and ovarian carcinoma are the most common, although other solid tumors may be associated with this entity. Antibodies against Purkinje cells have been demonstrated. Anti-Yo antibody is the best characterized and is associated with gynecologic malignancies.

8. With what is the anti-Hu antibody associated?

This antibody is commonly seen in the setting of oat-cell carcinoma with either a sensory neuronopathy or encephalomyelitis.

9. Retinal degeneration is associated with which tumor and antibody?

Retinal degeneration may occur with oat-cell carcinoma. The anti-Ri antibody is associated with this entity.

10. Opsoclonus-myoclonus is associated with which neoplasm?

This syndrome of myoclonic jerks and abnormal eye movements is seen with neuroblastoma in children, but in adults lung cancer is the usual underlying neoplasm.

11. Excluding spinal cord compression, what other common conditions may present with acute weakness in patients with cancer?

A myriad of conditions may present as acute weakness. The most common are stroke, metabolic insult such as severe hypokalemia, Guillain-Barré syndrome, hemorrhage or necrosis within a CNS mass, or an acutely expanding mass lesion. Myasthenia gravis occurs in roughly half of patients with a thymoma.

12. What situations that are relatively unique to patients with cancer may result in acute altered mental status?

Altered mental status may occur as a complication of chemotherapy with agents such as ifosfamide, procarbazine, 5-fluorouracil, methotrexate, cytosine arabinoside, and methylmelamine. Leptomeningeal disease may result in chronic, subacute, or abrupt changes in mental status. A common cause of abrupt mental obtundation in a patient with leptomeningeal disease is hydrocephalus. Subclincal seizures or status epilepticus also may occur.

13. Stroke and other cerebrovascular complications are the third most common problem in the CNS in patients with cancer. What are the differences between cancer and noncancer populations with regard to stroke presentation? Which complications are relatively unique to patients with cancer?

Patients with cancer present with many other CNS diseases, such as metastasis, meningitis, and opportunistic infections, which overshadow the cerebrovascular events. **Symptomatic** atherosclerotic and hypertensive cerebrovascular complications are actually less common in patients with cancer than in the general population.

Stroke may occur as a result of **disseminated intravascular coagulation with or without accompanying sepsis. Venous occlusion** may arise from dehydration, direct tumor invasion, or side effects of treatment such as L-asparaginase. **Embolic complications** include nonbacterial thrombotic endocarditis (NBTE), a disorder characterized by sterile platelet-fibrin debris on endocardium and valves. **Septic emboli** are due to pathogens such as fungi, staphylococci, and gram-negative agents and occur most frequently in patients who have indwelling lines and are neutropenic or in bone marrow recipients. **Tumor emboli** most commonly result from atrial myxoma but may occur with lung tumors. Serial neuroimaging is often required to confirm that a tumor embolus is present. **Sludging due to leukostasis** may result in altered mental status, seizures, and waxing and waning focal/multifocal signs secondary to leukemic crisis. **Multifocal cerebral hemorrhage** may be seen with acute promyelocytic leukemia. Necrotizing infections such as *Mucor* may cause a stroke by **direct invasion of the artery.**

14. What is progressive multifocal leukoencephalopathy (PML)?

PML is a multifocal demyelinating disease caused by JC or SV40 virus infection. It is a progressive disorder most commonly found in immunocompromised hosts such as patients with cancer or AIDS and transplant recipients. Strokelike events are common.

Berger JR, Pall L, Lanska D, Whiteman M: Progressive multifocal leukoencephalopathy in patients with HIV infection. J Neurovirol 4:59–68, 1998.

15. What are the three most common neurologic complications related to cytomegalovirus (CMV) infection?

CMV may cause Guillain-Barré syndrome, retinitis, and encephalitis.

16. Is cryptococcal meningitis restricted to patients with AIDS or cancer or other immunocompromised patients?

No. Although it is more common in such patients, it may occur in immunocompetent people.

17. How common is varicella zoster infection in patients with lymphoma?

The incidence is estimated to be about 15%. Dissemination is relatively common in patients with cancer. Rarely, stroke or a necrotizing CNS lesion may result from varicella zoster infection.

Pruitt AA: Central nervous system infections in cancer patients. Neurol Clin 9:867–888, 1991.

PRIMARY BRAIN TUMORS: DIAGNOSIS AND MANAGEMENT

18. Are supratentorial brain tumors more common in adults or children?

Two-thirds of the brain tumors in adults present supratentorially; in children the reverse is true.

19. What is the most common category of brain tumors?

Gliomas account for 50–60% of primary brain tumors. Low-grade glioma is most common in the first decade and decreases progressively with age. Astrocytoma peaks in incidence in the third decade. Anaplastic astrocytoma has a bimodal peak in the first and third decades. Glioblastoma multiforme (GBM) becomes progressively more frequent with age, representing only 1% of gliomas in the first decade but over 50% after the age of 60.

Surawicz TS, McCarthy BJ, Kupelian V, et al: Descriptive epidemiology of primary brain and CNS tumors: Results from the Central Brain Tumor Registry of the United States. Neuro-Oncology 1:14–25, 1999.

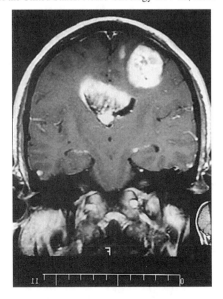

Gadolinium-enhanced T1-weighted MRI of the brain showing a malignant glioblastoma multiforme, with characteristic extension across the corpus callosum.

20. What is the customary total radiation dose administered to the brain for primary tumors such as gliomas?

The usual dose is 5500–6000 rads delivered in fractions over 6 weeks.

21. The nitrosoureas are the most active chemotherapeutic agents for astrocytoma, malignant oligodendroglioma, and glioblastoma multiforme. How are these agents used?

BCNU is administered intravenously in doses of 225 mg/m^2 as a single dose or 80 mg/m^2 for 3 days. CCNU is delivered orally once every 6 weeks at 110 mg/m^2. These are the most commonly used nitrosoureas in brain tumor therapy. They may be combined with other agents such as procarbazine, vincristine, or hydroxyurea. Bone marrow, hepatic, pulmonary, and renal toxicity may occur as dose-limiting side effects.

22. What is the mean survival rate associated with various gliomas?

Mean Survival Rate for Gliomas

TUMOR TYPE	TREATMENT MODALITY	MEAN SURVIVAL
Low-grade glioma*	Gross total resection	5–7 yr
	Biopsy/subtotal surgery	35% at 5 yr
	Subtotal surgery + x-ray therapy	46% at 5 yr
Cerebellar microcystic astrocytoma	Surgery	High cure rate
Optic glioma	Surgery	> 10 yr
	Surgery + x-ray therapy	> 10 yr
Anaplastic astrocytoma	Surgery alone	1 yr
	Surgery + x-ray therapy	2–3 yr
	Surgery + x-ray therapy + chemotherapy	3–5 yr
Glioblastoma	Surgery	4 mo
	Surgery + x-ray therapy	9 mo
	Surgery + x-ray therapy + chemotherapy	12 mo
Oligodendroglioma	Surgery	30% at 5 yr
	Surgery + x-ray therapy	85% at 5 yr
		55% at 10 yr
		10 yr
Ependymoma (differentiated) (anaplastic)	Surgery + x-ray therapy	2–5 yr[†]

* Location and resectability dictate survival.
[†] Malignant ependymoma with subtotal resection and CSF spread dictates a poor prognosis, whereas gross total resection of a supratentorial ependymoma with negative CSF findings dictates longer survival.
Adapted from Levin VA, Sheline GE, Gutin PH: Neoplasms of the central nervous system. In DeVita VT, Hellman S, Rosenberg SA (eds): Cancer: Principles and Practice of Oncology. Philadelphia, J.B. Lippincott, 1989, pp 1557–1611; and Forsyth PAJ, Roa WHY: Primary central nervous system tumors in adults. Curr Treat Opt Neurol 1:377–394, 1999.

23. What are the most common primitive neuroectodermal tumors (PNETs) in children?

Medulloblastoma and ependymoblastoma are two PNETs seen more commonly in children. Others include pineoblastoma, neuroblastoma, medulloepithelioma, and spongioblastoma.

24. What prognostic indices determine poor chance for survival with a diagnosis of medulloblastoma?

Poor prognostic features include (1) subtotal resection, (2) malignant cells in CSF, (3) documented spinal cord metastasis on neuroimaging, and (4) age less than 4 years.

25. What is the 5-year survival rate for good-risk patients with medulloblastoma?

Survival for good-risk patients (i.e., negative CSF, > 75% resection, over 4 yr of age, no metastases) is 70% with maximal treatment. The 5-year survival rate for poor-risk patients is only 25%.

26. Which CNS tumors are more likely to metastasize?

PNETs such as medulloblastoma have a high propensity to metastasize within the CSF pathway and may metastasize outside the CNS (e.g., bone marrow invasion).

27. What population is most at risk for ependymoma?

These tumors are most common in the first decade, and the frequency drops significantly after age 30. Ependymoma is the most common intraventricular tumor in children. In adults it is virtually confined to the spinal cord.

28. The incidence of meningioma increases with age. True or false?

True. Meningioma is rare in the first two decades and increases progressively thereafter.

29. What are the sites of predilection for meningiomas?

The parasagittal and convexity region has the highest incidence, followed by sphenoid ridge, olfactory groove, suprasellar region, posterior fossa, spine, periorbital region, temporal fossa, and falx—in that order.

30. What is the treatment of choice for meningioma?

If the tumor is resectable, surgery is the treatment of choice. Radiation and chemotherapy are of limited value. Unresectable, large meningiomas can be irradiated, and shrinkage may occur, but transformation to a sarcoma or higher malignant grade is a risk. Chemotherapy is limited to the treatment of meningeal sarcoma.

31. Which tumors have a high incidence of calcification on neuroimaging?

Calcifications are seen in over 50% of oligodendrogliomas and with high frequency in craniopharyngiomas and meningiomas. Metastatic melanoma and renal cell carcinoma are hemorrhagic tumors that may exhibit exuberant calcific changes on neuroimaging.

32. Neurofibromatosis is associated with what types of CNS tumors?

Acoustic neuroma and optic glioma.

33. Which tumors occur in the pineal area?

Tumors in the pineal region include astrocytoma, embryonal carcinoma, teratoma, choriocarcinoma, and pineoblastoma.

34. Alpha-fetoprotein and human chorionic gonadotropin (HCG) are markers for tumors in what area of the brain?

Tumors in the pineal region may secrete HCG if they are of trophoblastic origin and alpha-fetoprotein if they are of yolk sac origin.

35. What is primary CNS lymphoma?

Primary CNS lymphoma is a histiocytic lymphoma in the CNS without evidence of systemic lymphoma. Much controversy surrounds its site of origin. More than half of these tumors present in the hemispheres, with a periventricular predilection. One-third are multicentric. Males are affected more than females. Because of the higher prevalence in patients with AIDS, what was once a rare tumor is now increasingly common. The incidence of primary CNS lymphoma has also increased in immunocompetent people by approximately threefold. CNS lymphoma has a high predilection to affect the leptomeninges. Most CNS lymphomas have a large B-cell histology; few are T-cell types.

36. What staging tests help to exclude systemic lymphoma in patients with CNS lymphoma?

Chest radiograph, abdominal CT scan, and bone scan.

37. Are pituitary tumors more likely to produce hormone when they are intrasellar or extrasellar in extent?

Intrasellar tumors are more likely to be hormone-producing, whereas chromophobe adenoma, the most common pituitary tumor, is large, extends outside the sella frequently, and seldom produces hormone.

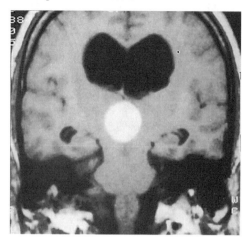

T1-weighted MRI showing a cystic craniopharyngioma, producing hydrocephalus.

38. What oral medication is commonly used to treat prolactinoma?

Bromocriptine reduces prolactin secretion and is used in many instances to shrink an intrasellar pituitary prolactinoma.

39. What are the most common tumors of the foramen magnum and skull base?

Meningioma, glomus jugulare, and nasopharyngeal carcinoma.

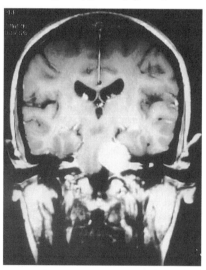

T1-weighted MRI shows a gadolinium-enhancing tumor of the left glomus jugulare, arising at the skull base and compressing the brainstem.

40. Which tumor is likely to present in the region of the clivus with evidence of bony erosion?

Chordomas occur in the region of the clivus (or the sacrum). Bony erosion results from direct tumor invasion and enzymatic digestion.

41. What are the most common tumors arising from the cerebellopontine angle?

The most common tumors in this area include acoustic neuroma and meningioma; others seen in this region include cholesteatoma and metastatic diseases.

42. What is von Hippel-Lindau syndrome?

This autosomal-dominantly inherited condition includes hemangioblastoma of the cerebellum or retina and associated systemic disorders—polycystic kidney/hypernephroma, pheochromocytoma, pancreatic cysts, or polycythemia.

43. What types of tumors are found in the intradural, extramedullary region of the spinal cord?

Schwannoma and meningioma.

44. Which tumors arise in the intradural intramedullary region of the spinal cord?

By far, the most common tumors occurring within the substance of the spinal cord parenchyma are astrocytomas and ependymomas. Ependymomas also may occur in the cauda equina, although the primary site of origin is in the spine.

METASTATIC DISEASE AFFECTING THE NERVOUS SYSTEM

45. What are the clinical features of epidural spinal cord compression? How is it diagnosed and treated?

The most common presentation is acute or subacute back pain, which occurs in over 90% of cases. The pain may even be radicular, such as a shooting dermatomal pain or a bandlike aching in the trunk. A sensory level is a strong indicator of a myelopathy. Paraparesis and bowel/bladder dysfunction usually indicate a more serious cord compression (with a worse prognosis).

Plain films should be obtained in patients with cancer who present with any of the above signs or symptoms. MRI of the spine or myelogram/CT is indicated in any patient whose presenting symptoms include back pain with corresponding x-ray or bone scan lesions or neurologic deficits consistent with radiculopathy or myelopathy.

Patients whose deficits are minimal and who are ambulatory at the time of diagnosis of epidural cord compression have the best prognosis following institution of treatment. In contrast, only 13% of patients who were paraplegic at the time of diagnosis demonstrated significant neurologic improvement with radiation therapy or surgery. Most studies indicate that surgery is no better than radiotherapy for epidural cord compression; therefore, oncologists regard radiation therapy as the treatment of choice with two exceptions: Patients with radioresistant tumors and patients who have previously received radiation at the involved site are candidates for surgery.

When the diagnosis of acute epidural cord compression is entertained as a significant possibility, IV dexamethasone, 100 mg, should be given immediately over $\frac{1}{2}$ to 1 hour and subsequently 4 mg every 6 hours if the diagnosis is confirmed by neuroimaging.

Posner JB: Spinal metastases. In Posner JB: Neurologic Complications of Cancer. Philadelphia, F.A. Davis, 1995, pp 111–142.

46. Most tumors that result in epidural spinal cord compression do so by direct extension from bone metastasis. How does lymphoma gain access to the epidural space?

In contrast to lung, breast, colon, and other solid tumors, lymphoma may extend via the foramina into the epidural space. Normal plain radiographs of the spine in the face of epidural lymphoma are not uncommon.

47. How can the clinician distinguish between radiation-induced plexopathy and cancerous invasion of the plexus?

Radiation-induced plexopathy is far less likely to present with pain, whereas weakness occurs early. Also, more than half of the reported cases of radiation plexopathy have myokymic discharges on EMG in contrast to none of the cancerous cases.

48. Metastatic disease accounts for what percentage of CNS tumors?

It is estimated that 20–40% of tumors in the CNS are metastatic.
Patchell RA: Metastatic brain tumors. Neurol Clin 13:915–926, 1995.

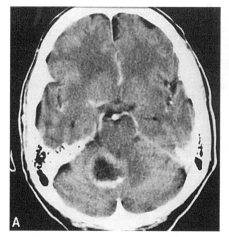 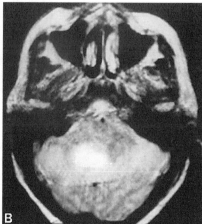

Small-cell carcinoma of the lung metastatic to the cerebellum shown on contrast-enhanced CT scan *(A)* and proton-density MRI *(B)*.

49. Solitary metastasis to the brain occurs in what percentage of brain metastases?

Approximately 50% of patients have one metastasis. However, the majority of these have evidence of systemic disease after investigation, which means that the single brain lesion is not the solitary focus of disease.

50. Does gross total resection of a solitary metastasis improve survival?

Surgical resection followed by radiotherapy improves survival in a selected subpopulation. Reasonable candidates are patients who have no evidence of disease elsewhere, who are ambulatory, and in whom gross total resection can be achieved without significant risk of inducing major neurologic deficits.

51. Without radiation therapy, what is the usual life expectancy of a patient with brain metastasis?

The mean life expectancy with steroids alone is 1 month. Radiation therapy extends the mean survival time to 4–6 months.
Patchell RA, Tibbs PA, Regine WP, et al: Postoperative radiotherapy in the treatment of single metastases to the brain: A randomized trial. JAMA 280:1485–1489, 1998.

52. Which solid tumors most commonly metastasize to the brain?

The lung is the most common, followed by breast and colon.

LEPTOMENINGEAL CARCINOMATOSIS

53. What is the clinical presentation of leptomeningeal carcinomatosis?

Leptomeningeal carcinomatosis (also known as carcinomatous or neoplastic meningitis) may present in a myriad of ways. Altered mental status is common, as are seizures, multiple cranial and root signs, and headache. The onset may be fulminant, as in lymphoblastic leukemia, or subacute, with stuttering multifocal deficits and deterioration of cognitive function, as in some patients with breast cancer and leptomeningeal carcinomatosis. The prognosis is poor, especially in metastasis from solid tumors.

54. Which cancer is the most common cause of leptomeningeal disease in children?
Leukemia.

55. Which solid tumor has the greatest prevalence of leptomeningeal carcinomatosis?
Breast cancer is the most common source in adults, followed by lung cancer and melanoma.

56. What is the diagnostic yield of CSF examination to establish the diagnosis of lepto-meningeal disease?
The first tap has a 50% yield, but by the third tap the yield increases to 85%. The CSF may show elevated protein, increased cells, or positive cytology.

57. What ancillary testing may help to determine the presence of leptomeningeal disease other than CSF examination?
Enhanced CT scan of the brain or MRI may reveal leptomeningeal deposits, meningeal enhancement, or hydrocephalus.

58. Name two chemotherapeutic agents used for the treatment of leptomeningeal disease.
Methotrexate and cytosine arabinoside are used intrathecally to treat leptomeningeal carcinomatosis. Systemic chemotherapy is also often effective.
    Glantz MJ, Cole BF, Recht L, et al: Methotrexate for patients with nonleukemic leptomeningeal cancer. J Clin Oncol 16:1561–1567, 1998.

CANCER PAIN

59. What percentage of patients with cancer die unrelieved of pain?
It is estimated that 25% of patients with cancer die without adequate pain relief.

60. What factors preclude adequate treatment of cancer pain?
Ironically, it is not lack of treatment options or technology that hampers pain treatment, but factors such as opiophobia (fear to use narcotics), inadequate understanding of the origin of the pain (is it nociceptive or neuropathic?), and failure to prioritize pain and suffering as an urgent symptom requiring treatment.

61. What is the difference between nociceptive pain and neuropathic pain?
Nociceptive pain arises from injury or disease in soft-tissue or other somatic structures. Neural structures are not affected. Pain emanating from neural injury or dysfunction is **neuropathic pain**. Neuropathic pain usually has bizarre or unfamiliar qualtities, such as intense burning provoked by light innocuous touch (allodynia). The pain may extend beyond the confines of injury (spatial summation or extension). Paroxysmal, lancinating pain may occur. Itchy, creepy, crawly, intense tingling or icy hot sensations may be experienced (dysesthesia).

62. How is nociceptive pain treated?
Nonsteroidal antiinflammatory drugs (NSAIDs) and acetaminophen can adequately relieve mild nociceptive pain. Opiates work well for severe pain.

63. How may neuropathic pain develop in patients with cancer?
Patients may experience neuropathic pain from invasion of neural structures by tumor (brachial and lumbosacral plexus, epidural space), as a byproduct of treatment such as surgical severance (e.g., thoracotomy, mastectomy, amputation), or as a side effect of chemotherapy such as cisplatin.

64. What types of treatment are available for neuropathic pain?
Neuropathic pain may respond to tricyclic antidepressants such as amitriptyline, protriptyline, and doxepin. Anticonvulsant medications such as phenytoin, carbamazepine, gabapentin, and clonazepam may relieve lancinating paroxysmal pain. Oral anesthetic drugs such as mexiletine may provide relief when tricyclics and anticonvulsants fail. Steroids are sometimes useful as a temporizing measure, and in conditions such as acute causalgia, they may be curative if begun

early in the course. Nerve blocks may be used if there is a focal source amenable to this measure. Chronic epidural infusion may be used in cases of lumbosacral plexopathy, intractable neuropathic limb pain, or postthoracotomy pain.

65. For a patient who is taking morphine, 30 mg every 4 hours, what would be the equivalent effective dose (equianalgesic dose) of hydromorphone?

The correct dose is 7.5 mg every 4 hours. Because hydromorphone is available in 4-mg tablets, a dose of 8 mg every 4 hours is appropriate.

Opiate Dose Conversion

DRUG	ROUTE	EQUIANALGESIC DOSE (MG)	CONVERSION FROM IV TO PO	CONVERSION TO MORPHINE
Morphine	IV/IM	10	3	=
	PO	30		=
Levorphanol	IV/IM	2	2	5
	PO	4		7.5
Methadone	IV/IM	10	2	=
	PO	20		1.5
Fentanyl	IV	0.1 (100 μg)	—	100
Hydromorphone	IV/IM	1.5	5	6.7
	PO	7.5		4
Meperidine	IV/IM	75	4	0.13
	PO	300		0.1
Oxycodone	IV/IM	15	2	0.67
	PO	30		=
Codeine	IM	130	1.5	0.8
	PO	200		0.15
Pentazocine	IM	60	2.5	6
	PO	150		
Butorphanol	IM	2	=	0.2
Nalbuphine	IM	10	=	1

IM, intramuscular; IV, intravenously; PO, orally; =, no conversion needed.

66. Patient-controlled analgesia (PCA) is an effective parenteral method of delivering analgesics. How does PCA work?

Patients with cancer who cannot tolerate oral medication because of nausea and vomiting, bowel obstruction, postoperative status, or marked moment-to-moment fluctuation in pain are candidates for PCA. A computerized pump delivers opiate analgesics in a variety of permutations: continuous-drip rate (basal rate), intermittent boluses (PCA doses) without a basal drip, or PCA doses superimposed on a basal rate. The physician predetermines the limit of PCA doses allowable per hour and the basal rate (continuous-drip dosage). Patient satisfaction with this modality is high because of self-empowerment, immediate access to medication rather than waiting for medication upon request, and flexible dosing.

Edmondson E: Advances in pain control for cancer patients. Clin Consult Obstet Gynecol 3:122–128, 1991.

67. What types of pain syndromes are relatively opiate-resistant?

Patients with metastatic bone pain and those with neuropathic pain are more apt to experience suboptimal relief from opiates.

68. What are the alternatives for patients with opiate-resistant cancer pain?

Metastatic bone pain may respond to combination therapy consisting of NSAIDs or corticosteroids in conjunction with an opiate drug. Radiation therapy frequently alleviates metastatic bone pain. Patients with neuropathic pain may require tricyclic antidepressants, anticonvulsants, or oral anesthetic agents (e.g., mexiletine). In some instances, chronic epidural infusion of anesthetic and opioids is necessary.

69. Is intravenous administration of opioid medication superior to the oral route?

Generally, oral medication is just as effective as parenteral injections if the dose is adequately titrated. Intravenous medications work faster but their duration of action is shorter. Intravenous dosing has an advantage in the patient with intractable nausea and vomiting, obstruction, or hyperacute pain who requires delicate but aggressive dose adjustments.

70. What types of pharmacologic agents are infused intrathecally for pain control?

Intraspinal opioid administration is approved by the FDA for the treatment of cancer pain and intractable chronic noncancer pain. The most commonly used drugs are morphine, fentanyl, and sufentanil. Nonopiate regimens for pain control also include intrathecal clonidine.

COMPLICATIONS OF CANCER THERAPY

71. What are the potential neurologic complications of chemotherapy and biologic response modifiers?

Side Effects of Chemotherapy and Immunotherapy

SIDE EFFECTS	COMMENTS
Drugs causing encephalopathy	
Alpha-interferon	
Cytosine arabinoside	
Cisplatin	Commonly from electrolyte imbalance
5-Fluorouracil	
Hexamethylmelamine	
Ifosfamide	
Interleukin-2	
L-asparaginase	Can cause hemorrhage or thrombotic insults as well as reversible encephalopathy without parenchymal insult
Methotrexate	
Nitrogen mustard	
Procarbazine	
VP-16 (high dose)	
Drugs causing neuropathy	
Adriamycin	Rare
Cytosine arabinoside	Rare
Cisplatin	Ototoxicity and sensory neuropathy
Procarbazine	
Taxol	
Vincristine	
Drugs causing myelopathy	
Cytosine arabinoside	Administered intrathecally
Methotrexate	Administered intrathecally
Thiotepa	Administered intrathecally
Drugs causing cerebellar dysfunction	
Cytosine arabinoside	
5-Fluorouracil	
Ifosfamide	
Procarbazine	

Adapted from Paleologos NA: Complications of chemotherapy. In Biller J (ed): Iatrogenic Neurology. Boston, Butterworth-Heinemann, 1998, pp 439–461.

72. Name two chemotherapeutic agents that may cause parkinsonism.
The interleukins (alpha-interferon and IL-2) and hexamethylmelamine.

73. Which hormonal drug may cause retinopathy?
Tamoxifen may result in retinopathy after prolonged use.

74. Name three chemotherapeutic agents that may induce TTP.
Seizures and encephalopathy are commonly seen in thrombotic thrombocytopenic purpura (TTP), which is accompanied by renal failure, hemolysis, schistocytes, fever, and thrombocytopenia. Bleomycin, cisplatin, and mitomycin-C have been reported to trigger TTP.

75. Name two drugs that enhance leukoencephalopathic changes induced by radiation therapy.
Methotrexate and cytosine arabinoside may enhance leukoencephalopathy. Both drugs may induce this problem without prior radiation therapy.

76. What is the peak time course to note radiation myelopathy?
Delayed progressive myelopathy peaks at 9–18 months after radiation therapy, although a transient myelopathy may occur within the first month to first 2 years. Progressive myelopathy increases in incidence as the radiation dose increases and is much more common with doses > 4400 rads.

77. What are early side effects of cranial radiation therapy?
Within the first few days of radiation treatment, cerebral edema occurs and may result in headache, lethargy, nausea, vomiting, and exacerbation of preexisting neurologic deficits. Dexamethasone ameliorates these symptoms and should be started prophylactically to minimize early ill effects from radiation.

78. How soon may delayed symptoms of cranial radiation occur?
Delayed signs may appear as soon as 1–4 months after completing radiation therapy and resemble early symptoms—somnolence, worsening of preexisting deficits, headache.

79. When is the peak incidence for focal cerebral radionecrosis?
Radionecrosis peaks at 18 months after radiotherapy but may occur many years later.

80. Name two tumors induced by radiation therapy.
The peripheral nerves and plexus within the radiation port can develop painful nerve sheath tumors years after radiation therapy. Children treated with whole-brain radiation for lymphoblastic leukemia are at risk for developing gliomas if they are long survivors.

BIBLIOGRAPHY

1. Levin VA (ed): Cancer in the Nervous System. New York, Churchill-Livingstone, 1996.
2. Posner JB: Neurologic Complications of Cancer. Philadelphia, F.A. Davis, 1995.
3. Schold SC (ed): Primary Tumors of the Brain and Spinal Cord. Boston, Butterworth-Heinemann, 1997.
4. Wen PY, Black PM: Brain tumors in adults. Neurol Clin 13:701–975, 1995.
Websites
www.azbta.org
www.braintumor.org
www.btfc.org

19. PAIN SYNDROMES

Steven B. Inbody, M.D.

CLASSIFICATION AND CHARACTERISTICS OF PAIN

1. What is the difference between pain and nociception?

The subcommittee on taxonomy of the International Association for the Study of Pain defines **pain** as an unpleasant sensory and emotional experience associated with actual or potential tissue damage. The sensation of pain is one of the vital functions of the nervous system, providing a signal to alert the organism to potential injury. **Nociception** is a response specific to tissue damage and stimulation. Pain perception is the conscious experience of nociception which, like other perceptions, can be influenced by psychosocial factors. Distinguishing between nociception and the more global construct of suffering (impairment in quality of life), helps to clarify the major goals of pain management, usually conceptualized as both comfort and function.

Merskey H, Bogduk N (eds): Task Force on Taxonomy: Classification of Chronic Pain. International Association for the Study of Pain, 1994.

2. What are the differences between acute and chronic pain?

Acute pain is recent in onset and often expected to end in days or weeks. Pain that persists or recurs frequently is ultimately considered **chronic**. Although the distinction was previously based solely on time criteria ranging from 3–6 months, a more recent definition includes biologic function. Pain is now defined as chronic if it (1) persists for 1 month beyond the usual course of an acute illness or healing injury, (2) is associated with a chronic pathologic process, or (3) recurs at intervals of months or years. Unlike acute pain, chronic pain appears to fulfill no adaptive biologic function and, for many patients, becomes the primary disease process.

3. How is chronic pain classified?

Three distinct pathophysiologic mechanisms predominate and are broadly categorized as (1) nociceptive, (2) neuropathic, and (3) idiopathic (psychogenic).

Portenoy RK, Kanner RM: Definition and assessment of pain. In Portenoy R, Kanner R (eds): Pain Management: Theory and Practice. Philadelphia, F.A. Davis, 1996, pp 3–18.

4. How do nociceptive, neuropathic, and psychogenic pain differ?

The three major categories of pain are defined by their respective pathophysiologic mechanisms but also can be distinguished by their clinical symptoms.

Nociceptive pain arises from the normal activation of peripheral nociceptors located at the site of tissue injury and is transmitted to the CNS via normally functioning sensorineural pathways dedicated to noxious stimuli. Nociceptive pain is generally believed to be commensurate with the presumed degree of tissue damage.

Neuropathic pain bypasses the normal nociceptive pathways and is usually precipitated by direct injury to neural tissue. Neuropathic pain appears to be sustained by aberrant somatosensory processing in the peripheral or central nervous system.

Idiopathic pain (psychogenic) persists in the absence of an identifiable organic pain source or is believed to be in excess of a documented organic lesion.

5. What are the abnormal sensations of neuropathic pain?

Spontaneous pain: burning, shooting, or lancinating without provocation.

Paresthesias: abnormal nonpainful sensations that may be spontaneous or evoked (tingling) and may accompany loss of sensory function.

Dysesthesias: abnormal pain that may be spontaneous or evoked (unpleasant burning or tingling).

Hyperalgesia: an exaggerated pain response evoked by a noxious stimulus.

Hyperpathia: an exaggerated pain response evoked by a noxious or nonnoxious stimulus (a particularly unpleasant evoked dysesthesia).

Allodynia: a painful (typically dysesthetic) response to a nonnoxious stimulus.

6. What are the fundamental aspects of chronic pain assessment?

Temporal features: acute vs. recurrent vs. chronic; onset, duration, daily variation, course; constant, paroxysmal, "colicky."

Sensory qualities: lancinating, stabbing, burning, aching, cramping, throbbing.

Intensity: pain on average, at its worst or least, or right now.

Topography: focal vs. multifocal; local vs. referred vs. radiating (i.e., radicular); superficial vs. deep.

Exacerbating/relieving factors: volitional (provoked pain) vs. nonvolitional.

Inferred pathophysiology: nociceptive pain vs. neuropathic pain vs. psychogenic pain.

Etiology: trauma, ischemia, inflammation, infection, other process.

Physical functioning: specific impairments (e.g., paresis); ability to perform activities of daily living; limitations in ambulating, lifting, or other functions; sleep quality, appetite, weight.

Psychologic functioning: affective symptoms; past and present psychiatric illness; personality variables (coping styles and adaptability); secondary gain issues.

Social functioning: family dynamics; social isolation; involvement in litigation or compensation issues.

Role functioning: ability to engage in vocational or avocational (i.e., recreational or housekeeping) activities; parenting responsibilities.

Other considerations: history of drug use/abuse; history of chronic pain; family history of chronic pain or illness, psychiatric disease, or substance abuse.

MYOFASCIAL PAIN SYNDROME AND FIBROMYALGIA

7. What are the two most common chronic muscular pain syndromes?

Over the past 100 years the literature has distinguished two primary types of musculoskeletal pain: myofascial pain syndrome (MPS) and fibromyalgia. At one end of the spectrum is MPS, a local syndrome characterized by abnormalities involving one or sometimes a few muscles. Cervical whiplash is a common example. Although in theory it is an acute, nonchronic, and localized disorder without systemic manifestations, in practice it often has a more complex presentation. Unlike fibromyalgia, MPS has no universally agreed-upon definition.

At the opposite end of the spectrum, fibromyalgia is a chronic systemic condition that affects general pain sensitivity and muscle function. The World Health Organization established fibromyalgia as an officially recognized syndrome in 1993, defining it as a painful but not articular condition predominantly involving muscles. It is the most common cause of chronic widespread musculoskeletal pain.

Inbody SB: Myofascial pain syndromes. In Evans R (ed): Neurology and Trauma. Philadelphia, W.B. Saunders, 1996, pp 458–495.

8. What is the role of trigger points in MPS?

MPS involves pain referred from trigger points within myofascial structures, either local or distant from the pain. A trigger point is defined as a localized tender area within a taut band of skeletal muscle or its associated fascia. These points occur most frequently in the head, neck, shoulders, and lower back. The mechanisms that produce the symptoms are largely speculative. Generally no neurologic deficits are associated with MPS.

9. What are the diagnostic criteria for fibromyalgia?

The American College of Rheumatology in 1990 set criteria for the diagnosis of fibromyalgia that includes at least 3 months of widespread pain and the presence of at least 11 of 18 specific tender points on examination.

10. What are the clinical features of fibromyalgia?

Fibromyalgia is a common muscular pain disorder consisting of a central set of core features that are essential for diagnosis and superimposed on a variable number of ancillary manifestations. The core features are generalized pain, decreased pain threshold, and widespread tenderness typically involving discrete anatomic foci known as fibrositic tender points (FTPs). Ancillary features have been divided into two groups based on their frequency of occurrence. Symptoms that are considered almost characteristic because they occur in over 75% of patients include fatigue, nonrestorative sleep pattern, and morning stiffness. Less common ancillary features (approximately 25% of cases) include irritable bowel syndrome, Raynaud's phenomenon, headache, subjective swelling, nondermatomal paresthesia, psychological distress, and marked functional disability.

11. How do MPS and fibromyalgia compare?

The distinction between MPS and fibromyalgia is important with respect to diagnostic criteria, treatment approach, and prognosis.

Myofascial Pain vs. Fibromyalgia

	MYOFASCIAL PAIN	FIBROMYALGIA
Sex	Male and female	Predominantly female
Age	All	Age 40–60 years primarily
Pain	Focal	Diffuse
Mediation	Endorphin	Substance P
Duration	Acute or chronic	Chronic
Twitch response	Present	Absent
Pain areas	Distinct reference zones	Nonradiating
Etiology	Generally mechanical	Internal, environmental
Prognosis	Good with elimination of perpetuating factors	Guarded

From Goldman LB, Rosenberg NL: Myofascial pain syndrome in fibromyalgia. Semin Neurol 2:274–280, 1991, with permission.

12. What treatments are recommended for MPS?

First, trigger points that stimulate a portion of the patient's pain complaints must be identified, and then all pertinent underlying or perpetuating conditions must be addressed. The clinician may then proceed with specific myofascial interventions. Techniques include loosening of the trigger points by spray-and-stretch counterstimulation, myofascial massage, and trigger-point injections. Completion of trigger-point therapy should be followed by a stretching and restrengthening program to restore optimal function to the injured muscle and to minimize the risk of reinjury.

13. What treatments are recommended for fibromyalgia?

Numerous treatments may be used for fibromyalgia, including physical therapy, acupuncture, and transcutaneous nerve stimulation. Behavioral therapies include biofeedback and psychotherapy. Medications such as tricyclic antidepressants and NSAIDs have been the most extensively studied; the tricyclic medications appear to be the most effective. Although all of these therapies may produce some initial improvement, long-term benefit in most patients has been disappointing.

COMPLEX REGIONAL PAIN SYNDROMES
(Reflex Sympathetic Dystrophy and Causalgia)

14. What are the standardized diagnostic criteria for complex regional pain syndome (CRPS) according to the International Association for the Study of Pain (IASP)?

The IASP defines CRPS with four criteria, the last three of which are required for the diagnosis: (1) the presence of an initiating noxious event or a cause of immobilization; (2) continuing pain, allodynia, or hyperalgesia with pain disproportionate to any inciting event; (3) evidence at some time of edema, changes in skin blood flow, or abnormal sudomotor activity in the region of pain; and (4) absence of conditions that otherwise would account for the degree of pain and dysfunction. CRPS is divided into types I and II to distinguish the inciting event or injury.

Wasner G, Backonja MM, Baron R: Traumatic neuralgias; complex regional pain syndromes (RSD and causalgia); clinical characteristics, pathophysiologic mechanisms and therapy. Neurol Clin 16:851–868, 1998.

15. How does CRPS correspond to reflex sympathetic dystrophy (RSD) and causalgia?

In CRPS type I, previously called RSD, minor injuries of the limb or lesions in remote body areas precede the onset of symptoms. CRPS type II, previously called causalgia, develops after injury of a major peripheral nerve.

16. Describe the typical clinical features and course of CRPS.

CRPS is characterized by burning pain, hyperesthesia, vasomotor changes, and dystrophic changes that usually begin gradually days or weeks after the injury but may manifest within a few hours. The patient suffers greatly and protects the affected area. This disorder progresses in stages that have variable lengths, lasting anywhere from weeks to years.

17. Describe the clinical stages of CRPS.

• **Stage I** (acute) is associated with pain that is disproportionate to the initial injury. The quality of pain is often burning or aching and is increased by dependency of the affected part, physical contact, or emotional upset. Edema, temperature inequality, or increased hair and nail growth may occur in the affected part.

• **Stage II** (dystrophic) is characterized by edematous tissue that becomes indurated and skin that is cool or hyperhidrotic with livedo reticularis or cyanosis present. Hair loss may occur, with nails becoming cracked or brittle. The pain is constant and increased by any stimulus to the affected part. Roentgenograms may reveal diffuse osteoporosis.

• **Stage III** (atrophic) is typified by paroxysmal spread of pain and irreversible tissue damage. The skin appear thin and shiny and the fascia becomes thickened, with flexion or Dupuytren's contractures. Roentgenograms show marked bony demineralization and ankylosis.

More commonly, CRPS fails to progress through classic stages and rather takes on a partial form in which severe pain is associated with a minimal degree of sympathetic hyperactivity, such as a slight or intermittent swelling and mottling in association with the characteristic burning pain. Decreased skin temperature also may occur early. When CRPS is precipitated by a peripheral nerve injury, the symptoms quickly spread outside the distribution of the damaged nerve. CRPS typically starts distally and spreads proximally, with some cases spreading into additional extremities without a new injury.

18. What precipitating events are associated with CRPS?

The frequency of CRPS after peripheral nerve injury ranges from 1–15%. The occurrence of CRPS after myocardial infarction has dropped to less than 1%. The frequency of CRPS after fractures, sprains, and trivial soft tissue injuries has not been ascertained, but these injuries are probably the most common precipitating causes. Central causes of CRPS include cerebral infarction, severe head injury, brain tumor, and cervical cord injury. Other associated causes include immobilization, such as prolonged bed rest or casting of injured limbs. CRPS seems to be idiopathic in 30–50% of cases.

19. How do emotional disturbance and CRPS interrelate?

Patients with CRPS seem emotionally unstable, anxious, and socially withdrawn. The combination of the emotional impact of the illness and the disparity between the degree of pain and the physical examination lead many physicians to think that the pain is psychogenic. Patients report that anxiety may exacerbate the pain. In patients observed before and after relief of CRPS, the emotional disturbance resolves with successful treatment of the condition. No significant differences have been found in the personality traits of patients with CRPS and patients with nerve injuries without CRPS.

20. What is the relationship between sympathetically maintained pain (SMP) and CRPS?

Several mechanisms can maintain a state of neuropathic pain; SMP is among them. SMP may be involved in neuropathies, shingles, neuralgias, and CRPS. The justification for replacing the old term RSD with CRPS is the significant clinical evidence that the sympathetic nervous system seldom plays a role in the pathogenesis of CRPS; few patients with CRPS appear to have SMP. CRPS is a clinical entity, whereas SMP is a pathogenic mechanism. Sympathetic dysfunction is a recognized component of CRPSs but only as the result of an abnormal neurobiologic response to injury—not as the cause. Sympathetic symptoms and signs include swelling and abnormalities of sweating and skin blood flow. When these symptoms, as well as pain, are relieved by specific sympatholytic procedures in a patient with CRPS, the patient is considered to have SMP as a component of CRPS.

21. What tests may aid in the diagnosis of CRPS?

The diagnosis of CRPS is primarily clinical. Although roentgenographic studies demonstrating patchy demineralization were the first to confirm this disorder, these changes often do not occur until later stages of the disease. Scintigraphy with agents containing technetium 99 demonstrate increased periarticular uptake in the involved extremity, but this finding also appears only late in the disease. The best diagnostic approach to confirm the presence of CRPS in the upper extremities is the use of differential neural blockade, often combined with placebo injections in the ipsilateral stellate ganglion. To ascertain successful sympathetic blockade, temperature monitoring and observation for the presence of Horner's syndrome are mandatory. Lumbar sympathetic blockade is used to evaluate lower-extremity CRPS. Some clinicians, however, favor epidural spinal blocks, titrating anesthetic agents in increasing increments to allow differentiation between primarily sympathetically maintained pain, which is abolished at low concentrations, and primarily peripheral nerve pain, which requires higher concentrations of anesthesia.

Roberts WJ: A hypothesis on the physiological basis for causalgia and related pains. Pain 24:297–311, 1986.

22. Which sympatholytic procedures are indicated in CRPS with SMP?

Paravertebral sympathetic ganglion blockade is now the most widely recommended treatment for CRPS. Serial sympathetic ganglion blocks lead to definite if transient improvement in most patients.

Paravertebral sympathetic ganglionectomy is recommended for patients in whom only transient relief occurs with ganglion blocks. Several major series have examined the results of paravertebral sympathectomy, with 58–100% of patients reporting complete relief of symptoms. Patients whose pain is not relieved by ganglionectomy usually have incomplete sympathetic denervation or severe longstanding disease.

23. What are the potential therapies for CRPS?

All effective therapies block the effects of sympathetic hyperactivity. The most important factors in the effective management of CRPS are early recognition and treatment. Physical therapy alone has been shown to be effective in the treatment of CRPS, with exercises directed toward improving the mobility of the affected extremity. Because of significant pain, however, patients are usually unable to participate in meaningful physical therapy. Studies of treatment with corticosteroids have shown variable benefit, and these agents are reserved for patients who refuse or cannot tolerate treatments that directly block sympathetic activity. Phenoxybenzamine, a sympathetic blocker, provides modest benefit, although most patients have recurrent pain after completing a tapering schedule. Orthostatic hypotension limits the use of this medication in many patients. Bier block, a technique used for regional anesthesia, is helpful in a subpopulation of patients whose symptoms have been present for 9 months or less.

NEUROPATHIC PAIN SYNDROMES

24. What are the clinical symptoms of painful polyneuropathy?

Despite the variability in the underlying pathophysiology of painful polyneuropathy, the spectrum of pain complaints is markedly uniform, at least among disorders characterized by a generalized axonopathy. Patients usually report a constellation of symptoms, including paresthesias and dysesthesias of the feet, distal legs, and sometimes the hands, often in association with paroxysmal lancinating pains (spontaneous or provoked), deep aching in the feet and legs, and muscle cramping. Some patients have severe allodynia or hyperpathia, which markedly impairs the ability to walk. They also may report the perception of gross swelling or squeezing of the feet, as if the shoes were too tight, paradoxical cold despite skin that may be red and warm, and a sense of walking on sandpaper or ground glass. Patients with significant dysesthesias typically manifest preserved reflexes, distal pain and temperature sensory loss, relative sparing of proprioception and vibratory sensibility, and an associated autonomic neuropathy. This pattern supports probable small-fiber involvement, because larger-fiber neuropathies, such as painless sensory neuropathies, tend to have areflexia with distal loss of proprioception and vibratory sense. Virtually all chronically painful neuropathies are distal axonopathies.

Asbury AK, Fields HL: Pain due to peripheral nerve damage: An hypothesis. Neurology 34:1587–1590, 1984.

25. What are the clinical features of postherpetic neuralgia (PHN)? How is it treated?

PHN is a common cause of severe neuropathic pain, especially in the elderly. PHN usually is defined as pain persisting beyond 3 months in the region of the cutaneous outbreak of herpes zoster (HZ). Destruction of the sensory ganglion neurons (i.e., dorsal root, trigeminal, or geniculate ganglion) and the severity of the inflammatory response are probably the proximate causes of the pathology of PHN. Chronic PHN occurs in approximately 10–15% of all patients with HZ and is seen in more than 50% of HZ-infected patients older than 50; the risk is > 80% in patients older than 80.

Patients with PHN describe three types of pain: (1) a constant deep aching or burning pain; (2) an intermittent spontaneous pain with a lancinating or jabbing qualilty; and (3) a dysesthetic pain provoked by light tactile stimulation (allodynia). The severity of pain and the response to adjuvant analgesic medications are determined in part by the mechanism of neuropathic pain. Irritation of the ganglion neurons causes primarily nociceptive pain, whereas neuronal injury often leads to a deafferent neuropathic pain.

Acyclovir is an effective analgesic agent for acute HZ. It results in rapid pain relief but does not prevent PHN. The lidocaine patch is the only treatment approved by the Food and Drug Administration (FDA) for PHN. Controlled clinical trials have shown that the lidocaine patch significantly relieves pain and allodynia in most patietnts when placed directly over the painful region. Intrathecal methylprednisolone and lidocaine were recently shown to provide astonishing benefit in patients with PHN; all but 4 of 255 patients improved significantly or were completely free of pain.

Cluff RS, Rowbotham MC: Pain caused by herpes zoster infection. Neurol Clin 16:813–832, 1998.

Kotani N, et al: Intrathecal methylprednisolone for intractable postherpetic neuralgia. N Engl J Med 343:1514–1519, 2000.

26. What are the dermatomal frequencies in PHN?

Thoracic dermatomes	55%
Trigeminal distribution	20%
Cervical dermatomes	10%
Lumbar dermatomes	10%
Sacral dermatomes	5%

27. What is phantom limb pain?

Phantom limb pain is a neuropathic deafferent pain syndrome seen after limb amputation. It is often delayed in onset and described as a sharp, shooting, or burning sensation. It develops after limb amputation in up to 80% of patients and may also complicate other traumatic nerve and nerve root lesions, such as nerve root avulsion or traction injuries of the brachial and lumbosacral plexus. Phantom pain may be triggered by touching cutaneous regions that are outside the deafferented zone or by visceral activities such as urinating or defecating. Phantom pain can also be aggravated by pain or discomfort in the stump of an amputee.

28. What is the central dysesthetic syndrome associated with spinal cord injury?
Spinal cord injury, whether due to trauma, demyelinating disease, necrotizing myelitis, syringomyelia, spinal cord ischemia, arteriovenous malformation, or spinal cord tumor, often interrupts the central connections of nociceptive neurons in the spinal cord. Despite differences in the site of injury in the central dysesthesia syndrome, phantom body sensations are often perceived below the level of injury, with intermittent lancinating pain against a background of continuous burning pain. Patients frequently have regions of hyperalgesia and allodynia in the deafferented zones. Electrophysiologic studies demonstrate changes in spinothalamic tract conduction with relative sparing of dorsal column conduction.

29. What are the clinical features of the thalamic syndrome of Dejerine and Roussy?
Dejerine and Roussy described a painful condition as a result of vascular injury to the ventral posterolateral (VPL) and ventral posteromedial (VPM) nuclei of the thalamus. This condition is characterized by persistent spontaneous burning and occasional sharp pain in the involved extremities as well as an altered response to cutaneous and deep painful stimuli. Vascular lesions reported to produce this thalamic pain syndrome include ischemic stroke and hypertensive vascular hemorrhage. Thalamic tumors, arteriovenous malformations, and surgical lesions of the VPM also may cause typical thalamic pain.

ATYPICAL FACIAL PAIN AND HEADACHE

30. What is trigeminal neuralgia?
Trigeminal neuralgia is characterized by recurring paroxysms of sharp, stabbing, burning, or electric shock-like pain in the distribution of one or more branches of the trigeminal nerve. Attacks last only a few seconds to minutes, with patients pain-free between attacks. It is most common in elderly patients and is due to paroxysmal firing of the trigeminal nerve, in some cases triggered by compression of the nerve from adjacent blood vessels.
Keller JT, Van Loresen H: Pathophysiology of the pain of trigeminal neuralgia and atypical facial pain: A neuroanatomical prospective. Clin Neurosurg 32:275, 1985.

31. What are the recommended treatments for trigeminal neuralgia?
Medical treatment should be the primary approach, with surgical intervention reserved for patients refractory or intolerant to currently available medications. Almost all patients with typical trigeminal neuralgia respond to carbamazepine, at least initially. Only 25% of patients obtain sustained relief with phenytoin; thus, its main use is as an adjuvant to carbamazepine. Baclofen, like carbamazepine and phenytoin, facilitates segmental inhibition and depresses excitatory transmission in the spinal trigeminal nucleus. Many investigators feel the treatment of trigeminal neuralgia should start with baclofen because it is so safe, even though it may not be as effective as carbamazepine.
Patients who become refractory to medications require neurosurgical intervention. Microvascular decompression and radiofrequency rhizotomy are currently the procedures of choice. Microvascular decompression has the advantage of attacking the presumed cause of trigeminal neuralgia, while preserving the trigeminal nerve and producing longer-lasting relief in most patients. Radiofrequency rhizotomy avoids the risk of craniotomy but lacks the long-term relief accomplished with microvascular decompression. Recurrent symptoms after surgical intervention should be rechallenged with another trial of medical therapy.
Jannetta PJ: Observations on the etiology of trigeminal neuralgia, hemifacial spasm, acoustic nerve dysfunction and glossopharyngeal neuralgia. Neurochirurgia 20:145, 1977.

32. What are the clinical features of glossopharyngeal neuralgia?
Patients describe severe paroxysmal jabs of pain in the neck or temporal area, radiating to the ear and mastoid. The pain may cause hypotension and syncopal episodes. Glossopharyngeal neuralgia has been reported in patients with leptomeningeal metastasis or the jugular foramen syndrome and as a presenting symptom of head and neck malignancy. Carbamazepine or phenytoin provides the best relief.

33. What are the most common causes of atypical facial pain?
1. **Odontalgia** is characterized by a dull aching, throbbing, or burning pain that is more or less continuous and is triggered by mechanical stimulation of one of the teeth. It is relieved by sympathetic blockade.
2. **PHN** affecting the first distribution of the trigeminal nerve is preceded by a vesicular eruption. The pain is usually described as a chronic burning feeling. Many patients may experience electric shock-like paroxysms on touching the elbow region on the affected side.
3. **Temporal arteritis** causes chronic aching over the affected artery, often with marked tenderness on palpation.
4. **Cluster headaches** cause a burning, boring, piercing, or tearing hemicranial pain lasting minutes to hours, often triggered by the ingestion of alcohol.
5. **TMJ dysfunction** causes aching pain that is triggered and exacerbated by jaw movement and may last for days, weeks, or months.
6. **Myofascial pain** similarly presents as an aching pain lasting from days to months and is elicited by palpation of trigger points in the affected muscle.
7. **Atypical facial neuralgia** causes chronic aching pain involving the whole side of the face or even the head outside the distribution of the trigeminal nerve. This condition is much more common in women than men and is often associated with significant depression.

PRINCIPLES OF PAIN MANAGEMENT

34. What are the primary categories of analgesic therapy?
Recent advances in basic and clinical pharmacology have yielded a large and diverse group of clinically useful analgesic drugs that can be divided into three broad categories: nonopioid analgesics, opioid analgesics, and adjuvant analgesics. Most opioid and nonopioid analgesics have been formally approved for the treatment of pain. The adjuvant analgesics have been approved for the treatment of other conditions but are analgesic in selected circumstances.

Opioid analgesics
• Agonists
• Partial agonists
• Mixed agonist-antagonist

Nonopioid analgesics
• Nonsteroidal antiinflammatory drugs (NSAIDs)
• Acetaminophen

Adjuvant analgesics
• Antidepressants
• Anticonvulsants
• Gamma aminobutyric acid (GABA) agonists
• Alpha$_2$-adrenergic agonists
• Sympatholytics
• Local anesthetics
• Benzodiazepines
• Muscle relaxants
• Corticosteroids
• Neuroleptics

35. What is the role of opioid therapy in chronic nonmalignant pain?
The persistent administration of opioid drugs to patients with chronic nonmalignant pain is controversial. Clinical experience suggests that some patients with painful polyneuropathy or other neuropathic pain syndromes can obtain partial and sustained analgesia without the development of either significant opioid toxicity or aberrant behaviors indicative of psychological dependence/addiction. A trial of regular doses of an opioid under close monitoring may be considered in patients for whom other treatments provide little relief.

36. What is "tolerance" in opioid-resistant pain?
The term **tolerance** refers to a phenomenon in which exposure to a drug results in diminution of effect or the need for a higher dose to maintain effect. Although acute analgesic tolerance or tolerance after 1 or 2 weeks of opioid dosing does occur, the ability to escalate opioid doses to high levels without serious toxicity suggests that tolerance to nonanalgesic side effects such as respiratory depression is also a clinically relevant phenomenon. Numerous longitudinal studies

that have demonstrated early tolerance to the analgesic effects of opioids also confirm that dose escalation typically stabilizes at a plateau that often extends for a prolonged period.

37. What is the role of NSAIDs in analgesia?

NSAIDs inhibit prostaglandin production, which normally mediates the inflammation that occurs after tissue damage. The analgesic benefit of NSAIDs is due to the inhibition of prostaglandin-mediated nociceptor sensitivity with lowered thresholds for receptor activation. Recent animal studies strongly suggest a central mechanism of analgesia for NSAIDs as well, supporting the clinical observation that the analgesic benefit is often disproportionately greater than the antiinflammatory effects. The central mechanism also explains the analgesic effects of NSAIDs in patients with no evidence of peripheral inflammation.

38. What are the primary drug types and classes used as adjuvant analgesics?

Currently almost every drug prescribed for the treatment of neuropathic pain is, by definition, an adjuvant analgesic. The antidepressants, anticonvulsants, sympatholytics, GABA agonists, alpha$_2$-adrenergic agonists, and local anesthetic antiarrhythmics are the primary therapeutic options available for the treatment of neuropathic pain. These drugs, of which only carbamazepine (Tegretol) has been approved by the Food and Drug Administration for the treatment of pain (trigeminal neuralgia), have been studied in a controlled fashion and have been shown to be safe and effective for some patients suffering from neuropathic pain:

Antidepressants
   Tricyclics: nortriptyline (Pamelor), desipramine (Norpramin), amitriptyline (Elavil)
   Selective serotonin reuptake inhibitors (SSRIs): fluoxetine (Prozac), paroxetine (Paxil)
   Other: trazodone (Deseryl), venlafaxine (Effexor)
Anticonvulsants: phenytoin (Dilantin), carbamazepine (Tegretol), gabapentin (Neurontin)
GABA agonists: baclofen (Lioresal)
Oral local anesthetics: mexiletine (Mexitil)
Sympatholytics: phenoxybenzamine (Dibenzyline)
Alpha$_2$-adrenergic agonists: clonidine (Catapres)

39. What is the mechanism of action of tricyclic antidepressants (TCAs) for chronic pain?

TCAs have been used for many years in the treatment of persistent pain. Their benefit does not come simply from treatment of depression caused by the pain. The TCAs prevent the reuptake of serotonin (amitriptyline, imipramine) or noradrenaline (desipramine), and their effect is probably through increasing the effectiveness of descending adrenergic and serotonergic modulation of spinal segmentation nociception. An additional effect, when they are given in combination with morphine, is the increase in the plasma concentration of free morphine by competition for protein binding. Sedation and cholinergic side effects may reduce the acceptability of treatment.

McQuay HJ: Pharmacologic treatment of neurologic and neuropathic pain. Cancer Surv 7:141–159, 1988.

40. How do the newer SSRIs and the selective norepinephrine and serotonin reuptake inhibitors (SNSRIs) compare in analgesic efficacy and side effects with the commonly prescribed TCAs?

Until 1995, the TCAs were considered the gold standard for the treatment of neuropathic pain. But after reports of the efficacy of gabapentin and the lidocaine patch and FDA approval of the lidocaine patch, the role of TCAs decreased rapidly. The SSRIs have shown variable benefits in clinical trials; insufficient data are available for the SNSRIs.

41. What is the role of anticonvulsant therapy in neuropathic pain?

Anticonvulsant medication is currently recommended as a second-line therapy when treatment with tricyclic antidepressants fails. Their mechanism of action appears to include suppression of excessive discharges from pathologically altered neurons and prevention of normal neurons from becoming involved in the process. Recent anticonvulsant trials in neuropathic pain suggest that carbamazepine appears effective in some patients with brief shooting pain and in patients with steady burning or muscular pain. Results of controlled trials with phenytoin are mixed, with several studies failing to demonstrate any analgesic effects. Two other anticonvulsant drugs, clonazepam and valproic acid, also may minimize lancinating neuropathic pains.

42. What is the current role of gabapentin in the treatment of neuropathic pain?

Gabapentin is recommended by most authorities as the first-line oral agent for all neuropathic pain because of its proven efficacy, relative good tolerability, and superior safety profile. Its mechanism for pain relief remains unknown. A clinical concern with gabapentin is its tremendously wide therapeutic dose range (100–6000 mg/day).

43. What other pharmacologic agents are useful as adjuvant therapy in chronic pain syndromes?

1. Baclofen's proved efficacy in trigeminal neuralgia suggests that it may be effective in the treatment of other lancinating neuropathic pains.

2. Clonidine relieves neuropathic pain in a subpopulation of patients with painful diabetic neuropathy. The hypothesized mechanism of action of this alpha$_2$-adrenergic agonist may involve direct inhibition of spinothalamic neurons or generalized inhibition of CNS sympathetic efferent activity.

3. Use of neuroleptics as independent analgesics has limited efficacy in neuropathic pain states. Although the combined use of an antidepressant and a neuroleptic in painful neuropathy can be beneficial, the minimal supporting data and the potential toxicity of these drugs relegate their use as analgesics to patients with pain that has been refractory to other classes of drugs.

4. Tizanidine is an alpha$_2$-adrenergic agonist, approved by the FDA for treatment of spasticity. Uncontrolled studies have shown that this novel agent may be of benefit to some patients with neuropathic pain. Sedative side effects require that it be initiated at low doses and at bedtime.

44. What is the mechanism of action of local anesthetics in neuropathic pain?

Various local anesthetics depress evoked discharges of spinal cord neurons activated by C fibers and may relieve burning pain by this central mechanism and by an effect on injured peripheral nerve. An orally available analog of lidocaine, mexiletine, is efficacious for the pain associated with diabetic neuropathy. Studies show that, like intravenous lidocaine infusion, mexiletine appears capable of ameliorating the continuous dysesthesias that usually characterize the pain associated with peripheral neuropathy.

45. What are the indications for topical analgesics?

Recently, there has been a renewed interest in topical agents—drugs that act locally within the skin and peripheral nerve—for the treatment of peripheral neuropathic pain. Because topical drugs have no significant systemic activity, they have the theoretical advantage of no systemic side effects. **Capsaicin ointment** has been used for peripherally mediated pain, including diabetic neuropathy, postherpetic neuralgia, and incisional or neuroma pain. **Lidoderm** is a new topical formulation of lidocaine produced as both gel and skin patch. Lidocaine serum levels after use of the topical formulation are an order of magnitude below antiarrhythmic serum levels and are thus quite safe. The lidocaine patch is the only drug approved by the FDA for PHN.

46. What are the recommended behavioral and cognitive therapies for chronic pain?

If the patient is amenable, referral to a professional to learn relaxation, imagery, hypnosis, or meditation can be a primary or adjuvant treatment for chronic pain. These techniques require practice, and the patient should be committed to work daily on the cognitive techniques for at least 1 month. Although specific data about the efficacy of these therapies are mixed, in the course of using these methods a patient's perspective on his or her situation may change and suffering may lessen.

47. Which neurostimulatory approaches are used for chronic pain?

Neurostimulatory approaches range from noninvasive counterirritation techniques, such as systematic rubbing of the painful part, to transcutaneous electrical nerve stimulation (TENS) and acupuncture. A number of invasive measures, such as dorsal column stimulation and deep brain stimulation have been used in patients for whom drug therapy was relatively contraindicated or failed to provide adequate relief. These invasive nerve stimulatory techniques should be considered only in patients with refractory disabling dysesthesias who have undergone extensive evaluation and treatment by practitioners experienced in chronic pain management.

48. What is the role of implantable drug pumps for the treatment of chronic pain?
Technologic advances have made possible the delivery of morphine to selected regions of the CNS. Support for this modality followed the identification of opiate receptors not only in brain regions but also in the spinal cord, where significant concentrations have been detected in substantia gelatinosa, which receives C fiber input from the dorsal roots. Morphine administered locally in this area can significantly reduce discharges from spinal nociceptive neurons. Local intrathecally applied morphine has been shown to raise the threshold of pain dramatically in the region of application only. Epidural administration of morphine has become more commonplace for control of postoperative pain. The most important observation has been that effective relief of pain can occur with regional morphine without central effects such as lethargy, confusion, and respiratory depression.

Choosing patients for implantation of drug pumps requires firm guidelines. The first indication is for patients who fail to control pain with supratherapeutic oral medication. A second indication is for patients who cannot tolerate narcotics because of mental confusion, lethargy, or nausea. The third indication is for patients who have good relief of pain from a single dose of intrathecally administered morphine or from chronically infused morphine by an external pump through an epidural catheter. Chronic infusion of intrathecal spinal morphine does not change the neurologic examination and tolerance has not been a major problem. It therefore appears that implantable morphine pumps may have a specific role in the management of pain when oral medications have failed.
Pawl RP: Surgery for pain. Semin Neurol 9:257–268, 1989.

49. What is the role of neural ablative procedures for chronic pain?
Cordotomy, or technically and more accurately spinal tractotomy, is an ablative procedure aimed at anesthetizing some significant portion of the body rendered painful from disease. Although popular a decade ago, its use has declined steadily. The procedure is performed stereotactically, using a radiofrequency current delivered through a needle or electrode, and resulting in coagulation of neural fibers. This procedure is most easily performed at the C1–2 interspace, where the fibers from the ventrolateral spinothalamic tract begin crossing from the anterior cord to the posterior lower brainstem. The presence of intermingled motor fibers at this level has led to unacceptable side effects, such as paresis or urinary incontinence.

Peripheral neuronectomy and rhizotomy are quite limited in scope, producing pain relief by anesthesia of the affected body part, and are no longer used regularly.

Stereotactic ablative and simulating procedures that target thalamic nuclei or frontal projections of the thalamus remain under study. Deep-brain stereotactic surgery has been advocated to treat patients with the chronic pain that accompanies cerebral damage. With the advent of magnetic resonance imaging, however, it has become apparent that cerebral injury outside the thalamus and even outside the nociceptive pain pathway may be associated with chronic pain.

50. What is the current spectrum of multimodality strategies for treatment of chronic pain?

General Treatment Strategies

STRATEGY	EXAMPLES
Analgesia	Opioid analgesics Local anesthetic nerve blocks
Sympathetic blockade	Alpha-adrenergic blockers Local anesthetic blocks

Table continued on following page

General Treatment Strategies (Continued)

STRATEGY	EXAMPLES
Pain modulation	Tricyclic antidepressants Antiepileptics
Other pain modulation	Systemic local anesthetics
Rehabilitation and physical medicine modalities	Customized rehabilitation programs Physical and occupational therapies
Relief of other symptoms	Tricyclic antidepressants Anxiolytics
Psychological therapy and social support	Antidepressants, anxiolytics Counseling, vocational training

Modified from Backorija M: Reflex sympathetic dystrophy/sympathetically maintained pain/causalgia: The syndrome of neuropathic pain with dysautonomia. Semin Neurol 14:263–271, 1994.

BIBLIOGRAPHY

1. Inbody SB: Myofascial pain syndromes. In Evans R (ed): Neurology and Trauma. Philadelphia, W.B. Saunders, 1996, pp 458–495.
2. Johnson RT, Griffin JW (eds): Current Therapy in Neurologic Disease, 5th ed. St. Louis, Mosby, 1997.
3. Merskey H, Bogduk N: Classification of Chronic Pain. Task Force on Taxonomy, International Association for the Study of Pain. Seattle, IASP Press, 1994.
4. Portenoy R, Kanner R (eds): Pain Management: Theory and Practice. Philadelphia, F.A. Davis, 1996.
5. Sindrup SH, Jensen TS: Efficacy of pharmacological treatments of neuropathic pain: An update and effect related to mechanism of drug action. Pain 83:389–400, 1999.
6. Wesselmann U, Reich SG: The dynias. Semin Neurol 16:63–74, 1996.
Websites
www.aapainmanage.org
www.pain.com/index.com

20. HEADACHES

Howard S. Derman, M.D.

1. What is the incidence of headaches of all types?

About 45% of adults report that at some time they have experienced a severe or disabling headache.

2. Are headaches more common in males or females?

Typically, 70% of migraines occur in females and 30% in males. Cluster headaches occur almost entirely in men (90%). Muscle contraction headaches have a slightly increased incidence in female patients, but they are seen almost equally in both genders.

3. Does the location of head pain help to differentiate headache types?

Typically, migraine occurs on half of the face, involving the frontal area, usually in and about the eye and cheek. Cluster headaches are more periorbital in location, and patients may report a boring, excruciating pain above and behind the eye. Muscle contraction headache is classically described as band-like pain in the temporal region, occasionally extending back to the occipital region and forward to the forehead.

4. Which cranial structures are sensitive to pain?

Certain pain-sensitive cranial structures are capable of producing headaches. The brain itself is insensitive to pain.

Pain-sensitive Cranial Structures

1. The scalp	5. Arteries of the meninges
2. Scalp blood supply	6. Larger cerebral arteries
3. Head and neck muscles	7. Pain-sensitive fibers of the fifth, ninth, and tenth cranial nerves
4. Great venous sinuses	8. Parts of the dura mater at the base of the brain

5. When is a headache a sign of a serious neurologic problem?

Some indications that a headache may be due to a serious underlying illness include:
1. Sudden onset of severe headache
2. Headache accompanied by impaired mental status, fever, seizures, or focal neurologic signs
3. New headaches beginning after age 50

6. What common, serious diseases may present as a headache?

Primary brain tumor	Meningitis
Metastatic brain tumor	Temporal arteritis
Abscess	Hypertension
Subdural hematoma	Hydrocephalus
Intracerebral hemorrhage	Glaucoma
Subarachnoid hemorrhage	

7. Is there a place for narcotic analgesics in treatment of headaches?

The use of narcotic analgesics for treatment of headaches should be strongly discouraged. For the most part, narcotic analgesics should not be be used. A talk with the patient about the issue of narcotic analgesia before starting therapy is often helpful.

MIGRAINE HEADACHES

8. What is the age of onset for migraine headaches?
Migraines typically begin in teenage years and seldom begin after age 40.

9. What is the frequency of attack in migraine headaches?
Migraines are highly variable but usually occur once or twice per month. Some migraineurs have headaches more sporadically, 3–4 times per year. Some women report a strong association with menstruation.

10. What are the common symptoms of migraine?
1. Unilateral headache (60% of cases). The pain may begin as a dull ache but then becomes throbbing and possibly incapacitating.
2. Visual or sensory loss
3. Anorexia, nausea, vomiting
4. Photophobia and phonophobia
5. Mood changes

11. What are the five phases of a complete migraine attack?
1. **Prodrome.** The prodrome occurs hours to days before the headache and consists of changes in mood, behavior, appetite, and cognition.
2. **Aura.** The aura occurs within 1 hour of the headache and is most commonly visual or sensory.
3. **Headache.** The headache itself is commonly unilateral and may be pulsatile.
4. **Headache termination**
5. **Postdrome.** After termination of the headache, the complete migraine attack is ended with the postdrome or hangover phase.

12. How often are migraines accompanied by an aura?
Approximately 35% of migraines are accompanied by an aura. This type of headache is known as a **classic migraine**. Migraine without an aura is known as **common migraine**.

13. What are the common auras of migraine?
Visual auras are the most common and include photopsias, flashing lights, scintillating scotomata, and fortification spectra. Sensory auras are the next most common, especially numbness or paresthesias in a limb. Motor weakness and aphasia are less common.

14. What are the characteristics of migraine with aura?
The patient must have two attacks with at least three of the following four characteristics:
1. One or more fully reversible aura symptoms, indicating focal cerebral, cortical, or brainstem dysfunction.
2. At least one aura symptom developing gradually over 4 minutes or two or more symptoms occurring in succession.
3. No aura symptom lasting more than 60 minutes.
4. The migraine headache must follow the aura within 60 minutes or less.

15. What are the characteristics of migraine without aura?
The patient must have attacks that fulfill the following criteria:
1. The duration of the headache must be 4–72 hours.
2. During the headache, the patient must suffer at least one of the following: nausea and vomiting or photophobia and phonophobia.
3. The headache must have at least two of the following characteristics: unilateral location, pulsating quality, moderate-to-severe pain that inhibits or prohibits daily activities, and aggravation by routine physical activity.

16. What is the vascular theory of migraine?

The vascular theory of migraine states that the migraine aura is due to cerebral vasoconstriction and that the headache itself is caused by vasodilatation. Recent cerebral blood flow studies cast some doubt on this theory. Cerebral blood flow is decreased during migraine with aura, but there is no change in cerebral blood flow during migraine without aura. The role of vascular changes in the pathogenesis of migraine thus remains controversial.

17. Does serotonin play a role in migraine?

Serotonin is widely distributed throughout the body, with 90% concentrated in the GI tract and the remainder in the brain and platelets. During a migraine attack, the blood level of serotonin may decrease, whereas urinary concentrations may increase. This shift in serotonin levels may trigger changes in blood vessels and blood flow and also alter pain perception in the brain. Serotonin thus may play a role (as yet incompletely understood) in the cause of migraine. Certain medications such as amitriptyline, nortriptyline, and sumatriptan, which have an effect on serotonin metabolism, are useful in treatment of migraine headache.

Peroutka SJ: Serotonin receptor subtypes: Their evolution and clinical relevance. CNS Drugs 4(Suppl 1):18–36, 1995.

18. Can certain foods bring on migraine?

Certain foods are known to precipitate a migraine, as some patients note during history taking, but the only food clearly associated with increasing frequency of migraine is red wine. Foods commonly identified as exacerbating migraine include:
- Foods rich in tyramine (cheese, red wine)
- Foods containing monosodium glutamate (Chinese and Mexican food)
- Foods containing nitrates (cold cuts—bologna, salami, smoked meats)
- Pickled, fermented, marinated foods (pasta salads)
- Alcoholic beverages (especially red wine)
- Caffeinated beverages (soft drinks, tea, and coffee)

19. What are the most useful drugs for acute, abortive therapy of migraines?

The most useful abortive migraine treatments are ergotamines, Midrin, or the triptans.

20. Is ergotamine helpful therapy for migraines?

Ergotamine derivatives can be helpful in patients who have migraine with a clear-cut prodrome. Ergotamine is available in oral, sublingual, suppository, injectable, and inhalation forms. Because of the extreme nausea and vomiting seen with migraines, the suppository and sublingual preparations are the most useful and tolerable. When using sublingual or suppository form, the usual dosage is 2 mg. The patient may take 3 doses per headache, separated by ½ hour, up to 9 doses per week.

21. What is Midrin? Is it useful in headaches?

Midrin is a combination medication that consists of dichloralphenazone (a muscle relaxant), isometheptene (a vasospasm agent), and acetaminophen. It may be used either as a prophylactic medication (1 pill 2–3 times/day) or as abortive therapy (2 pills with onset of headache and then 1 pill every hour after that, up to 5 pills total).

22. What is sumatriptan?

Sumatriptan (Imitrex) represents a new class of medications—the 5-hydroxytriptamine (5-HT) receptor agonists. It may be administered subcutaneously (6 mg), nasally (20 mg), or orally (50 mg) and provides relief in 70% of patients. The chief side effects are chest tightness and flushing. It should not be used concomitantly with ergotamines or in patients with heart disease.

23. What other 5-HT receptor agonists are beneficial for migraines?

Since the success of sumatriptan, several similar agents have been marketed, including zolmitriptan, rizatriptan, and naratriptan. The triptans differ somewhat in pharmacologic profile, but all are roughly comparable in effectiveness. They are generally preferred over ergotamines or Midrin as first-choice therapy for migraine.

24. Can different triptans be combined in abortive treatment of migraine?
In general, different drugs should not be combined (e.g., rizatriptan and sumatriptan), but different forms of the same medicine can be used (e.g., nasal sumatriptan followed in 2 hours by oral sumatritpan).

25. Are the triptans used only as abortive in migraine?
Because of its longer half-life, naratriptan (Amerge) is useful as a prophylactic agent in menstrual migraine. If a woman has headaches at a predictable time of the month, especially if she is taking birth control pills, use of naratriptan each morning 1–2 days before the period and through day 3 of the period may be helpful.

26. Are other anticonvulsants used in migraine prophylaxis?
Both gabapentin (Neurontin) and topirimate (Topamax) have been used in migraine and seem to be quite helpful.

27. Which group or groups of drugs represent first-line therapy for migraine prophylaxis?
Tricyclic antidepressants, beta blockers, calcium channel blockers, and sodium valproate are the drugs of choice for migraine prophylaxis.

28. What are the indications for prophylactic treatment of migraine?
When headaches occur at a frequency of two or more per month or, more importantly, when the headaches affect the patient's day-to-day life (causing absence from work or school), prophylactic therapy is indicated.

29. Which tricyclics are the most helpful prophylactic agents?
Tricyclic antidepressants work through an action independent of their antidepressant effect. Among the many tricyclic antidepressants, amitriptyline (Elavil) is most useful for migraine therapy. Other drugs that have been successful include doxepin (Sinequan), nortriptyline (Pamelor), and imipramine (Tofranil).

30. In prescribing a tricyclic antidepressant for migraine, what dosage should be considered?
In the case of amitriptyline, it is best to start at a dose of 25 mg at bedtime because patients often become lethargic with initial dosing. The level may be increased to a maximal dose of 200 mg by raising the dose slowly (25 mg/week over 3–4 weeks). However, doses greater than 100 mg are often associated with significant side effects, such as dry mouth, constipation, and urinary hesitancy. Patients also may become quite sedated. Finally, weight gain is often an intolerable side effect.

31. Are beta blockers useful as prophylaxis for migraine?
Beta blockers, especially propranolol, have been used effectively for migraine prophylaxis for many years. Propranolol is safe and has few side effects. The usual dose is 80 mg LA (long-acting); it may be increased to 160 mg LA, as indicated. Pulse monitoring is important, and the drug dose may be increased to 160 mg if the pulse stays greater than 60.

32. Are beta blockers well tolerated in migraineurs?
For the most part, beta blockers are well tolerated, but several issues need to be discussed with patients before starting the beta blocker. Bronchospasm is a concern in patients with asthma. In starting a beta blocker, find out whether the patient participates in an exercise program. The number of patients treated for migraine who are also enrolled in aerobic exercise classes is surprising. Patients often become irate when they see members of their exercise class achieving heart rates of 160 while they are on a drug that keeps their heart rate at 60. Patients often feel miserable during exercise while taking a beta blocker. Beta blockers thus should not be considered primary therapy in some groups of patients.

33. Which calcium channel blocker is most effective in migraine?

Calcium channel blockers are considered first-line therapy in migraine. Verapamil is the most useful in migraine and is usually started at a dose of 180 mg at night. The dose may be increased as necessary to 240 mg at night over a 4-week period. The drug is well tolerated and has efficacy in over 70% of migraineurs.

34. Are other calcium channel blockers useful in migraine?

Nifedipine started at 30 mg/day has proved to be useful in migraines; nicardipine, 20–60 mg/day, also has been efficacious in migraine prophylaxis. Both nifedipine and nicardipine should be started only after failure of verapamil.

35. Is sodium valproate successful in migraine prophylaxis?

Sodium valproate (Depakote) may be helpful in migraine prophylaxis. Its mechanism of action is unclear but seems independent of its anticonvulsant properties.

36. Is there a difference in treating seizures as opposed to migraine with valproate in terms of dosing and drug level?

Migraine usually responds to lower doses than seizures. Some migraineurs may respond to doses as small as 125 mg twice daily, and an average of 650 mg in divided doses is successful in 70% of patients. It is not necessary to monitor or follow drug levels in treating migraine.

37. How should you decide among a beta blocker, tricyclic antidepressant, calcium channel blocker, or valproate in migraine prophylaxis?

It is essential to consider patients' work habits and other factors, such as dosing schedule and exercise programs. Anecdotal reports seem to favor beta blockers for patients who have significant visual problems (flashing lights, zigzag lines, fortification spectra) with their headaches. In patients who are markedly anxious or depressed or who have a sleep problem, a tricyclic antidepressant may be more appropriate. The drugs are about equally effective, and studies have not identified any one as clearly superior to the others.

38. Is methysergide maleate a drug to consider for migraine?

Methysergide maleate (Sansert) is a selective vasoconstrictor and serotonin agonist. It is highly effective but is no longer considered a primary therapy in migraine because of serious side effects attending prolonged use. The most serious side effect is retroperitoneal fibrosis.

39. In using methysergide, what precautions should be taken?

Methysergide may still be used, despite major complications, if 5 months of drug therapy are followed by 1 month of drug holiday, repeated 2 times/year. However, because many other treatment options exist, methysergide should be used only when all other medications have failed.

40. How does pregnancy affect treatment of headache?

When pregnant patients must use some medication for their headaches, either acetaminophen or aspirin may be helpful. If these do not work, then and only then is the use of narcotics justified. Codeine is probably the safest medication to use judiciously for headaches during pregnancy. Finally, a tricyclic antidepressant or cyproheptadine (Periactin) may be used.

41. Are any drugs clearly contraindicated in pregnant patients?

Ergotamine derivatives and any drug with a vasospastic component are contraindicated. Usually, after a heart-to-heart talk, most pregnant patients are willing to proceed during their entire pregnancy without medication if they are convinced that drugs may in some way harm the fetus.

CLUSTER HEADACHES

42. What is the age of onset for cluster headaches?
Cluster headaches typically start at age 25 and may occur as late as age 45.

43. What symptoms are associated with cluster headaches?
The headache strikes abruptly, without any aura, around and behind one eye. The pain is extremely severe and lasts 20–60 minutes. Patients report nasal stuffiness, rhinorrhea, and redness of the eye ipsilateral to the head pain. There also may be partial Horner's syndrome with ptosis and miosis on the side of the head pain.

44. Why are cluster headaches called cluster headaches?
The headaches occur during a short time span; this cluster then recurs periodically. A typical cluster of headaches may last 4–8 weeks, with 1–2 headaches per day during the cluster. Patients may go 6 months to 1 year before another cluster occurs.

45. Are all cluster headaches associated with this episodic pattern?
Sixty-seven percent of patients with cluster headaches report an episodic pattern, but 33% have 1–4 headaches every month without a quiescent period.

46. What is the differential diagnosis of cluster headaches?
- Trigeminal neuralgia
- Cyclical migraine
- Sinus infection
- Raeder's paratrigeminal neuralgia

47. How are acute attacks of cluster headaches managed?
- Oxygen inhalation
- Locally applied anesthetic agents
- Ergotamine
- Dihydroergotamine (DHE) injections
- Sumatriptan

48. How is oxygen used in cluster headaches?
The average dose of oxygen is 8 L/min for 10 minutes, which relieves pain in approximately 80% of patients. Oxygen therapy must be instituted very early in the head pain, and some patients have a rebound headache once the oxygen is stopped.

49. What prophylactic medications may be considered for patients in the midst of a cluster?
Calcium channel blockers, particularly verapamil, have been used in cluster attacks at doses starting at 180 mg at night and increased to 360 mg as tolerated. Steroids, lithium, and topirimate also may provide relief.

50. Are steroids helpful in cluster headaches?
Steroids can be quite useful in two ways. For acute attacks, a tapering dose of 60 mg, 40 mg, and 20 mg of prednisone over 3 days may be helpful. If the patient is in the midst of a cycle, a tapering course starting at 60 mg, decreasing to 0 mg over a 3-week period, is recommended.

51. Is lithium useful in cluster headache?
Lithium carbonate is an excellent prophylactic treatment of cluster headaches. Patients usually benefit from a dose of 600–900 mg/day, maintaining a therapeutic level of 0.4–0.8 mEq/L.

52. What is the treatment for rhinorrhea and lacrimation associated with clusters?
Cyproheptadine (Periactin), a drug that works as an antihistamine and also has an effect on serotonin, may be useful. The dose is usually 2 mg by mouth 3 times/day. Side effects include sedation and appetite enhancement; these issues must be discussed with the patient before starting medication.

TENSION HEADACHES

53. What is a tension headache?
A tension headache is dull, persistent pain that occurs in the temporal region in a bandlike distribution and may radiate forward to the frontal region or posteriorly to the occipital region. It is also referred to as a muscle contraction headache.

54. What causes tension headache?
The cause of tension headaches is open to debate. It has not been possible to relate them very well to any particular psychological profile. They may arise from tight, tense muscles, but not all studies verify this association. Some authorities suggest that they are variants of migraine headaches.

55. What are the different types of tension headaches?
Episodic and chronic.

56. What are the characteristics of an episodic tension headache?
The patient must have at least 10 previous headache episodes fulfilling the following diagnostic criteria:
1. The headache must last from 30 minutes to 7 days.
2. A minimum of two of the following pain characteristics: pressing or tightening pain, mild-to-moderate intensity, bilateral location, no aggravation with physical activity.

57. What are the characteristics of a chronic tension headache?
1. Average headache frequency of 15 days per month for 6 months or 180 days per year.
2. Frequently associated with analgesic overuse.
3. Migrainous features may be superimposed intermittently.

58. What is the treatment for tension headache?
The treatment of muscle contraction headache is different from that of migraine. Treatment of the acute pain includes drugs that are primarily analgesics, such as nonsteroidal anti-inflammatory drugs. Chronic suppressive therapy is usually required, and the most effective agents are serotonergic tricyclics such as amitriptyline.

59. Is botulinum toxin (Botox) used in the treatment of tension headache?
Yes. Botox appears to be quite useful in the treatment of some muscle tension headaches when injected directly into trigger point areas in the head and neck.

60. What is analgesic rebound headache?
A well-described headache syndrome is associated with analgesic abuse, including over-the-counter medications such as aspirin and acetaminophen (Tylenol). Typically patients take from 10–20 pills/day and have headaches on a chronic basis, generally daily. Such patients must be switched to suppressive agents such as tricyclics and weaned from analgesics completely.

61. Are any nonpharmacologic treatments useful for tension headaches?
Nonpharmacologic approaches, including physical therapy to the head and neck regions and biofeedback, have been useful in tension headache. However, the benefits are generally short-lived, and long-term results are disappointing.

SPINAL TAP HEADACHES

62. Are headaches frequent after lumbar puncture?
Approximately 20–25% of patients have a headache after lumber puncture. Headaches occur whether or not the tap is traumatic and regardless of the amount of spinal fluid removed.

63. Do patients with postspinal tap headache have other complaints?

Patients are often severely disabled by nausea and vomiting along with the headaches. Characteristically, the headache is much worse when the patient is upright and improves dramatically when the patient lies flat in bed.

64. What is the treatment for postspinal tap headache?

The first step is to reassure the patient that the headache eventually will go away. The patient must remain flat in bed as much as possible. Simple analgesics are recommended. Finally, if the headache becomes disabling, blood patch therapy with a second spinal tap may be indicated.

POSTCOITAL HEADACHES

65. What is postcoital cephalgia?

Postcoital cephalgia refers to headaches that occur before and after orgasm. They occur with equal frequency in men and women. The pain is usually sudden in onset, pulsatile, and fairly intense; it involves the entire head.

66. Are headaches that occur with intercourse a sign of subarachnoid hemorrhage?

Less than 2% of patients who present with subarachnoid hemorrhage secondary to aneurysm leakage have leakage with intercourse. More often than not, headaches that occur with intercourse are either migraine or muscle contraction in origin.

67. What is the treatment for postcoital cephalgia?

There are two drugs of choice. If one believes the headaches are due to muscle contraction, a nonsteroidal anti-inflammatory drug is indicated. If the headaches are thought to be migraine, a beta blocker is most useful.

HEADACHES FROM BRAIN TUMORS OR MASS LESIONS

68. Are headaches associated with a brain tumor different from other types of headaches?

The headaches associated with a brain tumor may present in much the same fashion as headaches associated with muscle contraction. The headaches may be daily and are seldom severe.

69. What special features in the history and physical exam should be considered when brain tumor is a concern?

Patients who have headaches associated with brain tumor often awake early in the morning with headaches. Neurologic examination usually reveals focal abnormalities as well as papilledema on funduscopic examination.

PSEUDOTUMOR CEREBRI

70. What is pseudotumor cerebri?

Pseudotumor cerebri, also known as benign intracranial hypertension, is increased intracranial pressure without evidence of malignancy on neurologic testing. It is manifested primarily by headaches and visual obscuration.

71. How can one make the diagnosis of pseudotumor cerebri?

Patients are generally obese and female. The neurologic exam is normal. An MRI or CT scan is usually normal as well. The pressure is elevated on spinal fluid examination, which confirms the diagnosis.

72. What etiologic factors are associated with benign intracranial hypertension?

1. Mastoiditis and lateral sinus thrombosis
2. Head trauma
3. Oral progestational drugs
4. Marantic sinus thrombosis
5. Cryofibrinogenemia
6. Addison's disease
7. Hypoparathyroidism
8. Tetracycline therapy
9. Hypervitaminosis A

73. What are the visual complaints of patients with benign intracranial hypertension?

Visual acuity is usually normal, but patients may report transient obscurations of vision. Their visual fields may show enlargement of the blind spot, and examination may show optic disc edema.

74. What medicines are useful in benign intracranial hypertension?

Usually, treatment includes the use of acetazolamide at 500 mg 1 or 2 times/day or prednisone at 20–40 mg/day. Patients may need to be on treatment for up to 6 months at a time.

75. Aside from medication, what other treatments are used for benign intracranial hypertension?

Patients are generally treated with repeat spinal taps to maintain pressures in the normal range.

TEMPORAL ARTERITIS

76. What is temporal arteritis?

Temporal arteritis is a granulomatous arteritis affecting large and medium-sized arteries of the upper part of the body, including the temporal vessels. Histologic studies reveal intimal thickening and lymphocytic infiltration of the media and adventitia.

77. What is the clinical setting of temporal arteritis?

Patients generally present after age 60. The headaches are abrupt in onset, and patients also complain of pain and stiffness in the neck, shoulders, and back and sometimes in the pelvic girdle.

78. Describe the headache associated with temporal arteritis.

Severe pain may be experienced in one temple but often occurs in the occipital area, face, jaw, or side of the neck and may be associated with exquisite hypesthesia throughout the scalp. The pain may have a throbbing character.

79. Are there any serious complications of temporal arteritis?

The most severe complication is impairment of vision, which may result in loss of vision and may not be reversible.

80. How does one make a diagnosis of temporal arteritis?

In addition to clinical findings, ancillary data include an elevated sedimentation rate and positive temporal artery biopsy.

81. If temporal arteritis is suspected or diagnosed, is there any treatment?

Treatment involves immediate use of large doses (i.e., 40–60 mg) of prednisone daily for the first week, with gradual reduction over the next 4–6 weeks to a maintenance dose of 5–10 mg/day. Sedimentation rates can be followed, and when the sedimentation rate is normal for 4 months, further tapering of medication is justified.

BIBLIOGRAPHY

1. Goadsby PJ, Silberstein SD (eds): Headache. Boston, Butterworth-Heinemann, 1997.
2. Victor M, Ropper AJ (eds): Neurology, 7th ed. New York, McGraw-Hill, 2001.
Websites
www.achenet.org
ahsnet.org
www.migraines.org

21. SEIZURES AND EPILEPSY

Paul A. Rutecki, M.D.

DESCRIPTION AND CLASSIFICATION

1. What is a seizure?

Many behaviors are referred to as seizures, but the definition of a seizure should be restricted. Seizures are produced by the abnormal synchronization of cortical neurons that results in a change in perception or behavior. Seven to 10% of the population will have a seizure at some point in their lives.

2. What is epilepsy?

Epilepsy is the condition of recurrent seizures caused by an inherent brain abnormality. The underlying abnormality may result from a number of causes, including hereditary factors, developmental disorders, perinatal injury, cerebral infection, trauma, infarction, or neoplasm. Between 0.5 and 1% of the population has epilepsy.

3. How are seizures classified?

Seizures are classified according to their clinical and electroencephalographic (EEG) characteristics. The most recent classification of seizures is summarized below:

Classification of Epileptic Seizures

I. Partial seizures
  A. Simple partial seizures (consciousness not impaired)
  B. Complex partial seizures (consciousness impaired)
    1. Impairment of consciousness at onset
    2. Simple partial seizure onset followed by impaired consciousness
  C. Partial seizures evolving to generalized tonic-clonic convulsions (GTC)
    1. Simple partial evolving to GTC
    2. Complex partial evolving to GTC

II. Generalized seizures
  A. Absence seizures
    1. Typical
    2. Atypical, complex
  B. Myoclonic seizures
  C. Clonic seizures
  D. Tonic seizures
  E. Tonic-clonic seizures
  F. Atonic seizures (astatic)

Commission on the Classification and Terminology of the International League Against Epilepsy: Proposal for revised clinical and electroencephalographic classification of epileptic seizures. Epilepsia 22:489–501, 1981.

4. What is the difference between partial and generalized seizures?

Partial seizures start focally and have clinical and EEG changes that indicate onset from one brain region and in some cases one cerebral hemisphere. Impaired consciousness is the inability to respond normally to the environment because of altered awareness. Generalized seizures begin in both hemispheres at the same time. The clinician should try to classify all of the patient's seizure types because appropriate treatment depends on correct classification.

5. What causes primary generalized seizures? At what age do they usually start?

Primary generalized seizures (i.e., seizures that cannot be localized to one cerebral hemisphere at onset) usually have a genetic predisposition. The seizures usually begin before the age of 20. These seizures are not associated with well-defined auras (an aura is the first subjective symptom of the seizure).

6. What does the EEG show in primary generalized seizure?

The interictal EEG signature of generalized seizures is the frontocentral dominant spike and wave discharge or polyspike and wave pattern. There may be shifting asymmetry of voltage, but there is no consistent lateralizing feature.

7. What are the features of the different types of primary generalized seizures?

The shortest generalized seizures consist of a single myoclonic jerk during which consciousness is not lost. Associated with the jerk is a generalized spike or polyspike and wave discharge in the EEG. **Absence seizures** consist of 3-Hz spike and wave discharges in the EEG associated with a brief (usually less than 30 seconds) episode of unresponsiveness that may be accompanied by eyelid fluttering, decreased tone, increased tone, automatisms, autonomic components, or a combination of these elements. **Atypical or complex absence seizures** are longer in duration and are associated with more automatisms and motor signs. The EEG shows a 1.5–2.5-Hz spike and wave discharge during the seizure. **Tonic seizures** are associated with generalized 10-Hz or faster activity. **Generalized tonic-clonic seizures** begin with an initial tonic component that is followed by a clonic component. At the end of the seizure, the person is unresponsive and gradually regains consciousness. The EEG initially shows generalized 10-Hz activity during the tonic phase, followed by slow waves or sharp and slow waves during the clonic phase. **Atonic seizures** are associated with low-voltage fast activity, attenuation, or polyspike and wave discharges.

8. What are the characteristics of simple partial seizures?

The manifestations of partial seizures depend on the area of the brain involved. The more restricted the brain region involved, the more limited the symptoms and the less likely that consciousness will be impaired. Often simple partial seizures are referred to as auras, which may consist of an abnormal sensation (e.g., smells, flashing lights, somatosensory symptoms) or experiential phenomena (déjà vu, well-formed hallucinations). If the seizure is restricted to a small area of motor cortex, there is associated focal clonic activity. As the seizure activity spreads, the person may develop impaired consciousness and a complex partial seizure. Further elaboration of the seizure may include thalamocortical pathways and secondary generalization.

9. What are the characteristics of complex partial seizures?

Complex partial seizures are characterized by abnormal responsiveness to the environment, automatisms, autonomic features (pupillary dilatation, salivation), and amnesia for the seizure. Either simple partial or complex partial seizures may progress to a generalized tonic-clonic seizure.

10. How can complex partial seizures and absence seizures be differentiated clinically?

Three main features may help to differentiate complex partial from absence seizures:

1. Complex partial seizures, unlike absence seizures, may be preceded by a well-defined aura.

2. On average, complex partial seizures last 90 seconds, whereas absence seizures usually last only 10–15 seconds.

3. After complex partial seizures, the patient is usually confused or has some postictal cognitive problem. Absence seizures are not associated with a postictal state, and patients return to their baseline cognitive state at the end of the seizure.

Automatisms are common with both absence and complex partial seizures.

11. What are epileptic syndromes? How are they classified?

An epileptic syndrome is a composite of signs and symptoms that may be associated with certain pathologies or etiologies (symptomatic) or lack an identifiable pathology or etiology (idiopathic). Many of the idiopathic syndromes are inherited. Like seizures, epileptic syndromes are classified by localization or generalization of seizure activity. Syndromes may be associated with localized seizures that begin in one area of the brain (partial seizures) or generalized seizures that begin throughout the brain at onset. Syndromic classification of patients is useful because some of the syndromes have well-defined prognoses. In addition, more appropriate antiepileptic drug therapy can be guided by syndromic classification.

Classification of Epileptic Syndromes

I. Localization-related epilepsies and syndromes
  A. Idiopathic with age-related onset
    1. Benign childhood epilepsy with centrotemporal spike
    2. Childhood epilepsy with occipital paroxysms
  B. Symptomatic: related to area of onset and clinical and EEG features (encompasses most partial seizures)

II. Generalized epilepsies and syndromes
  A. Idiopathic, with age-related onset, listed in order of age
    1. Benign neonatal familial convulsions
    2. Benign neonatal convulsions
    3. Benign myoclonic epilepsy in infancy
    4. Childhood absence epilepsy (pyknoepilepsy)
    5. Juvenile absence epilepsy
    6. Juvenile myoclonic epilepsy (impulsive petit mal)
    7. Epilepsy with grand mal seizures (GTCS) on awakening
  B. Cryptogenic and/or symptomatic, in order of age
    1. West syndrome (infantile spasms)
    2. Lennox-Gastaut syndrome
    3. Epilepsy with myoclonic-astatic seizures
    4. Epilepsy with myoclonic absences
  C. Symptomatic-epileptic seizures as the presenting or dominant feature, i.e., malformations or degenerative diseases, with or without a metabolic etiology, that present with seizures as part of the clinical picture

III. Epilepsies and syndromes undetermined as to whether they are focal or generalized
  A. Both generalized and focal seizures
    1. Neonatal seizures
    2. Severe myoclonic epilepsy in infancy
    3. Epilepsy with continuous-spike waves during slow-wave sleep
    4. Acquired epileptic aphasia (Landau-Kleffner syndrome)
  B. Without unequivocal generalized or focal features—GTCS in which a focal or generalized onset cannot by determined by clinical or EEG features

IV. Special syndromes
  A. Situation-created seizures
    1. Febrile convulsions
    2. Seizures related to other identifiable situations such as stress, hormonal changes, drugs, alcohol, or sleep deprivation
  B. Isolated, apparently unprovoked epileptic events
  C. Epilepsies with specific modes of seizure precipitation, e.g., reflex epilepsies
  D. Chronic, progressive epilepsia partialis continua of childhood

Commission on the Classification and Terminology of the International League Against Epilepsy: Proposal for the classification of epilepsies and epileptic syndromes. Epilepsia 26:268–278, 1985.

12. What is Lennox-Gastaut syndrome?

This epileptic syndrome usually begins before age 5 and is characterized by tonic-axial, atonic, and atypical absence seizures. Most patients also have myoclonic, partial, and tonic-clonic seizures. The EEG is characterized by a slow (< 3 Hz) frontocentral dominant spike and wave pattern, and patients have mental retardation. The seizures are difficult to control, and status epilepticus associated with stupor, jerks, and changes in tone is common. About 60% of patients have a clear underlying cause of encephalopathy (symptomatic). The remaining cases are crypto-genic or idiopathic.

Motte J, et al: Lamotrigine for generalized seizures associated with the Lennox-Gastaut syndrome. N Engl J Med 337:1807–1812, 1997.

13. What are the four most common inherited epileptic syndromes?
1. Febrile convulsions
2. Benign childhood epilepsy with centrotemporal spikes
3. Childhood absence epilepsy
4. Juvenile myoclonic epilepsy

The first three syndromes usually are associated with seizures that remit spontaneously. Juvenile myoclonic epilepsy usually responds to treatment with valproate.

14. What are benign febrile convulsions?
Benign febrile convulsions are an inherited predisposition to developing a tonic-clonic seizure with a high fever. The description is limited to convulsions associated with high fever in persons under the age of 5 (usually between 6 and 36 months of age), with no cause for the seizure other than the fever. Benign febrile seizures are common, occurring in 3–5% of children under the age of 5. Most patients have only one or two seizures.

15. What is the consequence of a febrile seizure?
It is important to differentiate benign febrile convulsions from epilepsy. In general, if there are no other reasons to suspect recurrent seizures, the child is not treated. A single, isolated febrile seizure of short duration probably does not greatly influence the later development of epilepsy.

Risk Factors for Epilepsy

1. Underlying neurologic or developmental abnormality

2. Family history of nonfebrile seizures

3. Prolonged febrile convulsions

4. Multiple febrile convulsions

5. Atypical or focal features (complex febrile seizures)

16. Describe the syndrome of benign childhood epilepsy with centrotemporal spikes.
This syndrome accounts for about 15–20% of epilepsy under the age of 15 years. The seizures, which are mostly nocturnal, are associated with focal motor activity of the face and salivation and may generalize secondarily. Sensory symptoms may occur around the mouth in addition to motor components. Speech may not be possible. The EEG is characterized by a prominent centrotemporal sharp wave with otherwise normal background. The sharp waves occur more frequently during sleep. This epilepsy remits spontaneously after the age of 16, regardless of treatment. Treatment for partial epilepsy may be instituted, depending on how disruptive the seizures are.

17. What is juvenile myoclonic epilepsy?
This syndrome is characterized by myoclonic seizures that often occur shortly after wakening and generalized tonic-clonic seizures that tend to be precipitated by sleep deprivation. Interictally the EEG shows a generalized spike-wave pattern occurring at 4–6 Hz. The myoclonic jerks are associated with a spike-wave discharge, and usually consciousness is not lost. Valproate, lamotrigine, and primidone are effective therapies, and some of the newer antiepileptic drugs also may prove to be beneficial. Unlike the other common idiopathic epilepsies, juvenile myoclonic epilepsy does not remit with age.

18. What are channelopathies? Do they cause epilepsy?

A channelopathy is a disorder, usually inherited, of ion channels. Although first described in neuromuscular disorders (periodic paralyses), the following channelopathies may cause or predispose to epilepsy:

CHANNEL MUTATION	DISORDER
Potassium channels KCNQ2/KCNQ3	Benign familial neonatal convulsions
Sodium channels SCN1A/SCN1B	Generalized epilepsy with febrile seizures
Nicotinic acetylcholine receptor CHRNA4	Autosomal dominant nocturnal frontal lobe epilepsy

From Rogawski MA: KCNQ2/KCNQ3 K+ channels and the molecular pathogenesis of epilepsy: Implications for therapy. Trends Neurosci 23:393–398, 2000.

PHYSIOLOGY

19. What systemic physiologic changes occur during a seizure?

The systemic and CNS physiologic changes depend on the type of seizure. For both absence and complex partial seizures, the patient may have a variety of autonomic alterations, including changes in pulse rate, sweating, salivation, pupillary dilatation, and incontinence. The most dramatic systemic changes occur during generalized tonic-clonic seizures or prolonged tonic, myoclonic, or clonic seizures. Generalized tonic-clonic seizures are associated with an increase in blood pressure and pulse rate, increased autonomic nervous system activation, a metabolic acidosis, a drop in PO_2 and an increase in PCO_2 during the apneic tonic phase, and, rarely, hyperkalemia or rhabdomyolysis. After an isolated generalized tonic-clonic seizure, these abnormalities usually return to baseline within 1 hour. With prolonged generalized tonic-clonic seizures, systemic problems intensify and may have serious consequences.

20. What CNS physiologic changes occur during a seizure?

During a seizure, blood flow and glucose utilization in the brain are increased. Accompanying the neuronal activity may be an increase in lactate and a decrease in pH, alterations in the concentration of neurotransmitters, an increase in extracellular potassium, and a decrease in extracellular calcium. Generalized tonic-clonic seizures and most complex partial seizures activate the hypothalamus and increase serum prolactin, a finding that may help to differentiate epileptic from nonepileptic (psychogenic) seizures. Prolactin also may be elevated after syncope and hence cannot differentiate seizures from syncope.

Oribe E, Amini R, Nissenbaum E, Boal B: Serum prolactin concentrations are elevated after syncope. Neurology 47:60–62, 1996.

CAUSES

21. What are the identifiable causes of seizures as a function of age?

Common Causes of Seizures by Age

NEONATE TO 3 YR	3–20 YR	20–60 YR	OVER 60 YR
Prenatal injury	Genetic predisposition	Brain tumors	Vascular disease
Perinatal injury	Infections	Trauma	Brain tumors, especially
Metabolic defects	Trauma	Vascular disease	metastatic tumors
Congenital malformations	Congenital malformations	Infections	Trauma
CNS infections	Metabolic defects		Systemic metabolic
Postnatal trauma			derangements
			Infections

22. What are the metabolic causes of seizures?

1. Hypocalcemia	6. Anoxia
2. Hyponatremia	7. Nonketotic hyperglycemic states
3. Hypoglycemia	8. Inherited metabolic diseases
4. Liver failure	• Aminoacidurias
5. Renal failure	• Urea cycle disorders

23. What drugs are common causes of seizures?

Seizures may be caused by many drugs, both prescribed and illicit. Cocaine and amphetamines are the two drugs of abuse most commonly associated with seizures. Some drugs produce seizures at toxic levels, including penicillin, lidocaine, aminophylline, and isoniazid. Other drugs, such as phenothiazines and tricyclic antidepressants appear to lower seizure threshold and, in susceptible individuals, may produce seizures. Whenever a patient presents initially with a seizure, toxicology studies are indicated. The other setting associated with seizures is withdrawal from drugs, particularly alcohol, barbiturates, or benzodiazepines.

24. What are the characteristics of alcohol withdrawal seizures?

Chronic alcohol abuse may be associated with seizures during abstinence. Most seizures occur between 7 and 48 hours after the last drink. The seizures are usually generalized tonic-clonic, although multiple seizures or even status epilepticus may occur. A subset of patients with alcohol withdrawal seizures have epilepsy and require maintenance anticonvulsants. These patients usually have post-traumatic epilepsy. In patients with only alcohol withdrawal seizures, benzodiazepines appear to be the most efficacious therapy, whereas phenytoin does not appear to help.

Porter RJ, Mattson RH, Cramer JA, Diamond I (eds): Alcohol and Seizures: Basic Mechanisms and Clinical Concepts. Philadelphia, F.A. Davis, 1990.

25. What inherited diseases are associated with seizures?

Numerous genetic diseases, including many degenerative neurologic diseases, are associated with seizures. At least 25 autosomal dominant diseases are associated with seizures, including tuberous sclerosis and neurofibromatosis. Approximately 100 autosomal recessive diseases are associated with seizures, many of which have an inborn error of metabolism; for instance, the aminoacidurias and lipid storage diseases. Finally, some 20 X-linked diseases are associated with seizures, including adrenoleukodystrophy and Pelizaeus-Merzbacher disease.

26. Which factors predict the development of epilepsy after head trauma?

Open head trauma produced by bullets or shrapnel is associated with a 50% or greater chance of developing epilepsy. Closed head trauma, such as after automobile accidents or blunt injuries, carries a much lower risk (5% or less). Factors that predispose to the development of epilepsy after head trauma include a seizure within 2 weeks of injury, depressed skull fracture, loss of consciousness for longer than 24 hours, cerebral contusion, subdural hematoma, or subarachnoid blood, and age > 65.

Annegers JF, Hauser WA, Coan SP, Rocca WA: A population-based study of seizures after traumatic brain injuries. N Engl J Med 338:20–29, 1998.

27. What is the differential diagnosis of progressive myoclonus epilepsy?

The five main causes of progressive myoclonus epilepsy may be differentiated based on their clinical, pathologic, or laboratory features.

1. **Unverricht-Lundborg disease** is a clinical diagnosis. Affected patients begin having myoclonic seizures between the ages of 8 and 13 years. Dementia is not a prominent feature. The gene responsible for Unverricht-Lundborg disease has been discovered. The DNA codes for cystatin B, a small protein that functions as a cysteine protease inhibitor. Why this mutation leads to the syndrome is unclear.

2. **Lafora body disease** presents in persons 11–18 years of age. Dementia is a prominent

feature. The disease is named for Lafora bodies—eosinophilic inclusions present in skin, liver, or brain biopsies. The gene responsible for Lafora body disease codes for an intracellular protein, tyrosine phosphatase.

3. **Neuronal ceroid lipofuscinosis** may present at any age and is associated with dementia and visual loss, with characteristic funduscopic findings. It also is associated with inclusion bodies seen on electron microscopy of nerve, skin, or rectal mucosa.

4. **Sialidosis** is associated with dysmorphic features and funduscopic findings (cherry-red spot) and with α-N-acetylneuraminidase deficiency.

5. **Mitochondrial encephalomyopathy with ragged red fibers** (MERRF) on muscle biopsy is often associated with short stature, hearing loss, optic atrophy, neuropathy, and myopathy. Some patients have maternally inherited mitochondrial genome abnormalities.

Minassian BA, Lee JR, Herbrick JA, et al: Mutations in a gene encoding a novel protein tyrosine phosphatase causes progressive myoclonus epilepsy. Nat Genet 20:171–174, 1998.

Pennacchio LA, Lehesjoki A, Stone NE, et al: Mutations in the gene encoding cystatin B in progressive myoclonus epilepsy (EPMI). Science 271:1731–1734, 1996.

DIAGNOSTIC TESTING

28. What percentage of people with epilepsy has an abnormal EEG during the interictal period?

The answer depends on the type of epilepsy. One study found that only 35–40% of patients with the clinical diagnosis of epilepsy had interictal epileptiform activity on a single EEG. Most of these patients had partial seizures with or without secondary generalization. Multiple EEGs enhance the yield of positive EEGs to 60%. Untreated patients with absence seizures usually have an abnormal routine EEG. The diagnostic yield of EEG also may be increased by prolonged monitoring, including sleep. An important point is that epilepsy is a clinical diagnosis and cannot be ruled out by normal EEG.

29. Which patients with seizures should have MRI scans?

Patients with partial seizures or focal features on EEG should have MRI scans to look for a brain lesion associated with their seizures. Patients with clear-cut primary generalized epilepsy based on EEG and clinical features usually do not require MRI scanning.

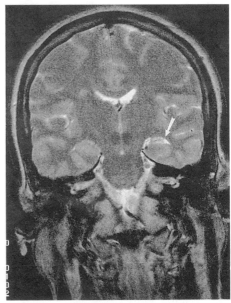

MRI scan in a patient with partial complex seizures. The arrow shows sclerosis in the hippocampus of the left temporal lobe (mesial temporal sclerosis).

30. What is the value of PET scanning in patients with epilepsy?

Positron emission tomography (PET) scans have helped us to understand some of the metabolic changes that occur during seizures. Most PET scans use 2-[^{18}F]fluoro-2-deoxyglucose to define cerebral glucose metabolism. PET scans demonstrate hypermetabolism or increased glucose uptake during the seizure. Most patients, however, are studied during the interictal period. In this setting, patients with epilepsy that have focal onset may show an area of hypometabolism in the region of seizure onset and a decrease in glucose uptake. PET scanning has been useful in helping to localize seizure onset in patients with intractable, complex partial seizures that are being evaluated for surgical therapy.

31. What is a SPECT scan? What role does it have in evaluating patients?

SPECT refers to single-photon emission computed tomography and usually uses a radioactive isotope that demonstrates blood flow. SPECT scans may identify areas of decreased blood flow interictally. If given at the start of a seizure or shortly thereafter, an increase in blood flow correlates with the area of seizure onset. SPECT scanning is primarily useful in the presurgical evaluation of patients with intractable epilepsy; it is most useful if an ictal scan can be obtained. Subtraction of the interictal scan from the ictal scan and superimposition on a MRI scan can provide an anatomic and physiologic picture of the epileptogenic zone.

O'Brien TJ, So EL, Mullan BP, et al: Subtraction peri-ictal SPECT is predictive of extratemporal epilepsy surgery outcome. Neurology 55:1668–1677, 2000.

THERAPY

32. When should antiepileptic treatment be initiated?

People should be treated with antiepileptic medication when the clinician thinks that the person will probably have another seizure without treatment. The seizure type or syndrome may help with this decision. For example, absence seizures are rarely isolated and so require therapy, whereas febrile seizures are often isolated and therapy is not indicated. Between 20 and 70% of people with an isolated, unprovoked generalized tonic-clonic seizure will never have another seizure. Ideally, it would be best not to treat these patients. Seizure recurrence is more likely if the patient has focal neurologic deficits, mental retardation, an EEG that demonstrates epileptiform abnormalities, or a structural brain lesion. In these patients it is reasonable to begin antiepileptic therapy. In patients with a well-defined provocative etiology, it is best to treat the underlying process rather than the seizures themselves, particularly in clear-cut cases of alcohol withdrawal seizures and drug-induced seizures.

33. When should antiepileptic treatment be stopped? What are the risk factors for recurrence of seizures?

Treatment should be stopped when it is the physician's opinion that the patient probably will not have seizures off medications. Certain seizure types and benign epileptic syndromes will remit. Patients with absence seizures usually "outgrow" their seizures, and therapy is no longer needed. Benign childhood epilepsy with centrotemporal spikes also remits. Recent studies suggest that approximately one-third of adult patients and one-fourth of children who are seizure-free for 2 years will relapse after termination of antiepileptic medication. Risk factors for recurrence include:

1. Prolonged period before seizures were controlled
2. High frequency of seizures before control
3. Neurologic abnormalities
4. Mental retardation
5. Complex partial seizures
6. Consistently abnormal EEGs

34. Which antiepileptic drugs (AEDs) are most appropriate for different seizure types?

The choice of AED is dictated by the types of seizures that the patient has. If possible, monotherapy should be used.

First- and Second-Line Drugs for Specific Seizure Types*

	PARTIAL SEIZURES AND LOCALIZATION-RELATED EPILEPSIES	GENERALIZED SEIZURES			
		TONIC-CLONIC	ABSENCE	MYOCLONIC	ATONIC/TONIC
First-line drugs	Carbamazepine Phenytoin Lamotrigine Valproate Oxcarbazepine	Valproate Lamotrigine Phenytoin Carbamazepine	Ethosuximide Valproate	Valproate Lamotrigine Topiramate	Valproate Lamotrigine Topiramate
Second-line drugs	Primidone Phenobarbital Felbamate	Topiramate Primidone Phenobarbital Felbamate	Topiramate Lamotrigine Clonazepam	Primidone Phenobarbital Clonazepam Ethosuximide Felbamate	Phenytoin Phenobarbital Primidone Clonazepam Felbamate
Add-on drugs[†]	Topiramate Levetiracetam Zonisamide Gabapentin Tiagabine	? Levetiracetam ? Zonisamide	? Zonisamide	? Levetiracetam ? Zonisamide	? Levetiracetam ? Zonisamide

* Listed in order of author's preference.
[†] May be effective as monotherapy but approved only as add-on agents.

The above selections are based on side effects as well as effectiveness. Phenobarbital and primidone are as efficacious as phenytoin and carbamazepine but are more likely to produce side effects. Tonic and atonic seizures are often resistant to therapy, and valproate seems to be most efficacious. Tonic and clonic seizures may be secondarily generalized, and phenytoin, carbamazepine, lamotrigine, topiramate, and felbamate can be helpful.

Mattson RH, Cramer JA, Collins JF, et al: A comparison of valproate with carbamazepine for the treatment of complex partial seizures and secondarily generalized tonic-clonic seizures in adults. N Engl J Med 327:765–771, 1992.

35. What AEDs have been released in the 1990s? What are their indications?
Since 1993, eight new AEDs have been released and four new preparations of old drugs have been approved. The eight new drugs are felbamate, gabapentin, lamotrigine, topiramate, tiagabine, zonisamide, levetiracetam, and oxcarbazepine. Felbamate was initially approved as an add-on drug or as monotherapy in adults with partial seizures alone or seizures that generalize secondarily and in children with partial or generalized seizures associated with Lennox-Gastaut syndrome. After its release, felbamate was found to cause a high incidence of aplastic anemia (about 1 in 5000) and hepatotoxicity (about 1 in 30,000). These serious idiosyncratic side effects have limited its use, and felbamate is used only in refractory patients in whom other AEDs have failed. The patient must be informed of the high frequency of potentially fatal side effects. Lamotrigine and oxcarbazepine are approved for monotherapy for partial seizures in adults. The other five new drugs have been approved as add-on therapy in adults with partial seizures and secondarily generalized seizures. Studies are ongoing to define their roles as monotherapeutic agents and their use in generalized seizures.

The four new preparations of old drugs include an osmotic slow-release form of carbamazepine (Tegretol-XR), a long-acting oral form of valproate (Depakote CR), an intravenous preparation of valproate (Depacon), and a phosphate preparation of phenytoin (fosphenytoin [Cerebyx]). Tegretol-XR may be given twice a day and should be used for patients with compliance problems and patients with peak-dose side effects on carbamazepine. Depacon can be used to administer valproate intravenously in patients with no oral intake. It should not be given intramuscularly. Fosphenytoin can be given intramuscularly or intravenously and is useful in patients with no oral intake or IV access. Fosphenytoin also may be given more rapidly and with fewer complications than the conventional propylene glycol preparation of phenytoin. These properties make it the preferred method of giving phenytoin to treat status epilepticus.

Brodie MJ, Richens A, Yurn AW: Double-blind comparison of lamotrigine and carbamazepine in newly diagnosed epilepsy. Lancet 345:476–479, 1995.

Dichter MA, Brodie MJ: New antiepileptic drugs. N Engl J Med 334:1583–1590, 1996.

36. How are the new AEDs started?

Gabapentin is the easiest new drug to use. It is excreted by renal clearance and has no interactions with other AEDs. The drug should be started at 300 mg/day and increased by 300 mg/day to 1200–2400 mg/day given in 3 divided doses. Further dose escalation to 3600–4800 mg/day is often well tolerated with potential improvement in efficacy.

Topiramate should be started at 25 or 50 mg/day. The dose should be increased slowly— by either 25 or 50 mg/day each week. A slower escalation of 25 mg/day each week may reduce side effects. Target dose according to the package insert is 400 mg/day given in 2 divided doses, but some epileptologists have observed efficacy at 200 mg/day. Phenytoin and carbamazepine increase topiramate metabolism, and topiramate may cause a slight increase in phenytoin concentrations.

Lamotrigine needs to be introduced slowly to prevent rash. Valproate inhibits lamotrigine metabolism, whereas phenytoin, carbamazepine, and phenobarbital increase lamotrigine metabolism. For patients taking valproate, lamotrigine is started at 12.5 mg/day or 25 mg every other day and increased to 25 mg/day after 2 weeks. The 25-mg/day dose is given for another 2 weeks; then the dose is increased by 25 mg/week to a maximal dose of 100–200 mg/day. If the patient is taking an enzyme-inducing AED, the initial dose is 50 mg/day for 2 weeks followed by 100 mg/day in 2 divided doses for 2 weeks. Thereafter the dose is increased by 100 mg/week to a target dose of 400–500 mg/day.

Tiagabine may be useful as an add-on drug for partial seizures. It must be introduced slowly to avoid sedation, and it requires dosing 3 times daily. The half-life is only 2–3 hours in patients whose liver enzymes have been induced by other anticonvulsant drugs. It is highly protein-bound. The chief side effect is sedation.

Felbamate is begun at 1200 mg/day in 2 divided doses. The dose is titrated to a total dose of 1800–5000 mg/day given in 3 or 4 divided doses. Dose increases of 600 mg every 2 weeks are reasonable. Because of its toxicity profile, felbamate should be reserved for use in intractable patients.

Levetiracetam is approved for add-on therapy in patients with partial seizures and secondarily generalized seizures. It may be effective in myoclonic and other generalized epilepsies. The usual starting dose is 250–500 mg twice daily. Efficacy may increase with doses up to 1500 mg twice daily, increasing by 1000 mg every 2 weeks. Because levetiracetam is excreted renally with minimal metabolism and is without protein binding, there are no significant drug interactions. It may cause sedation, especially with initiation of therapy.

Oxcarbazepine, a carbamazepine derivative, is approved for monotherapy and adjunct therapy for partial seizures. It is metabolized rapidly to an active monohydrated metabolite with a half-life that allows twice-daily dosing. In general, the dosing equivalent compared with carbamazepine is 1.5 times. The initial dose is 300 mg twice daily, with increases of 300–600 mg/day every week to target doses of 1200–2400 mg/day. Hyponatremia is a more common side effect than with carbamazepine. Oxcarbazepine induces metabolism of oral contraceptives, although it has fewer drug interactions than carbamazepine.

Zonisamide is a sulfonamide derivative that is approved as an adjunct therapy for partial seizures. It also may be effective in myoclonic and other primary generalized seizures. The usual starting dose is 100 mg/day with an increase of 100 mg/day every 2 weeks to a target dose of 200 mg twice daily. Renal stones are a potential complication, and the drug should be used cautiously in patients with sulfa allergies.

Leach JP, Brodie MJ: Tiagabine. Lancet 351:203–207, 1998.

37. What are the mechanisms of action of AEDs?

Phenytoin, carbamazepine, lamotrigine, gabapentin, topiramate, oxcarbazepine, zonisamide, and valproate block sodium channels and impair generation of high-frequency action potentials. At higher than therapeutic concentrations, phenobarbital also may decrease repetitive firing. Some of these drugs also may reduce high-threshold calcium currents, although this effect often is in the supratherapeutic range. In the therapeutic range, the barbiturates and diazepam derivatives enhance GABA responses. Diazepam derivatives increase the binding of GABA to the GABA receptor. The barbiturates appear to favor channel opening of the chloride ionophore associated with the GABA receptor. Topiramate may enhance GABAergic inhibition. Gabapentin may promote nonsynaptic GABA release. Felbamate has inhibitory effects on N-methyl-D-aspartate (NMDA) channel function. Topiramate antagonizes glutamate activation of AMPA/KA channel function. Tiagabine enhances the action of GABA by blocking GABA uptake. Lastly, ethosuximide and zonisamide appear to act by reducing the low-threshold calcium current that is responsible for burst behavior in thalamic neurons.

38. In general, how often should AEDs be given?

AEDs should be given at least every half-life. Some medications may need to be given more frequently because of peak-dose side effects. For example, patients tolerate twice daily or 3 times daily dosing of ethosuximide better than a single daily dose. In some cases, pharmacokinetics (drug metabolism, half-life) may not match pharmacodynamics (drug effect), and medication is given at intervals longer than the half-life. For example, levetiracetam has a half-life of 6–8 hours but is given twice daily. Steady state serum concentrations are reached in about five half-lives.

Half-life Frequencies for AEDs*

DRUG	HALF-LIFE (HR)
Carbamazepine	12–18
Ethosuximide	30–60
Felbamate	14–24
Gabapentin	5–7
Lamotrigine[†]	15–60
Levetiracetam	6–8
Oxcarbazepine (monohydroxylated derivative)[‡]	10
Phenobarbital	96
Phenytoin[§]	10–60
Primidone	8–12
Tiagabine[†]	7–9
Topiramate	19–23
Valproate	8–12
Zonisamide[#]	25–70

* Values represent adult half-lives and may vary depending on whether the patient is on monotherapy or polytherapy.
† The half-life of lamotrigine and tiagabine depends on other AED therapy. When used alone, lamotrigine has a half-life of 24 hours. If lamotrigine is taken with an enzyme inducer, the half-life is 15 hours; if taken with valproate, 60 hours. The half-life of tiagabine is 2–3 hours in enzyme-induced patients.
‡ Oxcarbazepine is metabolized quickly to a monohydroxylated derivative whose half-life is 10–15 hours.
§ The half-life of phenytoin depends on the serum concentration; a higher concentration is associated with a longer half-life because of nonlinear kinetics.
# The half-life is reduced to 25–40 hours in the presence of enzyme inducers.

39. What are the advantages of monotherapy?

(1) In most situations, one drug controls seizures as well as two drugs; (2) monotherapy prevents interactions between antiepileptic medications; (3) monotherapy is less expensive; and (4) monotherapy improves compliance.

40. What is rational polytherapy? Is it rational?

With the approval of new AEDs as add-on agents, a new view of polytherapy is evolving. Traditionally, polytherapy with AEDs was associated with increased side effects, poor compliance, and drug interactions that made it difficult to achieve therapeutic serum levels. Rational polytherapy is considered to be the combination of AEDs with different mechanisms of action or different side-effect profiles. AEDs known to block sodium channels (phenytoin, carbamazepine, lamotrigine) are not used together but are combined with AEDs that have other mechanisms of action (i.e., drugs that potentiate GABA, such as tiagabine, or have mixed mechanisms of action, such as gabapentin or valproate).

It is unclear whether a rational polytherapy works better than monotherapy. With conventional AEDs, the Veterans Affairs Cooperative Study found that only 11% of patients became seizure-free with a combination of drugs, although of patients in whom monotherapy failed, 40% had improved seizure control with more than one drug. What is rational is a therapeutic regimen that minimizes side effects and best controls seizures. In some cases, more than one AED may be required.

41. What are the main side effects of commonly used antiepileptic medications?

Side effects may be dose-dependent or dose-independent. In general, most anticonvulsants can have sedative properties and interfere with motor performance in a dose-dependent manner.

Side Effects of Anticonvulsants

CONCENTRATION-DEPENDENT		CONCENTRATION-INDEPENDENT	
Ataxia	Nausea, vomiting	Weight gain	Hirsutism
Phenytoin	Valproate	Carbamazepine	Phenytoin
Carbamazepine	Carbamazepine	Gabapentin	Dupuytren's
Phenobarbital	Ethosuximide	Valproate	contractures
Primidone	Phenytoin	Hair loss	Phenobarbital
Gabapentin	Headache	Valproate	Gingival hyperplasia
Lamotrigine	Ethosuximide	Behavioral	Phenytoin
Topiramate	Felbamate	Phenobarbital	Edema
Diplopia, blurred vision	Lamotrigine	Primidone	Gabapentin
Carbamazepine	Tremor	Ethosuximide	Valproate
Phenytoin	Tiagabine	Topiramate	Pancreatitis
Lamotrigine	Valproate	Gabapentin	Valproate
Sedation	Thrombocytopenia	Levetiracetam	Diarrhea
Phenobarbital	Valproate	Rash	Carbamazepine
Phenytoin	Weight gain	Carbamazepine	Topiramate
Carbamazepine	Valproate	Phenytoin	
Valproate	Cognitive problems	Lamotrigine	
Lamotrigine	Phenobarbital	Oxcarbazepine	
Levetiracetam	Primidone	Phenobarbital	
Gabapentin	Topiramate	Primidone	
Topiramate	Topiramate	Zonisamide	
Zonisamide	Paresthesias		
Hyponatremia	Topiramate		
Carbamazepine	Zonisamide		
Oxcarbazepine	Renal stones		
Anorexia	Topiramate		
Felbamate	Zonisamide		
Topiramate	Insomnia		
Zonisamide	Felbamate		

42. What are the main drug interactions among AEDs?

The answer is complex but can be simplified by understanding drug metabolism. Both gabapentin and levetiracetam are water-soluble and are excreted renally; thus, the dose should be adjusted downward with a reduction in creatinine clearance. Neither drug is protein-bound. There are no pharamacokinetic interactions with the other AEDs.

All of the other available drugs undergo hepatic metabolism, which may influence their own pharmacokinetics as well as the metabolism and pharmacokinetics of other AEDs. Hepatic pathways include the cytochrome P450 system (CYP), UDP-glucuronosyl transferase (UGT), and epoxide hydrolase (EH). The most common site for drug interactions is the CYP system, which is composed of a number of isoenzymes that may be induced or inhibited.

Enzyme Induction

EH	UGT	CYP1A2	CYP2C	CYP3A4
Carbamazepine	Carbamazepine	Carbamazepine	Carbamazepine	Carbamazepine
PB/PRM	Lamotrigine	PB/PRM	PR/PRM	Felbamate
Phenytoin	Oxcarbazepine	Phenytoin	Phenytoin	Oxcarbazepine
	PB/PRM			PR/PRM
	Phenytoin			Phenytoin
				Topirmate

EH = epoxide hydrolase, UGT = UDT-glucuronosyl transferase, PB/PRM = phenobarbital/primidone.

Enzyme Inhibition

2C9	2C19	EPX/GT
Phenytoin	Felbamate	Valproate
Valproate	Oxcarbazepine	
	Topiramate	
	Valproate	

The effects on hepatic enzymes dictate drug interactions. The CYP enzyme inducers (carbamazepine, phenobarbital, primidone, and phenytoin) cause an increase in dose requirements for many drugs, including all other AEDs metabolized in the liver. Valproate decreases carbamazepine epoxide formation and lamotrigine metabolism. Felbamate, oxcarbazepine, and topiramate inhibit phenytoin metabolism via inhibition of the hepatic enzyme 2C19.

The other main mechanism of drug interaction is protein binding. Phenytoin, valproate, and tiagabine are highly bound (> 90%) to plasma proteins and can compete for binding sites. Valproate protein binding displaces phenytoin or tiagabine so that free phenytoin and tiagabine levels increase.

43. Summarize the main effects of add-on drugs on original drug levels.

Effects of Add-on Drugs on Original Drug Levels

ORIGINAL DRUG	ADD-ON DRUG							
	CBZ	FBM	LTG	OXC	PB/PRM	PHT	TOP	VPA
Carbamazepine (CBZ)		↓ ↑ epx			↓ ↑ epx	↓ ↑ epx		↑ epx
Ethosuximide (ETH)	↓				↓	↓		↓ ↑
Felbamate (FBM)	↓				↓	↓		↑
Lamotrigine (LTG)	↓			↓	↓	↓		↑
Oxcarbazepine (OXC)†	↓				↓	↓		↓
Phenobarbital/primidone (PB/PRM)	↑PB	↑		↑				↑

Table continued on following page

Effects of Add-on Drugs on Original Drug Levels (Continued)

ORIGINAL DRUG	ADD-ON DRUG							
	CBZ	FBM	LTG	OXC	PB/PRM	PHT	TOP	VPA
Phenytoin (PHT)	↓↑	↑		↑	↑↓		↑	↓*
Tiagabine (TGB)	↓				↓	↓		↑*
Topiramate (TOP)	↓				↓	↓		
Valproate (VPA)	↓	↑	↓		↓	↓	↓	
Zonisamide (ZON)	↓				↓	↓		

↑↓ = may increase or decrease; epx = carbamazepine 10,11-epoxide; blank space = no known interaction.
* Valproate increases the unbound fraction of phenytoin or tiagabine and may result in toxicity.
† Monohydroxylated derivative.

44. What are the main interactions between AEDs and other commonly used medications?
Whenever there is a change in seizure control or development of toxic symptoms without a change in dosage of the AED(s), drug interactions should be considered.

Drugs That Increase the Effects of AEDs

PHENYTOIN	CARBAMAZEPINE	PHENOBARBITAL	VALPROATE
Amiodarone	Azide antifungals	Antihistamines	Erythromycin
Cimetidine	Cimetidine	Corticosteroids	Fluoxetine
Chloramphenicol	Clarithromycin	Isoniazid	Isoniazid
Clofibrate	Diltiazem	Propoxyphene	Salicylates
Diltiazem	Danazol	Tricyclic anti-	
Disulfiram	Erythromycin	depressants	
Fluconazole	Fluoxetine		
Fluoxetine	Isoniazid		
Imipramine	Lithium		
Isoniazid	Omeprazole		
Metronidazole	Propoxyphene		
Omeprazole	Verapamil		
Propoxyphene			
Salicylates			
Sulfonamides			
Ticlopidine			
Trazodone			
Tolbutamide			

Drugs That Decrease the Effects of AEDs

PHENYTOIN		GABAPENTIN	OXCARBAZEPINE
Antacids	Folate	Antacids	Verapamil
Bleomycin	Pyridoxine		
Ciprofloxin	Rifampin		
Cisplatinum	Sucralfate		
Diazoxide	Theophylline		
Enteral feedings	Vinblastine		

Commonly used drugs also are affected by AEDS. The enzyme inducers (carbamazepine, felbamate, oxcarbazepine, phenobarbital, primidone, phenytoin, and topiramate) make the low estrogen-containing oral contraceptives ineffective. A higher-dose estrogen pill may be effective. The inducers also result in a higher dose requirement for warfarin, cyclosporine, antipsychotics, steroids, theophylline, and other drugs metabolized by the cytochrome P450 enzymes (CYP).

45. What are the idiosyncratic reactions to AEDs?

The most common is skin rashes, which may be relatively severe, leading to exfoliative dermatitis or Stevens-Johnson syndrome. Skin rashes are most common with phenytoin, lamotrigine, carbamazepine, zonisamide, and barbiturates. Most AEDs can also suppress the bone marrow and cause aplastic anemia, agranulocytosis, or thrombocytopenia. Another idiosyncratic reaction consists of drug-induced hepatitis and, at times, full-blown serum sickness. Valproate hepatic toxicity is most common in patients under the age of 2 who are taking other medications. Phenytoin, phenobarbital, ethosuximide, and carbamazepine may produce vasculitis. Valproate has also been implicated as a cause of pancreatitis.

46. When and how often should blood levels of AEDs be checked?

Monitoring of AED levels is indicated when the patient is initially loaded with the medication and when the drug reaches a steady-state concentration, usually after approximately 5 half-lives. Monitoring of drug levels is helpful in determining patient compliance and in documenting high levels when the patient has toxic symptoms.

47. Which screening blood tests should be performed for patients taking AEDs? How often should they be done?

Many AEDs may affect the ability of the bone marrow to produce blood cells or may cause liver dysfunction. It is reasonable to use CBC and liver function tests as baseline studies to identify predisposing problems. After this initial screening, it is usually not necessary to perform these studies routinely unless the patient is symptomatic. The exceptions are young children and mentally retarded patients who cannot communicate their toxic syndromes. Another special situation is the use of felbamate, which requires hematologic and hepatic function monitoring.

Pellock JM, Willmore LJ: A rational guide to routine blood monitoring in patients receiving antiepileptic drugs. Neurology 41:961–964, 1991.

48. Should AEDs be used after head trauma to prevent the development of epilepsy?

There is no definitive answer to this question. The most recent study assessing phenytoin concluded that therapy was useful only during the first week after head trauma. At later dates, the side effects produced by phenytoin appeared to be detrimental to patients with severe neurologic damage after head trauma. Valproate also has been found to be ineffective as a prophylactic agent after head trauma. At present, no drug clearly has been shown to be effective prophylaxis against post-traumatic epilepsy.

Dikmen SS, Machamer JE, Winn HR, et al: Neuropsychological effects of valproate in traumatic brain injury: A randomized trial. Neurology 54:895–902, 2000.

Tempkin NR, Dikmen SS, Wilensky AJ, et al: A randomized, double-blind study of phenytoin for the prevention of posttraumatic seizures. N Engl J Med 323:497–502, 1990.

49. What are the teratogenic risks of AEDs?

All AEDs have teratogenic features. Furthermore, carbamazepine, phenytoin, phenobarbital, and primidone may interfere with the effectiveness of oral contraceptives, making pregnancy a possibility, especially with breakthrough bleeding. In general, taking a single AED increases the risk of birth defects by 3-fold. Teratogenic effects are more likely when more than one AED is used. The physician should try to treat the patient with only one AED during pregnancy. The patient and her family should be counseled about potential teratogenic effects, but rarely is pregnancy contraindicated because of antiepileptic therapy. Folate (1 mg/day) may help to prevent some teratogenic effects and should be taken by all women of childbearing age who are treated with AEDs.

50. What are the primary teratogenic effects of AEDs?

Most are relatively minor, such as cleft lip or cleft palate abnormalities, hypertelorism, hypoplastic fingernails, or hypoplastic distal phalanges. Major defects include congenital heart abnormalities, urogenital malformations, and neural tube defects. Valproate has been associated with approximately a 1% risk of neural tube defect. Recent information suggests that carba-mazepine may increase the risk of neural tube defects.

Rosa FW: Spina bifida in infants of women treated with carbamazepine during pregnancy. N Engl J Med 324:674–677, 1991.

51. What are other uses for AEDs?

Several AEDs are used for treatment of psychiatric and pain conditions. Both carbamazepine and valproate are used for bipolar disorders, particularly for mania or hypomania. Lamotrigine also appears to be effective in bipolar disorders. Carbamazepine and phenytoin are used for trigeminal neuralgia and painful peripheral neuropathy. Carbamazepine often helps paroxysmal symptoms associated with multiple sclerosis. Gabapentin is effective for pain associated with diabetic neuropathy and is developing a following for treatment of restless leg syndrome and alcohol withdrawal. Valproate now has an indication for migraine prophylaxis. Low-dose primidone is helpful for essential tremor.

STATUS EPILEPTICUS

52. What is status epilepticus? How is it classified?

Status epilepticus is a state of continuous seizures without return of normal neurologic function between them. Any of the classified seizures types may progress to status epilepticus. Another way to classify status epilepticus is convulsive or nonconvulsive. Convulsive status epilepticus is a medical emergency that can be produced by either primary generalized or secondary generalized tonic-clonic seizures. Nonconvulsive status epilepticus refers to either absence or complex partial status epilepticus. In either case, the patient does not have major motor seizures but is abnormal cognitively and may appear to be in a fugue state. Absence status appears to have no morbidity (unless injuries occurs during the status), but complex partial status may lead to permanent cognitive deficits.

53. What are the most common causes of status epilepticus?

1. AED noncompliance or withdrawal (most common in emergency department)
2. Alcohol withdrawal
3. Metabolic abnormalities
4. Brain tumors
5. Cerebral infarction
6. Cerebral hemorrhages
7. Meningitis
8. Undetermined (10–15% of patients)

Lowenstein DH, Alldredge BK: Status epilepticus at an urban public hospital in the 1980s. Neurology 43:483–488, 1993.

54. How is absence status epilepticus treated?

Absence status is treated with intravenous diazepam or derivatives—not with phenytoin or the barbiturates. Intravenous valproate also can be an effective therapy.

55. How is complex partial status epilepticus treated?

Complex partial status is usually not associated with life-threatening systemic complications but may result in impairment of memory function and should be treated aggressively, similar to generalized tonic-clonic status.

56. How is convulsive status epilepticus treated?

Generalized tonic-clonic or convulsive status epilepticus is a medical emergency, and every effort should be made to stop the seizures within 1 hour. Initial therapy using lorazepam, 0.1 mg/kg IV at 1–2 mg/min, often stops seizures so that the cause can be evaluated further. If seizures continue after lorazepam, intravenous fosphenytoin should be given at a rate up to 150 mg/min. If the patient continues to have seizures after the phenytoin load, phenobarbital should be given or anesthesia induced. If the patient has had benzodiazepines, the addition of intravenous phenobarbital is more likely to cause respiratory arrest and the patient should be intubated. If the patient is resistant to phenytoin, phenobarbital, and lorazepam, anesthesia should be administered, preferably with propofol. An outline for the treatment of status epilepticus is presented below.

Protocol for Treatment of Generalized Tonic-Clonic Status Epilepticus

0–5 min	Provide for maintenance of vital signs. Maintain airway. Give oxygen. Observe and examine patient.
6–10 min	Obtain 50 ml of blood for glucose, calcium, magnesium, electrolytes, blood urea nitrogen, liver functions, anticonvulsant levels, CBC, and toxicology screen. Begin normal saline IV and give 50 ml of 50% glucose and 100 mg of thiamine. Monitor EKG, blood pressure, and, if possible, EEG.
11–30 min	Use intravenous lorazepam to stop seizures, 0.1 mg/kg at 1–2 mg/min.
11–30 min	If seizures continue, load with phenytoin using fosphenytoin 20 mg phenytoin equivalents (PE)/kg at 150 mg PE/min. If cardiac arrhythmias or hypotension occurs, slow the infusion rate.
31–60 min	If seizures persist 10–20 minutes after administration of phenytoin, give an additional 10 PE/kg. If seizures continue, intubate patient and give phenobarbital at a rate of 50–100 mg/min until seizures stop or 20 mg/kg is given.
After 60 minutes of status	Review laboratory results and correct abnormalities. Arrange for anesthesia, neuromuscular blockade, and EEG monitoring. Inhalation anesthesia (isoflurane) or barbiturate anesthesia (pentobarbital, 6–15 mg/kg loading dose, then 0.5–5 mg/kg/hr) may be used. Pentobarbital often causes circulatory collapse, so be prepared to administer a pressor agent such as dopamine. Other options include midazolam (0.15–0.2 mg/kg load, then 0.06–1.1 mg/kg/hr) or propofol (1–2 mg/kg load, then 3–10 mg/kg/hr).

Epilepsy Foundation of America: Treatment of convulsive status epilepticus: Recommendations of the Epilepsy Foundation of America's Working Group on Status Epilepticus. JAMA 270:854–859, 1993.
Lowenstein DH, Alldredge BK: Status epilepticus. N Engl J Med 338:970–976, 1998.

57. What is fosphenytoin? How is it used?

Fosphenytoin, a water-soluble prodrug of phenytoin, is a disodium phosphate ester converted to phenytoin by phosphatases. The preparation may be given intramuscularly and is less irritative than phenytoin to veins and soft tissue when given intravenously. It is packaged as phenytoin equivalents (PE), and dosages should be given as phenytoin equivalents. It may be given intravenously at up to 150 mg PE/min; blood pressure as well as EKG needs to be monitored during infusion. If blood pressure drops or cardiac arrhythmias develop during infusion, the infusion should be stopped until the abnormalities resolve, then restarted at a slower rate. Fosphenytoin allows quicker intervention for patients in status epilepticus.

58. What is epilepsia partialis continua? How is it treated?

Epilepsia partialis continua is simple partial motor status epilepticus, which consists of rhythmic contractions of a restricted region of the body, usually the face and hand or fingers. These brief jerks are intermittent but occur at least every few seconds and may intensify or secondarily generalize. The patient is usually fully conscious during these seizures, but there may be associated weakness in the affected limbs. The most common causes include nonketotic hyperglycemic states, cerebral infarction, encephalitis, and cerebral neoplasms. Treatment is directed at correcting metabolic abnormalities. AEDs are used, but epilepsia partialis continua may be resistant to drug therapy short of anesthesia.

59. Does continuous seizure activity cause nervous system damage?

Certain seizure types, such as absence seizures, are not known to have any significant sequelae. In other settings, after a certain duration of epileptiform activity, there is irreversible neuronal loss. A number of mechanisms probably mediate this neuronal death, including calcium loading of neurons and and excitotoxicity produced by excessive glutamate release. Because continuous seizure activity can cause neuronal death, it is important to monitor the patient's EEG during the treatment of status, particularly if the patient is paralyzed by neuromuscular blockade. It is also important to try to prevent any neuronal death by controlling the patient's status within the first 60 minutes.

EPILEPSY SURGERY

60. When should patients be considered for epilepsy surgery?

Approximately 20% of patients with epilepsy have seizures that are not completely controlled despite adequate antiepileptic therapy and good patient compliance. These patients should be considered for epilepsy surgery.

Devinsky O: Patients with refractory seizures. N Engl J Med 340:1565–1570, 1999.

61. What types of epilepsy surgery are available?

There are basically three types of epilepsy surgery: (1) focal resection of areas of epileptogenesis; (2) disconnecting procedures, usually corpus callosotomy; and (3) implanted stimulators. Corpus callosotomy may be indicated in severe generalized seizures, usually associated with atonic or tonic seizures that produce falling. Resective surgeries should be considered in partial seizures, particularly those that seem to begin exclusively from one circumscribed area of the brain. A new FDA-approved treatment for refractory partial seizures is stimulation of the vagus nerve.

62. Which patients are good candidates for epilepsy surgery?

The actual criteria for choosing patients depend on a number of variables. First and foremost, the patient has seizures that are intractable to medical therapy. Second, the patient will derive significant benefit from becoming seizure-free. Third, seizure onset can be localized. Fourth, the potential morbidity of the surgery is acceptable and less than the morbidity of the seizures. The recent NIH Consensus Statement estimates that in the United States, 2000–5000 patients per year who develop epilepsy could benefit from epilepsy surgery.

63. What is hippocampal sclerosis? How is it diagnosed?

Hippocampal sclerosis is a common disorder associated with complex partial seizures of temporal origin. The term describes the pathology of the hippocampus that includes a loss of neurons in the dentate hilus, CA3, and CA1 regions and associated gliosis. In addition, sprouting of the mossy fibers that arise from granule neuron axons creates a new set of synaptic connections in the inner molecular layer of the dentate gyrus. MRI scans may demonstrate hippocampal sclerosis (see figure in question 29). Unilateral hippocampal sclerosis associated with intractable complex partial seizures is important to identify because it is a surgically curable syndrome.

EPILEPSY AND DRIVING

64. What recommendations about driving should a physician make to patients with epilepsy?

It depends on the state where the physician is practicing. Basically, states either require the physician to report any patient with a seizure or require the patient to report any medical condition that may interfere with the ability to operate a motor vehicle. In general, physicians should caution against driving if the seizures are not controlled and involve impairment of consciousness or motor function. It is usually appropriate to have the patient's case evaluated by the state's driver-licensing authorities. Of interest, drivers with epilepsy have only a slightly increased risk of an accident.

Krumholz A, Fisher RS, Lesser RP, Hauser WA: Driving and epilepsy: A review and reappraisal. JAMA 265:622–626, 1991.

ACKNOWLEDGMENT

The author thanks Michael Collins and Barry Gidal for helpful comments and suggestions.

BIBLIOGRAPHY

1. Engle J, Pedley TA: Epilepsy: A Comprehensive Textbook. Hagerstown, MD, Lippincott-Raven, 1997.
2. Levy RH, Dreifuss FE, Mattson RH, et al: Antiepileptic Drugs, 4th ed. New York, Raven Press, 1995.
3. Wyllie E (ed): The Treatment of Epilepsy, 3rd ed. Baltimore, Williams & Wilkins, 2001.
Websites
www.aesnet.org
www.efa.org
www.pslgroup.com/epilepsy.htm

22. SLEEP DISORDERS

James D. Frost, Jr., M.D.

1. What is sleep?

Sleep is a complex physiologic state that occurs periodically in most vertebrate species, and similar states are often observed in invertebrate organisms. It is characterized by relative quiescence, immobility, and greatly decreased responsiveness to external stimuli. In mammals, two distinct sleep states are recognized: rapid-eye-movement (REM) sleep and non-REM sleep. REM sleep is characterized by pronounced muscular atonia, phasic twitches, and bursts of rapid eye movements. During this state, the EEG is relatively low in amplitude and often is similar to that seen during drowsiness, although people in REM sleep appear deeply asleep by behavioral criteria. Most dreaming apparently occurs during the REM stage. Non-REM sleep is further subdivided into stages 1, 2, 3, and 4, which are characterized by progressively increasing amplitude and decreasing frequency on EEG. Muscle tone tends to be higher than that seen during REM, and phasic movements are not typical. People normally exhibit a fairly regular alternation of non-REM and REM sleep during the sleep period, with cycle times of approximately 90 minutes. There are relatively few awakenings (typically fewer than 10 per night), and the various stages of sleep are present in consistent amounts. In the typical adult, the total sleep time is divided as follows: stage 1, less than 5%; stage 2, 40–60%; stages 3 and 4, 10–20%; and stage REM, 18–25%.

2. How is normal sleep regulated by the brain?

Essentially every area of the brain is involved in sleep, as demonstrated by various experimental manipulations. Although no discrete "sleep center" exists, several regions appear to subserve crucial roles that govern the timing and sequencing of the sleep process. The suprachiasmatic area of the hypothalamus is directly involved in the regulation of circadian cycles that determine when sleep occurs within the 24-hour day. On the other hand, a group of nuclei in the pontomesencephalic region (including locus ceruleus, dorsal raphe, and several cholinergic areas) are critical for the alternating sequence of REM and non-REM cycles normally observed during sleep. Neurons of the basal forebrain and anterior hypothalamus also appear to play a primary role in control of sleep onset.

3. What are sleep disorders?

At present, more than 50 entities are classified as sleep disorders. In addition, many other medical and psychiatric conditions produce disturbed sleep as a secondary manifestation. Disordered sleep may be manifested in several ways: insomnia (difficulty with initiating or maintaining sleep), excessive sleepiness (hypersomnia), and atypical motor or behavioral events occurring in a particular relationship to sleep states or sleep-wake transitions.

4. How are sleep disorders classified?

1. **Dyssomnias** are associated with difficulty in initiating/maintaining sleep or excessive sleepiness. This group is subdivided into intrinsic, extrinsic, and circadian disorders.

2. **Parasomnias** are motor, behavioral, or autonomic events that occur in a particular relationship to the sleep process but are not necessarily associated with disrupted sleep or excessive sleepiness. This group include arousal disorders, sleep-wake transition disorders, REM-associated disorders, and a miscellaneous category.

3. **Sleep disorders associated with mental, neurologic, or other medical disorders** are essentially secondary sleep disorders that accompany many recognized medical entities.

5. What specific conditions are included within the dyssomnia category?

Intrinsic disorders	Extrinsic disorders	Circadian disorders
Obstructive sleep apnea syndrome	Hypnotic-dependent sleep disorder	Time zone change
Central sleep apnea syndrome	Limit-setting sleep disorder	syndrome (jet lag)
Psychophysiologic insomnia	Insufficient sleep syndrome	Shift work sleep
Idiopathic insomnia	Inadequate sleep hygiene	disorder
Narcolepsy	Environmental sleep disorder	Delayed sleep phase
Idiopathic hypersomnia	Altitude insomnia	syndrome
Periodic limb movement disorder	Adjustment sleep disorder	Irregular sleep-wake
Restless legs syndrome	Food-allergy insomnia	pattern
Central alveolar hypoventilation	Nocturnal eating (drinking) syndrome	Advanced sleep
syndrome	Toxin-induced sleep disorder	phase syndrome
Post-traumatic hypersomnia	Sleep-onset association disorder	Non–24-hr sleep-
Recurrent hypersomnia	Stimulant-dependent sleep disorder	wake disorder
Sleep state misperception	Alcohol-dependent sleep disorder	

6. What conditions are classified as parasomnias?

Arousal disorders	REM-associated parasomnias	Sleep-wake transition disorders
Confusional arousals	Nightmares	Rhythmic movement disorder
Sleepwalking	Sleep paralysis	Sleep starts
Sleep terrors	REM sleep behavior disorder	Sleep talking
	REM sleep-related sinus arrest	Nocturnal leg cramps
	Sleep-related painful erection	
	Impaired sleep-related penile erection	
Other parasomnias		
Bruxism	Nocturnal paroxysmal dystonia	Sudden infant death syndrome
Enuresis	Sudden unexplained nocturnal death	Benign neonatal sleep myoclonus
Primary snoring	Congenital central hypoventilation	Sleep-related abnormal
Infant sleep apnea	syndrome	swallowing syndrome

7. How reliable are patients' reports of sleeping difficulties?

Subjective reports of sleep quality and quantity are often grossly incorrect. For example, people with significant hypersomnic conditions are sometimes unaware of the fact that they fall asleep at inappropriate times. Motor vehicle accidents may be attributed to "blackouts" or seizures. Impaired job performance may be related solely to poor memory function. Patients with certain conditions (such as sleep apnea or periodic limb movements) may awaken literally dozens of times throughout the night and have both a low total sleep time and atypical sleep-stage distribution yet report to the physician that they fall asleep quickly every night and sleep soundly with few or no arousals. The opposite is also common, and many people who report severe insomnia later prove (during sleep laboratory testing) to have normal sleep times and few awakenings. Because this phenomenon is common, the physician must be wary of all subjective reports of sleep characteristics and seek independent verification whenever evidence suggests a clinically significant condition.

8. How much sleep is required for normal daytime function?

Most normal people average between 6 and 8 hours of sleep per night, but there is a great deal of individual variability. As a general rule, if daytime performance is significantly impaired by excessive sleepiness and this condition persists despite adherence to a regularly scheduled nocturnal sleep period of at least 8 hours, more definitive diagnostic tests are indicated. A significant change in apparent sleep requirements is also often an indication of an underlying sleep disorder.

9. Is total sleep time the only determinant of the ability to maintain a normal level of daytime alertness?

No. The structure or architecture of the sleep pattern is also crucial for normal waking function. When sleep is fragmented by frequent brief arousals or other factors disturb the normal stage distribution, excessive daytime sleepiness sometimes results even if actual sleep time is not significantly reduced.

10. How can the physician objectively assess nocturnal sleep quality and quantity?
The most important diagnostic tool available to the physician dealing with sleep disorders is the sleep study or polysomnogram. By monitoring sleep-wake state throughout the night, concurrently observing multiple physiologic parameters, and continuously documenting behavioral status (video recording), it is possible to obtain diagnostic information that is highly reliable and objective. This test provides quantitative measures of total sleep time, number of awakenings, sleep-stage distribution, respiratory dysfunction, cardiac arrhythmias, atypical movements, nocturnal seizures, and character of parasomnias.

11. What variables are typically recorded during polysomnography?
1. Electroencephalogram (EEG)
2. Electrooculogram (EOG)
3. Electromyogram (EMG) from submental area
4. Electrocardiogram (EKG)
5. Leg movement (EMG or accelerometer)
6. Snoring/vocalizations (audio monitoring)
7. Respiratory effort (chest and abdomen)
8. Nasal and oral airflow
9. Oxygen saturation
10. End-tidal PCO_2
11. Body position
12. Behavioral/motor events (video monitoring)

12. Can daytime sleepiness also be measured objectively?
Yes. The multiple sleep latency test (MSLT) evaluates the presence and degree of daytime sleepiness. This procedure makes use of polygraphic monitoring (EEG, EOG, EMG, and EKG) during a series of 4 or 5 nap sessions spaced at 2-hour intervals throughout the day. Quantitative information is provided about both average sleep latency and abnormalities of sleep-onset transition. The MSLT must be performed the day after an overnight sleep study to permit meaningful analysis of the results.

13. What is the normal sleep latency during the MSLT?
Normal people have an average sleep latency (time from onset of the nap session until the first appearance of any stage of sleep) of 10 minutes or longer.

14. Do medications alter the results of polysomnography and multiple sleep latency testing?
Many drugs (e.g., hypnotics, sedatives, tranquilizers, and stimulants) significantly alter the results of polysomnographic and MSLT examinations. In particular, both periods of drug initiation and acute withdrawal are often associated with major alterations of sleep characteristics, and the resultant patterns may mimic other sleep disorders, including narcolepsy. Consequently, whenever possible, CNS active drugs should be discontinued for 2 weeks or longer before diagnostic studies. When this is not possible, such drugs should be administered at constant and stable levels for at least 2 weeks before polysomnography and MSLT studies. Patients should never be told simply to refrain from taking a medication on the night of a study or for several nights before the examination. This approach may invalidate the results.

15. What is the most common condition associated with excessive daytime sleepiness and sleep at inappropriate times?
Obstructive sleep apnea syndrome. Sleep onset is typically associated with increased upper airway resistance, and partial or complete airway obstruction often occurs. The patient is usually aroused within a short period by ensuing hypoxia or hypercapnia as well as by the increased effort associated with attempts to breathe. These events typically recur throughout the sleep period, and the resultant sleep deprivation or fragmentation is presumably the basis for the daytime sleepiness. Pronounced oxygen desaturation may occur and cause potentially life-threatening cardiac arrhythmias. The polygraphic characteristics permit a conclusive diagnosis of this condition.

16. What is the treatment for obstructive sleep apnea?

Therapy must be directed toward correction of the airway obstruction (which may result from anatomic factors or abnormal relaxation of musculature in the oropharynx, causing increased upper airway resistance to air flow). Administration of continuous positive airway pressure (CPAP) by means of a nasal mask is currently the most frequently used therapeutic modality. Surgical procedures are effective in some cases, particularly when a discrete anatomic factor producing airway obstruction can be demonstrated. In some people, significant improvement is achieved by preventing assumption of the supine position during sleep. Tongue-retaining devices are beneficial in a small number of instances, particularly when the respiratory disturbance is mild.

17. What is the classic narcoleptic tetrad?

Narcolepsy is the most familiar condition associated with episodes of sleep at inappropriate times, although it is clear that many people diagnosed with this condition in the past actually had sleep apnea (or one of the other conditions associated with disturbed nocturnal sleep). The classic narcoleptic tetrad is
   1. Excessive sleepiness
   2. Cataplexy
   3. Sleep paralysis
   4. Hypnagogic hallucinations
The tetrad is observed in no more than 50% of patients meeting current criteria for the diagnosis of narcolepsy, and 90% lack at least one of the primary symptoms.

18. What is cataplexy?

Cataplexy is a condition characterized by episodes of muscular weakness or paralysis, without loss of consciousness, precipitated by emotional changes such as laughter, excitement, or anger. Episodes typically last from a few seconds to several minutes and sometimes are terminated by a direct transition to sleep.

19. What is sleep paralysis?

This condition is characterized by a transient inability to move during onset of sleep or during arousal from sleep. Episodes usually last no more than several minutes and may be associated with hallucinations.

20. What are hypnagogic hallucinations?

Hallucinations involving various sensory modalities (most commonly visual) that occur during sleep-wake transitions. Although this entity is typically observed in association with narcolepsy, it occasionally occurs in normal people.

21. How is narcolepsy diagnosed?

An unambiguous diagnosis of narcolepsy requires that all of the following criteria be met:
   1. History of recurrent daytime naps or episodes of sleep at inappropriate times for at least 3 months.
   2. History of cataplexy.
   3. Excessive degree of daytime sleepiness demonstrated during MSLT (average sleep latency less than 5 minutes).
   4. At least two episodes of stage REM sleep documented during the MSLT.
   5. Documentation of an adequate total sleep time and relatively normal sleep stage distribution during nocturnal polysomnography immediately preceding the MSLT.
The diagnosis is further strengthened by the presence of sleep paralysis, hypnagogic hallucinations, and HLA DQB1*0602 or DR2 positivity.

22. How is narcolepsy treated?

Excessive daytime sleepiness is usually managed with stimulant medications (e.g., methylphenidate, pemoline, dextroamphetamine, and modafinil). The requirement for stimulants can sometimes be reduced by prescribing several (typically 2 or 3) regularly scheduled short (1 hour or less) naps during the day. Cataplexy and sleep paralysis are often treated successfully with tricyclic antidepressants (e.g., imipramine, protriptyline) or selective serotonin reuptake inhibitors (e.g., fluoxetine).

23. What other disorders, in addition to narcolepsy and obstructive sleep apnea, may present as excessive daytime somnolence?

1. Periodic limb movements (nocturnal myoclonus)
2. Insufficient nocturnal sleep syndrome
3. Circadian rhythm disorders (e.g., jet lag)
4. Drug or alcohol dependency
5. Central sleep apnea
6. Toxin-induced sleep disorder
7. Mood disorders (depression)
8. Cerebral degenerative disorders
9. Dementia
10. Trypanosomiasis
11. Idiopathic hypersomnia
12. Recurrent hypersomnia (e.g., Kleine-Levin syndrome)
13. Posttraumatic hypersomnia

24. Is the occurrence of sleep paralysis pathognomonic of narcolepsy?

No. Although sleep paralysis is most commonly encountered as one of the ancillary manifestations of narcolepsy, it is sometimes seen as an independent entity in the absence of other signs of narcolepsy. It may occur sporadically or in a familial form. It is characterized by a transient (usually from less than 1 minute to several minutes) inability to move voluntarily either at the time of onset of sleep or during an arousal from sleep. Consciousness is maintained, and the person may experience severe anxiety and fear as well as hallucinatory images or dreamlike mentation. Eye and respiratory movements are not impaired. The condition disappears spontaneously but may be terminated immediately if the person is stimulated externally. A transition to sleep may occur during the event. In some people, this phenomenon may occur more frequently in the presence of sleep deprivation or other sleep disturbance. Although sleep paralysis is typically identified by its symptoms, a sleep study may be required to rule out narcolepsy or the presence of another sleep disorder that triggers sleep paralysis through sleep disruption. Treatment is usually not required, although if the condition is frequent or results in a high degree of anxiety, treatment may be indicated. Tricyclic antidepressant medications are often effective.

25. Is HLA typing useful in the diagnosis of narcolepsy?

It is of very limited value. Nearly 100% of narcoleptic patients have been found to be HLA-DR2- and DQ1 (including DR15 and DQ6)-positive in several studies. The DQB1*0602 marker (a subtype of DQ6) has been reported to be the most specific such marker for narcolepsy among various ethnic populations, and patients with narcolepsy/cataplexy are nearly always positive. However, the HLA test is of limited diagnostic value because 10–35% of the general population is also positive for these markers. Conversely, negativity for these HLA subtypes, although rare, does not entirely exclude the presence of narcolepsy.

26. What is the most significant risk factor common to all conditions associated with excessive daytime sleepiness?

People with hypersomnic conditions are at a significantly increased risk for death or serious injury as a result of motor-vehicle and job-related accidents.

27. How is insomnia defined?

Insomnia is a subjective symptom characterized by the perception that sleep is inadequate or otherwise abnormal. It includes complaints of a low total sleep time, difficulty in falling asleep, frequent awakenings, or unrefreshing sleep. It is a common symptom and is associated with a wide spectrum of underlying medical conditions as well as with specific sleep disorders.

28. What are the most common causes of insomnia?
1. Circadian rhythm disturbances (time zone change syndrome, shift work)
2. Psychophysiologic insomnia
3. Underlying medical or psychiatric disorders
4. Periodic limb movement disorder
5. Drug or alcohol dependency
6. Irregular or improper sleep habits (poor sleep hygiene)
7. Sleep apnea

29. What is the appropriate treatment for psychophysiologic insomnia?
1. Establish a regular and fixed sleep period, with a consistent bedtime and time of arousal. The sleep period should be long enough to permit adequate sleep time (typically 8 hours for an adult) but no longer.
2. Avoid daytime napping.
3. Minimize concern about inability to sleep.
4. Establish a regular, daily program of exercise, but do not exercise immediately before bedtime.
5. Avoid excessive consumption of caffeine and alcohol, and exclude these substances entirely during the evening before bedtime.
6. Ensure that the sleeping environment is optimal with regard to noise and temperature.
7. Avoid use of medication to induce sleep.
8. Obtain behavioral treatment (e.g., relaxation) if indicated.

30. What is the time zone change syndrome?
This condition, also known as jet lag, consists of symptoms of insomnia that begin immediately after rapid travel across several time zones. It results from loss of proper synchronization between the endogenous circadian timing system of the brain and external environmental cues (primarily day and night cycles).

31. What is the best way to manage insomnia resulting from a time zone change?
Some people adapt without difficulty, whereas others (particularly those older than 50 years) experience a prolonged period of disturbed sleep. Symptoms can be minimized by
1. Immediately adopting a sleep-wake schedule appropriate for the new environment.
2. Avoiding prolonged napping immediately after arrival in a new location. A mild degree of sleep deprivation the first day facilitates adaptation to the new environment.
3. Spending some time outdoors in bright light during the daytime on the first few days after arrival. This facilitates resetting of the circadian clock.
4. Avoiding excessive use of caffeine and alcohol.
5. Avoiding use of sleep medications.

32. What are sleep terrors (parvor nocturnus)?
Sleep terrors are episodes of apparent intense fear, often associated with crying or screaming, that occur during arousal from non-REM (typically stages 3 and 4) sleep. These events are characteristically accompanied by elevated heart and respiratory rates, and the patient may exhibit confusion and disorientation. Amnesia is most common, although some people report brief dreamlike images. This condition is most common in children between 4 and 12 years of age but may persist into the adult years. Drug treatment is usually unnecessary, but benzodiazepines may be effective for short-term use, especially when episodes become frequent.

33. What are the major characteristics of the periodic limb movement disorder?
Periodic limb movement disorder (nocturnal myoclonus) is characterized by frequent clusters of extremity movements (typically the legs, but occasionally the arms) that tend to recur periodically at intervals of 10–90 seconds for an extended time. When these events produce arousal,

as they often do, sleep may be disrupted, although the patient is typically unaware of the condition. This condition is readily apparent during sleep laboratory evaluation, and its severity can be quantitatively assessed. The periodic limb movement disorder is typically resistant to therapy, but daytime symptoms are often relieved by medications (e.g., clonazepam) that reduce the number of nocturnal arousals associated with the limb movements. Additional medications that have been reported to be useful include other benzodiazepines (e.g., diazepam, temazepam, and triazolam), opiates (e.g., codeine, propoxyphene, and oxycodone), dopaminergics (e.g., L-dopa, bromocriptine, and pergolide), carbamazepine, and clonidine.

34. Which conditions other than epilepsy may be associated with paroxysmal episodes of atypical, often complex, motor activity during the sleep period in adults?
1. Sleepwalking and other arousal disorders
2. Nocturnal paroxysmal dystonia
3. REM sleep behavior disorder

35. What are the key clinical and polysomnographic features of sleepwalking?
Sleepwalking consists of complex and usually inappropriate behavior beginning during non-REM sleep (typically stages 3 and 4). It occurs most frequently early in the night but may occur at other times on occasion. Although walking is common, other behavior such as sitting up in bed or talking is also frequent. The patient is difficult to awaken, may be confused, and usually is amnesic for the event. It occurs most commonly in children (3–10 years) but may occur in older people. Some medications and other medical conditions can induce or potentiate sleepwalking. Because serious accidental injury may result during these episodes, patients of all ages should be protected by appropriate safety precautions. Although drug treatment is usually not necessary, benzodiazepines (e.g, diazepam) are often effective, especially for short-term use.

36. What are the characteristics of nocturnal paroxysmal dystonia?
Nocturnal paroxysmal dystonia is a disorder of unknown etiology characterized by repeated dystonic or dyskinetic episodes during or immediately after arousal from non-REM sleep or, more rarely, during wakefulness. Episodes typically last less than 1 minute but in some cases are much more prolonged (reportedly up to 1 hour) and often occur several times per night. Movements are often relatively violent and may result in injury to the patient or bed partner. Patients typically do not recall these events after arousal. This condition has been reported in both children and adults, can be isolated or familial, and is apparently long-lasting. Nocturnal paroxysmal dystonia may be indistinguishable clinically from frontal lobe epilepsy, although episodes are not associated with evident epileptiform EEG activity or other abnormal EEG findings. The possibility that this condition is actually of epileptic origin is also suggested by the fact that carbamazepine is efficacious in many instances.

37. Which features distinguish the REM sleep behavior disorder from other conditions associated with atypical nocturnal events?
The REM sleep behavior disorder is typified by repeated episodes of complex, often violent, motor activity during periods of REM sleep. These episodes appear to represent enactment of dream mental activity as a result of loss of normal inhibitory mechanisms originating in the brainstem (specifically, in the perilocus ceruleus region of the pons). Patients often kick or punch repeatedly and may jump from the bed and run through the bedroom, frequently colliding with furniture or walls. Injuries to the patient and bed partner are common. Although full-blown episodes may occur infrequently, atypical movements and abnormally increased EMG tonic activity are typically present during all REM periods, as demonstrated during polysomnographic testing. Patients often recall the dream content after the event is over. Most cases are idiopathic, but a significant number are associated with specific neurologic disorders (e.g., Parkinson's disease, ischemic cerebrovascular disease, olivopontocerebellar degeneration, multiple sclerosis, brainstem neoplasm). Clonazepam is often efficacious. Patients should be advised to take safety precautions to minimize injury if an occasional episode does occur.

38. What is the restless legs syndrome?

The restless legs syndrome is characterized by unpleasant sensations in the lower legs before sleep onset (and sometimes at other times as well) that produce a strong urge to move the legs. This sensation is typically described as a "crawling" or "creeping" feeling, and it disappears temporarily when the lower extremities are moved, only to recur within a few seconds. The symptoms last from minutes to several hours and can significantly delay sleep onset, with resultant sleep deprivation. Many patients also experience periodic limb movements during sleep. The cause is unknown, and the condition is typically long-term, although gradual improvement is sometimes observed. Both idiopathic (presumably genetic) and symptomatic forms are recognized. Common symptomatic forms include those associated with iron deficiency, pregnancy, and metabolic dysfunction, such as renal failure. Medications reported to be beneficial include dopaminergics (e.g., L-dopa, bromocriptine, and pergolide), opiates (e.g., codeine, propoxyphene, and oxycodone), and benzodiazepines (clonazepam, diazepam, triazolam, temazepam, and nitrazepam).

BIBLIOGRAPHY

1. Culebras A: Clinical Handbook of Sleep Disorders. Boston, Butterworth-Heinemann, 1996.
2. International Classification of Sleep Disorders, Revised (ICSD-R). Rochester, MN, American Sleep Disorders Association, 1997.
3. Kryger MH, Roth T, Dement WC: Principles and Practice of Sleep Medicine, 2nd ed. Philadelphia, W.B. Saunders, 1994.
4. Poceta JS, Mitler MM: Sleep Disorders: Diagnosis and Treatment. Totowa, NJ, Humana Press, 1998.
Website
www.asda.org

23. NEUROLOGIC COMPLICATIONS OF SYSTEMIC DISEASE

R. Glenn Smith, M.D., Ph.D., and Loren A. Rolak, M.D.

CARDIAC DISEASE

1. What is the major neurologic complication of cardiac disease?

By far, stroke is the most common neurologic sequela of cardiac disease. The risks for embolic, thrombotic, and hemorrhagic stroke are all elevated in the presence of cardiac disease. Nonvalvular atrial fibrillation, followed by ischemic heart disease and valvular heart disease are the most common types of cardiac abnormalities causing embolic ischemic strokes. Infective endocarditis is most frequently associated with hemorrhagic strokes.

Vahedi K, Amarenco P: Cardiac causes of stroke. Curr Treat Opt Neurol 2:305–317, 2000.

2. What is the association between transient ischemic attack (TIA) and MI?

Patients who suffer a TIA are more likely to have an MI than a stroke in the subsequent 5 years. All patients who have suffered a mild stroke or TIA should undergo careful cardiac assessment as soon as possible.

Scheinberg P: Transient ischemic attacks: An update. J Neurol Sci 101:133–140, 1991.

3. What is the association between sleep, MI, and stroke?

In the stage of sleep associated with rapid eye movements (REM sleep), profound changes in centrally mediated sympathetic activity occur. These large changes in autonomic output are manifest by smaller increases in blood pressure and heart rate, skin conductance changes, momentary restorations in muscle tone, mesenteric and renal vasodilation, and skeletal muscle vasoconstriction. In the elderly, it is hypothesized that large fluctuations in sympathetic activity associated with REM sleep also cause increased rates of arrhythmias and increased risk for cardiac vasospasm. This, in turn, may increase the risk for embolic stroke and MI, respectively.

Somers VK, et al: Sympathetic nerve activity during sleep in normal subjects. N Engl J Med 328:303–307, 1993.

4. What are the non–stroke-related neurologic complications of cardiac disease?

Cardiac arrhythmias (especially sick sinus syndrome) may produce decreased cardiac output, causing syncope, and, rarely, encephalopathy. Cardiac failure may likewise impair cardiac output and produce encephalopathy. Cerebral blood flow is not directly altered in patients with cardiac failure or arrhythmias, except with major reductions in cardiac function. Instead, there appears to be a change in cerebral autoregulation caused by abnormal autonomic vagal activity. Persistent decreased brain perfusion may lead to laminar necrosis of the cerebral cortex or hippocampus, even in the absence of stroke. Delayed demyelination leading to coma and death may also occur after apparent recovery from hypotension or cardiac failure.

GASTROINTESTINAL DISEASE

5. What is the major cause of neurologic symptoms associated with gastrointestinal (GI) disease?

Most known neurologic complications of GI disease are the consequence of malabsorption. This is likewise true of neurologic problems arising after GI trauma or surgical resection. Although in many cases the specific absorptive deficiencies are unclear, the consequences of some nutrient deficiencies have been well described, including those involving thiamine, folate, cyanocobalamin, niacin, vitamin D, and vitamin E.

6. What are the neurologic manifestations of celiac disease?

Celiac disease, or gluten enteropathy, produces chronic small bowel malabsorption, often with iron deficiency anemia, osteoporosis and osteomalacia, and hypoalbuminemia. At least 10% of affected patients also have neurologic complaints, the most notable being cerebellar dysfunction secondary to chronic fat malabsorption. Patients may also have tremor, intranuclear ophthalmoplegia, symptoms suggesting Wernicke's encephalopathy or subacute combined degeneration, seizures, or myopathy. The observed myopathy is often treatable by vitamin D replacement.

Beyenburg S, Scheid B, Deckert-Schluter M, Lagreze H-L: Chronic progressive leukoencephalopathy in adult celiac disease. Neurology 50:820–822, 1998.

7. What is the triad of neurologic complaints commonly ascribed to Whipple's disease?

In Whipple's disease, a multisystem granulomatous infection, neurologic complaints develop in 10% of afflicted patients. The common triad of findings associated with this disease includes ocular disturbance (often ophthalmoparesis), gait ataxia, and dementia. Other abnormalities sometimes associated with this disease include seizures, myelopathy, meningoencephalitis, autonomic dysfunction, and steroid-unresponsive myopathy. Untreated, most patients die within 1 year of the onset of neurologic symptoms. Caused by *Tropheryma whippeleii*, this disease responds dramatically to antibiotic treatment.

8. What is the triad of neurologic complaints commonly ascribed to Wernicke's encephalopathy?

Thiamine deficiency may manifest as Wernicke's encephalopathy, whose clinical symptoms include the triad of ocular disturbance (with nystagmus), gait ataxia, and disturbances of mental function. The similarity of this triad to that found in Whipple's disease has suggested to some that thiamine uptake or utilization is altered in that disease. An axonal sensorimotor neuropathy appears in half of patients with this deficiency state, and Korsakoff's psychosis (dementia associated with profound amnesia and confabulation) is also variably present. The mortality associated with Wernicke's encephalopathy is still greater than 10%, although this is more due to concomitant infections and malnutrition than to the neurologic disorders.

9. What is Strachan's syndrome?

Strachan described a triad of sensory spinal ataxia, optic nerve atrophy, and sensorineural deafness that is partially responsive to high-dose thiamine therapy.

10. What is known about the etiology of nervous system impairment associated with B12 malabsorption?

The deficiency of methionine synthetase activity secondary to absence of its cofactor (B12) leads to accumulation of homocysteine. The resulting impairment in DNA synthesis is responsible for the megaloblastic anemia associated with B12 deficiency, while neurologic abnormalities are the result of failure to maintain methionine biosynthesis.

11. What are the neurologic manifestations of vitamin B12 deficiency?

Psychiatric symptoms fall into several clinical categories. Many patients manifest slowed cerebration, dementia, or delirium (with or without delusion), while others exhibit depression, amnesia, or acute psychotic states. Rarer are those patients whose B12 deficiency results in reversible manic or schizophreniform states. Nonbehavioral findings in B12 deficiency include myelopathy that affects the dorsal and lateral columns, and sensorimotor neuropathy.

So YT, Simon RP: Deficiency diseases of the nervous system. In Bradley WG, et al (eds): Neurology in Clinical Practice, 3rd ed. Boston, Butterworth-Heinemann, 2000, pp 1495–1509.

12. Which vitamin deficiencies cause different neurologic syndromes in children than in adults?

Lack of absorption of vitamin D from the intestinal tract leads to rickets in children and osteomalacia in adults. In children with rickets, neurologic sequelae include head shaking, nystagmus, and increased irritability that may evolve into tetany with a sufficient fall in serum calcium concentrations. **Malabsorption of folate** in infants leads to mental retardation, seizures, and athetotic movements, whereas in adults, polyneuropathy and depression are the primary complications. **Pyridoxine deficiency** leads to seizures in infants, but a sensory polyneuropathy in adults.

13. Malabsorption of which vitamins will lead to an increased risk for subdural hematoma?
Malabsorption of vitamin C or vitamin K results in an increased tendency for hemorrhage, especially following trauma. Lack of thiamine, vitamin B12, or vitamin E all can result in ataxia, with an increased tendency for falls and head trauma.

14. Besides thiamine, malabsorption or dietary lack of which vitamin may produce a syndrome resembling Korsakoff's dementia?
Nicotinic acid deficiency results in pellagra, whose major and often sole manifestation is psychiatric disturbance, sometimes mimicking Korsakoff's psychosis. Although vitamin B12 deficiency can also produce disturbances of cognitive function, the concomitant presence of other neurologic deficits usually serves to separate pernicious anemia from Korsakoff's psychosis.

HEPATIC DISEASE

15. What are the six major neurologic syndromes associated with hepatic dysfunction?
1. Encephalopathy
2. Acquired hepatocerebral degeneration
3. Wilson's disease
4. Reye syndrome
5. Intracranial hemorrhage
6. Hemochromatosis

16. What causes hepatic encephalopathy?
This complication may occur with hepatic failure or with portal or hepatic circulatory dysfunction, as caused by acute or chronic hepatitis, hepatic necrosis, cirrhosis, or portocaval anastomosis. No single cause has been identified for the production of neuropsychiatric manifestations associated with this syndrome. Ammonia is considered an important toxin, precipitating encephalopathy by increasing glutamine and gamma-aminobutyric acid (GABA) synthesis. Other undefined endogenous toxins appear to affect central neurotransmission, especially of the dopaminergic and GABA-nergic systems. Reduction in the serum concentration of ammonia, or addition of centrally acting GABA antagonists may temporarily improve hepatic encephalopathy, although correction of the precipitating causes of hepatic dysfunction are necessary for ultimate recovery.
Lockwood AH: Hepatic encephalopathy. In Aminoff MJ (ed): Neurology and General Medicine, 2nd ed. New York, Churchill-Livingstone, 1995.

17. How is hepatic encephalopathy treated?
Acute therapy for hepatic encephalopathy requires removal or blockade of neurologically-acting toxins produced in the gut. Reduction of protein intake, associated with lactulose therapy to enhance ammonia excretion and reduce ammonia absorption, is the mainstay of therapy. Oral antibiotics that are poorly absorbed from the gut, such as neomycin, are used as second-line agents to reduce gut bacterial levels and ammonia formation. Long-term treatment of hepatic encephalopathy by medical therapies has only limited success, depending in part upon whether the hepatic damage is reversible, static, or progressive. "Cure" of hepatic encephalopathy requires reversal of hepatic failure, and surgical shunting procedures and liver transplantation have been successful treatments for selected individuals.
Lockwood AH, Weissenborn R, Butterworth RF: An image of the brain in patients with liver disease. Curr Opin Neurol 10:525–533, 1997.

18. What is Reye syndrome?
Reye syndrome is a rare acute noninflammatory encephalopathy that primarily affects children and adolescents. An epidemiologic correlation has been found between this disease and immediately preceding viral infection (especially influenza and varicella) treated with salicylates,

although apparently it may be precipitated by other toxic, metabolic, or hypoxic insults. Hyper-ammonemia, hypoglycemia, coagulopathy, and cerebral edema with hypoxia may be present. Treatment is supportive, including administration of intravenous glucose to prevent hypo-glycemia, and in severe cases, hyperventilation, mannitol, etc., to reduce intracranial pressure.

Smith TC: Reye's syndrome and the use of aspirin. Scott Med J 41:4–9, 1996.

19. In addition to hepatic encephalopathy, what other diseases cause asterixis?

Asterixis, or flapping tremor, is best elicited by the extension of outstretched, opened hands. This sign is encountered in many metabolic encephalopathies, including uremia, malnutrition, severe pulmonary disease, and polycythemia rubra vera.

20. In addition to hepatic encephalopathy, what other diseases cause the electroencephalographic (EEG) abnormality of slow triphasic waves?

This abnormal EEG pattern, although commonly used to diagnose hepatic encephalopathy, may also accompany head trauma (especially with subdural hematoma), acute cerebral anoxia, uremia, or electrolyte imbalance.

21. What are the neurologic manifestations of Wilson's disease?

In almost half of patients with Wilson's disease, neurologic sequelae predominate. Signs in-clude gait instability and clumsiness, chorea, rigidity, tremor, dystonia, and seizures. The cere-bellar manifestations tend to involve the upper extremities earlier and more severely than the lower extremities, unlike those seen with Wernicke's syndrome and alcoholism. Psychiatric symptoms, including those of dementia, mania, depression, or schizophrenia, may dominate the presentation in up to 20% of patients.

22. What is the treatment for Wilson's disease?

Early diagnosis and copper chelation therapy are the mainstays of therapy. The chelation therapy of choice is 250 mg of penicillamine given by mouth 4 times per day between meals. Penicillamine should be administered concomitantly with pyridoxine to prevent vitamin B6 defi-ciency. Side effects of this treatment include rash, fever, thrombocytopenia, relative eosinophilia with total leukopenia, and reversible lupus-like and myasthenia-gravis-like syndromes. Zinc ac-etate is an alternative oral maintenance agent with few side effects; it eventually may supplant penicillamine.

23. What are the neurologic complications of hemochromatosis?

Encephalopathy, truncal ataxia, neuritis, and rigidity may all complicate hemochromatosis. Hepatomegaly and liver failure in these patients are due to cirrhosis, resulting from massive iron deposition in the liver. CNS abnormalities, including demyelination, are caused by the liver dis-ease. Neuritis is either a complication of the diabetes mellitus that accompanies most cases of he-mochromatosis, or is a result of local iron deposition.

Treatment requires serial phlebotomies four to six times per year. Lifetime treatment with phlebotomies is currently the treatment of choice, although newer therapies using growth factor control over red blood cell production are being tested.

24. Which porphyrias are associated with primarily neurologic manifestations?

So-called hepatic porphyrias, such as acute intermittent porphyria (AIP) and variegate (South African) porphyria, can be distinguished from the rare "erythropoietic" forms that pro-duce dermatologic symptoms without neurologic disease. In AIP, clinical symptoms develop during crises, most often precipitated by ingestion or administration of drugs that adversely affect porphyrin metabolism. Manifestations of AIP during crisis may include (1) abdominal pain with vomiting, constipation or diarrhea, and often a previous history of exploratory abdominal surgery; (2) psychiatric disorder, with symptoms suggesting conversion reactions, delirium, or psychosis; (3) peripheral neuropathy, primarily motor, often with autonomic abnormalities, that may be severe or fatal and mimic Guillain-Barré syndrome; and (4) central abnormalities, such as SIADH or convulsions.

Greer M: Neurologic manifestations of the porphyrias. In Samuels MA, Peske S (eds): Office Practice of Neurology, 2nd ed. New York, Churchill Livingstone, 2001.

25. Chronic ingestion of what substance may produce a condition similar to AIP?

Lead poisoning produces a condition (termed saturnism) that closely resembles AIP clinically, and also appears to share heme synthetic dysfunction with accumulation of delta-aminolevulinic acid. Increased levels of superoxide dismutase and glutathione reductase are also reported, presumably in response to the toxic effects of free radical–associated cellular damage.

Graeme KA, Pollack CV: Heavy metal toxicity. J Emerg Med 16:45–56, 1998.

26. What is the treatment for neurologic crises in acute intermittent porphyria (AIP)?

Therapy is directed at modifying the biochemical abnormalities found in the disease, including overproduction of the neurotoxin delta-aminolevulinic acid (which has been proposed as a source for free radical formation) and heme deficiency. Intravenous administration of hematin increases available heme and downregulates the patient's abnormal heme biosynthetic pathway, thus reducing delta-aminolevulinic acid levels. Prevention of crises is the primary goal in treating patients with AIP. Education of the patient to the many precipitants of acute attacks is necessary for their survival.

RENAL DISEASE

27. What are the most common neurologic complications of renal disease?

Typical neurologic complications of renal disease are peripheral neuropathy and metabolic encephalopathy.

28. What are the characteristics of uremic neuropathy?

Uremic neuropathy appears as a symmetric distal sensorimotor axonal neuropathy and is almost invariably present in patients by the time they require dialysis. Because conditions that predispose to renal failure (e.g., diabetes and vasculitis) may also produce neuropathy, symptoms can result from several different etiologies. The presence of mononeuritis multiplex or of autonomic dysfunction suggests nonuremic pathology, whereas a pattern of stocking-and-glove numbness without severe paresthesias is consistent with uremic neuropathy. Uremic neuropathy is at least partially reversible by repeated dialysis or by kidney transplantation.

29. What are the characteristics of uremic encephalopathy?

Patients with uremia often develop a metabolic encephalopathy. The mechanisms responsible for this encephalopathy remain unclear, but presumably involve the retention of inorganic and organic acids, fluid alterations among cerebral cellular compartments, and abnormalities caused by hypertension, hypocalcemia, hyperkalemia, hypernatremia, hyperphosphatemia, and hypochloremia. Uremic encephalopathy is unusual because of the coexistence of signs of neuronal depression (lethargy, coma) with those of neuronal excitation (agitation, muscle cramps, myoclonus, tetany, asterixis, and seizures).

30. Name three neurologic complications associated with dialysis.

Dialysis disequilibrium, dialysis dementia, and intracranial hemorrhage.

31. What is the dialysis disequilibrium syndrome?

Dialysis disequilibrium is the name given to the cerebral edema produced by too-rapid removal of urea and other osmoles, with resultant fluid and electrolyte shifts. Symptoms of dialysis disequilibrium may be mild, such as persistent headache or fatigue, or may be sufficiently severe to produce seizures, coma, and death. Recognition of this problem has led to newer protocols using more frequent, but less vigorous dialysis.

32. What is dialysis dementia?

Dialysis dementia refers to a rarer but much more serious syndrome of irreversible progressive dementia with apraxias, dysarthria, hyperreflexia, myoclonus, and multifocal seizures. Aluminum present in the dialysate is thought to be the primary agent causing CNS toxicity, and removal of aluminum with ion exchange resins prior to dialysis has significantly reduced the problem.

33. What causes intracranial hemorrhage in patients undergoing dialysis?

Because of the need for anticoagulation during dialysis, the incidence of trauma-related hemorrhage is elevated. Chronic hypertension is also associated with renal failure, further increasing the incidence of intracranial hemorrhage.

34. What neurologic complications are associated with renal transplantation?

Neurologic sequelae of renal transplantation are primarily the result of immunosuppression. *Listeria monocytogenes* and Cryptococcus and Aspergillus species account for 90% of the nonviral CNS infections in these patients. Cytomegalovirus, varicella zoster, and herpes simplex are more common viral infective agents that cause clinical nervous system involvement following renal transplantation. Malignancies, such as primary lymphomas, are also seen. The overall risk of developing cancer following renal transplantation is approximately 6%, or about 100-fold greater than that expected for the general nonimmunosuppressed population.

Amato AA, Barohn RJ: Transplantation and immunosuppressive medication. In Rolak LA, Harati Y (eds): Neuro-Immunology for the Clinician. Boston, Butterworth-Heinemann, 1997, pp 341–376.

PULMONARY DISEASE

35. What are the neurologic signs and symptoms of respiratory insufficiency?

Neurologic features of this medical emergency result from hypoxemia and acute hypercapnia. Initial symptoms may be those of a nocturnal or early morning headache, associated with lethargy, drowsiness, inattentiveness, and irritability. Motor signs at this stage include tremor and twitching, caused by hypercapnia-induced stimulation of sympathetic nervous system output. More severe levels of hypoxia result in somnolence, confusion, and asterixis. Prolonged severe hypoxia results in coma and generalized seizures. Ocular findings include papilledema in 10% of patients, probably from hypercapnia-induced increases in intracranial pressure. However, isolated chronic hypercapnia with PCO_2 measurements of up to 110 mmHg may exist without apparent neurologic symptoms or signs.

36. What neurologic diseases may result in respiratory insufficiency?

Various neuromuscular diseases may either acutely or insidiously result in respiratory insufficiency or failure:

1. Myotonic dystrophy
2. Limb-girdle muscular dystrophy
3. Nemaline myopathy
4. Centronuclear myopathy
5. Inclusion body myositis
6. Acid maltase deficiency
7. Hexosaminidase A deficiency
8. Myasthenia gravis
9. Congenital myasthenic syndromes
10. Postpolio syndrome
11. Spinal muscular atrophy
12. Amyotrophic lateral sclerosis
13. Duchenne muscular dystrophy
14. Guillain-Barré syndrome
15. Polymyositis

37. Describe the clinical features of prolonged hyperventilation.

Anxious patients with acute psychogenic hyperventilation usually complain of lightheadedness, dyspnea, circumoral and acral paresthesias, and the presence of visual phosphenes. Visual blurring, tremor, muscle cramps, carpopedal spasm, and chest pain are found with prolonged hyperventilation. In addition to psychogenic etiologies, prolonged hyperventilation may be the result of drug effects, metabolic acidosis, CNS damage or edema, or response to heat stroke or overexercise.

38. What causes high-altitude sickness? How is it treated?

Cerebral hypoxia results from the lower partial pressure of oxygen at high altitudes. A shift of water and sodium into neurons may also occur as the result of the failure of glycolysis-dependent cellular enzymes and transporters, such as the Na/K pump. Exercise in the cold temperatures encountered at high altitude worsens cerebral edema by further increasing cerebral blood flow. Treatment prophylactically with dexamethasone will prevent most cases of acute mountain sickness. The use of high pressure oxygen, removal to lower altitudes, and acetazolamide therapy may reduce symptoms in patients with preexisting high-altitude sickness.

Aminoff MJ: Neurologic complications of systemic disease. In Bradley WG, et al (eds): Neurology in Clinical Practice, 3rd ed. Boston, Butterworth-Heinemann, 2000, p 1020.

HEMATOLOGIC DISEASE

39. Name the most common symptoms associated with anemia.

Regardless of cause, headache, lightheadedness, and fatigue are the most commonly reported neurologic complaints of the anemic patient.

40. What is the most serious neurologic complication of sickle cell anemia?

Ischemic stroke, often affecting patients in childhood or adolescence, is the most frequent serious sequela of a vascular crisis in sickle cell disease. Intimal hyperplasia and stenosis of proximal cerebral vessels have been described in the pathogenesis for medium- and large-vessel stroke in these patients. Hyperventilation (with associated vasoconstriction) is thus a common precipitating event for stroke in the young patient with sickle cell disease. Recurrence rates for stroke in patients with sickle cell disease exceed 67%. Intracranial hemorrhage (ICH) may also be seen in patients with sickle cell disease. Rupture of intracranial aneurysms is the usual cause for ICH in affected individuals.

Adams RJ, McKie VC, Hsu L, et al: Prevention trial in sickle cell anemia: Study results. N Engl J Med 339:5–11, 1998.

41. What are the primary neurologic manifestations of hyperviscosity states?

Hyperviscosity states are conditions in which red blood cells, white blood cells, or serum proteins are increased to a sufficient degree that impedance of blood flow and/or oxygen delivery results. Neurologic manifestations include symptoms of chronic or acute vertebrobasilar insufficiency (tinnitus, lightheadedness, and headache), paresthesias, problems with mentation, visual/auditory disturbances, seizures, stroke, stupor, or coma.

42. What red cell diseases can produce a hyperviscosity state?

Polycythemia rubra vera and "secondary" or "relative" polycythemia increase the hematocrit or the red cell volume/plasma volume ratio, respectively. This increases blood viscosity, producing symptoms. Chronic reduction in hematocrit by phlebotomy or acute expansion of the plasma volume both reduce symptoms and may decrease the risk for serious sequelae.

43. What diseases produce elevated serum proteins and cause hyperviscosity states?

Paraproteinemias may be first detected by the onset of neurologic symptoms. Multiple myeloma and Waldenström's macroglobulinemia are the most common causes of increased serum viscosity, which appears to produce the complications of this state. Treatment usually requires plasmapheresis and therapy for the underlying condition.

44. What are the neurologic complications of hemophilia?

Intracranial hemorrhage is the most serious consequence of factor VIII deficiency. A history of head trauma is often obtained, preceding symptoms of a subdural hemorrhage by days. Subarachnoid and intraparenchymal hemorrhages cause more rapid progression of symptoms, and carry increased mortality. Intraspinal hemorrhage, while rare, rapidly produces cord compression and paralysis, while soft-tissue hematomas may cause focal compressive neuropathies.

45. Which platelet disorders produce neurologic disease?

Neurologic complications may arise from having too few or too many platelets, sometimes associated with platelet dysfunction. Thrombocytopenia-caused neurologic manifestations may be due to primary acute or chronic immune thrombocytopenia purpura (ITP), disseminated intravascular coagulation (DIC), thrombotic thrombocytopenic purpura (TTP), dysimmune thrombocytopenia (DIT) secondary to rheumatic disease (associated with anticardiolipin antibodies) or hyperviscosity states, and heparin-associated thrombocytopenia (HAT). TTP produces a microangiopathic hemolytic anemia with prominent neurologic symptoms of headache, encephalopathy, or seizures, whereas DIC and (less commonly) ITP may produce larger intracerebral hemorrhages. HAT and DIT more commonly cause stroke. Thrombocytosis usually results from essential thrombocythemia, which produces symptoms of a hyperviscosity state when platelet counts exceed 600,000–1,000,000/µl. Cerebrovascular complications—TIAs and stroke—are the serious consequences of this disease.

46. How are antiphospholipid antibodies related to neurologic disease?

Antibodies directed against phospholipids are associated with thrombotic states and are found with a high frequency in patients with retinal vascular thrombosis, amaurosis fugax, ischemic optic neuropathy, and stroke in the young. The most common antibodies, lupus anticoagulant and anticardiolipin antibody, probably induce thrombosis via multiple mechanisms.

Jacobs BS, Levine SR: Antiphospholipid antibody syndrome. Curr Treat Opt Neurol 2:444–458, 2000.

47. What are the nonischemic symptoms of the antiphospholipid antibody syndrome?

The presence of these antibodies has been associated with migraine, chorea, myelopathy, and orthostatic hypotension. Nonneurologic features may include miscarriages, livedo reticularis, and pulmonary hypertension. The pathophysiology of these symptoms is poorly understood.

48. What is the treatment for the antiphospholipid antibody syndrome?

Few controlled trials have been conducted, and there is no consensus about the optimal treatment for patients with antiphospholipid antibodies. Most authorities favor use of the antithrombotic agent warfarin, but plasmapheresis combined with immunosuppression and intravenous immunoglobulin (IVIG) increasingly is being used in severe cases. IVIG is the treatment of choice for pregnant women.

Valesini G, Pittoni V: Treatment of thrombosis associated with immunological risk factors. Ann Med 32(suppl 1):41–45, 2000.

ENDOCRINE DISEASE

49. Which endocrine diseases are commonly associated with neurologic complications?

1. Diabetes mellitus	4. Hyperparathyroidism	7. Adrenal insufficiency
2. Hyperthyroidism	5. Hypoparathyroidism	8. Glucocorticoid excess
3. Hypothyroidism	6. Acromegaly	9. Diabetes insipidus

50. Which endocrine diseases are complicated by seizures?

Seizures most commonly occur after an acute change in endocrine function and usually result from electrolyte imbalance. They occur in 50% or more of patients with hypoparathyroidism because of the hypocalcemia. Although seizures are usually generalized, partial or absence seizures may also complicate hypoparathyroidism. Seizures do not occur in hyperparathyroidism.

Seizures may be the presenting sign in 20% of all hypothyroid patients, and are nearly always generalized. In contrast, the incidence of seizures in thryotoxicosis is only 5–10%.

In Addison's disease, seizures follow the rapid onset of serum hyponatremia (< 115 mEq/L), and carry a subsequent mortality of greater than 50%. Seizures are seen in diabetes insipidus (DI) only with rapid elevation of serum sodium (usually to greater than 160 mEq/L). In DI, seizures are often partial and may occur as a result of brain shrinkage with focal hemorrhage, or during rehydration.

Seizures are observed with other endocrine causes of brain shrinkage, such as in nonketotic hyperosmolar states from diabetes mellitus (DM). In this setting, up to 25% of patients develop partial or generalized motor seizures that may evolve into epilepsia partialis continua or generalized status epilepticus. Seizures may also be seen in DM as the result of hypoglycemia from insulin therapy, but are distinctly uncommon in diabetic ketoacidosis. Seizures are not typically associated with Cushing's disease or acromegaly.

51. Which endocrine diseases may cause coma?

Coma is a rare and life-threatening complication of both hypothyroidism and hyperthyroidism. In the latter case, coma is almost always associated with thyroid storm. Coma is also found in hyperparathyroidism when serum calcium is greater than 19 mg/dl, in adrenal hypofunction with severe hyponatremia, and in diabetes mellitus.

52. What are the most common neurologic complications of hypothyroidism? What are several rare complications?

In more than 90% of tested patients, hypothyroidism causes headache, fatigue, slowness of speech and thought, apathy, and inattention. These symptoms are often mistaken for early dysthymia or depression. Reversible sensorineural hearing loss, with or without tinnitus, develops in 75% of hypothyroid patients, while 60% of patients have reversible ptosis as a result of diminished sympathetic tone. Sleep apnea occurs in up to half of hypothyroid patients and usually results from obstructive problems due to associated obesity and myxedema. Seizures may be found in 20% of patients, often as the presenting neurologic sign. Prolonged relaxation time for deep tendon reflexes can be elicited in many hypothryoid patients, but similar changes are noted in many other diseases.

More rare are findings of demonstrable muscle weakness, limb ataxia, nystagmus, carpal tunnel syndrome or demyelinating polyneuropathy, optic neuropathy, myxedematous constriction of extraocular movements, papilledema from pseudotumor cerebri, trigeminal neuralgia, Bell's palsy, reversible dementia, or overt psychosis (myxedema madness).

Abend WK, Tyler HR: Thyroid disease and the nervous system. In Aminoff M (ed): Neurology and General Medicine. New York, Churchill-Livingstone, 1995, pp 333–348.

53. What are the most dangerous neurologic complications of hypothyroidism? How are they treated?

Although myxedema coma develops in only 1% of hypothyroid patients, its often-rapid onset with associated bradycardia, ventricular arrhythmias, hypotension, hypopnea, hypothermia, hypoglycemia, electrolyte disturbance, and seizures make it life-threatening. Treatment is supportive, with correction of metabolic abnormalities, rewarming, ventilatory and/or cardiovascular support, and adequate replacement of thyroxine and corticosteroids. In utero and in the newborn period, undiagnosed and untreated hypothyroidism leads to cretinism. Treatment requires early screening prior to the onset of symptoms and thyroid hormone replacement before permanent damage occurs.

54. What is the spectrum of neurologic symptomatology in hyperthyroidism? Do symptoms resolve after correction of hyperthyroidism?

Thyrotoxicosis may manifest with reversible behavioral and cognitive changes, including emotional lability, euphoria, irritability, mania, and psychosis. Delirium may be observed as a manifestation of thyroid storm. Apathetic hyperthyroidism may appear as fatigue, with symptoms suggesting depression or dementia. Other features of thyrotoxicosis are tremor of the hands, eyelids or tongue, chorea, spasticity (sometimes with clonus and Babinski signs), thyrotoxic periodic paralysis, and myopathy.

Neurologic problems usually resolve after treatment of the underlying thyrotoxicosis, but thyroid ophthalmopathy often requires surgical orbital decompression. Additionally, bulbar palsies and motor weakness may not recover following correction of hyperthyroidism secondary to autoimmune disease, and may result from coincident affliction with other associated diseases, such as acute myasthenia gravis or amyotrophic lateral sclerosis.

55. Which psychiatric diseases have been mistakenly diagnosed in cases of parathyroid dysfunction?

Up to 25% of patients with hyperparathyroidism have prominent psychiatric symptoms resembling mania, schizophrenia, or acute confusional state. An additional 50% of hyperparathyroid patients may have symptoms suggesting depression. Interestingly, 80% of patients with hypoparathyroidism also exhibit psychological manifestations of their disease, including symptoms resembling depression, pseudodementia, mania, schizophrenia, and toxic delirium.

56. Which neurologic sequela of parathyroid disease pose serious health threats to afflicted patients?

In hyperparathyroidism, hypercalcemia-induced coma and spinal cord or root compression caused by collapse of decalcified vertebrae are the major nonpsychiatric symptoms that threaten a patient's health. Myopathy, which at times may be severe, is also a common finding in hyperparathyroidism. In contrast, hypocalcemia resulting from hypoparathyroidism is more closely associated with seizures and tetany. Seizures are often difficult to control with correction of the electrolyte imbalance. Latent tetany, which may become apparent as laryngeal spasm, can be evoked by mechanical stimulation of the facial nerve (Chvostek sign), by hyperventilation, or by occlusion of venous return from an arm, producing carpopedal spasm (Trousseau sign).

57. How may adrenal insufficiency lead to weakness?

Up to 50% of patients with Addison's disease have a glucocorticoid-sensitive myopathy with associated cramping. Adrenal insufficiency results in decreased blood flow to the muscle, reduced muscle carbohydrate metabolism, and altered Na/K pump function and potassium homeostasis with resulting reduced muscle intracellular potassium and altered muscle contractility. Decreased adrenergic sensitivity in patients with Addison's disease also results in reduced exercise tolerance and exercise-related hypotension. Abnormalities in potassium homeostasis may additionally result in the episodic appearance of extreme weakness, resembling hyperkalemic periodic paralysis.

Horak H, Pourmand R: Endocrine myopathies. Neurol Clin 18:203–214, 2000.

58. How does prolonged glucocorticoid excess lead to weakness?

Most patients with Cushing's disease have frank weakness and demonstrable myopathic findings on electromyography and selective type IIb atrophy on muscle biopsy. Chronic treatment with glucocorticoids, especially with the fluorinated steroids, will reproduce these effects on ectopic ACTH production in 10–20% of patients. Glucocorticoids produce an insulin-resistant state in myotubes, in which both glycolytic (nonoxidative) carbohydrate metabolism and protein synthesis are adversely affected. Type IIb fibers, which are least able to compensate for this reduction of glycolytic metabolism, are most affected.

59. Does acromegaly (excess growth hormone production) directly cause neurologic damage?

Sustained excessive growth hormone (GH) appears to directly produce myopathy. GH-induced changes in the myotube include impaired glycolytic carbohydrate metabolism, increased fatty acid oxidation, and increased protein synthesis with reduced protein degradation. The more highly oxidative type I and type IIa muscle fibers typically are most affected by GH. Myotube hypertrophy from abnormal protein synthesis produces weakness in the face of increased muscle size. Although central sleep apnea may also be caused directly by excessive GH production, the obstructive sleep apnea, basilar impression, myelopathy, and compressive neuropathies reported in this disease are all indirect effects of bony, ligamentous, and soft-tissue hyperplasia with secondary compression of neural tissue.

60. How does diabetes mellitus affect the nervous system?

Damage to the peripheral nervous system accounts for the main neurologic manifestations of diabetes. Initially, a symmetric distal stocking-and-glove sensory neuropathy involving small, unmyelinated or thinly myelinated fibers appears and is often associated with painful, burning paresthesias. In more severe cases, larger proprioceptive fibers are also affected, leading to Charcot joints. Autonomic nerve damage causes atrophic skin changes, impotence, orthostatic hypotension, arrhythmias, gastroparesis, and sphincter incontinence. Motor fibers may also be damaged, leading to symmetric distal weakness, especially of the lower extremities. Focal destruction of nerves may cause cranial nerve palsies, diabetic amyotrophy, and thoracoabdominal neuropathy.

61. What are the potential causes of coma in diabetes mellitus?

1. Nonketotic hyperglycemic coma
2. Lactic acidosis
3. SIADH
4. Hypophosphatemia
5. Cerebral infarction
6. Hypotension
7. Disseminated intravascular coagulation
8. Uremia with hypertensive encephalopathy
9. Cerebral edema
10. Hypoglycemia or acidosis as complications of therapy

62. Which neurologic complications of diabetes mellitus result from vascular occlusive disease?

Most focal neurologic complications of diabetes result directly or indirectly from infarction. In diabetes, the risk of stroke is increased between two- and four-fold. This may be due to accelerated atherogenesis, as well as to autonomic dysfunction that leads to hypotension and infarction. Most CNS abnormalities observed with diabetes, including hemiparesis, aphasia, and dementia, are the result of such pathology. Mononeuropathies, including those affecting median, ulnar, peroneal, femoral, and cranial nerves, are also thought to be vascular in origin, as is the lumbosacral pathology observed in diabetic amyotrophy, and the thoracic root damage with severe visceral pain found in thoracoabdominal neuropathy. Focal infarction of the vasa nervorum may be responsible for these abnormalities.

FLUID AND ELECTROLYTE DISORDERS

63. How do changes in serum potassium affect the nervous system?

In vitro experimental alterations in neuronal intracellular potassium change both the cell resting potential and neuronal excitability. However, the presence of mechanisms for active potassium transport into neurons, combined with the local control of perineuronal extracellular potassium by glia, prevents significant fluctuations in neuronal potassium over wide ranges of serum potassium concentration. For these reasons, neurologic complications of hypokalemia or hyperkalemia are few and are typically nonneuronal.

64. Name the most common neurologic complications of hypokalemia.

Myalgias and weakness can be found with serum potassium concentrations of 2.5–3.0 mEq/L. Prolonged hypokalemia of less than 2.5 mEq/L will lead to rhabdomyolysis, myoglobinuria, and cardiac arrhythmias.

65. What are the most common neurologic complications of hyperkalemia?

Hyperkalemia (> 6.0 mEq/L) likewise causes functional and structural muscle abnormalities, including weakness and cardiac arrhythmias. Ventricular asystole or fibrillation are life-threatening and occur long before neurologic symptoms are usually manifested. The few previous reports of drowsiness, lethargy, and coma in hypokalemia may actually be the result of acid-base disequilibrium.

66. How do changes in serum sodium affect the nervous system?

Because extracellular fluid volume changes as a direct function of total body sodium, patients who are hyponatremic are usually hyposmolar, whereas hypernatremic patients are hyperosmolar. Neurologic manifestations of sodium dysregulation mainly result from shrinkage or swelling of the brain, and the degree to which these changes occur depend both on the amount and the rapidity of the sodium changes.

67. What are the most common neurologic complications of hyponatremia?

Alteration of mental status is the common neurologic alteration resulting from hyponatremia. This may occur after acute reduction of serum sodium to below 130 mEq/L, or with chronically depressed sodium concentrations of below 115 mEq/L. Seizures, seen in the presence of acute reduction of serum sodium to less than 125 mEq/L, are generalized in nature and prognostically signify mortality of greater than 50%.

68. What are the neurologic complications of therapy for hyponatremia?

The most devastating complication of rapid sodium replacement is **central pontine myelinolysis**. This disease causes myelinolysis throughout the brain and can result from rapid osmotic shifts. Symptoms of corticospinal and corticobulbar destruction are prominent, and patients may develop a "locked in" syndrome. Rapid dehydration of persons who are hyponatremic may result in hyperviscosity syndrome from plasma volume depletion, despite the presence of persistent tissue edema. **Strokes** are the primary complication of this treatment and are especially likely when fluid restriction is used as therapy for subarachnoid hemorrhage-induced hyponatremia.

69. Describe the most common neurologic complications of hypernatremia.

Hypernatremia (serum sodium > 160 mEq/L) may lead to an altered mental state, progressing to coma or to seizures. Focal cerebral hemorrhage resulting from the tearing of parenchymal vessels or bridging veins produces multiple neurologic symptoms, including hemiparesis, rigidity, tremor, myoclonus, cerebellar ataxia, and chorea, as well as signs of subarachnoid hemorrhage or subdural hematoma.

70. What are the neurologic complications of hypercalcemia?

Hypercalcemia (> 12 mg/dl) leads commonly to symptoms of progressive encephalopathy and coma, and more rarely to seizures or signs of corticobulbar, corticospinal, or cerebellospinal tract dysfunction. Elevated serum calcium may also produce weakness with reduced membrane excitability at the level of the neuromuscular junction, and may possibly cause a reversible myopathy.

71. Name common neurologic complications of hypocalcemia.

Hypocalcemia may present with seizures or with neurobehavioral changes and dementia. Some patients develop parkinsonism after prolonged hypocalcemia. Increased excitability at the neuromuscular junction with reduced serum calcium may manifest as tetany.

72. What are the most common neurologic complications of hypomagnesemia?

Because, like potassium, magnesium is an intracellular ion whose intracellular concentrations are tightly controlled, the presence of neurologic complications may not directly correlate with extracellular magnesium concentrations. Hypomagnesemia, however, appears to present in patients with essentially the same findings as hypocalcemia. Because serum ionized calcium concentrations are reduced in the presence of hypomagnesemia, some of these symptoms may in fact be the functional result of hypocalcemia.

73. What are common neurologic complications of hypermagnesemia?

Hypermagnesemia results in CNS depression and muscle paralysis. While the mechanism of CNS depression is still being addressed, muscle paralysis occurs as a result of direct neuromuscular blockade.

RHEUMATOLOGIC DISEASE

74. What are the neurologic effects of systemic lupus erythematosus (SLE) on the CNS?

Symptoms of central dysfunction include neuropsychiatric and behavioral changes, such as dementia, psychosis, and confusional states (the most common central manifestation of SLE).

Physical signs of this disease include such localizing neurologic findings as hemiparesis, chorea, tremor, cerebellar ataxia, cranial neuropathies and optic neuritis, and transverse myelitis. These signs and symptoms may be due to SLE vasculitis or to stroke and vascular dementia seen in patients with SLE and antiphospholipid antibodies. Aseptic meningitis, seizures, and signs of increased intracranial pressure may also develop in patients with SLE.

Boumpas DT, Austin HA, Bessler BJ, et al: Systemic lupus erythematosus: Emerging concepts. Ann Intern Med 122:940–948, 1995.

75. What are the neurologic effects of SLE on the peripheral nervous system?

Peripheral neuropathy may appear in SLE as a vasculitis mononeuropathy or mononeuritis multiplex, or as an ischemic symmetric distal sensorimotor deficit. Myositis occurs in 25% of patients with SLE, but is a serious complication only when the myocardium is involved.

76. Do the neurologic sequelae of SLE adversely affect patient survival?

Neurologic symptoms and signs appear as manifestations of SLE in 50% of afflicted patients. The mean 5-year survival for such patients is 30% less than that found for SLE patients without neurologic problems. Vasculitis with CNS hemorrhage accounts for a large portion of this difference.

77. What are the neurologic effects of rheumatoid arthritis (RA) on the peripheral nervous system?

The major sequelae of RA are limited to the peripheral nervous system. Neuropathy may be the result of nerve entrapment near inflamed joints, direct inflammation of the perineurium resulting in distal demyelinating sensory neuropathies, and vasculitic destruction of larger nerves, resulting in asymmetric sensorimotor neuropathies. Diffuse nodular polymyositis may occur in 30% of patients with RA, although classic polymyositis is rare (5%). Disuse muscle atrophy is a common finding in severely affected individuals who are bedridden. Focal ischemic myositis occurs as a result of vasculitis attack on the muscle vasculature.

Akil M, Amos RS: Rheumatoid arthritis: Clinical features and diagnosis. Brit Med J 310:587–591, 1995.

78. What are the neurologic effects of RA on the CNS?

Effects include a rare polyarteritis-nodosa-like vasculitis that may affect cerebral vasculature, an even rarer hyperviscosity syndrome that produces focal ischemic and hemorrhagic lesions throughout the CNS, and rheumatoid cervical disease with myelopathy.

79. What causes myelopathy in patients with RA?

Myelopathy may result from atlantoaxial subluxation, vertical subluxation of the odontoid into the foramen magnum, backward subluxation of the atlas on the axis, or subaxial subluxation, most commonly occurring at C4–C5. Compression or laceration of the spinal cord may be the direct result of odontoid impaction or subluxation of one or more vertebral bodies or rings against the cord. Vascular compression syndromes may also be found in RA patients with cervical disease, especially involving the anterior spinal artery. These syndromes lead to ischemic central gray destruction and to necrosis of the dorsal columns and corticospinal tracts.

80. Which neuromuscular diseases may be associated with Sjögren's syndrome?

Sjögren's syndrome is an autoimmune disease that combines connective tissue disease (often rheumatoid arthritis), xerostomia, and keratoconjunctivitis sicca. It is the second most common rheumatic disease (after rheumatoid arthritis). Most of its neurologic complications are the result of vasculitis, but it is also associated with several (probably autoimmune) neurologic diseases. Thus, increased incidence for myasthenia gravis, polymyositis, inclusion body myositis, and ALS have been noted in patients with Sjögren's disease.

81. Trigeminal neuropathy is found in which rheumatic diseases?

Isolated trigeminal neuropathy may be the presenting sign in 10% of patients with neurologic manifestations of scleroderma and occurs in 4–5% of all patients with scleroderma. Fibrosis with nerve entrapment is the likely cause for this and other cranial neuropathies in progressive systemic sclerosis. Vasculitis damage to the trigeminal nerve is found in SLE and less commonly in mixed connective tissue disorder (MCTD).

82. What is the most common neurologic manifestation of Behçet's disease?
CNS disease is found in 10–30% of patients afflicted with this disease. An initially relapsing and remitting focal meningoencephalitis that predominantly affects the brainstem is the most commonly finding in Behçet's disease. Cranial nerve and long tract signs may eventually lead to spastic quadriplegia and pseudobulbar palsy. Subcortical dementia, pseudotumor cerebri, vasculitis with cerebral infarction, and peripheral neuropathy have also been reported in this disease.
   Siva A, Izzet F: Behçet's disease. Curr Treat Opt Neurol 2:435–448, 2000.

VASCULITIDES

83. Which vessels are affected by primary vasculitic disease?
Although all vessels may be damaged in vasculitis, different vasculitides affect different vessel types. The aorta is selectively damaged in Takayasu's arteritis, whereas giant cell arteritis more commonly affects the temporal, vertebral, and carotid arteries. Medium-sized muscular intracerebral arteries are affected in polyarteritis nodosa (PAN), allergic granulomatosis, and granulomatous angiitis, whereas small muscular arteries are thrombosed in Wegener's granulomatosis. Hypersensitivity angiitis selectively involves capillaries and venules, sparing the arterial system.

84. What are the peripheral nervous system effects of PAN?
Half of patients diagnosed with polyarteritis nodosa have evidence of peripheral neuropathy. Five different peripheral neuropathy syndromes have been identified: (1) mononeuritis multiplex, involving both sensory and motor nerves; (2) extensive mononeuritis multiplex, with severe, primarily distal weakness and sensory deficits; (3) isolated small cutaneous sensory nerve involvement; (4) distal symmetric sensorimotor neuropathy; and (5) radiculopathy. Myalgias have also been reported in 25% of patients with PAN, usually associated with weakness. Histologic assessment of muscle biopsies acquired from these patients reveals evidence of inflammatory myopathy in roughly half of the affected individuals.

85. What are the CNS effects of PAN?
CNS manifestations of vasculitic disease can be found in 40–45% of patients with PAN. Central neurologic complications may be grouped into those producing a diffuse encephalopathy, usually with seizures (40%), and those leading to focal deficits that are suggestive of infarction of the cerebrum, cerebellum, or brainstem (50%). Additionally, 15% of patients present to their physicians with isolated cranial neuropathies, most commonly involving cranial nerves II, III, and VIII. Hypertensive CNS changes with papilledema and focal hemorrhages are observed in 10% of patients with an acute confusional state, and often signify a poorer prognosis. Peripheral neuropathy is a common and early finding of PAN, whereas CNS sequelae are often late manifestations of this disease, occurring 2–3 years after the initial diagnosis.

86. Does Churg-Strauss syndrome cause neurologic damage?
Two-thirds of patients with allergic granulomatosis (Churg-Strauss syndrome) have CNS manifestations similar to those seen in PAN, commonly including encephalopathy, seizures, and coma, and almost all patients have mononeuritis multiplex. Hemorrhage is more common in this disorder than in PAN, but the clinical distinction between these two diseases rests on the almost invariable presence of pulmonary involvement with asthma in patients with Churg-Strauss syndrome, and the tremendous eosinophilia and elevated IgE levels found in this latter disease.

87. Are the neurologic sequelae of hypersensitivity angiitis usually central or peripheral?
Hypersensitivity vasculitides include cutaneous vasculitis, drug-induced allergic vasculitis, postinfectious vasculitis, serum sickness, Henoch-Schönlein purpura, hypocomplementemic

vasculitis, cryoglobulinemia, neoplastic angiitis, connective tissue disease-associated vasculitis, and Zeek angiitis. Neurologic complications are rare in hypocomplementemic vasculitis and in Henoch-Schönlein purpura, although both stroke and intracranial hemorrhage have been reported in the latter disease. With the exception of the hypersensitivity angiitis of Zeek and serum sickness, only peripheral nerve involvement is typically observed with the other forms of hypersensitivity angiitis.

In all forms of hypersensitivity angiitis, biopsy of the skin lesions will provide the diagnosis, and treatment of the underlying disorder with identification and removal of any sensitizing agent, combined with immunosuppression (when there is evidence of progression), usually cures the disease.

88. What are the neurologic effects of Wegener's granulomatosis?

Wegener's granulomatosis presents as a triad of focal segmental glomerulonephritis, granulomas of the respiratory tract, and necrotizing vasculitis. Neurologic complications occur in 25–50% of affected individuals, with peripheral vasculitis mononeuritis multiplex being the most common sign. CNS manifestations of the disease are more often the result of granulomatous invasion from the sinuses or nasal passages, and may appear as exophthalmos, pituitary disease, or basilar meningitis with cranial neuropathies. Up to 5% of patients will have intracranial hemorrhages secondary to either focal vasculitis or intragranulomatous hemorrhage.

Nishino H, Rubino FA, DeRemee RA, et al: Neurological involvement in Wegener's granulomatosis: An analysis of 324 consecutive patients at the Mayo Clinic. Ann Neurol 33:4–8, 1993.

89. Describe the triad of clinical findings often found in temporal arteritis.

Headache, jaw claudication, and constitutional symptoms compose the triad of clinical symptoms often found in temporal arteritis. The headache is typically boring, throbbing, or lancinating, radiating from one or both temples to the neck, jaw, tongue, or back of the head. Fever, malaise, nightsweats, and anorexia with weight loss usually present early in the disease. Patients with temporal arteritis are almost invariably over 50 years of age, and half will have evidence of concomitant polyarthralgia rheumatica. Mononeuritis multiplex may occur in 10% of afflicted patients, but should always suggest the possibility of PAN or an overlap syndrome.

90. What are the neurologic complications of temporal arteritis?

Untreated, one-third of patients will develop amaurosis fugax, monocular or binocular blindness, diplopia, or ophthalmoplegia. Cerebral infarctions or transient ischemic attacks that often involve the vertebral distribution are likewise common late complications of the disease.

91. How is temporal arteritis diagnosed and treated?

Evidence of an elevated sedimentation rate (> 60 mm/hr by the Westergren method) and characteristic findings of arteritis on biopsy of the temporal artery are helpful in making the diagnosis, but biopsy is frequently negative (70% diagnostic after bilateral biopsy). Treatment of temporal arteritis is with steroids and should not await biopsy (biopsy should be performed within the first few days of therapy). Treatment should continue at least 2 years, with regulation of steroid therapy usually on the basis of sedimentation rates.

92. What are four vasculitides whose effects are localized to the CNS?

Cogan's syndrome produces vestibular and/or auditory dysfunction with episodic acute interstitial keratitis, scleritis, or episcleritis. **Eale's syndrome** is an isolated peripheral retinal vasculitis. Both of these rare syndromes tend to afflict young adults. **Spinal cord arteritis** is a diagnosis of exclusion, since many diseases may present with myelopathy. Among those diseases is **granulomatous angiitis of the nervous system (GANS)**, the most severe isolated CNS vasculitic syndrome.

93. What are the nervous system manifestations of granulomatous angiitis?

GANS is also called isolated angiitis of the CNS, because the disease is almost always restricted to the CNS. This syndrome is likely a collection of vasculitides. A spinal tap reveals an elevated opening pressure in 30% of patients, CSF pleocytosis in 65% of patients, and increased protein in 80% of patients. Cerebral angiography and brain biopsy may each be diagnostic in 50% of cases. The differential diagnosis includes other vasculitides, tuberculosis, MS, strokes due to emboli, sarcoidosis, syphilis, Lyme disease, drug abuse associated CNS vasculopathy, neoplasm, and lymphomatoid granulomatosis.

Goldberg JW: Primary angiitis of the central nervous system. In Rolak LA, Harati Y (eds): Neuro-immunology for the Clinician. Boston, Butterworth-Heinemann, 1997, pp 177–186.

PREGNANCY AND SEXUAL DYSFUNCTION

94. What is the most common neurologic symptom found during pregnancy?

Headache is the most common neurologic symptom. Although pregnancy is generally thought to have a somewhat protective effect against headache in patients with an established diagnosis, it is still the most common neurologic complaint of the pregnant patient.

Headaches beginning during pregnancy are a cause for concern about serious underlying illnesses that occur with higher frequency in pregnant women. These include subarachnoid hemorrhage, rapid expansion of a tumor, cortical venous thrombosis, pseudotumor cerebri, *Listeria monocytogenes* meningitis, or preeclampsia and eclampsia. History and physical examination can usually exclude serious problems. Other headaches that may begin during pregnancy include migraines, even though the majority of female migraneurs improve during pregnancy. Onset of benign bifrontal nonmigranous headaches is also seen in pregnancy, and is most common during the first trimester. Postpartum headache is the most common self-limited headache of the puerperium and occurs in up to 40% of all women.

Shaner DM: Neurological problems of pregnancy. In Bradley WG, et al: Neurology in Clinical Practice, 3rd ed. Boston, Butterworth-Heinemann, 2000, pp 2257–2268.

95. What is eclampsia?

Eclampsia, which means "to shine forth," is a state characterized by the neurologic complications of seizures and/or coma, presenting in a pregnant patient with preeclampsia (i.e., with signs of hypertension and proteinuria with or without edema). It occurs in 0.05–0.2% of all pregnancies extending beyond the 20th week of gestation. Seizures or coma develop in 50% of eclamptic patients prior to the onset of labor, with an additional 25% becoming symptomatic during labor. The remaining 25% of eclamptic patients have onset of symptoms after delivery, usually within the first 24 hours postpartum. The differential diagnosis for eclampsia includes cerebrovascular accidents, hypertensive encephalopathy, epilepsy, brain neoplasms and abscesses, meningitis/encephalitis, and metabolic diseases such as hypoglycemia or hypocalcemia.

Fox MW, et al: Selected neurologic complications of pregnancy. Mayo Clin Proc 65:1595–1618, 1990.

96. What is the cause of associated mortality in eclampsia?

If present, eclampsia results in a maternal mortality of up to 14%, with associated fetal mortality of up to 28%. Maternal death from eclampsia is caused by complications of sustained intracranial and systemic hypertension. Death can be due to intracerebral hemorrhage, vasospasm, pulmonary edema, disseminated intravascular coagulation, abruptio placentae, the HELLP syndrome (hemolysis, elevated liver enzymes, and low platelet count), or renal or hepatic failure from decreased organ perfusion. Fetal mortality results from decreased uteroplacental perfusion.

97. How is eclampsia treated?

Because the maternal morbidity and mortality of eclampsia derive from complications of loss of cerebral autoregulation due to sustained hypertension, the primary objective of treatment is to reduce blood pressure without compromising uteroplacental or maternal renal perfusion. Intracranial hypertension is usually present in patients with encephalopathy or coma, and thus ICP should be monitored in such persons, with treatment by intubation and hyperventilation. These patients should also be imaged by CT to check for intracranial hemorrhage or the degree of cerebral edema.

Because eclamptic seizures result in high fetal mortality and further increases in intracranial pressure, they must be aggressively controlled. Diazepam may be used in doses of 5 or 10 mg. Phenytoin or phenobarbital are usually given concomitantly to provide longer-term prophylaxis. Intravenous administration of magnesium sulfate is effective as well.

However, the definitive treatment for eclampsia occurring before birth is termination of the pregnancy by delivery of the fetus. Therefore, preparations for immediate cesarean section should begin while attempting to control hypertension and seizures. The risk of recurrent seizures decreases within 24 hours following delivery, and long-term prophylaxis of eclampsia-induced seizures is unnecessary. Although hypertension resolves more slowly, normalization of blood pressure occurs in the first postpartum week.

98. Is the risk for stroke altered in pregnancy?

Cerebrovascular ischemic events occur 13 times more frequently in pregnant patients than in age-matched nonpregnant women, with an overall stroke risk of 1 in 3000 pregnancies. Stroke accounts for 10% of all maternal deaths during pregnancy, and 35% of all strokes in female patients aged 15 to 45 years occur during pregnancy or in the puerperium. Atherosclerotic disease is less commonly a cause for stroke in this population than is arterial embolus or cerebral venous thrombosis.

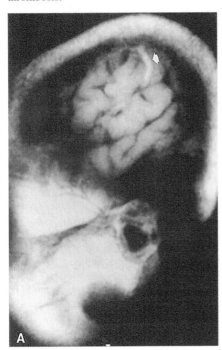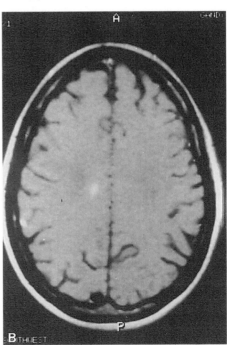

T1-weighted sagittal view of the superficial cerebral cortex of the parietal lobe, showing a cerebral vein thrombosis (A, arrow). The axial T1 view (B) shows the small hemorrhagic infarction caused by the venous thrombosis.

99. How does the physician clinically distinguish puerperal cerebral venous thrombosis from arterial thrombosis?

Central venous thrombosis usually occurs in the first three postpartum weeks and commonly presents with headache, focal or generalized seizures, stupor or coma, transient focal deficits, and/or signs of increased intracranial pressure. Rare thromboses include superior sagittal sinus thrombosis, which may present with paraplegia and sensory deficits of the leg with associated bladder dysfunction, and rolandic vein thrombosis, which causes sensory and motor deficits of the leg, hip, and shoulder, sparing the face and arm. Mortality in sagittal sinus thrombosis approaches 40% when diagnosis is delayed, but may be reduced to 20% with intensive care and, in some cases, anticoagulants. Recovery of survivors is usually complete.

Arterial thrombosis is more rare than arterial embolus or venous thrombosis, is more likely to occur in the second or third trimester than in the puerperium, and commonly presents with persistent focal deficit, such as hemiparesis, without alteration of consciousness, seizures, or signs of increased intracranial pressure.

Recently an immune mechanism has been hypothesized for a significant percentage of pregnancy-related venous and arterial thromboses. The presence of antiphospholipid antibodies should be sought, especially when a history of previous miscarriages or preeclampsia is obtained.

100. What is the differential diagnosis for seizures during childbirth?

As cause for seizures, **eclampsia, HELLP syndrome**, and **thrombotic thrombocytopenic purpura** are most commonly observed during the third trimester. **Amniotic fluid embolism, water intoxication, autonomic stress in patients with upper spinal cord injury**, and **toxicity from local anesthetics** are all intrapartum causes for seizures. **Cerebral vein thrombosis** usually occurs postpartum and may present with seizures.

Subarachnoid hemorrhage may occur at any time during pregnancy to produce seizures, although aneurysms most commonly rupture during the third trimester, with greatest risk for rebleeding in the postpartum period. Arteriovenous malformations are more likely to rupture in the second trimester and rebleed during delivery or with subsequent pregnancies. **Epilepsy** may manifest at any time before, during, or after pregnancy, and may require lifelong therapy. However, such patients must be distinguished from those with **gestational epilepsy**, which requires therapy only during pregnancy.

101. How should therapy of epilepsy change during pregnancy?

First, all anticonvulsants have some potential to be teratogenic or in some other way harmful to the fetus, and complications to the fetus increase as the number of therapeutic agents used to control seizures increases. Thus, in patients who require pharmacologic anticonvulsant therapy, monotherapy at the lowest functionally effective dose is best.

Second, a number of physiologic changes occur in pregnant patients that alter the pharmacokinetics of anticonvulsants. Effective pre-pregnancy anticonvulsant levels should be used as the target levels during pregnancy. Drug levels should be measured as soon as pregnancy is diagnosed, since blood concentrations of anticonvulsants may drop precipitously during the first trimester, as a result of alterations in drug absorption, metabolism, or protein binding. This is especially true for phenytoin, with its nonlinear kinetics, in which doses may need to be increased by 50–100% during pregnancy to maintain pre-pregnancy levels. Routine drug levels should be measured each trimester, and more frequently if seizure control worsens, or if patients have a history of previous alterations in drug levels during pregnancy. Since drug clearance returns to pre-pregnancy norms within 3–6 weeks postpartum, pre-pregnancy anticonvulsant doses should be gradually introduced during this period.

102. What neuropathies are commonly associated with pregnancy and childbirth?

Whether due to peripheral edema, birth trauma, or other causes, certain neuropathies occur more commonly in pregnancy. Prior to birth, carpal tunnel syndrome is most common. This neuropathy is usually treated conservatively with wrist splinting, since it commonly resolves within 3 months postpartum. Meralgia paresthetica (numbness or dysesthesia of the anterolateral thigh due to compression of the lateral femoral cutaneous nerve along the pelvic wall or obturator canal) occurs as the fetus enlarges, and is also a self-limited process, typically resolving within 3 months of delivery. Bell's palsy is seen with increased frequency in pregnant women. The use of corticosteroids during pregnancy for treatment of Bell's palsy is still controversial.

Traumatic mononeuropathy usually occurs during childbirth. Trauma involving the obturator nerve may result from compression by the fetal head, from misplaced forceps, or from hyperflexion in the lithotomy position. Compression injuries during delivery have also been reported involving the femoral, saphenous, common peroneal, or sciatic nerves. Postpartum foot drop is an interesting example of traumatic mononeuropathy with generally excellent prognosis, most typically observed in short primigravid women with large infants.

103. Is male impotence caused by neurologic disease?

Organic disease is responsible for about half of all cases of impotence assessed by physicians. Of patients with organic disease, primary or secondary neurologic causes can be identified in an additional half. Although neuropathy (especially diabetic neuropathy) is the most common neurologic explanation for impotence, other causes may include spinal stenosis, myelopathy, cerebrovascular accident, multiple sclerosis, or neoplasm of the brain, pituitary gland, or spinal cord. In 85% of these cases, the underlying neurologic cause was unsuspected until the evaluation for impotence.

104. Is female sexual dysfunction caused by neurologic disease?

This question has unfortunately not been addressed by a significant number of clinician researchers. However, because both male and female sexual response and behaviors have been shown to involve activation of specific portions of the neuroendocrine axis, it must be assumed that a woman who reports dyspareunia or loss of ability to achieve orgasm should have a similar risk for organic cause of her complaints as is found in the male population. A search for similar neurologic etiologies as identified for male impotence would thus seem appropriate in the assessment of these complaints.

BIBLIOGRAPHY

1. Aminoff MJ: Neurology and General Medicine, 2nd ed. New York, Churchill-Livingstone, 1995.
2. Bradley WG, Daroff RB, Fenichel GM, Marsden CD: Neurology in Clinical Practice, 3rd ed. Boston, Butterworth-Heinemann, 2000.
3. Rosenbaum RB, Campbell SM, Rosenbaum JT: Clinical Neurology of Rheumatic Diseases. Boston, Butterworth-Heinemann, 1996.
4. Samuels MA, Feske S (eds): Office Practice of Neurology. New York, Churchill-Livingstone, 1996.
Websites
www.wilsonsdisease.org
www.sjogrens.com
www.neuropathy.org
www.ninds.nih.gov/health.htm

24. INFECTIOUS DISEASES, INCLUDING AIDS

Maria E. Carlini, M.D., and Richard L. Harris, M.D.

BACTERIAL INFECTIONS

1. What clinical findings differentiate meningitis from encephalitis?

Patients with meningitis have nuchal rigidity, headache, photophobia, and fever. Patients with encephalitis have disruption of cognitive function that may include altered consciousness, disorientation, behavioral or speech difficulties, and focal neurologic signs such as seizures or hemiparesis. In reality, the majority of infections cause a combination of symptoms and thus lead to meningoencephalitis. In classic presentations, however, bacterial meningitis leads to predominantly meningeal symptoms and processes, whereas herpes encephalitis produces predominantly cerebral symptoms.

Whitley RJ: Viral encephalitis. N Engl J Med 323:242–250, 1990.

2. When may a bacterial infection produce CSF results identical to aseptic meningitis?

Aseptic meningitis is often a viral infection and typically produces lymphocytic pleocytosis, normal glucose, mildly elevated protein, negative Gram stain, and sterile bacterial cultures. Similar cerebrospinal fluid (CSF) findings may occur in partially treated bacterial meningitis or parameningeal foci such as epidural, subdural, or brain abscesses.

3. Bacterial meningitis is the most common cause of hypoglycorrhachia. What are the other common causes?

1. Cryptococcal meningitis
2. Tuberculous meningitis
3. Syphilitic meningitis
4. Neurosarcoidosis
5. Meningeal carcinomatosis

4. A patient presents with probable acute bacterial meningitis, but you are unable to obtain informed consent for lumbar puncture until after a CT scan. You wisely decide to start antibiotics immediately and not wait for the lumbar puncture. What tests can you still perform that may identify the etiologic agent?

1. Blood cultures should be obtained before antibiotics are given. Approximately 50% of patients with bacterial meningitis have a positive blood culture.

2. Serologic studies, such as latex agglutination or counter immunoelectrophoresis (CIE), for *Streptococcus pneumoniae, Neisseria meningitidis, Hemophilus influenzae,* and *Listeria monocytogenes* may be positive in blood, urine, and CSF (even after antibiotics).

3. Culture of CSF, even after antibiotics are given, will probably be positive for hours.

5. Who should receive prophylaxis after contact with a patient with meningitis?

Prophylaxis depends on the organism and the age of the exposed person:

1. *H. influenzae,* **type B**—all children who have close contact with the patient and who have not been vaccinated.

2. *Neisseria* **meningitis**—all close contacts, regardless of age.

Rifampin is usually considered the drug of choice for prophylaxis. Quinolones such as ciprofloxin are also effective.

6. What are the most common gram-negative bacilli causing meningitis after the neonatal period?

Klebsiella spp., *Escherichia coli,* and *Pseudomonas* spp. account for 75–90% of gram-negative bacillary meningitis after the neonatal period. Eighty percent of gram-negative meningitis occurs in conjunction with head trauma or neurosurgical procedures.

7. Which organisms are most likely to cause meningitis after neurosurgical procedures?

Gram-negative bacilli and staphylococci are the most common organisms, but virtually any kind of bacteria and even fungi such as *Candida* spp. can gain access to the subarachnoid region.

Morris A, Lowe DE: Nosocomial bacterial meningitis, including central nervous system shunt infections. Infect Dis Clin North Am 13:735–750, 1999.

8. In a patient with a ventriculoatrial or ventriculoperitoneal shunt, what is the most common cause of bacterial meningitis?

Coagulase-negative staphylococci account for > 50% of cases of meningitis in patients with ventricular shunts, followed by *Staphylococcus aureus, Propionibacterium acnes,* gram-negative bacilli, and enterococci.

9. What bacteria is the most common cause of meningitis in patients with a CSF leak?

Streptococcus pneumoniae.

Durand ML, Calderwood SB, Weber DJ, et al: Acute bacterial meningitis in adults. N Engl J Med 328:21, 1993.

10. What is the most common cause of meningitis after blunt head trauma?

Streptococcus pneumoniae.

11. What are the most common clinical settings in which brain abscesses develop?

1. Contiguous suppurative foci such as otitis media or sinusitis
2. Hematogenous spread from a distant focus
3. Penetrating cranial injuries or neurosurgical procedures
4. Cryptogenic (20% of cases)

Mathisen GE, Johnson JP: Brain abscess. Clin Infect Dis 25:763–781, 1997.

12. Describe the presentation of a brain abscess.

A brain abscess often presents with symptoms similar to those of a brain tumor, but they are more rapidly progressive. Headache, focal neurologic signs dependent on the site of the lesion, and signs of increased intracranial pressure are present. Fever and elevated white blood cell count are *not* common.

13. How does an abscess appear on CT scan?

An abscess appears as a hypodense lesion surrounded by a contrast-enhancing ring. A thin-walled ring is more common in an abscess, whereas a thick-walled, irregular ring is more characteristic of tumor.

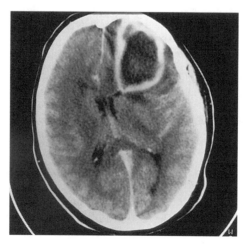

CT scan of the head showing a contrast-enhancing ring around a large frontal lobe brain abscess.

14. What is the most common bacterial agent involved in spinal epidural abscess?

S. aureus accounts for approximately 62% of cases; aerobic gram-negative rods for 18%; aerobic streptococci for 8%; and *Staphylococcus epidermidis* and anaerobes for about 2% each. Unknown or other organisms (1%) cause the remainder. Empirical antibiotics must include an antistaphylococcal agent. Gram-negative coverage may be warranted in patients with a history of a spinal procedure, intravenous drug abuse, or recent gastrointestinal or genitourinary infection. Antibiotic therapy is required for 4–6 weeks, and prompt surgical drainage may be needed.

    Wheeler D, Keiser P, Rigamonti D, Keay SL: Medical management of spinal epidural abscesses. Clin Infect Dis 15:22, 1992.

15. Describe the clinical course of an untreated spinal epidural abscess.

The first symptom noted is usually focal vertebral pain, followed by root pain, then deficits of motor, sensory, or sphincter function, and finally paralysis.

16. What conditions predispose to recurrent bacterial meningitis?

    1. Anatomic communications with paranasal sinuses, nasopharynx, middle ear, skin (such as congenital midline dermal sinus tracts), or prosthetic devices such as ventriculoperitoneal shunts.

    2. Parameningeal foci may either drain into the meninges or lead to repeated inflammatory reactions and meningeal signs or symptoms.

    3. Immunologic defects such as hypogammaglobulinemia, splenectomy, leukemia and lymphoma, sickle cell anemia and other hemoglobinopathies, or complement deficiencies.

17. Name conditions that predispose to polymicrobial meningitis.

    1. Infections at contiguous foci

    2. Tumors in close proximity to the central nervous system

    3. Fistulous communications

    4. Disseminated strongyloidiasis (enteric organisms carried "piggy-back" from the gut through the bloodstream to the subarachnoid space)

18. A 72-year-old man was hospitalized 1 week ago for stroke. He has dense right hemiplegia and is incontinent of bowel and bladder. Today he developed a fever of 101° F, along with shaking chills. What sources are most likely responsible?

The cause of fever is probably a nosocomial infection. A lower urinary tract infection is most likely—whether he has a Foley catheter, a condom catheter, or a neurogenic bladder that does not fully empty. Other good possibilities include pneumonia (especially aspiration pneumonia) or venous catheter-related infection.

19. An elderly man taking steroids chronically for lung disease presents with a history and physical exam consistent with meningitis and new-onset seizures. The laboratory tells you that the "preliminary" exam of the CSF shows "diphtheroids" on the Gram stain. What organism is probably responsible for the infection?

Listeria spp. may be mistaken for diphtheroids on Gram stain; both are gram-positive bacilli. Listerial infection often occurs in immunocompromised patients. Risk factors include cirrhosis, neoplastic disease, renal failure, pregnancy, chronic steroid therapy, and extremes of age (i.e., very young and elderly). Some outbreaks have been traced to food-borne sources, and the disease has been classically associated with animal exposure. CSF cell counts, protein, and glucose are variable and do not distinguish listerial infection from other forms of meningitis. Monocytosis is not common. Common treatment is with ampicillin and an aminoglycoside. Cephalosporins are not effective.

    Mylonakis E, Hohman E, Caldewood B: Central nervous system infection with *Listeria monocytogenes.* Medicine 77:313–316, 1998.

20. A 14-year-old boy whose only medical problem is acne presents with diplopia, photophobia, and right periorbital edema. His neurologic examination reveals a midposition, fixed right pupil, decreased sensation over the upper face, right ophthalmoplegia, and papilledema on the right. What is wrong?

The symptoms and signs are consistent with an infectious cavernous sinus thrombosis on the right, most likely from squeezing a pimple. Untreated, he may develop progressive exophthalmos, loss of corneal reflex, retinal hemorrhage, and visual loss. As the infection spreads to the contralateral cavernous sinus, similar findings appear in the opposite eye. Cranial nerves III, IV, V, and VI are affected as they pass through the cavernous sinuses.

21. A 57-year-old diabetic man presents with a right facial nerve palsy, otalgia, and otorrhea. What is the most likely organism?
The condition is most often due to *Pseudomonas aeruginosa*, producing the syndrome of necrotizing or "malignant" external otitis.

22. In what clinical situations does a CNS infection merit the use of systemic steroids?
1. An infant with *H. influenzae* meningitis
2. A severely ill adult with tuberculous meningitis
3. A patient with neurocysticercosis and increased intracranial pressure

ANTIBIOTIC TOXICITY

23. What is the clinical presentation of a patient receiving excessive doses of beta-lactam antibiotics?
Toxicity may cause confusion, jitteriness, myoclonic jerks, and seizures.

24. In addition to aminoglycosides, what other drugs cause ototoxicity?
1. Ethacrynic acid—probably the highest risk
2. Furosemide
3. Erythromycin—usually reversible hearing loss with high-dose therapy
4. Vancomycin—listed as ototoxic, but if so, rarely

25. Which conditions predispose to peripheral neuropathy in patients who take isoniazid?
Peripheral neuropathy is especially likely to occur in patients who are slow acetylators, are poorly nourished, or have an underlying neuropathy secondary to diabetes, uremia, or alcoholism. Concomitant administration of pyridoxine (vitamin B6) may prevent the neuropathy.

TOXINS

26. What three bacteria produce exotoxins that affect peripheral nerves either directly or indirectly?
1. The B subunit of diphtheria toxin binds to cell membranes and allows the A subunit to enter nerves, where it inhibits protein synthesis and causes a noninflammatory demyelination. Cranial nerves are affected more frequently than peripheral nerves.
2. Tetanus toxin is transported up the axon and binds to the presynaptic endings on motor neurons in the anterior horns of the spinal cord. Inhibitory input is blocked, resulting in muscle spasms.
3. Botulinum toxin binds to the presynaptic axon terminal of the neuromuscular junction, preventing acetylcholine release and producing a flaccid paralysis.

27. What are the manifestations of ciguatera? How does one acquire this illness?
Patients ingest ciguatoxin, produced by the dinoflagellate *Gambierdiscus toxicus*, when they eat large, carnivorous reef fish such as grouper or snapper. Within about 6 hours, GI symptoms of nausea, vomiting, diarrhea, and cramps begin. Bizarre neurologic symptoms may appear early or after the GI complaints and resolve in 24–48 hours. Neurologic manifestations include numbness and tingling of lips and extremities, reversal of hot-cold sensation, and tooth pain. Paresthesias may not follow dermatomal patterns. Vertigo, hypersalivation, blurred vision, tremor, ataxia, and coma may occur.

28. What illness is caused by eating puffer fish?
Tetrodotoxication occurs within 3 hours of eating a tetrodotoxic fish such as puffer fish, porcupine fish, ocean sunfish, blue-ringed octopus, and some species of newts and salamanders.

Symptoms include lethargy, paresthesias, hyperemesis, salivation, weakness, ataxia, and dysphagia. Ascending paralysis, respiratory failure, hypotension, and bradycardia may occur. Diagnosis is clinical, and treatment is supportive. Gastric lavage, activated charcoal, and anticholinesterase inhibitors may be helpful.

29. What are the symptoms of scombroid poisoning?

Symptoms of scombroid poisoning begin within minutes to hours of ingestion of toxic fish. The fish are usually of the family Scombridae, which includes tuna, mackerel, and jacks, but cases are also reported from nonscombroid fish. Victims experience flushing and a hot sensation of the skin, headache, dizziness, burning sensation in the mouth and throat, and palpitations. Nausea, diarrhea, and occasionally vomiting occur. A sunburn-like skin rash appears. In severe case, bronchospasm, palpitations, supraventricular arrhythmias, and occasionally mild hypotension may occur. The diagnosis is clinical. Treatment is supportive. Deaths have not been reported.

30. What is the scombrotoxin?

The scombrotoxin is formed when surface bacteria (*Proteus* and *Klebsiella* spp.) proliferate on the flesh of the fish because of improper refrigeration. Free histidine, present in increased quantities in dark meat fish, is degraded to histamine by the bacteria. The exact role of histamine is unclear because orally ingested histamine is degraded in the gastrointestinal tract, but a histamine-like substance such as saurine produces the clinical effects. Another substance in the fish may prevent degradation or increase absorption of histamine.

Clark RF, et al: A review of selected seafood poisonings. Undersea Hyperbar Med 26(3):175–185, 1999.

SPIROCHETAL INFECTIONS

31. What serologic laboratory tests are used to assist in the diagnosis of syphilis? How should they be interpreted?

Two general classes of lab tests are used: nontreponemal antigen tests and treponemal tests. The nontreponemal tests use extract of normal tissues (i.e., beef cardiolipin) as antigens to measure antibodies formed in the blood. The commonly used nontreponemal tests are the rapid plasma reagin (RPR) and Venereal Disease Research Laboratory (VDRL) tests. Both become positive in the early stages of the primary lesion and are almost always positive by the secondary stage. They decline in later stages of the disease. False-positive results occur in autoimmune illness, malaria, mononucleosis, and pregnancy, among others. The nontreponemal tests, therefore, should be used as a screening test for the more specific treponemal tests. They also may be used to follow response to treatment because they decline with time after successful treatment. The treponemal tests use live or killed *Treponema pallidum* as antigen to detect treponemal antibody directly. The commonly used treponemal tests are the microhemagglutination test for antibody to *T. pallidum* (MHA-TP) and the fluorescent treponemal antibody absorption test (FTA-ABS). These tests remain positive even after appropriate treatment.

If a patient has strongly positive serum RPR or VDRL and MHA-TP or FTA-ABS tests and symptoms consistent with neurosyphilis, most experts agree that the patient should undergo a lumbar puncture, if feasible, to look for a positive VDRL and/or MHA-TP in the CSF, which helps to confirm the need for treatment for neurosyphilis. These tests may be falsely negative even in CSF. If clinical suspicion is high enough, most clinicians treat for neurosyphilis. Obtaining documentation of prior treatment for syphilis is important, because it can obviously shorten the evaluation considerably.

32. How frequent are abnormalities in the CSF of patient with primary or secondary syphilis?

Abnormalities in the CSF are found in 15–40% of patients who have primary or secondary syphilis and are usually asymptomatic.

Musher DM, Hamill RJ, Baughan RE: Effects of human immunodeficiency virus (HIV) infection on the course of syphilis and on the response to treatment. Ann Intern Med 113:872–881, 1990.

33. At what stage of syphilis (primary, secondary, or tertiary) does neurosyphilis occur?

Neurosyphilis may occur in any stage of syphilis. CNS invasion by *T. pallidum* occurs in nearly one-third of patients with primary and secondary syphilis.

Simon RP: Neurosyphilis. Neurology 44:2228, 1994.

34. What circumstances predispose to early neurosyphilis?

Inadequate treatment of early syphilis and HIV infection predisposes to early neurosyphilis.

Musher DM, Hamill RJ, Baughan RE: Effects of human immunodeficiency virus (HIV) infection on the course of syphilis and on the response to treatment. Ann Intern Med 113:872–881, 1990.

35. Which cranial nerves are most often involved in syphilitic meningitis?

Syphilis affects the seventh and eighth cranial nerves most often (40%) and the second, third, and fourth cranial nerves less frequently (25%).

36. What are the neurologic complications of Lyme disease?

Early in the course, meningitis, cranial neuritis, Bell's palsy, motor or sensory radiculoneuritis, subtle encephalitis, mononeuritis multiplex, myelitis, chorea, or cerebellar ataxia may occur. Chronically, patients may develop encephalitis, spastic paraparesis, ataxic gait, subtle mental disorders, chronic axonal polyradiculography, or dementia.

Pfister HW, Wilske B, Weber K: Lyme borreliosis: Basic science and clinical aspects. Lancet 393:1013, 1994.

Halperin JJ: Nervous system Lyme disease. Neurol Sci 133(2):189–191, 1998.

37. What is the most likely clinical presentation of infection with *Borrelia burgdorferi* (Lyme disease)?

A 10-cm erythematous lesion with central clearing on the patient's back. The presence of the typical tick-bite wound is a more reliable guide to infection than serologic titers or (often vague) clinical symptoms.

38. What is the clinical presentation of leptospirosis?

Leptospirosis often develops after a camping trip and may present as aseptic meningitis (with normal CSF glucose), bulbar conjunctivitis, erythematous rash, adenopathy, hepatosplenomegaly, and renal insufficiency.

FUNGAL, PARASITIC, AND OTHER PROCESSES

39. Describe the clinical presentation of infection with *Acanthamoeba* or *Naegleria* spp.

Both infections usually present as severe persistent frontal headache after swimming in a fresh-water lake.

40. What neurologic abnormalities occur with cerebral malaria? What does the spinal fluid show?

Neurologic abnormalities include disturbances of consciousness, acute organic brain syndromes, seizures, meningismus, and, rarely, focal neurologic signs. A lumbar puncture usually reveals an elevated opening pressure with normal CSF. Occasionally CSF protein is elevated. Low-level pleocytosis occurs, but hypoglycorrhachia does not. Therapy is with quinine, chloroquine, and dexamethasone.

41. What is the epidemiology of neurocysticercosis?

Infection with eggs of the pork tapeworm, *Taenia solium*, can lead to neurocysticercosis. In the intermediate stage, it is referred to as *Cysticercus cellulosae*, but *T. solium* and *C. cellulosae* are the same parasite. Ingestion of measled (infected pork) → intestinal tapeworm (often asymptomatic) → fecal excretion → human fecal-oral contamination → egg ingestion and penetration of intestinal wall → oncospheres → larvae that encyst → neurocysticercosis. Therapy is with praziquantel, 50 mg/kg for 15–30 days.

The clinical presentation of neurocysticercosis depends on the number and location of the cysts but usually includes seizures. Headache, altered mental status, or symptoms of hydrocephalus may occur. Disease may be active or inactive; this distinction guides further evaluation and treatment.

White AC Jr: Neurocysticercosis: Updates on epidemiology, pathogenesis, diagnosis and management. Annu Rev Med 51:187–206, 2000.

42. A 21-year-old archeology student complains of headache, fever, lethargy, and difficulty with concentrating in class. He had been well until 2 months previously, when he had a brief illness with fever, arthralgia, cough, and sputum production just after he returned from a dig in Arizona. He was again well until his current symptoms began 2 weeks ago. What is his probable diagnosis? How should he be treated?

The most likely diagnosis is coccidioidomycosis meningitis. He needs intrathecal amphotericin B as well as small doses of systemic amphotericin. Treatment will be long-term, and relapses are common. Other drugs that may have a role are fluconazole and itraconazole.

43. Which antifungal agents are most useful in CNS infections because of their good spinal fluid penetration?

Amphotericin B and fluconazole enter the CSF adequately. Ketoconazole has poor penetration.

44. What are the side effects of treatment with amphotericin?

Amphotericin may produce fever, chills, hypotension, nausea, headache, and tachypnea during or shortly after administration. Premedication with antipyretics and supplemental intravenous hydration may reduce these effects. Meperidine has been used to reduce discomfort secondary to severe chills. Renal impairment may occur, chiefly in the form of decreased glomerular filtration rate and increased blood urea nitrogen and creatinine. But hypokalemia and hypomagnesemia also result from renal wastage and renal tubular acidosis. Hydration may lessen renal side effects.

45. Describe the presentation of tuberculous meningitis.

The onset of symptoms is usually gradual, and behavioral changes may precede more classic symptoms of headache, vomiting, seizures, and cranial nerve abnormalities. A focus of tuberculosis may be found in another organ system. Meningitis follows rupture of subependymal lesions (Rich foci) into the subarachnoid space. Basilar inflammation with cranial nerve entrapment and severe arteriolitis with subsequent thrombosis (commonly of middle and anterior cerebral artery territory) is characteristic.

CSF shows increased protein, decreased glucose, increased opening pressure, and 50–1000 WBC (polymorphonuclear cells predominate early, lymphocytes predominate late). Acid-fast stains and cultures are often negative in the presence of disease. Treatment with antituberculous drugs should be initiated if clinical suspicion is high. Initial concurrent treatment with steroids is controversial.

46. A patient in whom you are about to begin high-dose steroids has a purified protein derivative test (PPD) that is positive at 17 mm with a known negative PPD 1 year ago. What should you do before beginning steroids?

The patient should have a chest radiograph to exclude evidence of active pulmonary tuberculosis. If the chest radiograph is positive, the patient needs treatment for pulmonary tuberculosis. If no evidence of active infection is found, the patient needs isoniazid prophylaxis for tuberculosis because of the recent and strongly positive conversion and immunosuppression by steroids.

47. An 82-year-old woman presents with fever, sweats, generalized body aches, weakness, severe headache, and weight loss. She describes intermittent cough and painful jaw muscles while chewing food. Her laboratory studies show anemia, elevated alkaline phosphatase, and sedimentation rate of 92 mm/hr. What is the diagnosis?

Temporal arteritis. This granulomatous arteritis often mimics an infectious disease.

48. A patient whom you diagnosed 1 year previously with temporal arteritis has done well on her therapy. She returns for an office visit and complains of dysphagia and weight loss. What do you suspect?

Infectious esophagitis. *Candida* spp. or perhaps herpes simplex virus is the most likely pathogen in a patient who has taken long-term steroids.

49. What is Vogt-Koyanagi-Harada syndrome?

This syndrome consists of subacute meningoencephalitis with severe, protracted granluomatous uveitis and depigmentary skin changes. The cause is unknown, but it is noninfectious. Other noninfectious lymphocytic meningitides include Behçet's disease and CNS vasculitides.

50. What is neuroleptic malignant syndrome (NMS)?

NMS is a noninfectious cause of fever characterized by autonomic and extrapyramidal dysfunction as a consequence of neuroleptic drug use (e.g., haloperidol, chlorpromazine, fluphenazine). Major clinical findings include fever, hyperreflexia, tachypnea, diaphoresis, altered mental status, labile blood pressure, tremor, and rigidity. Laboratory findings include elevated creatine phosphokinase (CPK), leukocytosis, myoglobinuria, and metabolic acidosis. Therapy involves immediate discontinuation of neuroleptics and treatment with dantrolene and bromocriptine.

Caroff SN, Mann SC: Neuroleptic malignant syndrome. Med Clin North Am 77:185–202, 1993.

51. What is Whipple disease? Describe the central nervous system (CNS) manifestations.

Whipple disease is a systemic illness caused by *Tropheryma whippelli*, a gram-positive bacillus. Gastrointestinal signs and symptoms are usually primary components of the illness and include weight loss, diarrhea, and malabsorption. Arthralgias, pleural effusions, and fever also may be present. CNS involvement can include upper motor neuron signs, hypothalamic dysfunction, supranuclear gaze palsy, and cognitive and psychiatric aberrations. CNS findings are rare in the absence of systemic illness but have been reported.

Mandell K, Tranel D, Cooper G: Cognitive and behavioral abnormalities in a case of central nervous system Whipple disease. Arch Neurol 57:399–403, 2000.

PRIONS

52. What is a prion? Why is it important in neurologic disease?

A prion is a small proteinaceous infectious particle that resists inactivation by procedures that modify nucleic acids. The concept of an infectious agent that does not require DNA or RNA is novel. This type of agent is thought to be responsible for scrapie, Creutzfeldt-Jakob disease, and kuru.

Haywood AM: Transmissible spongiform encephalopathies. N Engl J Med 337:1821–1827, 1997.

53. A 45-year-old man presents with myoclonus and dementia that have progressed rapidly over the past 6 months. CSF is normal. What is the likely diagnosis? What does his EEG show?

The patient has findings characteristic of Creutzfeldt-Jakob disease. Dementia progresses rapidly over months, and death usually occurs in less than 1 year. The EEG characteristically (but not always) has periodic-appearing, biphasic or triphasic, high-amplitude sharp waves. CSF is usually normal, although a mild elevation in protein is occasionally found.

54. What is the pathologic lesion in Creutzfeldt-Jakob disease?

The pathologic lesion is spongiform encephalopathy characterized by loss of neurons, with astrocytic proliferation and gliosis, swelling, and intracytoplasmic vacuolization of neuronal and astroglial processes.

55. What infection control measures should be observed for a patient with Creutzfeldt-Jakob disease?

Blood, brain, cornea, visceral organs, and CSF are infectious. Autoclaving for 1 hour at 250°F and 15 psi, exposure to 1 N or 0.1 N sodium hydroxide for 1 hour at room temperature, or exposure to 0.5% sodium hydrochlorite will kill the causative agent. Of note, the agent is not destroyed by boiling, ultraviolet radiation, ionizing radiation, 70% ethyl alcohol, formaldehyde, glutaraldehyde, or 10% formalin. The patient need not be isolated, but blood and body fluid precautions should be observed.

56. What is "mad cow" disease?

Mad cow disease is the sobriquet of bovine spongiform encephalopathy (BSE), a variant of Creutzfeldt-Jakob disease recently described in a series of young patients in the United Kingdom. It is believed to be transmissible by consumption of contaminated beef. Studies are under way to determine the scope of the problem and measures needed for containment.

Weihl C, Ross R: Creutzfeldt-Jakob disease, new variant Creutzfeldt-Jakob disease, and bovine spongiform encephalopathy. Neurol Clin 17:835–854, 1999.

57. What is kuru? How is it transmitted?

Kuru, another disease caused by prions, is transmitted by cannibalism. New Guinea natives practicing ritualistic consumption of dead kinsmen (including their brains) as a rite of mourning developed this illness. Clinically, kuru presents as a progressive fatal dementia with severe ataxia.

VIRAL INFECTIONS

58. When may aseptic meningitis be confused with bacterial meningitis? How do you resolve the confusion?

Early in viral meningitis, the spinal fluid may have a predominance of polymorphonuclear (PMN) leukocytes. The Gram stain is negative, and CSF glucose is normal. Because the PMN predominance quickly changes to a mononuclear cell predominance, a repeat lumbar puncture 6–12 hours later will clarify the issue.

59. Other than culture results, which of the routine studies performed on CSF is the most useful for distinguishing between meningitis due to tuberculosis and that due to a virus, such as ECHO 9? What does ECHO stand for?

The glucose test is most useful. Glucose is usually low in tuberculous infection, but normal in viral infections. ECHO = enteric cytopathic human orphan [virus].

60. Worldwide, what is the most common cause of epidemic encephalitis?

Japanese B encephalitis is the most common epidemic infection outside North America. It is a major medical problem in China, Southwest Asia, and India.

61. What is the most common sporadic encephalitis in the United States?

Herpes simplex causes encephalitis most frequently.

Whitley RJ: Viral encephalitis. N Engl J Med 323:242–250, 1990.

62. What are the common arthropod-borne viral encephalitides in the United States?

1. **St. Louis encephalitis** occurs in the central, western, and southern U.S. and affects older adults.

2. **La Crosse encephalitis:** La Crosse, a type of California encephalitis, is a common arthropod-borne encephalitis in the United States. It occurs in the central and eastern U.S. and primarily affects children. It has a mortality of < 1%, and sequelae are rare.

3. **Venezuelan equine encephalitis** occurs in the South, affects adults, and has low mortality and sequelae rates.

4. **Western equine encephalitis** occurs in the West and Midwest, affecting people at extremes of age. Mortality is 5–15%, and sequelae are more common in infants than in older survivors.

5. **Eastern equine encephalitis** affects children in the East, South, and Gulf Coast. Mortality is 50–75%, and 80% of survivors have sequelae.

Johnson P: Acute encephalitis. Clin Infect Dis 23:219–226, 1996.

63. What are the major differences between Western, Eastern, and Venezuelan equine encephalitis?

1. **Eastern:** a summertime disease that causes less than 15 human cases per year but has a 50–75% mortality rate. It strikes mainly in the Gulf/Atlantic states.

2. **Venezuelan:** occurs in epidemics that have caused tens of thousands of cases but with a fatality rate of only 0.6%; mainly in Central and South America.

3. **Western:** occurs in the summer months also, usually in states west of the Mississippi. It causes 0–200 cases/year, and infants are most susceptible. The risk is greatest in rural areas. The case fatality rate is 3–5%.

64. What is West Nile encephalitis?

West Nile encephalitis is caused by a flavivirus endemic in Africa, West Asia, and the Middle East. It is related to St. Louis encephalitis. Recently cases of West Nile encephalitis have been reported in New York, and the virus has been isolated in the local mosquito population. Symptoms are usually mild and include headache, fever, and myalgias, but severe forms of the illness also occur.

Centers for Disease Control and Prevention: Update: West Nile activity in the Northeastern United States. MMWR 49(31):714–718, 2000.

65. A patient presents with aphasia, right-sided weakness, fever, and confusion. A lumbar puncture reveals CSF with 400 RBC/mm³, 30 WBC/mm³ (predominantly mononuclear cells), glucose of 70 mg/dl, and protein of 60 mg/dl. EEG shows periodic high-voltage spike wave activity from the left temporal region. What is the most likely causative agent?

Herpes simplex encephalitis. The main clue to herpes vs. other causes of viral encephalitis is focality, especially to the temporal lobe.

66. What are typical CSF findings in herpes encephalitis?

Normal CSF cell counts and chemistries are occasionally seen in herpes simplex virus (HSV) encephalitis. Typical CSF findings are lymphocytic predominance, elevated protein, and the presence of RBCs. In most cases, HSV cannot be cultured from the CSF. Diagnosis may be made with polymerase chain reaction (PCR) for herpes DNA in CSF.

67. What histopathologic finding is pathognomonic for herpes encephalitis?

The Cowdry type A inclusion body, an eosinophilic, intranuclear particle.

68. What is the recommended therapy for HSV encephalitis?

Treatment requires acyclovir, 10 mg/kg every 8 hours for at least 14 days. Because acyclovir is cleared by the kidney, the dose requires adjustment for renal insufficiency, and patients with normal renal function should be encouraged to drink generous amounts of free water each day.

69. A 32-year-old woman presents with painful genital vesicular lesions, urinary retention, and severe headache. CSF shows lymphocytic pleocytosis. The neurologic examination is otherwise unremarkable. What is the probable diagnosis?

Herpes simplex virus II meningitis. Genital lesions usually recur, but the meningitis usually does not. It has an excellent prognosis neurologically. This benign form of "aseptic" meningitis should not be confused with the potentially fatal, necrotizing form of HSV 1 encephalitis.

70. What is Ramsey-Hunt syndrome?

Herpes zoster infection involving cranial nerves VII and VIII. Patients present with vertigo, ipsilateral hearing deficit, and facial palsy plus vesicles in the external auditory canal.

71. What are the most important neurologic complications of primary varicella infections?

1. Reye syndrome. This acute, noninflammatory encephalopathy is characterized by fatty destruction of the liver, hypoglycemia, and increased intracranial pressure. It has a 20% fatality rate. Aspirin use with varicella and influenza has been associated with Reye syndrome in children.

2. Aseptic meningitis
3. Transverse myelitis
4. Guillain-Barré syndrome
5. Cerebellar encephalitis. In children, it results in ataxia, nausea, and rigidity, but most make a full recovery. In adults, it results in altered sensorium, seizures, focal signs, and a mortality rate up to 35%.

72. Which two viruses enter the CNS by peripheral intraneural routes to cause encephalitis?

Herpes simplex and rabies viruses enter the nervous system by peripheral intraneuronal routes. One route for HSV may be the olfactory tract.

73. Who should receive postexposure rabies prophylaxis?

Postexposure prophylaxis for rabies is recommended for all persons bitten or scratched by wild or domestic animals that may be carrying the disease or who have an open wound or mucous membrane contaminated with saliva or other potentially infectious material from a rabid animal. It is also recommended for persons who report a possibly infectious exposure to a human with rabies. Potentially rabid animals include (but are not limited to) dogs, cats, skunks, raccoons, foxes, and bats.

74. Which infections may lead to a postinfectious encephalomyelitis?

Immune-mediated inflammation following an infection, sometimes called acute disseminated encephalomyelitis, usually presents with multifocal lesions of the brain and spinal cord that may closely resemble multiple sclerosis. This demyelinating syndrome is most common after infections with varicella, influenza, and measles virus.

Johnson R: Acute encephalitis. Clin Infect Dis 23:219–226, 1996.

75. What clinical features characterize postpolio syndrome?

The main symptoms of postpolio syndrome are the new onset of weakness, pain, and fatigue years after acute poliomyelitis. About 25% of survivors of polio are affected. EMG and muscle biopsy show evidence of both chronic and recent denervation, although these changes are nonspecific; asymptomatic survivors of polio also exhibit these changes.

76. What virus appears to be the most common cause of Bell's palsy?

Recent studies implicate herpes simplex as the cause of Bell's palsy. Some studies have shown superior response to treatment with acyclovir and prednisone as opposed to prednisone alone; however, clear benefit has not been shown in all studies.

Adour KK, et al: Bell's Palsy: Treatment with acyclovir and prednisone compared with prednisone alone: A double blind randomized, controlled trial. Ann Otol Rhinol Laryngol 105:371–378, 1996.

AIDS

77. Which antiretroviral drug may cause myopathy and myositis?

Zidovudine (AZT) may cause both myopathy and myositis, especially with long-term therapy. It is often difficult to distinguish this entity from myopathy due to HIV itself, but a drug holiday usually makes the distinction. In addition, muscle biopsy shows abnormal mitochondria in AZT-induced myopathy.

78. Which mediations used to treat HIV may cause peripheral neuropathy?

D4T (Zerit), ddI (Videx), ddC (Hivid), and 3TC (lamivudine) have been shown to cause neuropathy. The first three medications may have added toxicity when combined.

79. What is the most common type of peripheral neuropathy in patients with HIV infection?

A chronic, distal, symmetric polyneuropathy is most common. It is predominantly sensory with painful dysthesias, numbness, and paresthesias. Weakness or autonomic dysfunction is less frequent. Occasionally, a chronic or acute inflammatory demyelinating polyneuropathy is seen.

80. How is the acute, inflammatory, demyelinating neuropathy of HIV infection distinguished from Guillain-Barré syndrome?

In the HIV-related disorder, CSF pleocytosis ranges from 10–50 cells/mm³ along with CSF protein elevation. In Guillain-Barré syndrome, pleocytosis generally does not occur.

81. What CSF findings do you expect in a patient with HIV-associated aseptic meningitis?

Like other causes of viral meningitis, HIV infection may produce a mononuclear pleocytosis with 20–300 cells/mm³ and a protein elevation in the range of 50–100 mg/dl. Meningeal signs, headache, fever, and cranial nerve palsies, especially of the fifth, seventh, and eighth cranial nerves, also occur.

Hollander H, McGuire D, Burack JH: Diagnostic lumbar puncture in HIV-infected patients: Analysis of 138 cases. Am J Med 96:223–228, 1994.

82. What are the most common causes of new-onset seizures in patients with HIV infection?

Toxoplasmosis, HIV encephalopathy, cryptococcus, and lymphoma.

83. A patient treated with phenytoin for many years was seizure-free until initiation of treatment of HIV. What medication may the patient be taking?

AZT may decrease serum phenytoin levels so that the patient now requires a higher dose to achieve therapeutic levels.

84. What clinical feature distinguishes AIDS dementia complex from Creutzfeldt-Jakob disease?

In AIDS dementia, a normal level of consciousness is usually maintained, even late in the disease, unless some other systemic disease intervenes. This is not true in Creutzfeldt-Jakob disease, which otherwise is clinically similar to AIDS dementia.

Simpson DM, Tagliati M: Neurologic manifestations of HIV infection. Ann Intern Med 121:769–785, 1994.

85. A patient with known AIDS complains of decreased visual acuity. What infectious agents are most likely responsible?

Cytomegalovirus (CMV) retinitis is most common, occurring in about 30% of patients with AIDS. Toxoplasmosis is probably the second most common retinal infection, accounting for only 4% of retinitis cases. Ocular syphilis may manifest as iridocyclitis, neuroretinitis, optic perineuritis, and retrobulbar neuritis. HIV infection itself may cause cotton-wool spots that usually are not visually significant. A rare cause of retinitis is tuberculosis.

de Smet MD, Nussenblatt RB: Ocular manifestations of AIDS. JAMA 266:3019–3022, 1991.

86. What are the diagnostic features of toxoplasma encephalitis in patients with AIDS?

Most patients have elevated IgG antibodies to toxoplasma. The absence of toxoplasma IgG in a patient with suspected toxoplasma encephalitis militates strongly against the diagnosis. Routine analyses of the CSF may be normal. Contrast-enhanced CT scans demonstrate nodular or ring-enhancing lesions in more than 90% of patients. The treatment of choice is high-dose pyrimethamine and sulfadiazine.

87. What is PML? How does it present?

Progressive multifocal leukoencephalopathy (PML) is an opportunistic infection caused by a polyomavirus called the JC virus (JCV). It occurs in HIV-infected patients and other immunocompromised hosts. It is characterized by patchy areas of demyelination in the white matter of the cerebral hemispheres. The clinical presentation is diverse, reflects the scattered areas of demyelination, and progresses rapidly. Motor weakness, personality changes, dementia, ataxia, and cortical blindness occur and may culminate in coma. Survival after diagnosis is often less than 6 months.

88. How does cryptococcal meningitis present in an HIV-positive patient?
The common presentation includes fever, altered mentation, headache, and meningismus. Papilledema may result from increased intracranial pressure. CSF cell counts and chemistries may be minimally altered. Cryptococcal antigen is the most sensitive marker of infection. India ink stain may be positive but has a high rate of false negatives. Initial treatment is with amphotericin B with or without flucytosine. Chronic suppressive treatment must be continued with fluconazole, and relapses are common.

89. Numerous patients with AIDS are sulfa-allergic. In patients with sulfa allergy, what is the treatment of choice for toxoplasma encephalitis?
Clindamycin, 600 mg intravenously every 6 hours, plus pyrimethamine, 200 mg, then 75–100 mg/day orally, plus folinic acid, at least 10 mg/day orally.
Dannemann B, McCutchan A, Israelski D, et al: Treatment of toxoplasmic encephalitis in patients with AIDS. Ann Intern Med 116:33–43, 1992.

90. What are the most common presentations of neurosyphilis in patients with HIV infection?
1. Acute meningitis
2. Cranial neuropathy
   Optic neuritis
   Eighth cranial nerve palsy
3. Meningovascular, causing strokes

91. How does HIV infection affect the diagnosis of syphilis?
Patients with HIV infection, especially with a very low CD4 lymphocyte count, may lose reactivity to treponemal tests for syphilis. Both FTA-ABS and MHA-TP tests may be negative in patients with prior syphilis infection and HIV infection.
Haas JS, et al: Sensitivity of treponemal tests for detecting prior treated syphilis during human immunodeficiency virus infection. J Infect Dis 162:862–866, 1990.

92. How does HIV affect the course of syphilis?
HIV infection may cause failure to respond to treatment within the expected time frame, a higher rate of false-negative serologic tests, relapse of infection after treatment, and frequent appearance of early neurosyphilis. Conventional doses of penicillin may not be adequate. Three doses of benzathine penicillin, 2.4 million units at weekly intervals, has been suggested for treatment of primary or secondary infection. Alternative regimens have been suggested—amoxicillin (up to 6 gm/day) or supplementing three doses of benzathine penicillin with oral penicillin or amoxicillin for a 2- to 3-week period, or ceftriaxone, 500 mg or 1 gm, given daily or every other day for 5–10 days.
Musher DM, Hamill RJ, Baughn RE: Effect of human immunodeficiency virus (HIV) infection on the course of syphilis and on the response to treatment. Ann Intern Med 113:872–881, 1990.

BIBLIOGRAPHY

1. Mandell GI, Douglas RG, Burnett JE: Principles and Practice of Infectious Disease, 5th ed. New York, Churchill Livingstone, 2000.
2. Price RW: Neurological complications of HIV infection. Lancet 348:445–452, 1996.
3. Samuels MA, Feske S (eds): Office Practice of Neurology, 2nd ed. New York, Churchill Livingstone, 2001.
Websites
www.cdc.gov/ncidod/dbmd/diseaseinfo/meningococcal_g.htm
www.postgradmed.com/issues/1998/03_98/guti.htm
www.nmia.com/%7emdibble/prion.html

25. PEDIATRIC NEUROLOGY

Angus A. Wilfong, M.D., F.R.C.P.C.

NORMAL NEUROLOGIC GROWTH AND DEVELOPMENT

1. In addition to the routine questions asked during a neurologic interview, what additional questions are important for a complete pediatric neurology history?

Pediatric Neurology History

I. Antenatal
  A. Maternal parity
  B. Previous miscarriages or abortions
  C. Illnesses during the pregnancy
  D. Maternal nutrition and supplementation
    1. Weight gain
    2. Uterine size
  E. Medications taken during the pregnancy
    1. Prescription
    2. Over-the-counter
  F. Illicit drug abuse
  G. Alcohol use
  H. Cigarette use
  I. Toxic exposures
    1. Occupational
    2. Industrial
    3. Agricultural
    4. Irradiation
  J. Accidents and trauma
  K. Travel abroad
  L. Fetal movements
  M. Premature labor contractions
  N. Vaginal spotting or bleeding
  O. Premature rupture of the membranes

II. Perinatal
  A. Spontaneous or induced labor
  B. Duration of labor
  C. Fetal monitoring during labor
  D. Type of delivery
    1. Vaginal
      a. Vertex
      b. Breech
      c. Forceps or vacuum assisted
        (1) failure to progress
        (2) fetal distress
    2. Cesarean section
      a. Repeat
      b. Failure to progress
      c. Fetal distress

II. Perinatal *(Cont.)*
  E. Type of anesthesia, if any
    1. Local
    2. Spinal
    3. Epidural
    4. General
  F. Estimated gestational age at time of delivery
  G. Infant's appearance at birth and need for resuscitation—Apgar score if recalled
  H. Birth weight, length, frontooccipital circumference (FOC)

III. Neonatal Complications
  A. Jaundice
  B. Temperature
  C. Breathing
  D. Feeding: breast, bottle, tube
  E. How long in hospital until released home

IV. Neurodevelopment
  A. Progressing or regressing
  B. Development of handedness
  C. Attainment of major milestones
  D. Academic performance in school

V. Immunizations
  A. Diphtheria-pertussis-tetanus
  B. Measles-mumps-rubella
  C. Bacille Calmette-Guérin
  D. *Hemophilus influenzae* type B
  E. Varicella
  F. Hepatitis

VI. Behavior
  A. Peer relations
  B. Interpersonal skills
  C. Conduct

VII. Family History—Consanguinity

VIII. Social History
  A. Intrafamilial psychosocial stressors
  B. Pets

2. List important features of the physical examination of infants and young children that may not be included in the examination of adults.

1. Measurement of frontooccipital circumference (FOC) and comparison with previous values
2. Palpation of cranial sutures and fontanelles if open
3. Cranial and ocular auscultation
4. Documentation of any craniofacial dysmorphology
5. Funduscopic examination with careful attention to the retina, not just to the optic disc
6. Limb asymmetries and malformations (including dermatoglyphics)
7. Abnormal cutaneous lesions
8. Assessment of developmental reflexes
9. Evaluation of developmental progress
10. Motor tone—appendicular and axial
11. Gowers' maneuver

3. List the common developmental reflexes. When do you expect them to be present?

Developmental Reflexes

REFLEX	APPEARS	DISAPPEARS
Lateral incurvation of trunk	Birth	1–2 months
Rooting	Birth	3 months
Moro	Birth	5–6 months
Tonic neck reflex	Birth	5–6 months
Palmar grasp	Birth	6 months
Crossed adduction with knee jerk	Birth	7–8 months
Plantar grasp	Birth	9–10 months
Extensor plantar responses	Birth	6–12 months
Parachute response	8–9 months	Persists
Landau reflex	10 months	24 months

4. What is the average FOC for a term newborn? What is the rate of growth over the first year?

Average FOC for a term newborn is 35 cm.

Average FOC growth: 2 cm/month for first 3 months
1 cm/month for next 3 months
0.5 cm/month for the last 6 months

5. What are the important developmental milestones for the first 5 years of life?

Developmental Milestones

AGE	REFLEX	AGE	REFLEX
0–4 weeks	Flexed posture Brief visual fixation and following Preference for human face Active Moro, stepping, placing, grasping, rooting	12 weeks	Lifts head and chest off bed Head above horizontal with ventral suspension Listens to music
4 weeks	Legs extended Tonic neck posture when supine Follows moving objects	16 weeks	Symmetric posture Reaches and grasps for objects Hands in midline
8 weeks	Head level with ventral suspension Tonic neck posture Follows through 180° Social smile, coos, listens	28 weeks	Rolls over, sits briefly Transfers objects hand to hand Babbles, enjoys mirror

(Table continued on following page.)

Developmental Milestones (Continued)

AGE	REFLEX	AGE	REFLEX
40 weeks	Pulls to stand Crawls, pincer grasp "Mama," "dada" Peek-a-boo, pat-a-cake	3 years	Walks up stairs alternating feet Rides tricycle Stands momentarily on one foot Tower of 9 cubes and bridge of cubes Knows name and sex Counts 3 objects Parallel play and washes hands
12 months	Cruises or walks with one hand held 2 or 3 single words		
15 months	Walks independently Tower of 2 cubes Makes line with crayon 2 word sentences	4 years	Hops on one foot Throws ball overhand Uses scissors Copies cross and square on paper Draws man with 2–4 parts Counts 4 pennies accurately Role playing Goes to toilet alone
18 months	Runs, walks up stairs with one hand held Explores drawers, wastebaskets Tower of 3 cubes 10 single words, names pictures Identifies 1 or 2 body parts Feeds self with fingers		
2 years	Runs well, walks up and down stairs alone Tower of 6 cubes Imitates horizontal strokes on paper 3-word sentences Holds spoon well	5 years	Skips Copies triangle, names 4 colors Counts 10 pennies Dresses and undresses self

PRENATAL DISEASES AND DEVELOPMENTAL DEFECTS

6. What is the Apgar score?

The Apgar score is a clinical vitality rating scale applied to newborn infants in an attempt to identify those at risk for certain neonatal complications. Apgar is an eponym (Virginia Apgar, U.S. anesthesiologist), although it is often used as an acronym.

Apgar Score

SIGN		SCORE		
		0	1	2
A	Appearance (color)	Blue, pale	Acrocyanosis	Pink
P	Pulse (heart rate)	Absent	< 100	> 100
G	Grimace (reflex irritability in response to nasal suctioning)	No response	Grimace	Cry
A	Activity (muscle tone)	Limp	Some flexion of limbs	Active motion
R	Respiration (respiratory effort)	Absent	Slow and irregular	Strong crying

Infants are routinely scored at 1 and 5 minutes after birth. Further scores may be made at 10 and 20 minutes if the infant appears to have been compromised.

7. Is the Apgar score useful in determining neurologic prognosis?

The 1-minute Apgar score reflects whether the newborn requires cardiopulmonary resuscitation and correlates little with long-term neurologic outcome. Five-minute Apgar scores of less than 5, particularly in infants with hypotonia, apnea, or feeding difficulties, raise the possibility of neurologic disability. One-third of infants with Apgar scores of 3 or less beyond 10 minutes will have severe neurologic sequelae, one-fifth will not survive the neonatal period, and the remainder will have milder disabilities or be normal.

8. **How is neonatal intraventricular hemorrhage (IVH) classified?**

Grade I   Localized subependymal hemorrhage into the germinal matrix

Grade II Subependymal hemorrhage with extension into the ventricles (less than 50% of the ventricular volume filled with blood)

Grade III Subependymal hemorrhage with extension into the ventricles and acute ventricular dilatation (greater than 50% of the ventricular volume filled with blood)

Grade IV Subependymal, intraventricular, and extension into the surrounding cerebral parenchyma

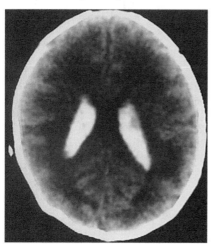

Unenhanced axial CT: grade III, IVH in a premature newborn (32 weeks' gestation). Note acute ventricular distention with blood filling more than 50% of the ventricular volume. There is no parenchymal extension of the hemorrhage.

9. **What risk factors are thought to play a role in the genesis of IVH?**

The most important risk factor for the development of an IVH is prematurity. Approximately 40–50% of neonates weighing less than 1500 gm experience an IVH. Other risk factors include mechanical ventilation, pneumothoraces, rapid expansion of intravascular volume (large or rapid IV infusions), rapid or wide fluctuations in blood pressure, hypoxic-ischemic injury, hypernatremia and hyperosmolality, and administration of certain medications such as indomethacin.

10. **What complications may arise secondary to an IVH?**

The most common complications of IVH include posthemorrhagic hydrocephalus, seizures, and the parenchymal cerebral injury associated with grade IV bleeds.

11. **Does the neurologic prognosis correlate with the different IVHs?**

Long-term follow-up studies of neonates grouped with all grades of IVH who reached kindergarten age revealed that 40% survived and 60% were neurologically abnormal. Approximately 30% now have a static encephalopathy (cerebral palsy); 30% have hydrocephalus, most of which required a shunting procedure; and 30% are multi-handicapped with combinations of blindness, paresis, spasticity, delayed fine motor and language skill, hydrocephalus, hearing loss, and seizures. Generally, grades I and II IVH are relatively benign, grade III has more significant hydrocephalus and seizures, and grade IV has by far the greatest likelihood of severe neurologic sequelae such as spastic quadriparesis, blindness, and mental retardation.

12. **What is the clinicopathologic classification for perinatal hypoxic-ischemic brain injury?**

Neuropathologic findings associated with perinatal asphyxia are of four principal types. Each type has a rather characteristic clinical presentation:

1. **Neuronal necrosis**—may be restricted to certain regions of the brain or may be more widespread and multifocal. This is typically the most severe form of insult, and children who survive are left with quadriplegia or hemiplegia, mental retardation, and seizures.

2. **Status marmoratus**—occurs only in term infants and is characterized by gliosis and hypermyelination of the basal ganglia. Clinically this is associated with choreoathetoid cerebral palsy.

3. **Watershed infarction**—in term infants results in neuronal injury in the border zones between anterior, middle, and posterior cerebral arteries and often involves the motor cortex, resulting in hemiparesis.

4. **Periventricular leukomalacia**—a form of watershed infarction that occurs in premature infants and involves the white matter adjacent to the lateral ventricles. Clinically this is associated with a spastic paresis of the lower extremities termed spastic diplegia.

13. What are the common antenatal risk factors for developing a static encephalopathy?

1. Hypoxic-ischemic encephalopathy
2. Intrauterine infections
3. Exposure to teratogens, including illicit drugs, alcohol, and smoking
4. Congenital malformations
5. Genetic anomalies
6. Multiple gestations
7. Maternal factors
   • Diabetes
   • Malnutrition
   • Toxemia

14. What are the most common perinatal/neonatal risk factors for developing a static encephalopathy?

1. Prematurity
2. Hypoxic-ischemic encephalopathy
3. Kernicterus
4. Trauma
5. Sepsis, including meningitis

15. What is TORCH?

This acronym refers to the agents most commonly responsible for intrauterine infection:

TO = **To**xoplasmosis
R = **R**ubella
C = **C**ytomegalovirus (CMV)
H = **H**erpes simplex virus

16. Damage of which neuroanatomic structures may result in infantile hypotonia (floppy baby)?

Differential Diagnosis of a Floppy Baby

STRUCTURES	EXAMPLES
Muscle	Congenital myopathies, congenital myotonic dystrophy, type II glycogenosis (Pompe's disease)
Neuromuscular junction	Congenital myasthenic syndromes, transient neonatal myasthenia gravis, botulism, hypermagnesemia
Peripheral nerve	Giant neuroaxonal dystrophy, familial dysautonomia (Riley-Day syndrome), hypomyelinative neuropathy
Anterior horn cell	Type I spinal muscular atrophy (Werdnig-Hoffmann disease)
Spinal cord	Myelodysplasias (meningomyeloceles, diplomyelia, diastematomyelia), traumatic transection
Cerebellum, brainstem, basal ganglia, cerebral hemispheres	Malformations, infections, toxic encephalopathies, metabolic encephalopathies, hypoxic-ischemic encephalopathies, genetic and chromosomal anomalies, neurodegenerative disorders

17. What are the most common causes of a floppy baby? What are the least common?

By far the most frequent are the central causes involving the cerebellum, brainstem, basal ganglia, and cerebral hemispheres. The least common causes of infantile hypotonia afflict the peripheral nerves.

18. Which syndromes are associated with agenesis of the corpus callosum?

Formation of the corpus callosum takes place over days 60–120 of gestation, but myelination continues after birth. Agenesis of the corpus callosum may be partial or complete. Many cases of this malformation appear to be sporadic; however, autosomal dominant and X-linked recessive inheritance has been described. In addition, agenesis of the corpus callosum is a feature of Aicardi's syndrome, which only affects females (X-linked dominant inheritance) and also includes infantile spasms with a hypsarrhythmic EEG pattern, severe psychomotor retardation, and characteristic chorioretinal lacunae.

19. What is the difference between macrocephaly and megalencephaly?

Macrocephaly refers to a large head, whereas megalencephaly refers specifically to a large brain.

20. What is the differential diagnosis of macrocephaly in an infant?

1. Hydrocephalus
   - Obstructive
   - Communicating
2. Extra-axial fluid collections
   - Subdural effusions
   - Subdural hematomas
3. Thickened skull
   - Anemia with increased marrow space
   - Osteopetrosis
   - Rickets
   - Osteogenesis imperfecta
4. Megalencephaly

21. What is the differential diagnosis of megalencephaly?

Toxic/metabolic
- Cerebral edema
  Lead
  Pseudotumor cerebri
- Canavan's disease
- Alexander's disease
- Tay-Sachs disease
- Metachromatic leukodystrophy
- Mucopolysaccharidoses

Structural
- Cerebral gigantism
  (Sotos' syndrome)
- Familial megalencephaly
- Neurofibromatosis
- Tuberous sclerosis
- Fragile X syndrome

22. In evaluating a child with microcephaly, what are the most important questions to ask in the history?

Is the microcephaly congenital or acquired? Serial measurements of FOC are helpful. Is the FOC getting progressively worse (Rett's syndrome in girls), returning to normal (catch-up growth after a serious illness or prematurity), or remaining on the same percentile line (static process)? Review the antenatal history carefully for evidence of intrauterine infection. Did the infant appear healthy at birth? Any postnatal central nervous system (CNS) infections or trauma? Family history of microcephaly?

23. What are some of the more important features of the physical examination to review in children with microcephaly?

Palpate the fontanelles and sutures for the presence of craniofacial dysmorphology suggestive of the craniosynostosis syndromes (premature closure of the cranial sutures), chromosomal anomalies (trisomy 13, 18, 21), or other nonchromosomal hereditary syndromes (Rubinstein-Taybi and Cornelia de Lange syndromes). The retinal exam may show chorioretinitis associated with the TORCH agents. Focal or lateralizing neurologic deficits suggest CNS damage or malformation.

24. Which laboratory tests, if any, would you order in a child with microcephaly?

Plain skull x-ray studies evaluate premature closure of the cranial sutures. A head computed tomography (CT) scan or cranial ultrasound (before closure of the fontanelles) surveys for evidence of CNS malformations, abnormal calcification (which may indicate infection with a TORCH agent or earlier hypoxic-ischemic injury), or massive destruction of the cerebrum as in hydranencephaly. Magnetic resonance imaging (MRI) gives greater anatomic detail of the brain but is rarely needed in this circumstance. The EEG is sometimes helpful in evaluating developmental characteristics and may also suggest the presence of certain malformations, encephaloclastic events, and chromosomal anomalies. In addition, TORCH titers may be measured if such an infection is suspected, or a chromosomal analysis may be used to evaluate genetic causes.

25. How would you evaluate and manage a newborn with spina bifida?

Perform a careful neurologic examination to estimate the level of spinal cord and nerve root involvement, including assessment of bowel and bladder function. Cranial neuroimaging (ultrasound, CT, MRI) is essential to determine the presence of other CNS conditions that are frequently present. Plain spine x-rays evaluate the bony extent of the lesion.

Immediately following birth, sterile saline–soaked gauze pads must be gently applied to the myelomeningocele membrane and all attempts should be made to keep the membrane intact during transfer to a tertiary center. Bladder catheterization may be necessary to ensure adequate drainage. Neurosurgical closure of the dysraphic defect should be performed within the first day or two of life.

26. What are the most common complications that may confront a child with myelomeningocele?

Virtually all children with lumbosacral myelomeningoceles have an associated type II Arnold-Chiari malformation that results in hydrocephalus. The hydrocephalus may be congenital or may occur following closure of the dysraphic defect. Many children will require a shunting procedure. CNS infectious complications are common and devastating. Infants at highest risk are those with

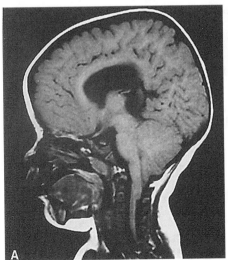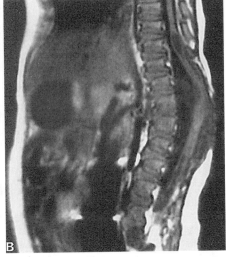

A, Unenhanced midsagittal T1-weighted MRI in a 6-month old boy with type II Arnold-Chiari malformation. Note "herniation" or downward displacement of the cerebellar tonsils through the foramen magnum to the level of C2 and the associated obstructive hydrocephalus. *B,* Unenhanced midsagittal T1-weighted MRI lumbosacral spine: extensive thoracolumbar myelomeningocele associated with the Arnold-Chiari malformation in *A.* Note the dorsal kyphosis, absence of posterior elements of the vertebrae, and the malformed spinal cord at the level of the defect. A small syrinx in the cord is present above the defect.

large defects, the covering membrane of which has been ruptured. Out of infancy, one of the most common causes of mortality in these individuals is renal failure due to chronic and repeated urinary tract infections and obstructive uropathy. Many children with myelomeningoceles experience seizures at some point, some of which may be related to the placement of ventriculoperitoneal shunts. Some children, after years of static neurologic deficits, experience progressive spasticity and weakness in their legs, worsening bladder and bowel function, progressive scoliosis, or increasing low back pain and stiffness. With CT myelography or MRI, these children are found to have a low-lying conus medullaris and are said to have a "tethered cord." Some of these children have improved neurologic function with surgical release of the filum terminale and freeing of the cord.

27. Classify the Arnold-Chiari malformations.

Type I—characterized by downward displacement of the cerebellum with elongation of the medulla such that the cerebellar tonsils egress through the foramen magnum into the cervical spinal canal. It is not associated with other nervous system malformations and clinically may be asymptomatic or may present with recurrent headaches, neck pain, and unsteady gait. The function of certain lower cranial nerves may be compromised, producing dysphagia and dysarthria. Cerebellar function may be affected, producing progressive ataxia and disordered ocular movements. The pyramidal tracts may be compressed, producing spasticity and extensor plantar responses. The posterior columns are often affected, resulting in impaired proprioception and vibratory sensation.

Type II—by definition, this type is associated with a lumbosacral myelomeningocele and with numerous other nervous system malformations. The posterior fossa is small and, as in Type I, there is downward displacement of the cerebellar tonsils through the foramen magnum. The medulla is elongated and thinned and often kinked so that it may lie beside the upper segments of the cervical cord. A characteristic beaking appearance of the quadrigeminal plate is present. Hydrocephalus frequently occurs, but its exact mechanism is unclear. Syringomyelia and occasionally syringobulbia also occur, along with a number of other malformations. These include a curious interdigitation of gyri along the interhemispheric fissure, polymicrogyria, gray matter heterotopias, craniocervical junction anomalies, and craniolacunia.

Type III—an occipital encephalocele with protrusion of cerebellar remnants into the overlying sac.

Type IV—isolated hypoplasia of the cerebellum not associated with other nervous system malformations.

28. What is Down syndrome?

A chromosomal anomaly characterized by trisomy 21. The majority of cases result from chromosomal nondisjunction, a phenomenon increasingly more likely to occur as maternal age advances. Clinically, it is characterized by marked infantile hypotonia with hyperflexibility of joints, mental deficiency, brachycephaly with flat occiput, upslanting palpebral fissures, late closure of fontanelles, flattened nasal bridge, epicanthal folds, speckling of iris (Brushfield's spots), fine lens opacities, small ears, hypoplastic teeth, short neck, brachydactyly with clinodactyly of fifth fingers, simian creases with distal axis triradius, wide space between first and second toes, congenital heart disease (in 40%), and hypogonadism.

NEURODEGENERATIVE DISORDERS

29. In general terms, how does a neurodegenerative disease affecting white matter present?

These diseases are classically described as presenting with loss of motor skills, spasticity, and ataxia.

30. In general terms, how does a neurodegenerative disease affecting gray matter present?

These diseases are classically described as presenting with loss of intellectual skills (dementia), seizures, and blindness.

31. What are the seven clinical variants of metachromatic leukodystrophy?

Metachromatic leukodystrophy (MLD) is an autosomal recessively inherited metabolic disorder of myelin due to a deficiency of arylsulfatase A. The disorder has been linked to chromosome 22. The seven clinical variants are

1. Congenital MLD—onset at birth with apnea, seizures, and weakness. Very rare.
2. Late-infantile MLD—most common and the classic form. Onset between 1 and 2 years of age.
3. Juvenile MLD—onset from 3–16 years of age, often presents with school or behavioral problems.
4. Adult MLD—onset in fourth decade with dementia and psychiatric disturbances.
5. Multiple sulfatase deficiency—clinically a combination of late-infantile MLD and Hurler's syndrome.
6. Pseudo-arylsulfatase deficiency—clinically asymptomatic but enzyme assays are positive for MLD. These patients have a mutated but functional variant of arylsulfatase A.
7. Activator protein deficiency—clinically, patients have late-infantile MLD but a normal enzyme assay. They have normal arylsulfatase A but lack a critical protein necessary for the enzyme to perform its function.

Polten A, Fluharty AL, Fluharty CB, et al: Molecular basis of different forms of metachromatic leukodystrophy. N Engl J Med 324:18–22, 1991.

32. Which leukodystrophy is virtually always associated with a particular endocrinologic deficiency?

Adrenoleukodystrophy, an X-linked recessive disorder, is one of the peroxisomal disorders. It is characterized by impaired beta-oxidation of the very long-chain (C26) fatty acids, leading to their accumulation. In addition to neurodegeneration typical of the leukodystrophies, patients also have adrenocortical insufficiency. Onset is usually between 4 and 6 years of age. An adult form of the disease called adrenomyeloneuropathy is characterized by progressive spastic paraparesis and peripheral neuropathy.

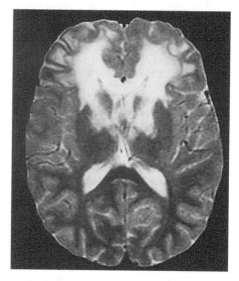

Unenhanced axial T2-weighted MRI in a 9-year-old boy with adrenoleukodystrophy. Note extensive dysmyelination involving the anterior centrum semiovale, subcortical white matter, genu of the corpus callosum, and internal capsule. The cerebral cortex, basal ganglia, and thalami are unaffected.

33. Which of the leukodystrophies is characterized in early infancy by hyperirritability with an exaggerated startle response, marked spasticity with *decreased* tendon reflexes, and a normal FOC?

Globoid cell leukodystrophy, or Krabbe's disease, is an autosomal recessive disorder due to a deficiency of galactocerebroside beta-galactosidase. Onset is between 3 and 8 months and clinical presentation is as outlined above.

34. Which leukodystrophies have prominent megalencephaly?

1. **Canavan's disease** (spongy degeneration)—autosomal recessive disorder recently shown to be secondary to a deficiency of aspartoacylase in the white matter of the brain, leading to an excess of *n*-acetyl-aspartate (NAA). The classic infantile form has its onset within the first few weeks of life and is characterized by initial hypotonia, followed at 6 months by hypertonia, megalencephaly, visual loss with optic atrophy, nystagmus, mixed seizures, choreoathetosis, vomiting, transient increases in intracranial pressure, and hyperpyrexia. Death occurs by 3–4 years of age. Rare neonatal-onset and juvenile-onset forms are described.

2. **Alexander's disease**—sporadic occurrence; etiopathogenetic origin unknown. Infantile or juvenile onset with spasticity, psychomotor retardation, seizures, ataxia, and prominent mega-lencephaly with or without hydrocephalus. The pathologic hallmark is prominent Rosenthal fibers throughout the brain.

Leone P, Janson CG, Bilianuk L, et al: Aspartoacylase gene transfer to the mammalian central nervous system with therapeutic implications for Canavan's disease. Ann Neurol 48:27–38, 2000.

35. Pathologically, most of the leukodystrophies are characterized by a process referred to as dysmyelination. Because of metabolic derangements, myelinogenesis is disturbed and the resulting myelin is defective in structure and function. Which leukodystrophy has virtual amyelination (absence of any myelin) as opposed to demyelination?

Pelizaeus-Merzbacher disease is an X-linked recessive disorder that is caused by a lack of proteolipid protein in myelin. Proteolipid protein is one of two principal structural components of myelin, the other being myelin basic protein. In addition to psychomotor retardation, spasticity, and ataxia, children with this disease also have marked choreoathetosis and pendular nystagmus.

Sistermans EA, de Coo RFM, De Wijs JJ, Van Oost BA: Duplication of the proteolipid protein gene is the major cause of Pelizaeus-Merzbacher disease. Neurology 50:1749–1754, 1998.

36. How often does multiple sclerosis occur in children?

Approximately 3–5% of all patients with multiple sclerosis (MS) have onset of symptoms in childhood. The majority of affected children (more than 90%) are greater than 10 years of age, but MS cases have been described in patients less than 3 years old. The clinical spectrum of disease is just as broad in children as it is in adults.

Ruggieri M, Polizzi A, Pavone L, Grimaldi LME: Multiple sclerosis in children under 6 years of age. Neurology 53:478–484, 1999.

37. What is a cherry-red spot?

It is the bright red appearance of the fovea centralis of the eye as seen by funduscopy in children with certain gray-matter storage diseases, classically Tay-Sachs disease. As the storage material accumulates in the nerve fiber layer, the retina takes on a grayish-white appearance. Because there are very few fibers traversing the fovea, it retains its normal color and continues to reflect the bright red vascular choroid underneath.

38. Tay-Sachs is often thought of as the prototypical gray-matter neurodegenerative disease. What are its principal clinical features?

Tay-Sachs is an autosomal recessive disorder due to a deficiency of hexosaminidase A. Until recently, the highest prevalence was in the Ashkenazi Jewish community. However, due to an aggressive and very successful screening program, most cases diagnosed today are in non-Jewish individuals. Onset is within 3–5 months of age with extreme irritability, hyperacusis, global developmental delay, and hypotonia. Often a hypsarrhythmia pattern develops on the EEG, and seizures are prominent within the first 6 months of life (usually myoclonic). Decreasing vision develops by 12 months of age and a cherry-red spot appears. Spasticity occurs late in the course and death is by 2–4 years of age. There are also juvenile-onset and adult-onset forms of the disease. The adult form may have an amyotrophic lateral sclerosis (ALS) type of presentation.

39. Which neurodegenerative diseases are associated with an enlarged liver and/or spleen?

Neurodegenerative Diseases with Hepatosplenomegaly

DISEASE	INHERITANCE	FEATURES
Niemann-Pick disease	Autosomal recessive	Deficiency of sphingomyelinase
Gaucher's disease	Autosomal recessive	Deficiency of glucocerebrosidase
Mucopolysaccharidoses Hurler's disease (severe expression)	Autosomal recessive	Deficiency of alpha-L-iduronidase
Mucopolysaccharidoses Hurler's disease (mild expression)	X-linked recessive	Deficiency of iduronate-2-sulfatase
Zellweger's syndrome	Autosomal recessive	Peroxisomal disorder
Wilson's disease	Autosomal recessive	Deficiency of ceruloplasmin, which leads to accumulation of copper in brain (predominantly basal ganglia) and liver causing cirrhosis
Galactosemia	Autosomal recessive	Deficiency of galactose-1-phosphate uridyltransferase

40. What are the neuronal ceroid lipofuscinoses (NCL)?

NCL is a group of autosomal recessively inherited disorders characterized by excessive neuronal accumulations of the lipid pigments, ceroid, and lipofuscin. These compounds are normally present in small amounts as cells become senescent. However, excessive and premature accumulation, as occurs in these diseases, leads to cell dysfunction and death.

Types of Neuronal Ceroid Lipofuscinoses

Infantile NCL (Santavuroi-Haltia) Onset 8–18 months, death 5–10 years Dementia, seizures, myoclonus, blindness	**Juvenile NCL** (Spielmeyer-Vogt-Sjögren) Onset 5–10 years, death 15–25 years Dementia, seizures, blindness
Late-infantile NCL (Jansky-Bielschowsky) Onset 3–4 years, death 9–12 years Dementia, seizures, myoclonus, blindness, ataxia	**Adult NCL** (Kuff's) Variable onset, slow course, variable age at death Extrapyramidal signs, ataxia, myoclonus, dysarthria, no dementia

41. What are ragged red fibers?

In some of the mitochondrial cytopathies, mitochondria become clumped beneath the skeletal muscle sarcolemmal membrane. When the muscle biopsy specimen is prepared with modified Gomori's trichrome stain and viewed by light microscopy, the clumps of mitochondria stain red and give the muscle fibers a ragged appearance—hence the term ragged red fibers.

42. What is the mode of inheritance and biochemical defect in each of the three principal mitochondrial encephalomyopathies?

1. **Kearns-Sayre syndrome** occurs sporadically and has dysfunction of complex I of the respiratory chain. The predominant clinical features include progressive encephalopathy, external ophthalmoplegia, pigmentary retinopathy, ptosis, weakness, sensorineural deafness, ataxia, spasticity, cardiac conduction abnormalities, and respiratory insufficiency. Laboratory study reveals elevated blood lactate and pyruvate, increased cerebrospinal fluid (CSF) protein, and ragged red fibers on muscle biopsy.

2. **M**yoclonus, **e**pilepsy, encephalomyopathy, and **r**agged **r**ed **f**ibers are characteristics of the **MERRF syndrome**. This disorder has a maternal pattern of inheritance (mitochondrial genetic defect) and affects complex IV of the respiratory chain.

3. **M**itochondrial encephalomyopathy with lactic acidosis and strokelike episodes occur in the **MELAS syndrome**. This syndrome has maternal inheritance and affects complex I.

Johns DR: Mitochondrial DNA and disease. N Engl J Med 333:638–644, 1995.

43. A fair-skinned, blue-eyed, and blonde-haired infant was normal at birth. He now presents at 6–8 months of age with progressive psychomotor retardation, infantile spasms, microcephaly, dystonia, vomiting, and has a "musty" odor. What would be first on your list of differential diagnoses?

This is a classic description of phenylketonuria (PKU); however, other aminoacidurias and some of the organic acidurias may present similarly. The three main types of PKU are (1) deficiency of phenylalanine hydroxylase; (2) deficiency of dihydropteridine reductase (DHPR); and (3) deficient synthesis of dihydrobiopterin (DH_2).

44. Which endocrinologic disorder may present as a gray matter neurodegenerative disease if it is missed on neonatal screening?

Congenital hypothyroidism (cretinism) is extremely difficult to detect clinically at birth and the diagnosis may not be suspected until it is too late for replacement therapy to be maximally efficacious. Left untreated, these children develop prolonged jaundice, abdominal distention with umbilical hernia, large fontanelles, hypotonia, impaired bony development, large tongue, psychomotor retardation, seizures, spasticity, ataxia, and deafness.

45. Which neurodegenerative disorder results in excessive accumulation of iron in the basal ganglia?

Hallervorden-Spatz disease is an autosomal recessive disorder due to a deficiency of cysteine dioxygenase. This deficiency leads to increased concentrations of cysteine, whose thiol group chelates iron. This promotes the formation of free radicals, which cause cell damage and death. Affected individuals present before 10 years of age with psychomotor regression, extrapyramidal signs followed by pyramidal signs, optic atrophy, and pigmentary retinopathy. Neuroimaging reveals dense deposits of iron in the basal ganglia.

Swaiman KF: Hallervorden-Spatz syndrome and brain iron metabolism. Arch Neurol 48:1285–1293, 1991.

NEUROCUTANEOUS SYNDROMES

46. What is the most common neurocutaneous syndrome? What are its clinical characteristics?

Neurofibromatosis (NF) type I (von Recklinghausen's disease of the nerves) has an incidence of 1/3,000–4,000 population. Inheritance is autosomal dominant and the spontaneous mutation rate is very high (30–50%). The mutation has been linked to chromosome 17. Clinical characteristics include café-au-lait spots, neurofibromas, axillary/inguinal freckling, optic gliomas, iridic Lisch nodules, megalencephaly, mental retardation, seizures, and characteristic bony lesions.

Neurofibromatosis type II is much less common (1/50,000) than NF-I. Inheritance is autosomal dominant and it has been linked to chromosome 22. The principal clinical manifestation is bilateral acoustic neurinomas.

Berg BO: Current concepts of neurocutaneous disorders. Brain Dev 13:9–20, 1991.

47. When evaluating an infant with hypsarrhythmia and infantile spasms, which neurocutaneous syndrome must be specifically sought?

Tuberous sclerosis (TS) is highly correlated with the occurrence of infantile spasms (more than 25% of infants with infantile spasms will later express other signs of TS). TS is an autosomal dominant disorder with genetic heterogeneity. Individuals with the same clinical phenotype have been shown to have different underlying genetic mutations. Some families with TS have been mapped to chromosome 9q and others to chromosome 16p. Its incidence is 1/10,000 with a high spontaneous mutation rate.

Clinical manifestations include mental retardation, seizures, adenoma sebaceum, ash-leaf spots, shagreen patches, café au lait spots, subungual and periungual fibromas (Koenen's tumors), gingival fibromas, dental enamel pits, retinal tumors (mulberry tumor of the optic disc), cardiac rhabdomyomata, renal angiomyolipomata, and CNS cortical tubers and subependymal hamartomas that calcify and occasionally become malignant (subependymal giant cell astrocytomas).

Crino PB, Henske EP: New developments in the neurobiology of the tuberous sclerosis complex. Neurology 53:1384–1390, 1999.

48. Of the more common neurocutaneous syndromes, which one has no clear pattern of inheritance?

Sturge-Weber syndrome (encephalofacialangiomatosis) has no clear pattern of inheritance. Prevalence and incidence is unknown, but it is less common than NF or TS. Patients have a characteristic congenital facial port-wine stain (nevus) that is usually unilateral and involves the V_1 segment of the trigeminal nerve (may be much larger and involve the entire side of the face and body). The nevus may involve the nasopharyngeal mucosa and ocular choroidal membrane, causing glaucoma. Other findings include iridic heterochromia, optic atrophy, progressive dementia, and steadily worsening partial motor seizures, with longer duration of postictal paralysis eventually leading to permanent hemiplegia and hemianopsia. Arteriography reveals extensive arteriovenous malformation involving the ipsilateral cerebral hemispheric dura. Vascular "steal" phenomenon leads to chronic ischemia of the underlying cerebral cortex. The characteristic "tram" or "railroad track" sign seen on skull films is due to mineralization of adjacent gyri from chronic ischemia.

49. In addition to brain and skin involvement, which neurocutaneous syndrome also has immunologic abnormalities, impaired DNA repair mechanisms, and a high propensity for various neoplasms?

Ataxia-telangiectasia. The responsible gene, called ATM, has recently been identified and is on chromosome 11q. Ataxia-telangiectasia is an autosomal recessive disorder with an incidence of 1/100,000. Affected individuals develop telangiectasias by 2–4 years of age on exposed areas of skin and conjunctiva. Other skin lesions include premature aging, frequent infections with poor healing, vitiligo, café au lait spots, and occasionally scleroderma-like lesions. Progressive cerebellar ataxia begins within the first few years of life. Muscle bulk becomes diffusely diminished and tendon reflexes are reduced. Choreoathetosis is common, but sensory changes are rare. Patients have decreased or absent IgA and IgE and decreased IgG_2 and IgG_4. Tonsils, lymphoid tissues, and thymus gland are abnormal or absent. Defective cellular DNA repair leads to increased spontaneous and radiation-induced chromosomal aberrations, inducing various neoplasia. Patients also have elevated alpha-fetoprotein levels, which can be used as a screening technique, including antenatal detection.

Spacey SO, Gatti RA, Bobb G: The molecular basis and clinical management of ataxia-telangiectasia. Can J Neurol Sci 27:184–191, 2000.

50. Which neurocutaneous syndrome has no skin lesions?

Von Hippel-Lindau disease has autosomal dominant inheritance and no skin lesions. It has an incidence of 1/36,000 live births and has been linked to chromosome 3p. Clinical manifestations include retinal and cerebellar hemangioblastomas, polycythemia, elevated CSF protein, pheochromocytomas, and cystic changes in the pancreas, liver, and epididymis.

Roach ES: Von Hipple-Landau disease. How does one gene cause multiple tumors? Neurology 53:7–8, 1999.

INFECTIONS AND INFESTATIONS

51. Infectious etiologies account for what percentage of prenatally and postnatally acquired cerebral palsy?

Infectious disease accounts for approximately 50–60% of postnatally acquired cerebral palsy (CP), as opposed to only 10–20% of prenatally acquired CP.

52. What are the most common bacterial pathogens responsible for meningitis at different ages?

Most Common Bacterial Pathogens

NEONATAL	CHILDHOOD
Group B beta-hemolytic streptococci	*Haemophilus influenzae* type B
Escherichia coli	*Streptococcus pneumoniae*
Listeria monocytogenes	*Neisseria meningitidis*
Klebsiella pneumoniae	

53. What are the usual signs and symptoms of neonatal meningitis?

1. Lethargy
2. Irritability
3. Apnea
4. Hypotonia or hypertonia
5. Opisthotonos
6. Poor feeding
7. Hypothermia or hyperthermia
8. Seizures
9. Bulging fontanelle
10. Cranial nerve palsies

54. What factors predict a poor outcome at the time of admission for neonatal bacterial meningitis?

1. Coma
2. Shock
3. Peripheral neutrophil count $< 2 \times 10^9/L$
4. Thrombocytopenia
5. High CSF protein
6. High concentration of type III capsular antigen in CSF
7. Birth weight < 2500 gm
8. Age at diagnosis < 1 day

55. What are the usual signs and symptoms in the older infant and child with bacterial meningitis?

1. Fever
2. Altered mental status
3. Meningismus
4. Headache
5. Nausea and vomiting
6. Irritability
7. Full or bulging fontanelle
8. Seizures
9. Focal neurologic signs
10. Papilledema
11. Syndrome of inappropriate secretion of antidiuretic hormone (SIADH)

56. How does herpes encephalitis in neonates differ from that in the older child or adult?

Two strains of herpes simplex virus (HSV) may infect the neonatal CNS, types I and II. In older children and adults, non-CNS disease caused by HSV-I usually manifests as a mucocutaneous infection (herpes labialis or ocular herpes), whereas non-CNS disease caused by HSV-II usually manifests as a genital infection. As a result, the vast majority of neonatal HSV encephalitis is due to type II infection. Neonatal HSV infection produces a panencephalitis with high mortality and morbidity. Neonates with HSV-II tend to present with a higher frequency of seizures, greater pelocytosis and protein concentrations in the CSF, and more frequent evidence of structural damage on neuroimaging studies than those with HSV-I infection. Recent widespread availability of the antiviral agent acyclovir has improved the outcome considerably. Children who survive neonatal HSV encephalitis will develop significantly disabling static encephalopathies in up to 64% of cases. HSV-I encephalitis tends to respond more favorably to acyclovir than does HSV-II encephalitis.

Cameron PD, Wallace SJ, Munro J: Herpes simplex virus encephalitis: Problems in diagnosis. Dev Med Child Neurol 34:134–140, 1992.

57. A child from Central America presents with a prolonged partial motor seizure. Neurologic examination the following day demonstrates no focal or lateralizing findings; however, funduscopic examination reveals early papilledema. CT scanning of the brain

discloses a number of small, densely calcified lesions scattered along the gray-white junction of the cerebral hemispheres. Contrast administration reveals two additional lesions that were not calcified and have bright ring enhancement and surrounding edema. What is the most likely diagnosis and how might you confirm your suspicions?

The pork tapeworm, *Taenia solium*, is endemic in Central America. When a human inadvertently becomes the intermediate host (rather than the pig), he may develop neurocysticercosis. This occurs when the ingested *T. solium* ova become partially digested, releasing oncospheres that gain access to the circulation and are carried throughout the body. They then become larvae (cysticerci) in subcutaneous tissue, muscle, and brain. The majority of the CNS cysticerci die spontaneously and become densely calcified. The most common clinical manifestation is seizures, although focal neurologic deficits, hydrocephalus, and meningitis are also encountered. Rarely, in disseminated cases, progressive massive cerebral edema with increasing intracranial pressure may occur, leading to coma and death. The diagnosis can be confirmed by serum or CSF antibody and antigen detection methods and in certain cases by tissue biopsy.

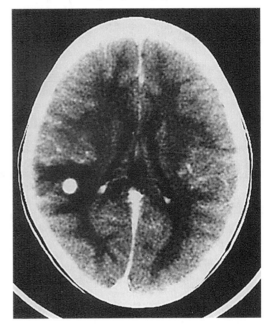

Enhanced axial CT: neurocysticercosis in a 7-year-old girl. Note the solitary, densely enhancing lesion with surrounding edema.

Carpio A, Escobar A, Hauser WA: Cysticercosis and epilepsy. A critical review. Epilepsia 39:1025–1040, 1998.

58. Which parainfectious neurologic diseases are known to result in cerebral palsy?
1. Acute disseminated encephalomyelitis
2. Acute hemorrhagic leukoencephalitis
3. Acute cerebellar ataxia (rarely)
4. Reye syndrome

59. What is the most commonly identified infection before the onset of acute cerebellar ataxia of childhood?

In children diagnosed with acute cerebellar ataxia, 26% had chickenpox, 52% other viral infections, 3% immunizations, and 19% no definite antecedent.

Conolly AM, Dodson WE, Prensky AL, Rurt RS: Course and outcome of acute cerebellar ataxia. Ann Neurol 35:673–679, 1994.

VASCULAR DISORDERS

60. Which laboratory investigations may be important in the evaluation of acute infantile hemiplegia (childhood stroke)?

Laboratory Evaluation of Childhood Stroke

I. CBC with differential and platelets
  A. Polycythemia, thrombocytosis, thrombocytopenia
  B. Leukemia
II. Prothrombin time, partial thromboplastin time, anticardiolipin antibodies, lupus anticoagulant, antithrombin III, protein S, and protein C for coagulopathies
III. Erythrocyte sedimentation rate, rheumatoid factor, antinuclear antibody, rapid plasma reagin test, serum protein electrophoresis for vasculitides
IV. Hemoglobin electrophoresis for hemoglobinopathies
V. Serum cholesterol, triglycerides, lipoprotein, electrophoresis for familial hyperlipoproteinemias
VI. Serum amino acids, especially homocystinuria

VII. Alpha-galactosidase A for Fabry's disease
VIII. Viral titers for postexanthem vasculitis and varicella
IX. CSF analysis
  A. Infection
  B. Vasculitis
X. EKG/echocardiography
  A. Septal defects
  B. Endocarditis
  C. Valvular disease
  D. Thrombus
XI. CT scan/MRI: infarct vs. hemorrhage
XII. Angiography
  A. Arteriovenous malformation
  B. Vasculitis
  C. Fibromuscular dysplasia
  D. Thrombosis/embolism

Lanska MJ, Lanska DJ, Horwitz SJ, Aram DM: Presentation, clinical course, and outcome of childhood stroke. Pediatr Neurol 7:333–341, 1991.
Lanthier S, Carmant L, David M, et al: Stroke in children. Neurology 54:371–378, 2000.

61. What is the most common hemoglobinopathy associated with cerebrovascular disease?
Approximately one-fourth of all patients with sickle cell disease experience cerebrovascular complications; the vast majority are children. When strokes occur in adults, they are more likely to be intracerebral hemorrhages as opposed to the infarctions that affect children. In addition to small vessel occlusion by sickled red cells, endothelial proliferation is also thought to be an important mechanism in the genesis of these strokes.

62. How does the prognosis for neurologic recovery following a stroke relate to age?
As a broad generalization, the younger a particular CNS insult occurs, the better is the prognosis for meaningful neurologic recovery. The developing brain can assume the function of areas that have been damaged. This has been quite convincingly demonstrated in children who develop a slow-growing neoplasm in a temporal lobe. For example, a patient may start out being right-handed, but as a tumor damages the left temporal lobe, he or she gradually becomes left-handed. Neuropsychological tests reveal either a transference of language and memory to the opposite side as well, or "crowding" within the left temporal lobe.

63. Describe the three common presentations of Galen malformations.
1. Newborns may present in florid high-output congestive cardiac failure due to direct shunting of blood from the carotid circulation into the vein of Galen, which becomes massively dilated. The majority of these infants have severe cerebral ischemic damage due to the "steal" phenomenon of blood being diverted into the AVM. Prognosis is extremely grave.
2. Another group of patients have less marked malformation and present in later infancy. They develop hydrocephalus due to the aneurysmal compression of the cerebral aqueduct. Prognosis in these patients is also poor because of progressive enlargement of the aneurysm and its propensity for rupture.
3. A third group of patients presents in later childhood with subarachnoid hemorrhages, hydrocephalus, or signs of brainstem compression.
Pavlakis SG, Gould RJ, Zito JL: Stroke in children. Adv Pediatr 38:151–179, 1991.

NEOPLASMS

64. Are infratentorial or supratentorial tumors more common in infants? Children? Adults?

In infants less than 1 year of age, supratentorial brain tumors predominate. In children older than 1 year, infratentorial tumors are more common. In adults, supratentorial tumors are again more frequently encountered.

65. What is meant by the term PNET?

PNET is an acronym for primitive neuroectodermal tumor. These are highly malignant, small, blue cell tumors. They are part of a newer classification of CNS tumors and replace the term "blastoma." If a PNET is completely undifferentiated and is in the midline posterior fossa, it would previously have been referred to as a medulloblastoma. PNETs may show varying degrees of differentiation along different cell lines, including glial, ependymal, pineal, and neuronal.

Pollack IF: Brain tumors in children. N Engl J Med 331:1500–1507, 1994.

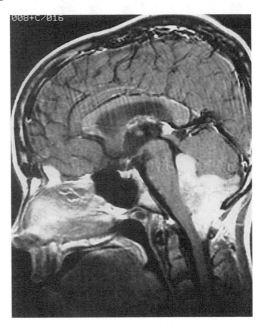

Enhanced midsagittal T1-weighted MRI reveals a posterior fossa primitive neuroectodermal tumor (PNET) in a 5-year-old boy. Note the brightly enhancing tumor mass extending upward through the fourth ventricle into the cerebral aqueduct and downward through the foramen magnum. There is compression of the medulla and marked displacement of the cerebellum. Early obstructive hydrocephalus is developing.

66. What are some of the common complications associated with PNETs?

PNETs have an extremely high propensity to metastasize along CSF pathways, which may lead to complete filling of the subarachnoid space over the surface of the cerebrum or cerebellum (so-called sugar coating), obstructive hydrocephalus, drop metastases along the spinal cord, and intra-abdominal spread through ventriculoperitoneal shunts.

67. A school-aged child complains of recurrent headaches and recent onset of marked polyuria and polydipsia. Examination reveals bitemporal homonymous hemianopsia and papilledema. Laboratory tests are consistent with diabetes insipidus. Where is the lesion? What is the differential diagnosis?

The anatomic location of this lesion must be in the parasellar region. The visual field defect is produced by compression of the optic chiasm. The diabetes insipidus is produced by compression of the pituitary stalk.

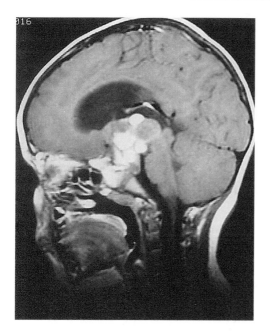

Enhanced midsagittal T1-weighted MRI demonstrates a craniopharyngioma in a 3-year-old girl. Note the large, multilobulated tumor extending from the parasellar region through the midbrain. The tumor has brightly enhancing solid areas and fluid-filled cysts. There is associated obstructive hydrocephalus.

Differential Diagnosis of Parasellar Lesions

Neoplasm	**Inflammatory: chronic basilar meningitis**
Craniopharyngioma	Tuberculosis with or without tuberculoma
Germ-cell tumor, including teratoma	Fungal
Pituitary tumor	Neurosarcoidosis
Optic glioma (astrocytoma) with or without	**Structural**
neurofibromatosis	Rathke's pouch cyst
Hypothalamic glioma	Enlarging arachnoid cyst
Meningioma	Aneurysm
Chordoma of the clivus	
Metastatic tumor	

68. What are the implications if a patient with a parasellar lesion also developed wasting of subcutaneous tissue despite apparently normal, or even increased, food intake, an unusually euphoric disposition, and Collier's sign (upper eyelid retraction)?

This constellation of features is typical of the diencephalic syndrome (Russell's syndrome) and implies dysfunction of the hypothalamus. Thus the lesion may have originated in the hypothalamus or may be invading or compressing it.

69. How do posterior fossa tumors commonly present in the younger child?

1. Irritability and altered mental status
2. Unsteadiness and ataxia
3. Headache, vomiting, progressive obtundation, and bulging fontanelle due to hydrocephalus
4. Head tilt
5. Cranial nerve palsies

70. Most posterior fossa tumors in children portend a grave prognosis. However, one particular posterior fossa tumor has an excellent prognosis. What is it?

Juvenile cerebellar pilocystic astrocytoma has virtually a 100% 50-year survival rate. This tumor develops in the cerebellar hemispheres of school-aged children. Histologically, the tumor cells are hairlike (pilocystic) and there is a microcyst formation and often Rosenthal fibers. The tumor is well circumscribed without local invasiveness. Neurosurgical resection is usually complete and recurrence is very uncommon.

71. An older child with medically intractable complex partial seizures has an MRI scan performed. The scan reveals a partially calcified mass in the right mesial temporal lobe without associated edema. What is the most likely diagnosis?

Gangliogliomas and oligodendrogliomas are slow-growing benign neoplasms that are increasingly being recognized as a cause for intractable seizures.

Olson JD, Riedel E, DeAngelis LM: Longterm outcome of low-grade oligodendrogliomas and mixed glioma. Neurology 54:1442–1448, 2000.

INJURY BY PHYSICAL AGENTS AND TRAUMA

72. Does age have any effect on whether or not cranial irradiation would be considered as treatment for cancer?

Children who received cranial x-ray therapy (XRT) prior to 3 years of age have significantly reduced intelligence quotients.

73. What are some of the other adverse effects that may be encountered in children who receive cranial XRT?

Many children experience transient somnolence, headaches, and anorexia 6–8 weeks after initiation of XRT. However, a severe and potentially life-threatening side effect may occur 1–3 years after the XRT has stopped, and is termed radiation necrosis (radionecrosis). This phenomenon may mimic a mass effect, and it may be difficult to distinguish tumor recurrence from radionecrosis. Pathologically the lesion involves hyalinization of blood vessels with massive infarction and necrosis of brain tissues.

Children may also experience hypothalamic-pituitary dysfunction following XRT. This usually involves decreased production of growth hormone and thyroid-stimulating hormone. The formation of cataracts is also common if the ocular globes were exposed to irradiation. Finally, XRT may induce a second malignancy that appears years later. These are usually meningiomas, sarcomas, thyroid tumors, and parotid gland tumors.

Duffner PK, Cohen ME: The long-term effects of central nervous system therapy on children with brain tumors. Neurol Clin 9:479–495, 1991.

74. Children with acute lymphoblastic leukemia receive CNS prophylaxis in the form of cranial XRT or intrathecal methotrexate and occasionally cytosine-arabinoside. What is the severe neurologic complication that some of the children experience?

Some of these children develop a leukoencephalopathy with progressive dementia, seizures, and focal neurologic deficits. Neuroimaging reveals cerebral atrophy, extensive white matter lesions, and scattered calcifications.

75. A 6-month-old infant presents to the emergency room with obtundation and a history of recent onset of seizures. Examination reveals no fever, anterior fontanelle slightly bulging, depressed level of consciousness, and hypotonia. A partial motor seizure is witnessed. On funduscopic examination, extensive, bilateral retinal hemorrhages and mild papilledema are observed. What is your leading diagnosis?

Child abuse, specifically the shaken-baby syndrome, needs to be first on the list of diagnostic possibilities. Because of the violent shaking of the body and head, these infants sustain massive subarachnoid hemorrhages and associated retinal hemorrhages. This commonly leads to seizures and may cause cortical infarctions as the cerebral vessels spasm.

76. What is a growing skull fracture?

This is a rather rare complication of linear skull fractures, usually occurring in children younger than than 3 years of age. Because of brain and CSF pulsations, the opposing edges of bone along the fracture do not fuse. Resorption of bone along the edges occurs so that the fracture opening progressively enlarges, producing a "growing skull fracture."

SEIZURES AND OTHER PAROXYSMAL DISORDERS

77. What is a simple febrile seizure?

A simple febrile seizure is a convulsion that occurs in a child between 6 months and 5 years of age in association with a fever greater than 38° C, but not in the presence of a CNS infection. The seizure must last less than 15 minutes, have no focal features, not recur within 24 hours, and be associated with no postictal neurologic abnormalities.

78. What is a complex febrile seizure?

The convulsion has focal features, lasts longer than 15 minutes or recurs within 24 hours, or occurs in a child younger than 6 months or older than 5 years of age.

79. Does having had a simple febrile convulsion increase the risk for later development of epilepsy (recurrent nonfebrile seizures)?

Yes, the risk of developing epilepsy increases to about 1%, double the risk for the general population.

Verity CM, Golding J: Risk of epilepsy after febrile convulsions: A national cohort study. Br Med J 303:1373–1376, 1991.
Knudson FU: Febrile seizures: Treatment and prognosis. Epilepsia 41:2–9, 2000.

80. What is the incidence of neonatal seizures? How do they usually present?

The incidence of neonatal seizures is approximately 0.5–1%. Because of maturational factors such as lack of myelination of commissural fiber tracts, neonates do not experience the bilaterally synchronous generalized tonic-clonic seizures common in older children and adults. Clinically, neonatal seizures can be classified into one of five main types:

1. Subtle seizures with eye deviation, eye fluttering, sucking, drooling, tonic posturing, or apnea
2. Multifocal clonic seizures that exhibit clonic activity of one or more extremities that often randomly and irregularly migrate to another part of the body
3. Focal clonic seizures
4. Tonic seizures with decerebrate posturing
5. Myoclonic seizures with rapid synchronous single or multiple flexion jerks of the extremities

81. An 18-month-old child is referred for evaluation of possible epilepsy. The mother relates a history of several paroxysmal spells that have occurred over the past month or so. Each spell has been similar in nature and consists of the child turning red, then blue in the face, and then passing out with a few clonic jerks of the extremities. Detailed questioning reveals that immediately preceding each spell, the child had been startled, frightened, or frustrated and began crying. This was soon followed by the sequence of events outlined earlier. What is the probable diagnosis?

This is a typical history of blue breathholding spells, a form of infantile syncope. Breathholding spells occur in 4–5% of children; there is a positive family history in 25% of cases. Two-thirds have cyanotic or blue breathholding spells, 20% have pallid breathholding spells, and the remainder have a mixture of the two. The peak incidence is between 1 and 2 years of age and resolution occurs by 6 years of age. The spells follow minor injuries, fright, or frustration. Twenty percent of these children will have syncope as older children or adults, but there is no increased risk for epilepsy.

DiMauro FJ Jr: Breath-holding spells in childhood. Am J Dis Child 146:125–131, 1992.

82. Other than syncope, what other spells may be confused with seizures?

- Classic and complicated migraines
- Pavor nocturnus (night terrors)
- Benign nocturnal myoclonus
- Motor tics and Tourette's syndrome

- Paroxysmal dyskinesias/dystonias
- Benign paroxysmal vertigo of childhood
- Narcolepsy/cataplexy

- Gastroesophageal reflux in infants
- Attention deficit disorder and daydreaming
- Pseudoseizures
- Munchausen's syndrome by proxy

Aicardi J: Differential diagnosis of nonepileptic paroxysmal events. Int Pediatr 9:55–81, 1994.

HEAD PAIN

83. What features of headache raise concern about the presence of an intracranial mass lesion?

1. Recent onset of headaches or change in character of chronic headaches
2. Headaches that awaken the patient from sleep or are present on awakening in the morning
3. Association with altered mental status, vomiting, constriction of visual fields (papilledema), or focal neurologic deficits

84. What are the clinical features of childhood migraine headaches?

Migraine headaches in children are common. Approximately 50% of all individuals who develop migraine had the onset of their attacks before 20 years of age. Boys are more frequently affected until puberty, after which time the incidence is considerably higher in girls. Younger children usually complain of a generalized or bifrontal or bitemporal headache, rather than the hemicranial pain characteristically present in the older child or adult. The pain may or may not be described as throbbing or pulsatile. Abdominal distress with nausea and sometimes vomiting is prominent. While experiencing a migraine, the child often appears pale and frequently stops all activities and lies down. Photophobia and acousticophobia are usually present. If the child is able to fall asleep, the headache is virtually always gone on awakening. The family history for migraine is positive in 70–90% of cases.

Maytal J, Young M, Shechter A, Lipton RB: Pediatric migraine and the International Headache Society Criteria. Neurology 48:602–607, 1997.

85. What are the different types of migraine headaches?

1. **Migraine without aura** (formerly common migraine)—accounts for up to three-quarters of all migraine attacks. Clinical manifestations are those listed in the preceding answer.

2. **Migraine with aura** (formerly classic migraine)—same as above except these individuals experience an aura just before the onset of the headache. The aura is usually visual but rarely can be somatosensory in nature.

3. **Complicated migraine**—migraine headache associated with various transient neurological phenomena. These include hemiplegic migraine, ophthalmoplegic migraine, vertebrobasilar migraine, and acute confusional migraine.

4. **Migraine variants or equivalents**—benign paroxysmal vertigo of childhood and cyclical vomiting of childhood are two syndromes thought to be related to migraine. Both are paroxysmal in nature and patients with these syndromes often develop typical migraine headaches in later life.

86. What is the syndrome of alternating hemiplegia?

A special subtype of hemiplegic migraine is the syndrome of alternating hemiplegia. Affected individuals present with recurrent episodes of hemiplegia which occur on each side of the body at different times. Each hemiplegic episode may last hours to days, and one may merge into the next. The headache component is usually not prominent. One clue to the diagnosis is that during a particular episode of weakness, the hemiplegia usually resolves during sleep, only to return moments after awakening.

87. What are some of the therapeutic strategies used in treating migraines?

Biofeedback and relaxation techniques seem to work well for some individuals. In addition, avoidance of particular foods that appear to precipitate migraines in a small percentage of patients is helpful. Foods that have been implicated include chocolate, caffeine, nitrites, monosodium glutamate, and sharp cheeses.

88. What are the most important pharmacologic agents used in treating migraine?

1. **Symptomatic treatments:** basically painkillers that have no action on the underlying cause of the migraine headache. Examples include aspirin, ibuprofen, acetaminophen, codeine, and meperidine. It is usually best to avoid narcotic preparations in the treatment of chronic illnesses if at all possible.

2. **Abortive therapies:** vasoactive agents that modify the vasculature so that the migraine headache is aborted before becoming fully developed. Examples include the ergotamine preparations, isometheptene mucate, and the serotonin receptor agonists (triptans).

3. **Prophylactic medications:** drugs that the patient takes every day in an attempt to prevent the migraine headaches. Examples include nonsteroidal anti-inflammatory agents (aspirin), beta blockers, calcium channel blockers, antiepileptic medications (sodium valproate and gabapentin), tricyclic antidepressants (amitriptyline), the serotonin antagonists (cyproheptadine and methysergide), and the selective serotonin reuptake inhibitor antidepressants (sertraline and paroxetine).

Silberstein SD, Goodsby PJ, Lipton RB: Management of migraine: An algorithmic approach. Neurology 55:546–552, 2000.

89. What is occipital neuralgia?

Occipital neuralgia is a childhood syndrome of recurrent occipital headaches. Clinical manifestations include pain and numbness in the C2 distribution, loss of the cervical lordotic curve, tenderness of the C2 spinous process, and limitation of cervical range of motion. The syndrome is thought to be due to C2 root irritation caused by excessive mobility of the C1 vertebra on the C2 vertebra.

NEUROMUSCULAR DISORDERS

90. What is the gene product of the Xp21 portion of the X chromosome?

The gene product is a protein called **dystrophin**. Dystrophin is a structural protein that is important in several tissues, including skeletal muscle, cardiac muscle, and brain. Certain mutations of the dystrophin gene lead to essentially no dystrophin production and result in Duchenne muscular dystrophy. Other mutations allow for the production of some dystrophin and cause the less severe and later-onset Becker muscular dystrophy.

Dickson G, Love DR, Davies KE, et al: Human dystrophin gene transfer: Production and expression of a functional recombinant DNA-based gene. Hum Genet 88:53–58, 1991.

91. What are the clinical manifestations of Duchenne muscular dystrophy (DMD)?

Estimates of the incidence of DMD range from 10–30 cases per 100,000 live male births. Affected children are normal through the first year of life. The first clue is that the child may walk later than expected, but detectable weakness is not present until 3–4 years of age. The pelvic girdle weakens first and gives rise to the characteristic Gowers' sign. Soon widespread weakness is apparent and relentless progression ensues. Most children become unable to walk by the end of their first decade. Once the patient is wheelchair bound, the disease seems to progress rapidly, with development of flexion contractures and progressive scoliosis. Cardiac involvement, as evidenced by EKG abnormalities, is invariable. Mild intellectual impairment is also common in these patients. Death from pulmonary infection, respiratory failure, or cardiac failure usually occurs by age 30 years.

92. How is the clinical diagnosis of DMD confirmed?

Electromyography and routine muscle biopsy can reveal the characteristic but nonspecific changes of a dystrophy. True confirmation can be obtained, however, with immunocytochemical studies of muscle biopsy specimens, in which the dystrophin levels are directly quantitated. In addition, molecular genetic analysis is possible, which can assay for the specific gene mutations.

93. What are some of the therapeutic strategies currently being investigated for DMD that hold promise for the future?

There are currently two active areas of research. The first is the myoblast transfer project. Here healthy myoblasts are injected into individual muscles of a DMD patient. Because skeletal muscle is a syncytium, the dystrophin produced by the donor cells should mix with the deficit cells and reverse disease progression in that particular muscle. The disadvantages are the impracticality of injecting all the muscles in the body, and the inability to affect the cardiac and CNS involvement. The second area of research is to introduce a normal copy of the dystrophin gene throughout the affected patient, theoretically by using a retrovirus vector.

Blau HM, Springer ML: Muscle-mediated gene therapy. N Engl J Med 333:1554–1556, 1995.

Mendell JR, Kissel JT, Amato AA, et al: Myoblast transfer in the treatment of Duchenne's muscular dystrophy. N Engl J Med 333:832–838, 1995.

94. What are the most common congenital myopathies?

(1) Central core disease, (2) centronuclear myopathy, (3) nemaline myopathy, (4) minimal change myopathy, and (5) congenital fiber type disproportion.

95. What are the clinical manifestations of myotonic muscular dystrophy?

Myotonic dystrophy is an autosomal dominant disease that has been linked to chromosome 19. Clinical manifestations usually begin in adolescence or early adult life; however, there is variable expressivity. Clinical features include distal muscle weakness and myotonia. Muscle wasting about the face and sternocleidomastoids, in combination with facial weakness, leads to the distinctive "hatchet-face" appearance. Patients have partial ptosis, swanlike posture of the neck, enlarged paranasal sinuses, early prominent male-pattern balding in both sexes, cataracts, cardiac conduction abnormalities, hypogonadism with testicular atrophy, and abnormal glucose tolerance.

Thorton CA, Ashizowa T: Getting a grip on the myotonic dystrophies. Neurology 52:12–13, 1999.

96. What is a common and potentially life-threatening complication that may befall neonates born to mothers with myotonic muscular dystrophy?

Some newborns who have inherited the myotonic dystrophy gene from their mothers experience profound weakness, with respiratory failure and bulbar insufficiency requiring endotracheal intubation and mechanical ventilation. The mortality rate may be as high as 30–40%. Should the neonate survive, the weakness resolves spontaneously. The occurrence of the neonatal syndrome has no effect on the severity of the adult expression of the disease.

97. What are the two types of myasthenia that may affect the newborn or young infant?

1. **Transient neonatal myasthenia gravis.** Affected neonates are born to mothers with autoimmune myasthenia gravis. The newborns experience transient weakness and hypotonia, which may be severe and life-threatening, due to the transplacental transfer of maternal antiacetylcholine receptor antibodies.

2. **Nonautoimmune congenital myasthenia syndromes**.

Younger DS (ed): Advances in the diagnosis and treatment of myasthenia gravis. Neurology 48(Suppl 5):51–581, 1997.

98. Which types of myasthenia are not due to autoimmune production of antibodies against the acetylcholine (Ach) receptor?

1. Defects in ACh synthesis or mobilization
2. End-plate acetylcholinesterase deficiency
3. Slow-channel syndrome
4. End-plate ACh receptor deficiency

Engel AG, Walls TJ, Nagel A, Uchitel O: Newly recognized congenital myasthenic syndromes. I. Congenital paucity of synaptic vesicles and reduced quantal release. II. High-conductance fast-channel syndrome. III. Abnormal acetylcholine receptor (AChR) interaction with acetylcholine. IV. AChR deficiency and short channel-open time. Prog Brain Res 84:125–137, 1990.

99. A school-aged child presents with a few days' history of progressive weakness in his legs. This "ascending paralysis" was first noted at his ankles and now has spread to involve his hips. List the differential diagnoses.

- Guillain-Barré syndrome
- Acute cerebellar ataxia
- Acute spinal cord lesion
- Tick bite paralysis
- Poliomyelitis
- Periodic paralysis
- Myasthenia gravis
- Botulism
- Poisoning

Felz MW, Smith CO, Swift TR: A six-year-old girl tick paralysis. N Engl J Med 342:90–94, 2000.

LEARNING DISABILITIES

100. What is meant by the term "learning disability"?

A learning disability is present when a child with overall normal intellect has a deficit in acquiring the skills needed to perform a specific cognitive task. For example, the most common learning disability is dyslexia, a disorder manifested by difficulty in learning to read despite conventional instruction, adequate intelligence, and sociocultural opportunity.

101. A school-aged child is referred for evaluation of possible absence epilepsy because of constant "day-dreaming" and worsening grades. The mother and teachers relate a history of short attention span for school work but not for television or video games, easy distractibility, impulsiveness, constant supervision needed to complete homework and chores, adventurous and risk-taking behavior, and constant physical activity (as if driven by a motor). What is the most likely diagnosis?

This is the usual presentation of a child with attention-deficit hyperactivity disorder (ADHD). Some children have the attention deficit without the hyperactivity. This is a troublesome disorder and not infrequently leads to conduct problems. Affected children have unusually short attention spans and are simply unable to concentrate for more than a few minutes for all but the most stimulating and enjoyable activities. Their constant distractibility and day-dreaming may be confused with the seizures of absence epilepsy.

If resources are available, many of these children do very well with individualized instruction. However, for most of the more severely affected children, pharmacotherapy is necessary and generally works very well. CNS stimulants, which greatly enhance the ability to concentrate and pay attention, such as methylphenidate (Ritalin), dextroamphetamine (Dexedrine), and pemoline (Cylert) are used.

102. What are the clinical manifestations of infantile autism?

The onset of autism usually occurs by the end of the first year of life and is manifested by social and language developmental regression and a relative lack of communication. Motor development is generally not affected. These children reject or ignore virtually all interpersonal interactions. They are often disturbed by even the slightest change in their environment, such as rearranging the furniture or books on a shelf. Repetitive self-stimulation behaviors are common and consist of rocking, head banging, whirling, and flapping of hands in front of face. Many of these children appear to have normal intelligence. The etiopathogenetic basis remains unknown and the prognosis for meaningful recovery is very poor.

DeLong GR: Autism: New data suggest a new hypothesis. Neurology 52:911–916, 1999.

BIBLIOGRAPHY

1. Behrman RE, Kliegman RM, Jenson HB (eds): Nelson's Textbook of Pediatrics, 16th ed. Philadelphia, W.B. Saunders, 1999.
2. Berg BO (ed): Principles of Child Neurology. Columbus, OH, McGraw-Hill, 1996.
3. Dubowitz V: Muscle Disorders in Childhood, 3rd ed. Philadelphia, W.B. Saunders, 2001.
4. Fenichel GM: Clinical Pediatric Neurology: A Signs and Symptoms Approach, 4th ed. Philadelphia, W.B. Saunders, 2001.
5. Jones KL: Smith's Recognizable Patterns of Human Malformation, 5th ed. Philadelphia, W.B. Saunders, 1997.
6. Menkes JH (ed): Textbook of Child Neurology, 6th ed. Philadelphia, Lippincott Williams & Wilkins, 2000.
7. Miller G, Ramer JC (eds): Static Encephalopathies of Infancy and Childhood. New York, Raven Press, 1992.
8. Swaimann KF, Ashwal S (eds): Pediatric Neurology: Principles and Practice, 3rd ed. St. Louis, Mosby, 1999.
9. Volpe JJ: Neurology of the Newborn, 4th ed. Philadelphia, W. B. Saunders, 2000.
Websites
www1.umn.edu/cns/index.htm
www.waisman.wisc.edu/child-neuro/index.html

26. ELECTROENCEPHALOGRAPHY

Richard A. Hrachovy, M.D.

1. What is believed to be the source of the electrical activity recorded by scalp electrodes in the electroencephalogram (EEG)?

The best available evidence indicates that surface- and scalp-recorded electrical activity results from extracellular current flow associated with summation of excitatory postsynaptic potentials and inhibitory postsynaptic potentials.

2. What are the different frequencies recorded on an EEG?

Four frequency bands are recorded: delta = < 4 Hz, theta = 4–7 Hz, alpha = 9–13 Hz, and beta = > 13 Hz.

3. What are the features of an EEG in an awake, normal adult?

The EEG reveals a dominant rhythm in the occipital leads bilaterally. The frequency of this rhythm in most adult individuals is between 9 and 11 Hz. This rhythm is variously referred to as the occipital dominant rhythm, the occipital dominant alpha rhythm, or simply the alpha rhythm. The occipital dominant rhythm is best seen with the eyes closed and the individual relaxed. This rhythm usually attenuates when the eyes are opened. In the anterior regions, alpha frequency activity is also present but is lower in voltage and generally less continuous than that in the posterior regions. There is also low-voltage 18–22 Hz activity present in the anterior leads.

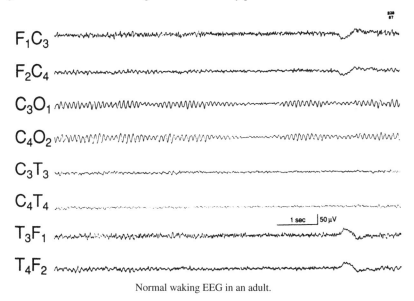

Normal waking EEG in an adult.

4. What are the EEG features of the various sleep stages in the adult?

Nonrapid eye movement (NREM) sleep

Stage 1: The first change in the EEG as an individual becomes drowsy is the disappearance of the occipital dominant alpha rhythm, followed by increasing amounts of theta frequency activity in all regions. During stage 1, diphasic sharp waves also appear in the EEG, occurring maximally at the vertex. These sharp waves are referred to as vertex transients.

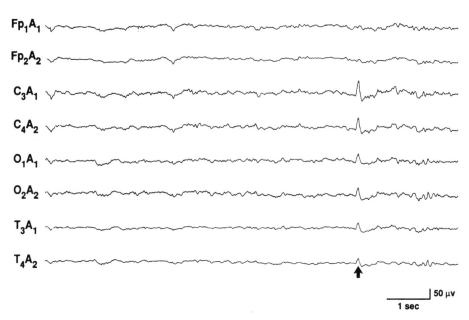

Stage 1 NREM sleep. Arrow denotes vertex transient.

Stage 2: The onset of stage 2 NREM sleep is characterized by the appearance of sleep spindles. Sleep spindles consist of bursts of 12–14 Hz activity, maximally expressed over the central regions of the head. These bursts generally last less than 2 seconds in the adult. The background activity during stage 2 sleep consists of relatively low-voltage, mixed frequency EEG background activity, with delta activity comprising less than 20% of the sleep period.

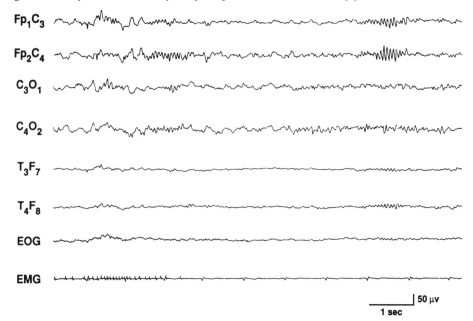

Stage 2 NREM sleep.

Stage 3: As the patient enters deeper NREM sleep, the amount of delta activity increases in voltage and quantity. During stage 3 NREM sleep, the amount of delta activity comprising the record varies between 20 and 50%. Sleep spindles persist into stage 3 sleep.

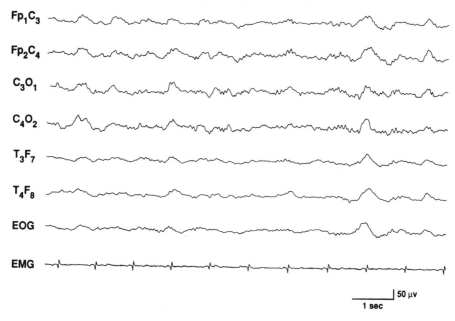

Stage 3 NREM sleep.

Stage 4: During stage 4 NREM sleep, the amount of delta activity comprises more than 50% of the record. Spindles persist into stage 4 NREM sleep.

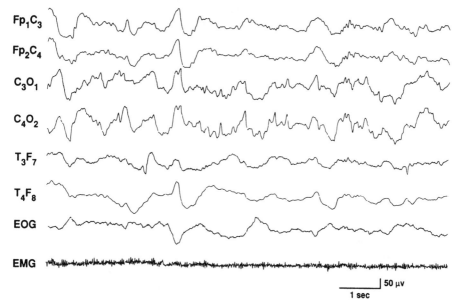

Stage 4 NREM sleep.

Rapid eye movement (REM) sleep

This state is also referred to as paradoxical sleep. The EEG during REM sleep reveals a generally lower voltage record similar in appearance to stage 1. However, in some individuals, runs of alpha frequency activity may appear in the occipital leads identical to the alpha rhythm in the awake tracing. During this stage of sleep, the individual has spontaneous rapid eye movements and tonic motor activity is suppressed.

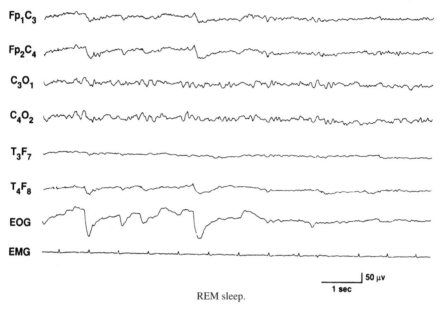

REM sleep.

5. What is a K complex?

A K complex is a high-voltage diphasic slow wave that may be preceded or followed by a spindle burst, maximally expressed in the frontocentral regions bilaterally. K complexes occur spontaneously during sleep but may be elicited by sudden sensory stimuli, such as loud noises.

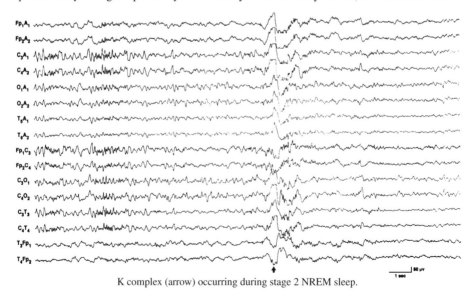

K complex (arrow) occurring during stage 2 NREM sleep.

6. What is the *tracé discontinu* pattern?

Tracé discontinu refers to the EEG pattern seen in premature infants. When the brain's electrical activity first appears, it is discontinuous, with long periods of quiescence or flattening. Initially, it is present in all states of waking and sleep. In early prematurity (26–28 weeks), the periods of flattening may last up to 20–30 seconds. As age increases, the periods of inactivity shorten, and, at 30 weeks' conceptional age, the EEG activity becomes continuous during REM sleep. At about 34 weeks, the EEG activity becomes continuous in the awake state. Continuity appears last in NREM, or quiet sleep, at about 37–38 weeks.

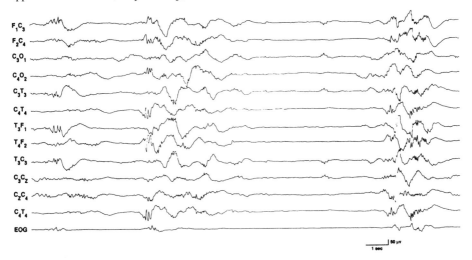

Tracé discontinu pattern in a premature infant.

7. What does the EEG show in an awake term infant?

The typical awake pattern in a term infant is characterized by a mixture of alpha, beta, theta, and delta frequencies, and is often referred to as a poly frequency record.

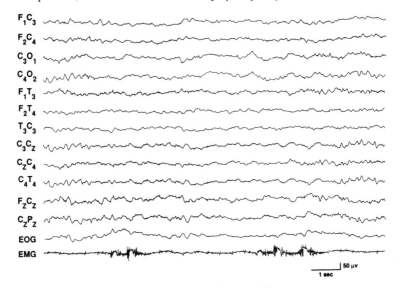

Normal awake pattern in a term infant.

8. What is the *tracé alternant* pattern? At what age is it seen?

The *tracé alternant* pattern is seen from about 37–38 weeks' conceptional age to about 5–6 weeks postterm. This pattern occurs during NREM sleep and is characterized by bursts of slow waves mixed with low-voltage sharp activity, separated by episodes of generalized voltage attenuation lasting from 3–15 seconds, but not absolute quiescence.

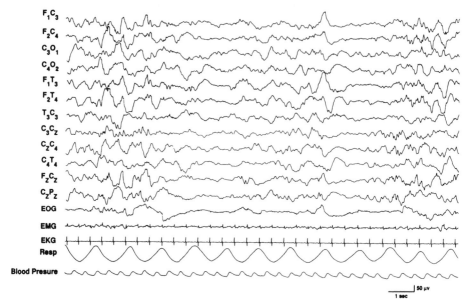

Tracé alternant pattern in a term infant.

9. At what age do vertex transients appear in the EEG? At what age are these transients synchronous? At what age are they symmetrical?

Vertex transients first appear in the EEG at 6–8 weeks postterm. They are synchronous and symmetrical from the time they first appear.

10. At what age do sleep spindles first appear in the EEG? At what age are they synchronous? At what age are they symmetrical?

Like vertex transients, sleep spindles first appear in the EEG at 6–8 weeks postterm. From the time they first appear, they are symmetrical on the two sides; however, spindle synchrony does not occur until approximately 12 months of age.

11. At what age does the occipital dominant rhythm first appear? At what age does the occipital dominant rhythm attain a frequency of 8 Hz?

At approximately 3 months of age, a rhythm that blocks with eye opening and disappears with drowsiness appears in the occipital leads bilaterally. The frequency of this rhythm when it first appears is 3–4 Hz. At 1 year of age, the occipital dominant rhythm is approximately 6 Hz. It does not reach 8 Hz until the age of 3 years.

12. What are the differences in the EEG of an awake child or young adolescent compared with an adult?

- The background activity in the child's EEG is usually higher in voltage.
- The occipital dominant rhythm in children is mixed, with slower fused waveforms referred to as slow waves of youth.
- There is more theta frequency activity in the anterior leads of a child's EEG.

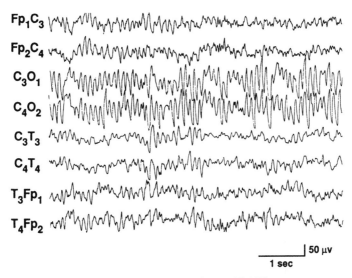

Normal waking EEG in a 9-year-old child.

13. What is the mu rhythm?

The mu rhythm is a normal central rhythm of alpha-activity frequency, usually in the range of 8–10 Hz, which occurs during wakefulness. This rhythm is detectable in approximately 20% of young adults, but is less common in older individuals and children. The mu rhythm is blocked or attenuated by movement, or thought of movement, of the contralateral extremity.

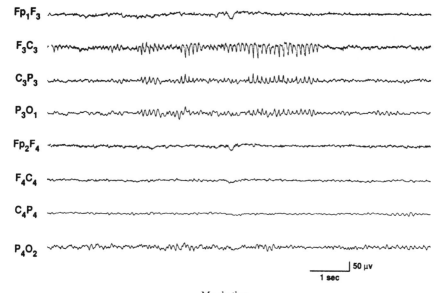

Mu rhythm.

14. What is a breach rhythm?

A breach rhythm typically refers to a high-voltage, sharply contoured rhythm appearing over an area of a skull defect. It is important to realize that this is an accentuated normal rhythm and should not be reported as a focal abnormality.

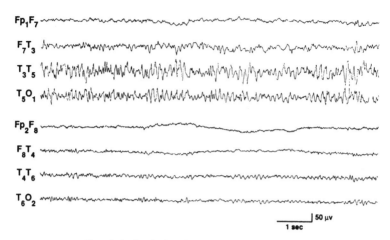

Breach rhythm in the left posterior temporal (T_5) region.

15. What is the most common finding in pseudotumor cerebri?

Although there may be a variety of nonspecific findings in patients with pseudotumor cerebri, the EEG is usually normal.

16. If you were recording the EEG at the time a patient experienced a middle cerebral artery infarction, what would be the sequence of EEG changes you would expect to see?

The initial change following an ischemic episode is depression of the background rhythms over the ipsilateral hemisphere, followed by the appearance of continuous polymorphic slow activity over this hemisphere, maximally expressed in the temporofrontal region.

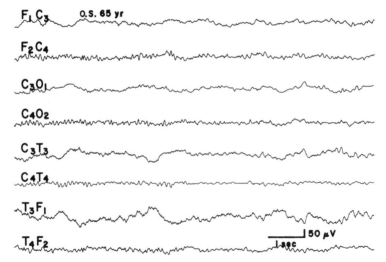

EEG of a patient with a left middle cerebral artery infarction. Note depression of activity over the left hemispheric leads and left temporal slowing.

17. An EEG is obtained 3 years after a person has experienced a hemispheric infarction. What EEG findings may be seen in this patient?

As in the acute state, the EEG recorded years after a hemispheric infarction may continue to show depression of background activity over the ipsilateral hemisphere. Focal slow-wave activity may also continue ipsilaterally. However, the focal slow-wave activity is not as continuous as it is in the acute state. The patient may continue to show depression of the occipital dominant rhythm on the side of the infarct. However, in many patients, the amplitude of the occipital dominant rhythm returns to normal ipsilaterally, and in some patients the occipital dominant rhythm becomes enhanced on the side of the infarction (so-called paradoxical enhancement of the alpha rhythm). A small number of patients may reveal a spike focus ipsilaterally. Finally, a large percentage of patients will show a normal EEG years after a hemispheric infarction.

18. What are the typical EEG changes seen with a small lacunar infarct?
Small lacunar infarcts usually produce no change in the background EEG activity; the EEG in such infarcts is usually normal.

19. What types of EEG findings may be seen with a subdural hematoma?
Depression of background activity over the ipsilateral hemisphere or focal slow-wave activity over the ipsilateral hemisphere are the findings most frequently seen with a subdural hematoma. Episodic bifrontal slow activity may also occur. However, it is important to remember that the EEG may be normal.

20. A 6-year-old child presents with headache and ataxia. A posterior fossa tumor is suspected. What EEG findings suggest this diagnosis?
The most common EEG finding associated with posterior fossa tumors in children is paroxysmal bioccipital delta activity.

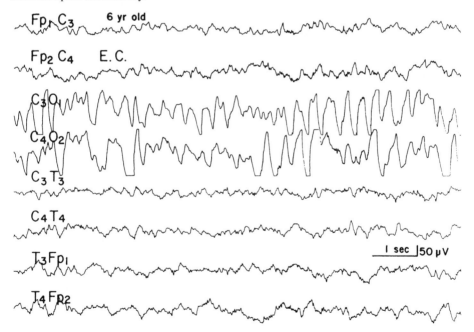

Rhythmic occipital slow activity in a child with a posterior fossa tumor.

21. What is the significance of triphasic waves in the EEG?
Triphasic waves usually appear in the EEG when there has been diffuse slowing of background rhythms. Although triphasic waves may be seen with a variety of encephalopathies (e.g., infectious, toxic, postanoxic), they most often are associated with metabolic encephalopathies, most commonly hepatic or renal.

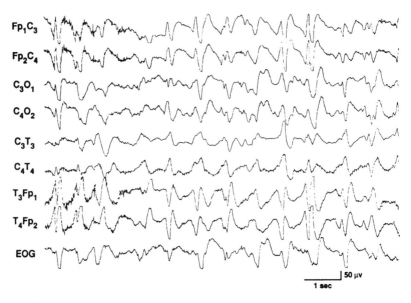

EEG in metabolic encephalopathy demonstrating triphasic waves in the frontal regions.

22. What is the relationship between clinical improvement and EEG improvement in children with various encephalopathies?

Although in older individuals with various types of encephalopathies, clinical and EEG improvement usually occur simultaneously, in children the clinical status of the patient may improve more rapidly than the EEG.

23. What is the usual progression of EEG changes in Alzheimer's disease (AD)?

During the early stages of AD, the EEG may be normal. As the disease progresses, the EEG initially shows slowing of the occipital dominant rhythm, which, in turn, is followed by increasing amounts of theta-frequency activity and then by the appearance of bifrontal and, in some patients, bioccipital delta activity. Occasional sharp waves may appear in the frontal and posterior head regions in severely demented patients; however, these sharp waves never develop the periodic character of the sharp waves seen with Creutzfeldt-Jakob disease. Marked asymmetries of the background activity and focal slow wave activity are not features of AD.

24. What are the major differences between the periodic pattern seen with Creutzfeldt-Jakob disease and that seen with subacute sclerosing panencephalitis (SSPE)?

Creutzfeldt-Jakob Disease vs. SSPE

	C-J	SSPE
Complex morphology	Di- or triphasic sharp waves	Slow waves or groups of slow waves; may have sharp component
Period	Classically, 1 sec	4–14 sec
Distribution	Generalized but may begin focally or lateralized to one hemisphere	Usually generalized but maximal in frontocentral leads
Background activity	Diffusely slow when complexes first appear	May be normal when complexes first appear

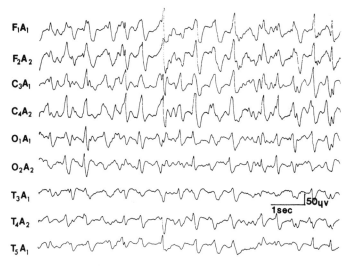

Periodic pattern in Creutzfeldt-Jakob disease.

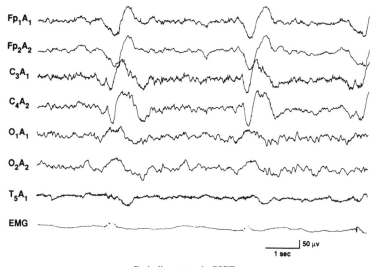

Periodic pattern in SSPE.

25. What other disease processes may produce a periodic pattern similar to that seen with Creutzfeldt-Jakob disease?

The periodic pattern consisting of generalized, high-voltage diphasic and triphasic sharp waves recurring with a period of 1 second is highly suggestive of Creutzfeldt-Jakob disease. However, a pattern indistinguishable from that seen in Creutzfeldt-Jakob disease may occur in the postanoxic state. Also, a similar type of pattern may be seen with lithium intoxication.

26. What is the significance of periodic lateralizing epileptiform discharges (PLEDs)? What is the most common etiology?

PLEDs signify the presence of a large destructive lesion involving one hemisphere. They may be seen with a variety of lesions, including tumors, abscesses, hematomas, and herpes encephalitis. However, the most common cause of PLEDs is acute cerebral infarction.

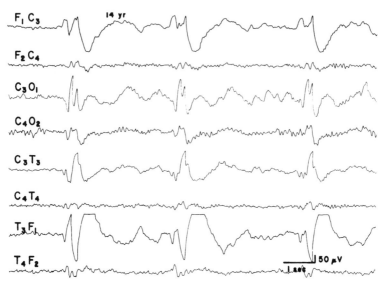

Periodic lateralizing epileptiform discharges (PLEDs).

27. What classes of drugs produce increased amounts of voltages of beta activity in the EEG at therapeutic doses?

The most common classes of drugs that produce increased fast activity in the EEG are the sedatives, anxiolytic agents, CNS stimulants, and antihistamines. Antidepressants may increase the amount of beta activity in the EEG at therapeutic doses but also result in an increase in the amount of theta-frequency activity.

Excessive beta activity in a patient receiving a benzodiazepine.

28. What is hypsarrhythmia?

Hypsarrhythmia is the interictal EEG pattern usually seen in infants who experience infantile spasms. The pattern consists of random, high-voltage slow waves mixed with high-voltage, multifocal spike and sharp waves arising from all cortical regions. The triad of infantile spasms, hypsarrhythmia, and mental retardation is often referred to as West's syndrome.

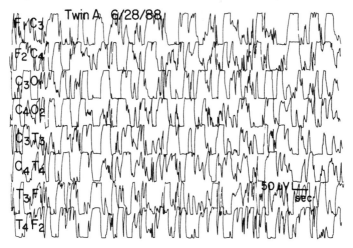

Hypsarrhythmia.

29. What are the characteristics of the 3 per second spike and slow-wave pattern?

This pattern is bilateral, symmetrical, and usually maximally expressed in the frontocentral regions. In some patients, however, the bursts of 3 per second spike and wave activity may be restricted to or maximally expressed in the occipital regions. The discharges appear and disappear suddenly. The frequency of the spike and wave complexes may vary slightly during the burst. The first few complexes of the bursts may occur at a frequency of 3.5–4.0 Hz, whereas the last few may slow to 2.5 Hz. As soon as the 3-Hz spike and wave bursts stop, the EEG returns to its interictal state immediately with no postictal depression or slowing.

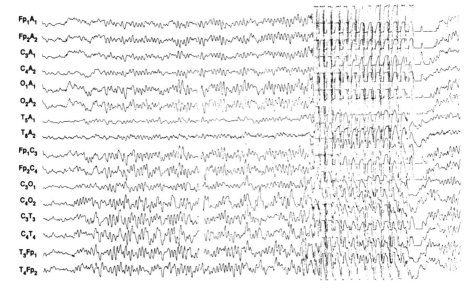

3-Hz spike and wave in a child with absence seizures.

30. A 10-year-old girl with staring spells is referred for an EEG. What routine activating procedures should be performed on this patient?

The common activating procedures usually performed on patients with suspected seizures are hyperventilation, photic stimulation, and sleep. Generalized spike and wave activity may be activated by any of these three activating procedures, whereas focal spikes are usually activated only by sleep.

31. Which two normal patterns are frequently confused with generalized spike and wave activity in children?

The first is **hypnagogic hypersynchrony**. This pattern appears at 3–4 months of age and persists until 10–12 years of age. It consists of paroxysmal rhythmic 3–5 Hz activity, maximally expressed in the central and centrofrontal regions. This activity may occur in long runs; however, it may also appear in brief paroxysms. Faster components may be mixed with the paroxysmal slower activity. The second pattern often confused with generalized spike and slow-wave activity is the **normal hyperventilation response**. Children, particularly between the ages of 5 and 15 years, often show a buildup of high-voltage, frontal dominant, generalized 3–4 Hz activity. This high-voltage, rhythmic slow activity may be continuous or occur in a paroxysmal fashion while the child is deep-breathing. This pattern may be easily confused by the novice electroencephalographer with the 3-Hz spike and slow-wave pattern, which may also occur during hyperventilation in children.

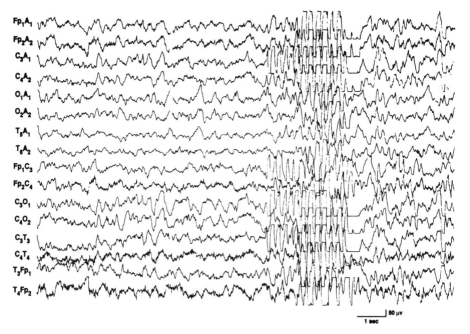

Hypnagogic hypersynchrony.

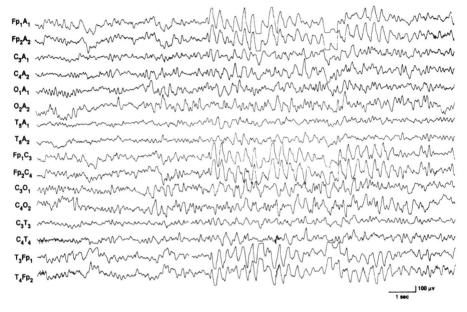

Hyperventilation response in a child.

32. What are the characteristics of focal epileptiform spikes?

A spike is an EEG transient with a duration of less than 70 ms. The transient may occur alone, but frequently a slow wave follows, forming a spike and slow-wave complex. The duration of the slow wave may last from 150–350 milliseconds. The spike transient may be monophasic or polyphasic. The polarity of most focal epileptiform spikes recorded at the scalp is surface negative. Surface positive spikes rarely occur in patients with epilepsy.

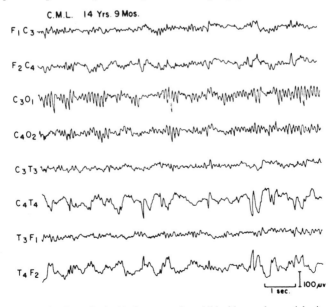

Right temporal spikes mixed with slow waves in a child with complex partial seizures.

33. Which three normal EEG patterns may be confused with focal epileptiform spikes in the EEG?

    1. Vertex transients = synchronous diphasic sharp waves that appear at the vertex.

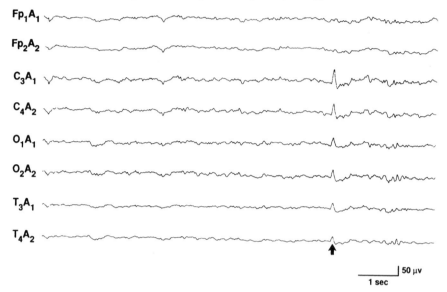

Stage 1 NREM sleep. Arrow denotes vertex transient.

    2. Lambda waves = multiphasic spikes that appear in the occipital leads, with eyes open, and are associated with saccadic eye movements when looking at geometric patterns.

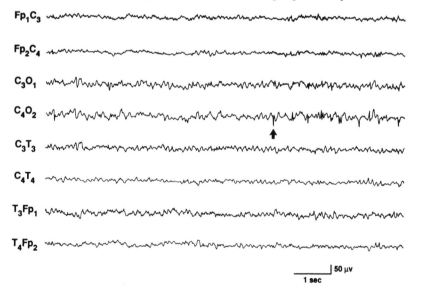

Lambda waves (arrow) in the occipital leads in an individual looking at a geometric design.

    3. Positive occipital sharp transients of sleep = positive sharp waves that appear in the occipital leads during NREM sleep.

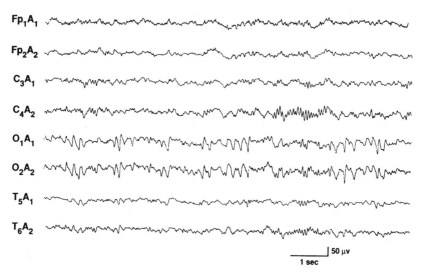

Positive occipital sharp transients of sleep.

34. What are the typical clinical characteristics of a patient whose EEG shows bursts of generalized 2-Hz spike and slow-wave activity?

They have varying degrees of developmental and mental retardation. These patients experience multiple types of seizures, most commonly atonic, tonic, atypical absence, and generalized tonic-clonic. Partial seizures may also occur. These seizures are generally refractory to anticonvulsant therapy, and such patients will often be treated with polytherapy. This constellation of clinical and EEG features is often referred to as the Lennox-Gastaut syndrome, or slow-spike and slow-wave syndrome.

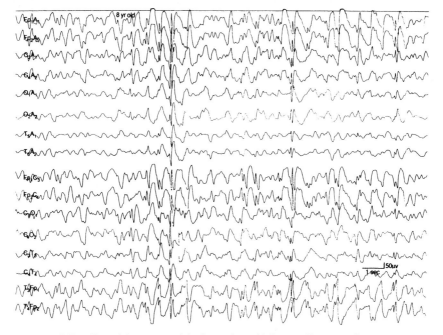

2-Hz spike and slow-wave activity in a patient with Lennox-Gastaut syndrome.

35. What are the usual effects of NREM and REM sleep on interictal generalized or focal epileptiform discharges?

In general, NREM sleep greatly enhances the frequency of interictal generalized spike and wave or focal spike activity, particularly the first NREM sleep episode of nocturnal sleep. On the other hand, REM sleep is usually associated with a marked attenuation or total abolishment of epileptiform activity.

36. What types of EEG changes may be seen postictally?

Immediately after a generalized tonic-clonic seizure, there is marked depression of background activity in all regions, followed by an increase in the voltage and frequency of the background activity, and a gradual return to the baseline state. Focal slowing may also occur postictally in a patient who has experienced a generalized tonic-clonic seizure. Following a partial seizure, the EEG frequently shows regional or hemispheric depression of the background activity over the ipsilateral hemisphere and/or focal slow-wave activity over the ipsilateral hemisphere. The duration that the postictal changes will persist in the EEG is highly variable. In general, the longer the duration of the seizure, the longer the postictal changes persist. This is particularly true in children, who may show diffuse or focal postictal changes for days following a prolonged seizure or an episode of status epilepticus.

37. What four EEG patterns with an epileptiform morphology are classified as patterns of uncertain diagnostic significance?

    1. The 14- and 6-Hz positive bursts (14 and 6 per second positive spikes)

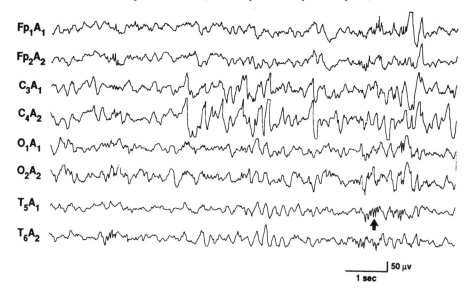

14 and 6 per second positive spike pattern.

2. The rhythmic temporal theta bursts of drowsiness (psychomotor variant pattern)

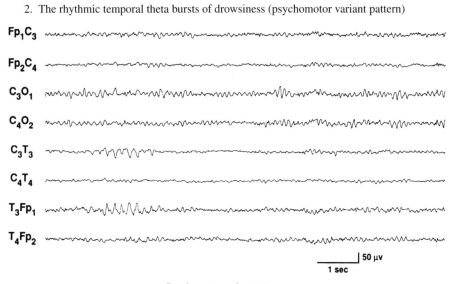

Psychomotor variant pattern.

3. The 6-Hz spike and wave pattern (phantom spike and wave pattern)

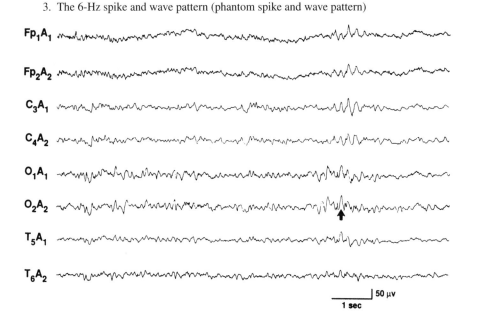

Phantom spike and wave pattern.

4. The small, sharp spike pattern (benign epileptiform transients of sleep)

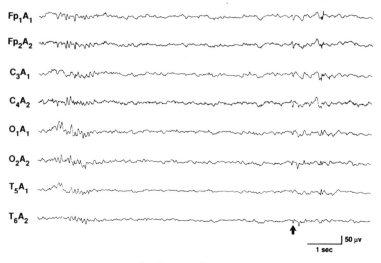

Small sharp spike pattern.

The 14 and 6 per second positive burst pattern is a pattern of childhood and adolescence, whereas the remaining three patterns are usually seen in adulthood.

38. What is the significance of a suppression-burst pattern? Which conditions may produce this pattern?

The suppression-burst pattern consists of brief paroxysms of activity occurring between periods of little or no discernible electrical activity. The activity during the bursts may consist of alpha, theta, or delta frequencies and/or sharp waves. The suppression-burst pattern indicates the presence of a severe diffuse disturbance in brain function. It may be seen in a variety of conditions, including anoxic insult, drug overdose, and severe head injury.

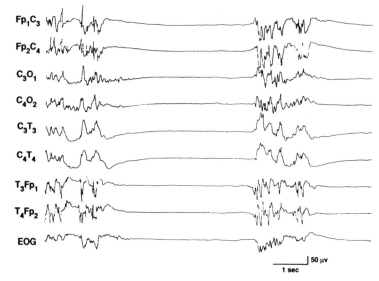

Suppression burst pattern in a comatose patient.

39. What are some of the patterns that may be seen following an anoxic insult?

Depending on the degree of the anoxic insult and the timing from the insult to the EEG, a variety of patterns may be seen. With mild insults, the EEG may be normal or show only slight diffuse slowing. As the severity of the insult increases, so does the degree of slowing of the background rhythms. In addition, periodic diphasic and triphasic sharp waves, superimposed upon a slow-background, alpha coma pattern, and suppression-burst patterns may all occur in the postanoxic state.

40. What are the three brainstem coma patterns? Which pattern generally has the best prognosis?

Alpha coma, spindle coma, and theta coma. Of these, spindle coma usually carries the best prognosis.

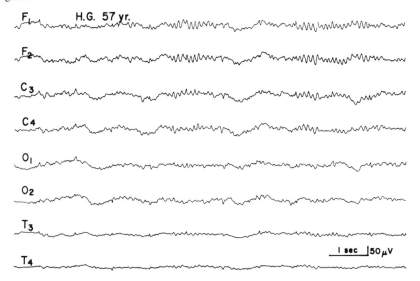

Alpha coma pattern in a comatose patient following a brainstem infarction. Note alpha frequency activity in frontal deviations.

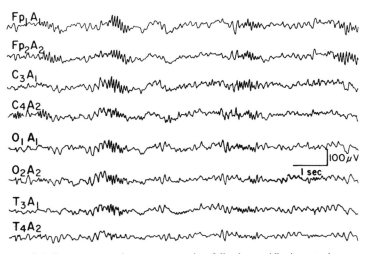

Spindle coma pattern in a comatose patient following a midbrain contusion.

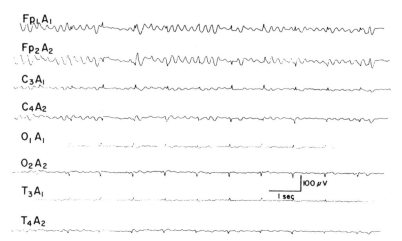

Theta coma pattern in a comatose patient following a cardiorespiratory arrest. Periodic low-voltage sharp waves represent EKG artifact.

41. What are the major criteria for recording a case of suspected brain death?
- A minimum of 8 scalp electrodes and earlobe reference electrodes should be used.
- The interelectrode impedances should be under 10,000 ohms but over 100 ohms.
- The interelectrode distances should be at least 0 cm.
- The sensitivity should be changed from 7 µV/mm to 2 µV/mm during most of the recording with inclusion of appropriate calibrations.
- A time constant of 0.3–0.4 seconds should be used during part of the recording.
- The integrity of the entire recording system should be tested.
- Monitoring techniques (e.g., EKG, ambient noise, respiratory, etc.) should be used as needed to identify other physiologic signals and artifacts as not being of brain origin.
- The EEG should be tested for reactivity by intense stimulation such as pain and loud sound.
- The EEG should be recorded for at least 30 minutes.
- The recording should be made only by qualified technologists.
- A repeat EEG should be performed if there is any doubt about electrocerebral silence.
- Telephone transmission of an EEG should not be used for determination of electrocerebral silence.

42. What are the two conditions that may produce temporary, reversible, electrocerebral inactivity?

The two conditions that may result in reversible electrocerebral inactivity are overdoses with CNS depressants and hypothermia.

BIBLIOGRAPHY

1. Daly DO, Pedley TA (eds): Current Practice of Clinical Electroencephalography, 2nd ed. New York, Raven Press, 1990.
2. Blume WT, Kaibara M: Atlas of Adult Electroencephalopathy. Philadelphia, Lippincott-Raven, 1995.
3. Fisch B (ed): Spehlman's EEG Primer, 2nd ed. Amsterdam, New York, Elsevier, 1991.
4. Hrachovy RA: Development of the normal electroencephalogram. In Levin KH, Lüders HO (eds): Comprehensive Clinical Neurophysiology. Philadelphia, W.B. Saunders, 2000, pp 387–413.
5. Niedermeyer E, Lopes da Silva F (eds): Electroencephalography: Basic Principles, Clinical Application, and Related Fields, 4th ed. Philadelphia, Lippincott Williams & Wilkins, 1999.

27. ELECTROMYOGRAPHY

James M. Killian, M.D.

1. What is an electromyogram (EMG)? How is it recorded?

An electromyogram is an electrical recording of resting and voluntary muscle activity. It is transmitted from a needle electrode through a preamplifier and amplifier to a loudspeaker and oscilloscopic or digital visual display. When an EMG is ordered, nerve conduction studies are included as part of the overall electrodiagnostic examination.

2. What are the clinical indications for ordering an EMG?

An EMG is usually ordered to determine the localization and severity of neurogenic disorders and to differentiate them from myogenic disorders. Focal neurogenic lesions are localized using the same logic as is used in the clinical muscle exam, but important subclinical information can be determined in muscles with indefinite weakness. Myogenic disorders are separated into inflammatory (myositis) and noninflammatory (myopathy).

3. What are the characteristics of normal voluntary motor unit potentials?

Normal muscle potentials appear as waveforms with a duration of 5–15 ms, 2–4 phases, and amplitude of 0.5–3 mv (depending on the size of the unit and type of recording needle electrodes).

4. What are polyphasic units? When are they seen on EMG?

These are voluntary motor units with more than four phases. They are seen in both myogenic and neurogenic disorders.

5. What are the characteristics of abnormal voluntary motor unit potentials?

Abnormal motor unit potentials are classified as either neurogenic or myogenic. Neurogenic motor units appear of longer duration and higher amplitude than normal potentials and are usually polyphasic. Myopathic potentials are just the opposite, with shorter durations and smaller amplitudes than normal potentials. They are also usually polyphasic.

6. What are the EMG characteristics of fasciculation potentials?

A fasciculation is an involuntary firing of a single motor neuron and all its innervated muscle fibers. It is displayed by EMG as a single motor unit and, if close to the surface, is visible as a brief irregular undulation of muscle.

7. What is the significance of fasciculations? When are they nonpathologic?

Fasciculations may be associated with pathology in the anterior horn cells or motor roots. However, fasciculations may be present with no evidence of any nerve or muscle disease and then are termed "benign fasciculations."

8. What are the EMG characteristics of fibrillation potentials?

Fibrillations are involuntary contractions of single muscle fibers and cannot be seen through the skin. Electrically, they appear as regular or irregular, short, small action potentials that sound like static or cooking bacon. Fibrillations are always abnormal and indicate loss of innervation of a single muscle fiber from a variety of causes.

9. What is the importance of insertional activity?

Insertional activity is the discharge of single muscle fibers during insertion of an EMG needle and does not indicate abnormality. The discharges look like fibrillations on the EMG. Increased insertional activity may indicate irritable muscle fibers, such as in early denervation, but it is often nonspecific.

10. What are positive sharp waves?

Positive sharp waves are spontaneous discharges from groups of denervated muscle fibers. They are larger than fibrillation potentials but have the same pathologic implication (i.e., denervation). They appear on the EMG screen as downward monophasic wave formations that indicate a positive polarity—hence the name.

11. What electrical activity can be measured from the endplate?

High-frequency, short-duration potentials can be seen when the EMG needle is close to or in the motor endplate. They are called endplate activity or endplate noise. This activity is not pathologic but may be confused with fibrillation potentials.

12. What are the two types of myotonia? Describe their appearance on an EMG?

Myotonia refers to a delayed relaxation of muscle after contraction or needle insertion. The two types of myotonia are true and pseudo. True myotonia occurs in the myotonic dystrophies and myotonia congenita and is seen as muscle action potentials that vary in amplitude and frequency and are heard on the loud speaker as "dive bombers." Pseudomyotonia has a more stable firing frequency that resembles an airplane in steady flight, with abrupt termination. Pseudomyotonia occurs in both muscle and nerve disorders, including myositis, glycogen storage diseases, hyperkalemic periodic paralysis, root disease, and anterior horn cell disorders.

13. What are the EMG characteristics recorded in a myopathy?

In myopathy, the motor unit potentials are smaller and shorter because of a reduction in the size of the muscle fibers. The discharging motor unit firing rate is unchanged; therefore, a full pattern of muscle activity on effort ("interference pattern") is still seen on the EMG screen.

14. What are the EMG characteristics of activity recorded from a denervated muscle?

Fibrillations and positive sharp waves begin in resting muscles 7–14 days after the onset of axonal denervation. When partially denervated muscle is voluntarily contracted, clinical weakness from axonal loss is seen on the EMG as a reduction in motor unit firing patterns proportional to the amount of axonal loss.

15. How soon do electrical changes develop after a nerve is transected?

Transection of a nerve is followed immediately by loss of voluntary activity; therefore, no electrical motor units are seen with attempted contraction. Spontaneous abnormal EMG activity consisting of fibrillation and positive sharp waves begins 7–10 days later and reaches maximum level at approximately 14–21 days.

16. After nerve transection, what happens to nerve conduction in the distal segment?

Nerve conduction in the distal segment is retained for 3 days after proximal transection of the nerve. Wallerian degeneration rapidly interferes with nerve conduction, and after 3–5 days, all conductibility is lost.

17. How do recruitment patterns differ in normal muscles, myopathies, and neurogenic disorders?

The pattern of motor activity on effort does not differ between normal muscles and those with myopathic abnormalities, because all motor units are intact and fire normally. However, neurogenic abnormalities show a dropout of motor units, which reduces the recruitment pattern according to the severity of axonal loss.

18. What are the clinical indications for ordering nerve conduction velocities?

Nerve conduction velocities (NCV) are ordered to demonstrate presence or absence of focal or generalized abnormalities of the peripheral motor and sensory nerves, to assess the severity of any abnormalities, and to determine whether the nerve pathology is axonal or demyelinative.

19. What is the normal NCV?

Normal motor nerve conduction velocity (MCV) in the arm is above 50 meters per second (m/s) and in the leg above 42 m/s. Distal latencies vary with the nerve studied, as do sensory nerve conduction (SCV) measurements.

20. What is a normal compound motor action potential (CMAP)?

A CMAP is the muscle contraction resulting from stimulation of a motor nerve and is a measure of the functioning motor axons in that nerve. The amplitude varies with the muscle that is stimulated, but in the hand it is above 6 mV, and in the foot it is above 1 mV.

21. What is a normal sensory nerve action potential (SNAP)?

A SNAP measures the conducting sensory axons after nerve stimulation with velocities similar to motor conduction in the arms (50 m/s) but slower than motor conduction in the legs (35 m/s). The SNAP amplitude depends on the size of the nerve studied but may range from 10 to 100 μV, which is small compared with the amplitude of CAMPs.

22. What is the H-reflex? How is it used clinically?

The H-reflex is the electrical counterpart of the ankle jerk; it gives clinical information about any pathology in the S1 afferent-efferent reflex arc. The H may be prolonged or absent in neuropathies, S1 radiculopathies, or sciatic mononeuropathies.

23. What is the F-wave? How is it useful clinically?

After motor nerve stimulation, the F-wave is seen as a late motor action potential that follows the initial compound muscles' action potential (M-wave). Retrograde (antidromic) transmission of stimulated motor axons causes a discharge of the motor neurons in the spinal cord, resulting in a late discharge of the distal muscle. An F-wave usually is tested on the median, ulnar, peroneal, and tibial motor nerves. The F-wave gives information about abnormal conductibility across both proximal and distal nerve segments and is useful in acute and chronic demyelinating neuropathies.

24. What is repetitive nerve stimulation (RNS)? How is it used clinically?

RNS measures the motor responses to slow rates of motor nerve stimulation. RNS is used as a diagnostic test for myasthenia gravis (MG) and Lambert-Eaton myasthenic syndrome (LEMS).

25. What does repetitive nerve stimulation show in a patient with MG?

About 65–85% of patients with MG show a decremental motor response of 10% or more to slow repetitive stimulation of a motor nerve at 2–3 Hz. The highest yield is in the proximal muscles, such as the trapezius, when the spinal accessory nerve in the neck is stimulated. The facial nerve also may be tested, but the results are often technically unsatisfactory because of patient discomfort. Prolonged neuromuscular blockade in intensive care patients may show findings similar to MG.

26. What does repetitive nerve stimulation show in a patient with LEMS?

Repetitive stimulation in LEMS shows pre-exercise low-amplitude compound muscle action potentials in distal muscles because of reduced release of acetylcholine (Ach) at the motor nerve terminal. The muscle potentials double or triple in size after exercise because of increased release of Ach at the motor nerve terminal (postexercise facilitation). Decremental responses similar to MG often are superimposed on the facilitated motor units. Botulism may show findings similar to LEMS.

27. What is the clinical utility of single-fiber EMG?

Single-fiber EMG measures the difference in transmission between two individual muscle fibers from the same motor unit (jitter). A delay beyond normal, known as prolonged jitter, indicates an abnormality in neuromuscular transmission at the motor endplate. Special needles and recording equipment are necessary for the procedure. Single-fiber EMG is used mainly in the diagnosis of early cases of MG, for which its accuracy is 90–95%. However, it is a nonspecific measurement and may show abnormal results in motor neuron disease and other neurogenic disorders.

28. Define neurapraxia and conduction block. How do they differ from axonal damage?

Neurapraxia is a reversible physiologic nerve lesion often seen after trauma. If the lesion is focal, distal motor conduction is normal but conduction proximal to the lesion is absent or slowed for up to 4–6 weeks. Axonal lesions have a longer recovery because of wallerian degeneration of fibers, which requires reinnervation. **Conduction block** is a pathologic focal lesion of myelin. In early stages, conduction block shows up only as decreased proximal motor amplitude compared with distal conduction amplitude. Conduction block is seen in demyelinating neuropathies of various causes and with focal trauma.

29. How can the EMG and nerve conduction studies help differentiate a demyelinating peripheral neuropathy from an axonal peripheral neuropathy?

Demyelinating neuropathies show moderate to severe slowing of motor conduction, with temporal dispersion of the CMAP, normal distal amplitudes, reduced proximal stimulation amplitudes (conduction block), and delayed distal latencies. Axonal neuropathies show a milder or borderline slowing in conduction velocity, with generally low CMAP amplitudes at both proximal and distal sites of stimulation because of axonal loss. The EMG shows denervation abnormalities early in axonal neuropathies and only late in demyelinating neuropathies, when axons begin to degenerate.

30. What does the EMG show in polymyositis?

Myopathic motor units, fibrillations, and pseudomyotonia are the classic triad of EMG findings in polymyositis.

31. Can inclusion body myositis (IBM) be differentiated from polymyositis by EMG?

Proximal myositic abnormalities may be seen in both conditions, but the EMG findings in IBM may show a concentration of focal myositic abnormalities in the forearm flexors and quadriceps muscles.

32. Describe the EMG findings in spastic (upper motor neuron) paresis.

No abnormal findings are noted if the anterior horn cells and roots are normal. EMG patterns on attempted maximum effort are reduced by lack of upper motor neuron control, but the patterns per se are nondiagnostic.

33. What EMG findings confirm the diagnosis of amyotrophic lateral sclerosis (motor neuron disease)?

The EMG should show widespread proximal and distal denervation with fasciculations and giant units in at least two extremities, plus denervation in either the tongue or thoracic paraspinous muscles. Cervical and lumbar spondylosis may show similar abnormalities in the extremities but normal tongue and thoracic paraspinous muscles.

34. What do EMG and nerve conduction studies show in Guillain-Barré syndrome? What is their prognostic utility?

In early Guillain-Barré syndrome, the EMG simply shows reduction in motor unit firing patterns, depending on the degree of paralysis. After 14–21 days, spontaneous denervation activity (fibrillations and positive sharp waves) indicates wallerian degeneration (axonal loss). The EMG is useful prognostically because greater axonal loss generally implies longer recovery time. Motor conduction velocities show marked slowing in proximal and distal motor conduction and other changes of demyelination, beginning 3–5 days after onset. Severe slowing may be delayed for 7–14 days. Sensory conduction studies often show normal results, but an early sign may be a reduction in amplitude of the median sensory potential compared with that of the sural sensory potential.

35. How is EMG useful in brachial plexus lesions?

The main value of the EMG is in delineating the presence and degree of denervation in the appropriate arm muscles and thus localizing damage in the roots, trunks, cords, or distal branches of the brachial plexus. When the plexopathy is diffuse, motor and sensory conduction studies in the arm are severely abnormal.

36. What is the role of EMG and nerve conduction studies in evaluating a patient with a suspected radiculopathy from cervical or lumbar disc disease?

EMG can confirm the root distribution of muscle weakness noted on clinical examination and give information about muscles that were not examined completely because of pain or lack of full effort. Nerve conduction studies have limited value unless multiple cervical or lumbar roots are involved, but such studies can exclude other focal peripheral nerve lesions.

37. Define carpal tunnel syndrome (CTS).

CTS consists of nocturnal hand paresthesias caused by compression of the median nerve at the wrist from thickening of the flexor retinaculum, possibly in conjunction with congenital narrowing of the carpal tunnel or, rarely, in association with other conditions that cause thickening of the median nerve.

38. What is the best test for an electrical diagnosis of CTS?

Sensory nerve action potential latencies of the median nerve are delayed twice as often as motor latencies. CTS is diagnosed electrically by a delay in sensory conduction latencies from the index finger or mid-palmar area to the wrist. The most sensitive is the palmar latency. Needle EMG, although of limited value, indicates denervation in the thenar muscles in more advanced cases.

39. What other conditions are associated with median nerve entrapment at the wrist?

The differential diagnosis of CTS includes (1) fluid retention secondary to pregnancy, (2) hypothyroidism, (3) diabetes, (4), amyloid deposits, and (5) hereditary hypertrophic neuropathies (Charcot-Marie-Tooth type IA and hereditary neuropathy with liability to pressure palsies).

40. How is CTS treated?

Wrist splints at night may be helpful for mild to moderate cases that show mainly sensory abnormalities on nerve conduction studies. More severe or persistent cases require surgical sectioning of the transverse carpal ligament (flexor retinaculum), which should be decompressed to the distal margin of the ligament in the upper palmar region.

41. What are the most common causes of ulnar nerve entrapment at the elbow?

External pressure over the nerve in its shallow groove, flexion dislocation of the nerve over the medial epicondyle, and compression of the nerve as it enters the aponeurosis of the flexor carpi ulnaris (cubital tunnel syndrome) may cause ulnar nerve lesions at the elbow. Arthritis from an old fracture (tardy ulnar palsy) and rheumatoid arthritis are less common causes.

42. Describe the role of EMG and nerve conduction studies in diagnosing ulnar nerve entrapment at the elbow.

Motor and sensory conduction studies can confirm ulnar nerve entrapment at the elbow in 60–80% of cases, with the EMG indicating the distribution and degree of denervation in the ulnar-innervated hand and forearm muscles.

43. What is the best conduction test for diagnosis of ulnar nerve entrapment at the elbow?

Both motor and sensory conduction studies are helpful. The motor conduction across the elbow segment may show the earliest motor delay or conduction block. The amplitude and velocity of ulnar sensory conduction may be affected more than motor slowing. In early cases, studies may be normal.

44. What is the best therapy for ulnar nerve entrapment at the elbow?

Therapy varies according to the underlying mechanism of entrapment. Elbow protectors are helpful for mild to moderate pressure lesions, but surgery is indicated for more persistent or severe entrapments. Surgery may involve sectioning of the flexor digitorum aponeurosis in cubital tunnel syndromes or medial epicondylectomy in flexion nerve dislocations and tardy ulnar palsies. Translocation of the nerve to the forearm may be necessary in rare cases.

45. How is a lesion in the C8 root differentiated from a plexus or ulnar nerve lesion?
    1. For a lesion in the C8 root, the EMG may show denervation in the following muscles: (1) extensor carpi ulnaris (radial); (2) abductor pollicis brevis (median); (3) first dorsal interosseous, abductor digiti quinti, and flexor carpi ulnaris (ulnar); and (4) C8 paraspinous muscles. Motor and sensory conductions are normal in the ulnar and median nerves unless multiple roots are involved.
    2. A lesion in the plexus (lower trunk or medial cord) involves denervation in all of the above muscles, except for normal C8 paraspinous muscles. Sensory conduction studies are abnormal in the ulnar and medial antebrachial cutaneous forearm nerves. Motor conduction is normal or minimally slow unless atrophy is severe.
    3. In ulnar nerve lesions, the EMG is normal in the radial and median-innervated C8 muscles but shows denervation in the ulnar-innervated muscles of the forearm and hand. Motor and sensory ulnar conduction studies also are abnormal, but the medial antebrachial cutaneous nerve is normal.

46. What is the key muscle in differentiating a radial nerve palsy from a C7 radiculopathy?
    Flexor carpi radialis, which is a C7–C8 muscle innervated by the median nerve.

47. How is a radial nerve palsy differentiated from a brachial plexus posterior cord lesion?
    Abnormalities in the deltoid muscle in addition to radial-innervated muscles indicate a lesion in the posterior cord of the brachial plexus.

48. How is a suprascapular nerve lesion differentiated from a C5–C6 radiculopathy?
    Preservation of the deltoid, biceps, and rhomboid muscles, with abnormalities in the supraspinatus and infraspinatus muscles, indicates a suprascapular nerve lesion.

49. Describe the difference between a long thoracic nerve palsy and a C5–C6 radiculopathy.
    A long thoracic nerve palsy causes winging of the scapula from weakness of the serratus anterior muscle, with normal C5–6 shoulder and arm muscles (e.g., deltoid, biceps supraspinatus). The serratus anterior muscle is not routinely studied by EMG. Long thoracic nerve conduction is slow or nonconductible when performed 3 days after onset.

50. How is a peroneal nerve palsy differentiated from an L4–L5 radiculopathy?
    The invertors of the foot (posterior tibial muscle) are abnormal in L4–L5 radiculopathies.

51. How does a femoral nerve lesion differ from an L3 radiculopathy?
    Abnormalities in the hip adductors and quadriceps muscles are present in L3 radiculopathies.

52. How does a femoral nerve lesion in the pelvis differ from an inguinal lesion?
    Weakness and denervation in the iliopsoas in addition to the quadriceps muscle indicates a femoral nerve lesion in the pelvis.

53. What is the value of motor conduction velocities in Bell's palsy?
    Facial nerve conduction studies 3–5 days after the onset of Bell's palsy may indicate the prognosis. Normal latencies and amplitudes at 5 days indicate an excellent prognosis for recovery. Loss of nerve conductibility indicates the onset of wallerian degeneration with a prognosis of incomplete or no recovery.

54. Describe the role of EMG and nerve conduction studies in critical care patients who develop neuromuscular weakness.
    These studies help to distinguish critical illness polyneuropathy (CIP) from critical illness myopathy (CIM) and prolonged neuromuscular blockade.

55. How does CIP differ from CIM (acute quadraplegic myopathy)?

CIP is an axonal polyneuropathy associated with sepsis. Nerve testing shows abnormal motor and sensory conduction. EMG shows distal denervation, more in the legs than arms. Results of direct muscle stimulation and repetitive nerve stimulation are normal. CIM is a muscle membrane disorder seen with use of nondepolarizing blocking agents and corticosteroids. EMG findings are limited by profound weakness, but motor nerve conduction studies and direct muscle stimulation are nonconductible.

56. Which tests are used to diagnose neuromuscular blockade in the intensive care unit?

Prolonged neuromuscular blockade occurs in patients with abnormal renal function who have been treated with nondepolarizing blocking agents. Repetitive nerve stimulation shows decrement similar to myasthenia gravis and distinguishes these patients from patients with polyneuropathy or myopathy.

57. Which drugs can cause myopathic EMG changes with chronic use?

Myopathic EMG abnormalities can be seen with long-term use of steroids, statin drugs and other cholesterol-lowering agents, chloroquine, amiodarone, and colchicine. The findings are usually mild but indistinguishable from other types of myopathies and are slowly reversible after cessation of the drug.

BIBLIOGRAPHY

1. Johnson EW, Pease WS: Practical Electromyography, 3rd ed. Philadelphia, Lippincott Williams & Wilkins, 1997.
2. Preston DC, Shapiro BF, Barber E: Electromyography and Neuromuscular Disorders. Boston, Butterworth-Heinemann, 1998.
3. Seth I, Thompson LL: The Electromyography Handbook, 2nd ed. Boston, Little, Brown, 1989.

28. NEURORADIOLOGY

Loren A. Rolak, M.D.

Care has been taken to include in this book representative examples of the most common radiographs and images that appear on examinations and boards. These are located in their appropriate place in the text, but they are specifically indexed here to facilitate a neuroradiologic review. The radiographs in this book, representing the major areas of neuroradiology, are cross-referenced below by chapter and page number.

Vascular Disease
1. Superior sagittal sinus thrombosis — ch. 30, p. 403
2. Superficial cortical vein thrombosis — ch. 23, p. 325
3. Brainstem ischemic stroke: Wallenberg syndrome — ch. 9, p. 127
4. Vertebral artery dissection — ch. 9, p. 127
5. Anterior inferior cerebellar artery (AICA) ischemic stroke — ch. 10, p. 139
6. Superior cerebellar artery hemorrhagic stroke — ch. 10, p. 139
7. Intracerebral hemorrhage — ch. 12, p. 192
8. Anterior cerebral artery ischemic stroke — ch. 17, p. 240
9. Gadolinium enhancement of an ischemic stroke — ch. 17, p. 240
10. Internal carotid artery stenosis — ch. 17, p. 241
11. Arteriovenous malformation — ch. 17, p. 246
12. Subarachnoid hemorrhage — ch. 17, p. 247

Spine Disease
1. Transverse myelitis — ch. 8, p. 115
2. Syringomyelia — ch. 8, pp. 115–116
3. Spinal cord astrocytoma — ch. 8, p. 117
4. Spinal cord neurofibroma — ch. 8, p. 118
5. Spinal cord compression from metastatic cancer — ch. 8, p. 118
6. Cervical spondylosis — ch. 7, p. 105
7. Herniated lumbar disc — ch. 7, p. 106
8. Myelomeningocele — ch. 25, p. 349

Demyelinating Disease
1. Multiple sclerosis — ch. 13, p. 204
2. Adrenoleukodystrophy — ch. 25, p. 351
3. Transverse myelitis — ch. 8, p. 115

Neoplastic Disease
1. Acoustic neuroma — ch. 10, p. 145
2. Primitive neuroectodermal tumor (PNET) — ch. 25, p. 359
3. Craniopharyngioma — ch. 25, p. 360
4. Craniopharyngioma (cystic) — ch. 18, p. 254
5. Glioblastoma multiforme — ch. 18, p. 251
6. Glomus jugulare tumor — ch. 18, p. 254
7. Metastatic small-cell lung cancer — ch. 18, p. 256
8. Astrocytoma of the spinal cord — ch. 8, p. 117
9. Neurofibroma of the spinal cord — ch. 8, p. 118
10. Metastatic cancer to the spinal cord — ch. 8, p. 118

Malformation
1. Arnold-Chiari I   ch. 8, p. 116
2. Arnold-Chiari II   ch. 25, p. 349
3. Syringomyelia   ch. 8, pp. 115–116
4. Myelomeningocele   ch. 25, p. 349

Other
1. Cysticercosis   ch. 25, p. 357
2. Neonatal intraventricular hemorrhage   ch. 25, p. 346

29. NEUROLOGIC EMERGENCIES

Loren A. Rolak, M.D.

A number of conditions affecting the nervous system may have a crippling or even fatal outcome. They often present abruptly and require rapid medical intervention. These illnesses have been discussed in their appropriate place in the text, but they are specifically indexed here to facilitate easy access and rapid review of neurologic emergencies. These particularly important conditions are cross-referenced below by chapter and page number.

1.	Coma	ch. 9, pp. 133–134
2.	Hepatic encephalopathy	ch. 23, p. 311
3.	Myxedema	ch. 23, p. 317
4.	Reye syndrome	ch. 23, pp. 311–312
5.	Respiratory insufficiency	ch. 23, pp. 314–315
6.	Botulism	ch. 5, p. 81
7.	Myasthenic crisis	ch. 5, p. 79
8.	Guillain-Barré syndrome	ch. 6, pp. 94–96
9.	Critical care neuropathy	ch. 6, p. 90
10.	Status epilepticus	ch. 21, pp. 298–299
11.	Eclampsia	ch. 23, pp. 324–325
12.	Cerebellar hemorrhage and herniation	ch. 10, pp. 144–145
13.	Subarachnoid hemorrhage	ch. 17, pp. 245–248
14.	Bacterial meningitis	ch. 24, pp. 329–331
15.	Herpes simplex meningitis	ch. 24, p. 338
16.	Spinal cord compression	ch. 8, pp. 117–118
17.	Neuroleptic malignant syndrome	ch. 24, p. 336

30. NEUROLOGY TRIVIA

Questions You Will Often Be Asked by Attendings, but That Are
Not Important for Understanding Science or Taking Care of
Patients, and You Should Not Have to Answer Them

Loren A. Rolak, M.D.

1. Who performed the first spinal tap?
Probably Dr. E. Wynter, in 1891, to drain cerebrospinal fluid from children with tuberculous meningitis. Dr. H. Quinke that same year developed the instruments and technique still used today.

Gorelick PB, Zych D: James Leonard Corning and the early history of spinal puncture. Neurology 37: 672–674, 1987.

Frederiks JAM, Koehler PJ: The first lumbar puncture. J Hist Neurosci 6:147–153, 1997.

2. Who suffered the first spinal tap headache?
The first post spinal tap headache was reported in 1899 by Dr. August Bier, who described it as a consequence of a spinal tap performed on himself by his laboratory assistant in the course of studies on spinal anesthesia. The fate of the assistant is unknown.

3. How do you pronounce the last name of Dr. Georges Guillain, the French neurologist who helped to describe the Guillain-Barré syndrome?
According to Dr. Joseph Rogoff, writing in the *Journal of the American Medical Association*, "The mispronunciation of Dr. George Guillain's name by English-speaking physicians has bothered me for many years. Even the medical dictionaries (e.g., Dorland's) give the pronunciation as "ge-yan," which is incorrect. I was Dr. Guillain's extern in 1939, and I never heard him called anything but "ghee-lain" (with the final 'ain' nasalized). If Guillain wanted his name pronounced thus, why should we insist on changing it?"

4. What is the smallest amount of light the human eye can detect?
The human eye has 125 million rods, each one containing 1000 folds in its photoreceptor membrane, with each fold containing 1 million molecules of photoceptor. This extraordinary light-sensing array can detect one single photon, which is 10^{-11} watts. (Wow!)

5. What does the word *myelin* mean?
Myelin is the Greek word for "marrow" and comes from the belief that the white matter was the marrow of the brain, much like the central portion of the bone is the marrow of the bone.

6. What is Baltic myoclonus?
It is another name for Unverricht-Lundborg disease. Does that help? (It is a type of progressive myoclonic epilepsy.)

7. Why are the zigzag, scintillating, shimmering lights that often precede classic migraine headaches referred to as fortification spectra?
They are called fortification spectra because of their resemblance to the star-shaped, zigzag fortifications constructed in Europe during the Renaissance to protect cities and military compounds.

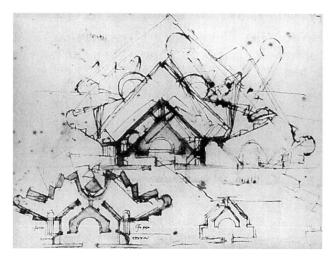

A drawing by Michelangelo for a proposed fortification, showing the triangular, zigzag defensive plan.

8. A lesion that transects the lateral half of the spinal cord will produce a Brown-Sequard syndrome of weakness and loss of proprioception ipsilaterally, with contralateral numbness. Who was Brown, and who was Sequard?

This is a trick question. Brown-Sequard was only one person, Charles Edward Brown-Sequard. His father was an American sailor, and his mother was of French descent, from the island of Mauritius. He took the unusual course of combining his mother's and his father's last names. He became one of the preeminent neurologists of the 19th century, holding professorships, at various times, in America, England, and France.

9. What happened to Charles Edward Brown-Sequard when he ate chocolate?

He developed gustatory perspiration and broke into a sweat.

Gooddy W: Charles Edward Brown-Sequard. In Rose FC, Bynum WF (eds): Historical Aspects of the Neurosciences. New York, Raven Press, 1985, pp 371–378.

10. Jules Dejerine was a brilliant contemporary of the great French neurologist Charcot and ultimately succeeded him at the Salpetriere. He described Dejerine's syndrome (medial medullary infarction) and collaborated with other colleagues of Charcot's to describe the syndromes of Dejerine-Landouzy (muscular atrophy), Dejerine-Roussy (thalamic pain), Dejerine-Thomas (cerebellar-brainstem atrophy), and Dejerine-Sottas (neuropathy and tremor). But who was Klumpke of Dejerine-Klumpke (lower brachial plexopathy)?

Sorry, wrong Dejerine. When Augusta Klumpke married Jules Dejerine, she hyphenated her last name, in a fashion now popular with some modern women. An accomplished physician herself, the syndrome of brachial plexus injury is named after her, not her husband. Like Brown-Sequard (sort of), Dejerine-Klumpke is one person.

11. A meningioma arising from the olfactory groove can extend to compress the optic nerve, producing anosmia, optic atrophy, and unilateral papilledema, a constellation of findings known as the Foster Kennedy syndrome. Who was Foster, and who was Kennedy?

This is another trick question. Dr. Foster (first name) Kennedy (last name) was a prominent American neurologist in the first part of the twentieth century, at one time president of the American Neurological Association. (To muddle things further, his real first name was Robert, although he never used it.) This use of first names is rare, but it gets even more confusing—the famous eponymic Marcus Gunn pupil comes from the *middle* name of the Scottish physician

Robert Marcus Gunn. Exactly how names are applied to diseases is one of medicine's great unsolved mysteries.

12. Who first used the word *neurology*?

The word first appears in Pordage's English translation of Thomas Willis's book *Cerebri Anatome* in 1664. Incidentally, Willis assembled a collaborative research team composed of the greatest minds of his time: Christopher Wren, Robert Hooke, Robert Boyle, Isaac Newton, and William Harvey. In a sense, these men formed the first "Circle of Willis."

13. What was the first description of a neurologic disease?

The first description of a neurologic disease appears in the Smith papyrus, which is the oldest known medical text. This ancient papyrus, translated by Edward Smith, consists of a number of "case reports" of different diseases, presented and discussed by an unknown Egyptian author, written about 3300 B.C. One of the cases is a person with a traumatic head injury, which is the earliest known description of a neurologic problem.

14. Neurology, more than most other specialties, abounds with eponyms and mellifluous phrases that roll off the tongue. For example, what is the torcular herophili?

It is the confluence of the straight, lateral, and sagittal sinuses, where much of the venous drainage occurs in the brain. A torcula is a cistern or well, sometimes used to collect liquor from a wine press, and Herophilus (335–280 B.C.) was the ancient Greek anatomist who described this region of the brain.

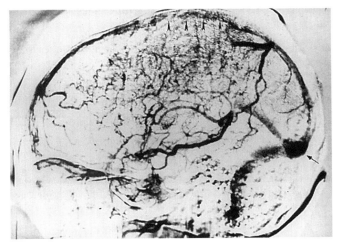

Venous phase of a cerebral angiogram, showing the venous drainage into the torcular herophili (arrow at the right of photo). This patient also has a thrombosis of his superior sagittal sinus (small arrowheads).

15. Refsum's disease is an inherited peripheral neuropathy with ataxia and accompanying retinitis pigmentosa, characterized by accumulation of phytanic acid. What is phytanic acid?

Phytanic acid is 3,7,11,15-tetramethyl-hexadecanoic acid.

16. If you place a human skull on the ground and begin piling weight on top of it, how much weight can you add before it cracks?

If the weight is applied slowly, the human skull can support 3 tons. (Wow!)

17. What does the word *carotid* mean?

It is derived from a Greek word meaning "to put to sleep," because pressure on the carotid arteries can cause loss of consciousness (as any fan of the World Wrestling Federation is aware).

18. What did Aristotle say was the function of the brain?
To cool the heart.

19. In 1909, Korbinian Brodmann divided the human cerebral cortex into 47 cytoarchitec- turally distinct regions and gave each one a "Brodmann's number." What is found in Brodmann's areas 13–16?
Nothing. For some reason, Brodmann left out numbers 13–16, which do not appear any- where on his cortical maps. The reason for the omission has never been discovered (*see figure on facing page*).

20. Who first described transient ischemic attacks (TIAs) and noted that they were warn- ing signs of a future stroke?
Hippocrates first described TIAs, noting that "unaccustomed attacks of numbness and anes- thesia are signs of impending apoplexy."

21. What are the five diagnoses neurologists most dread telling a patient (according to a recent survey of practicing clinical neurologists)?
The most distressing diagnoses to tell a patient, in order, are:
1. Amyotrophic lateral sclerosis   4. Multiple sclerosis
2. Malignant brain tumor   5. Epilepsy
3. Traumatic paraplegia

22. What are the four drugs most commonly prescribed by neurologists in America?
1. Acetaminophen   3. Phenytoin (Dilantin)
2. Aspirin   4. Amitriptyline (Elavil, Endep)

23. How many pounds of aspirin are consumed each year in the United States?
Americans ingest 30 million pounds of aspirin per year.

24. Why did Rene Descartes choose the pineal gland as the seat of the soul?
He believed it was the only unpaired structure in the brain and occupied the brain's exact center.

25. What was Gilles de la Tourette's first name?
George.

26. Who did Gilles de la Tourette believe was the greatest neurologist of the century?
Himself. He died of general paresis, at age 47, in a state of grandiose megalomania.
Guilly P: Gilles de la Tourette. In Rose FC, Bynum WF (eds): Historical Aspects of the Neurosciences. New York, Raven Press, 1985, pp 397–413.

27. What percentage of all visits to a doctor are visits to a neurologist?
One percent of all doctor visits are to a neurologist, which is reasonable because 1% of all doctors in America are neurologists.

28. Who described the first reflex, and what was it?
In 1662, Rene Descartes described the blink reflex, where a blow aimed at the eyes causes a person to blink. The word *reflex* derives from the sight of an approaching object causing a "re- flection" in the brain.

29. Why are cerebral infarctions called strokes?
According to the *Oxford English Dictionary*, a sudden, inexplicable cerebrovascular acci- dent was first likened to a "stroke of God's hand" in 1599. The relationship of a cerebral infarc- tion to an act of God exists in other cultures as well: the Greek verb "plesso" means to "stroke, hit, or beat," and the derivative "plegia" gives us our term hemiplegia.
Dirckx JH: Stroke. Stroke 17:559, 1986.

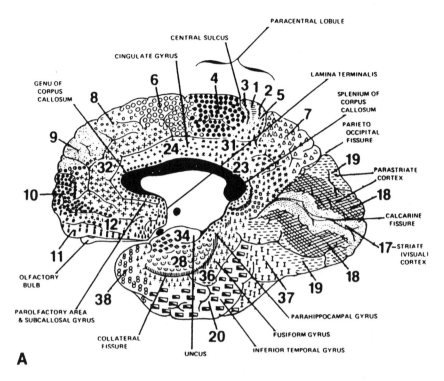

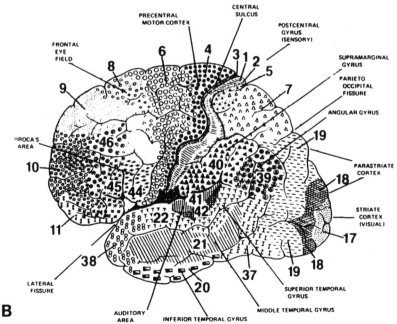

Diagram of Brodmann's areas of the brain—note the absence of numbers 13–16. (From Garoutte B: Functional Neuroanatomy, 2nd ed. Greenshore, CA, Life Press, 1990, with permission.)

30. The Babinski sign is produced by stroking the lateral aspect of the foot with a noxious stimulus and observing whether the great toe dorsiflexes. What did Babinski call the Babinski sign?

There is no more pompous figure in medicine than the posturing attending physician on rounds expounding pedantically on the supposed oxymoron of a "negative Babinski sign" and extolling the "extensor plantar reflex." In fact, in his original papers, Babinski referred to his sign as "the phenomenon of the toes," but on rounds with his pupils he always insisted it be called "the great toe sign." By the way, Babinski referred to the failure of the platysma to contract on the side of a hemiparesis as the "Babinski sign."

Babinski J: Sur le reflexe cutane plantiare dans certaines affections organiques du system nerveux central. C R Soc Biol (Paris) 48:207–208, 1896.

Babinski J: Du phenomene des orteils et de sa valeur semiologique. Semaine Medicale 18:321–322, 1898.

31. There are many minor, generally useless variations of the Babinski sign, most of them with eponymic names bestowed by egotistical neurologists (Chaddock, Oppenheim, etc.). But sometimes pyramidal tract lesions cause hyperactive plantarflexion of the toes, a movement opposite to the Babinski sign. How many variations of this reflex can you name?

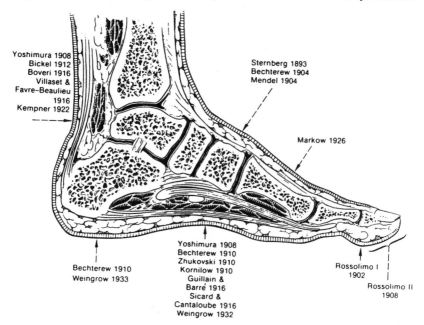

Yoshimura 1908
Bickel 1912
Boveri 1916
Villaset &
Favre–Beaulieu
1916
Kempner 1922

Sternberg 1893
Bechterew 1904
Mendel 1904

Markow 1926

Bechterew 1910
Weingrow 1933

Yoshimura 1908
Bechterew 1910
Zhukovski 1910
Kornilow 1910
Guillain &
Barré 1916
Sicard &
Cantaloube 1916
Weingrow 1932

Rossolimo I
1902

Rossolimo II
1908

Some variations of the Rossolimo sign of toe flexion ("grasp reflex of the foot") with pyramidal tract disease. (From DeJong RN: The Neurologic Examination, 4th ed. Hagerstown, MD, Harper & Row, 1979, p 462, with permission.)

32. What are crocodile tears?

After damage to the facial nerve, such as from Bell's palsy, regenerating fibers may become misdirected such that impulses to mouth and lip muscle instead stimulate the lacrimal gland. As a result, chewing food will cause the patient to weep. The expression comes from old African folklore that corcodiles felt compassion and remorse for their prey and wept with sorrow whenever they ate.

33. The first successful treatment for epilepsy was bromides. Why was an obstetrician the first person to recommend their use?

It was believed in the mid-19th century that excessive sexual activity, especially masturbation, contributed greatly to epilepsy. Because bromides are known to cause impotence, Sir

Charles Locock, personal obstetrician to Queen Victoria, proposed in 1857 that their suppression of sexual function (and menstruation) would result in suppression of seizure activity. He was right, for the wrong reason.

Scott DR: The discovery of anti-epileptic drugs. J Hist Neurosci 1:111–118, 1992.

34. Ondine's curse refers to a neurologic lesion, usually in the medulla or high cervical cord, that destroys the pathways for automatic, rhythmic breathing, thus forcing the patient to breathe voluntarily. Who was Ondine, and what was his curse?

Nobody, and nothing. Ondine is simply the French word for mermaid and refers to the (unnamed) mermaid in the French version of Hans Christian Andersen's fairy tale, "The Little Mermaid." In this story, based on old Germanic legends mermaids can assume human form, but only as part of a pact or bargain (not a curse) that requires them to return to the ocean if their human lover is unfaithful to them. The mangled approbation of Ondine's curse, referring to a neurologic deficit that interrupts automatic breathing, is derived from the 1939 play "Ondine" by the French author Jean Giraudoux, who embellished the story by having the mermaid's hapless knight punished for his infidelity by the cessation of all his automatic functions (not just breathing). The ondine (mermaid) loved (not cursed) her human prince and was always faithful. No Ondine, no curse, no one stops breathing.

Giraudoux J: Ondine. New York, Random House, 1954.

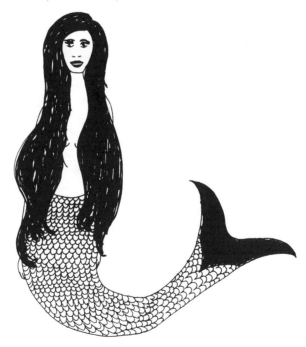

35. What are Finnish snowballs?

These are osmophilic, globular, intracellular inclusions seen with electron microscopy in patients with neuronal ceroid lipofuscinosis. They really don't look anything like Finnish snowballs.

36. What is the softest sound that can be detected by the human ear?

The decibel scale is set at 0 for the softest audible sound, which represents vibratory energy striking the eardrum at an intensity of 0.0002 dynes per square centimeter, which is a range of vibration scarcely larger than the width of several atoms.

37. What is the lowest form of life that sleeps?

Some insects sleep. The reason why animals sleep—its evolutionary or survival advantage—is unknown. There are many theories to account for the existence of sleep, but none of them really makes much sense.

38. Most humans have a clearly dominant hand (usually the right one). What is the lowest form of life that shows such a preference or dominance? Why are most people right-handed?

Birds, which have neuronal populations in the left hemisphere that regulate their song production, are the lowest phylum with a convincing laterality or dominance. The reason for dominance—its evolutionary or survival advantage—is unknown. There are many theories to account for the existence of dominance, but none of them really makes much sense.

39. What is the smallest concentration of a substance that can be smelled by the human nose?

The more than 10 million specialized neuroepithelial cells that make up the olfactory sensory receptors can detect some substances, such as musks, in concentrations of 10^{-12} moles, which is scarcely more than a few molecules.

40. What are the most common movements seen in dead people?

The Lazarus sign is a quick flexion of both arms up over the chest, beneath the chin, observed in brain-dead patients. It may represent spontaneous firing of hypoxic cervical spinal cord neurons.

Ropper AH: Unusual spontaneous movements in brain-dead patients.Neurology 34:1089–1092, 1984.

NEUROLOGIC BIOGRAPHIES

41. This shy, serious university mathematics professor had an alter ego. Using a pseudonym derived from a latinization of his own name, he wrote a series of playful "nonsense" books and poems, which, although ostensibly for children, were derived from chess games, mathematical logic, probability theory, and political satire. A neurologic syndrome of altered body image and time perception has been named after one of the characters in his books who suffered from similar bizarre distortions. **Who was this author, and what was his neurologic disease?**

Charles Lutwidge Dodgson, under the pseudonym of Lewis Carroll, achieved immortality with works such as *Alice's Adventures in Wonderland* and *Through the Looking Glass*. In the first book, Alice, trying to follow a white rabbit through an underground hallway and into an enchanted garden, must change sizes to accommodate various obstacles. She does this by drinking bottles marked "Drink Me," eating cakes marked "Eat Me," and swallowing magic mushrooms. Distortions of body size, which can be produced by lesions affecting the nondominant posterior parietal lobe, have been termed the Alice in Wonderland syndrome and are virtually pathognomonic for migraine headaches. Like many Victorians, Lewis Carroll kept a diary, and from this we know he suffered from classic migraine headaches, which he described as "bilious headaches," preceded by visual disturbances and fortification spectra. Although he never described body distortions accompanying his migraines, some experts speculate that he drew upon personal experiences for these scenes in his book and that "Alice trod the paths of a wonderland well known to her creator."

Rolak LA: Literary neurologic syndromes: The Alice in Wonderland syndrome. Arch Neurol 46:353, 1992.

42. The Tony award-winning Broadway musical *The Mystery of Edwin Drood* (later shortened to just *Drood*) tells of a love triangle and a mysterious murder. The play uses a gimmick of asking the audience to choose who they believe the murderer is and then substituting the appropriate ending based on the vote. **What is the neurologic reason why the playwrights have to use this trick?**

Charles Dickens, arguably the greatest novelist of all time, was writing his book, *The Mystery of Edwin Drood*, when he suffered a massive left hemisphere stroke and slumped forward on his desk, the pen sliding across the paper as he collapsed unconscious. He died shortly afterward, only 58 years old. Because he had never revealed his intended solution to the murder, audiences must now guess the identity of the villain.

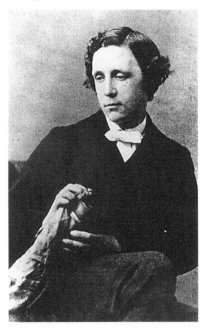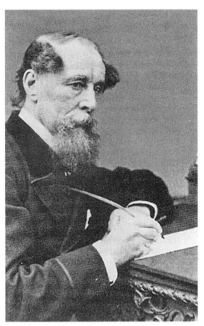

Lewis Carroll, a pioneer in early photography, took this photograph of himself polishing a camera lens.

Charles Dickens

43. This author, a minor French nobleman, was a brilliant observer of human foibles and was gifted with a phenomenal memory. He made his reputation almost entirely through his short stories, which tell isolated, small, but revealing anecdotes about human behavior. Many of his stories have an ironic twist, and the overall tone is often sardonic and misanthropic. One of his stories, "The Horla," is believed by many critics to be an autobiographical description of his own neurologic sufferings. **Who was this writer, and what was his neurologic disease?**

Guy de Maupassant is considered one of the greatest short story writers of all time. Some of his stories, such as "The Queen's Necklace," are among the most famous ever written. Unfortunately, he contracted syphilis at an early age and subsequently developed neurosyphilis and general paresis. Demented and delusional, he had to be institutionalized. "The Horla," an intense psychological thriller, tells of a man's mounting terror as he becomes increasingly obsessed with the conviction that his mind has been invaded by an evil demon. It is a gifted writer's description of his own paranoid delusions and progressing insanity. Guy de Maupassant finally died, in status epilepticus, at age 45.

44. This Russian writer, the son of a minor landowner, saw his father killed in a peasant uprising and was himself arrested and threatened with execution. His harsh life left him a friendless, embittered man through most of his adult years. His bleak books, considered among the first great Russian novels, frequently included characters with the same neurologic problem from which he himself suffered. **Who was this writer, and what was his neurologic problem?**

Fyodor Dostoyevsky established his talent with such works as *The Brothers Karamazov, The Idiot*, and *Crime and Punishment*. He had his first epileptic seizure at age 7 and suffered from complex partial seizures most of the remainder of his life. Of interest, his aura was one of ecstasy and extreme joy. He once wrote about his aura, "During a few moments I feel such a happiness that it is impossible to realize at other times, and other people cannot imagine it. I feel a complete harmony within myself and in the world, and this feeling is so strong and so sweet that for a few seconds of this enjoyment one would readily exchange ten years of one's life—perhaps even one's whole life."

Alajouanine T: Dostoiewski's epilepsy. Brain 86:209–218, 1963.

45. This French writer produced a number of notable works, but his reputation rests primarily on one supreme masterpiece, a single book that he spent much of his life writing, revising page by page, and even word by word, counting the number of syllables in each line. He was unpopular with many of his contemporaries, some of whom felt his great acclaim was due to sheer plodding work rather than talent, and some of whom were jealous of his extraordinarily beautiful mistress. His enemies even circulated the rumor that his neurologic problem was hysterical. Nevertheless, he remained generous and good humored, and when his masterpiece was condemned as being immoral and he was placed on trial for indecency, many of the leading artistic figures of his age rallied to this defense. **Who was this writer, and what was his neurologic disease?**

Gustave Flaubert's reputation rests on his novel *Madame Bovary*, which tells the story of a restless woman unfulfilled by her marriage to a provincial country doctor. The great French writer Emile Zola defended Flaubert and his use of realism during the trial against his book, at which Flaubert was acquitted. Beginning at age 22, Flaubert suffered from seizures, which had the unusual manifestation of visual phenomena. He described "a hundred thousand images jumping up and down together, like illuminated rockets during a firework display." Candles, flames, and Japanese lanterns danced before his eyes during his seizures. Modern authorities speculate that these seizures with visual symptoms arose from occipital lobe damage suffered when Flaubert fell backward off his horse as a young man. His death was also neurologic—he suffered an intracerebral hemorrhage, reportedly while making love to his young servant.

Gastaut H, Gastaut Y, Broughton R: Gustave Flaubert's illness: A case report in evidence against the erroneous notion of psychogenic epilepsy. Epilepsia 25:622–637, 1984.

46. This musician, a gifted "child prodigy" at the piano, achieved even more success as a composer than as a performer. He was at the height of his fame when he suffered an apparently trivial head injury but afterward experienced a decline in abilities. He noted speech difficulties, memory loss, and an inability to express any of his musical ideas in writing or performance. Indeed, he wrote essentially no further compositions. A bitter and public feud arose among the many physicians called in at various times to treat this famous patient, culminating when one of the doctors "kidnapped" the composer when his primary physician was on Christmas vacation. Surreptitious exploratory neurosurgery was performed, which the patient did not survive. **Who was this composer, and what was his neurologic disease?**

Maurice Ravel (1875–1937) was injured in Paris when a taxi cab carrying him from the theater to his hotel collided with another cab on October 10, 1932. He suffered facial injuries and the loss of two teeth but jokingly dismissed the trauma as minor. It was some months later that he began experiencing his mental decline and frustrating inability to compose. His neurologist, Theophile Alajouanine, believed that Ravel was suffering from a degenerative progressive aphasia, which today we would probably diganose as Alzheimer's disease. Many of Ravel's friends were convinced that this decline was caused by the automobile accident, possibly by enlarging subdural hematomas or hydrocephalus. They persuaded the famous neurosurgeon, Clovis Vincent, to operate on him; the surgery revealed only a shrunken, atrophic brain. Ravel did not survive the surgery.

47. This American composer began playing the piano and performing at age 12 and, using the media of American popular culture—Broadway musicals and Hollywood motion pictures—

became one of the wealthiest and best-loved American musicians. He was a critical success as well, winning a Pulitzer Prize for his music, and later composed America's first true opera. Wealthy and respected, with a huge Hollywood estate and series of beautiful lovers, he neverthe-less remarked at one point, "I am 38 years old, wealthy and famous, but I am still deeply un-happy." Indeed, his neurologic problem was long diagnosed as pyschiatric in nature; it was not recognized as organic until two days before it finally killed him. **Who was this composer, and what was his neurologic disease?**

George Gershwin won a Pulitzer Prize in 1932 for *Of Thee I Sing* and completed his opera *Porgy and Bess* in 1935. On February 11, 1937, while conducting his *Piano Concerto in F Major* with the Los Angeles Philharmonic Orchestra, he experienced a repulsive and nauseating smell of burnt rubber, followed by a 10–20-second alteration of consciousness. Although he re-mained upright, he stopped conducting for several bars while staring into space, a lapse that was quite noticeable to the audience. He had increasing headaches and mental apathy, diag-nosed as "hysteria" or "neurosis," until he collapsed on July 9, 1937 and was rushed to the hos-pital, comatose with a left hemiparesis. He was operated on for removal of a cystic right temporal lobe glioblastoma multiforme but died without regaining consciousness on July 11, 1937, at age 38.

Ljunggren B: Great Men with Sick Brains. Park Ridge, IL, American Association of Neurological Surgeons, 1990, pp 91–100.

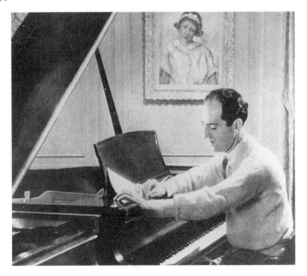

George Gershwin.

48. This wealthy, refined, witty, kind, and generous composer was the antithesis of the romantic conception of the impoverished artist suffering in his garret while pouring out his heart into his music. Instead, this privileged musician, whose very name means "happy," came from a re-spected and talented family, and his own music is generally bright and vivacious. His contribu-tions were unfortunately cut short by his sudden and early death from a neurologic problem—the same one that killed his grandmother, father, and sister (herself a child musical prodigy). **Who was this composer, and what was his neurologic problem?**

Felix Mendelsohn, the grandson of distinguished philosopher Moses Mendelsohn and the son of wealthy banker Abraham Mendelsohn, demonstrated considerable musical talent as a child, as did his sister Fanny. On May 14, 1847, Fanny suddenly became pale and nauseated, her upper ex-tremities numbed and paralyzed, and she mumbled incoherently. She slipped quickly into uncon-sciousness and was pronounced dead of an intracranial hemorrhage, the same condition thought to be responsible for the deaths of her father and grandmother. On November 1 and 2, 1847, Felix suffered a similar hemorrhage, with severe headaches, stuttering paralysis, unconsciousness, and death.

O'Shea J: Was Mozart Poisoned? Medical Investigations into the Lives of the Great Composers. New York, St. Martin's Press, 1990, pp 118–123.

49. These brothers, during 14 years of entertaining with the circus, achieved such fame that they literally became a household word. When they retired, they married sisters on adjoining farms and raised large families. Legendary for their closeness, when one of them died of a neurologic disease, the other died just hours later. **Who were these famous brothers, and what was their neurologic problem?**

Chang and Eng, Siamese twins, were joined at the thorax, with a common liver and diaphragm. Early on the morning of January 17, 1874, Chang suffered a fatal stroke (he had had a minor cerebral thrombosis in 1870). Eng, terrified and panic-stricken, was inextricably joined to his now dead brother. A physician was summoned to attempt a separation, but before he could arrive, Eng also died. Both brothers were autopsied, and it was believed that Eng had collapsed from massive sympathetic stimulation, with neurogenic pulmonary edema and cardiac arrhythmias—he had literally died of fright.

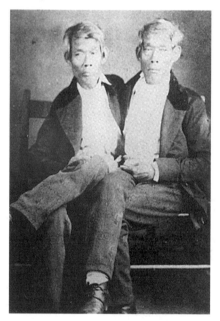

The Siamese twins Chang *(left)* and Eng *(right)*.

50. In 1951, Dr. Richard Asher published a paper in the *Lancet* entitled "Münchausen's Syndrome," describing patients who simulate physical illness for the sole purpose of obtaining medical treatment, with no other recognizable motive. Asher chose his name in honor of a famous teller of dramatic and untruthful folklore, Baron von Münchhausen. **What was von Münchhausen's neurologic problem?**

Karl Friedrich Hieronymous Freiherr von Münchhausen (1720–1797), a minor nobleman and country gentleman with a large estate near Hannover, Germany, was famous locally for his hospitality and clever storytelling. Several of his good-natured tales were plagiarized by a notorious rascal, Rudolf Eric Raspe, who published them anonymously in the 1785 monograph *Baron Münchhausen's Narrative of His Marvelous Travels and Campaigns in Russia*. Ironically, the real Baron von Münchhausen became an embittered and irascible old man as he unsuccessfully pursued a series of lawsuits and other actions to stop the plagiarism and protect his name. Approaching ruination at age 74, he tried to console himself by marrying an 18-year-old girl, Bernhardine Von Brunn, who was said to have her eye on the remainder of his estate. Three years later, in 1797, he died of a massive left hemisphere stroke.

51. What congenital neurologic problem almost cost James Buchanan the presidency?

James Buchanan, the 15th President of the United States, served just before Lincoln from 1856 to 1860. He had a habitual head tilt forward and to the left, which was probably caused by a congenital right superior oblique palsy (cranial nerve IV). This well-known head tilt was the focus for a rumor circulated by Buchanan's opponents in the presidential election. In 1819, at age 28, Buchanan (who was the only bachelor president America has ever had) was engaged to marry Annie Coleman of New York, when she broke off the wedding at the last minute because of gossip about Buchanan's philandering. Shortly afterward, she committed suicide. Although this unfortunate incident was true, Buchanan's adversaries fabricated a sequel stating that Buchanan's head tilt was the result of his own attempted suicide by hanging in an effort to escape the vengeance of his fiancée's brother. The abortive hanging attempt was supposed to have twisted Buchanan's neck for life. Buchanan overcame this early example of "negative campaigning" to win the election.

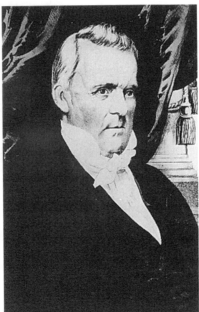

President James Buchanan.

52. This 39-year-old, right-handed white male civil servant described his neurologic problems in his own words: "I first had a chill in the evening which lasted practically all night. On the following morning, the muscles of the right knee appeared weak, and by afternoon, I was unable to support my weight on my right leg. That evening, the left knee began to weaken also, and by the following morning I was unable to stand up. This was accompanied by a continuing temperature of about 102° and I felt thoroughly achy all over. By the end of the third day, practically all muscles from the chest down were involved. Above the chest, the only symptom was a weakening of the two large thumb muscles., making it impossible to write. There was no special pain along the spine and no rigidity up the neck. For the following two weeks, I had to be catheterized and there was a slight, though not severe, difficulty in controlling the bowels. The fever lasted only six or seven days, but all the muscles from the hips down were extremely sensitive to the touch and I had to have my knees supported by pillows. This condition of extreme discomfort lasted about three weeks." **What is your diagnosis?**

This is Mr. Franklin Delano Roosevelt's own description of the onset of his polio on August 10, 1921. His physician initially diagnosed, "A clot of blood from a sudden congestion has settled in the lower spinal cord temporarily removing the power to move though not to feel." Subsequently the correct diagnosis of polio was established. Unfortunately, Roosevelt never regained any use of his lower extremities whatsoever and remained with complete flaccid paralysis for the rest of his life. Of interest, his disability was a well-kept secret, guarded by a press that considered it undignified to mention; the tenor of the times forbade such personal scrutiny. Photos of Roosevelt were always composed to conceal the disability (although a discerning eye can guess at the weakness and atrophy in the photo below, taken on his yacht in 1933, shortly after his first election to the presidency), and the general public never learned of his paralysis.

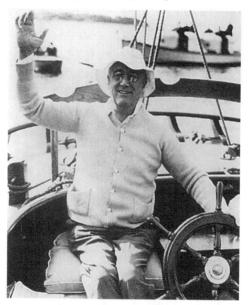

President Franklin Roosevelt, 1933.

53. The president of an Ivy League University, this man was one of America's most intellectual presidents and also one of the most liberal and socially minded. He was not any more reliable, however, because he ran for office with the slogan, "He kept us out of war," and then plunged the nation into war four months after his inauguration. One of his most visionary and potentially greatest achievements was never realized, however, because he developed a serious neurologic problem while in office. **Who was this president, and what was his neurologic disease?**

Woodrow Wilson, America's 28th President, was a pacifist who did not wish to become embroiled in World War I but felt compelled to do so by April of 1918. He suffered a variety of ailments throughout his life, including probably an intraocular hemorrhage, writer's cramp, and viral encephalitis. On September 1, 1919, he suffered a right hemisphere stroke with resultant left hemiparesis and considerable mental clouding. His wife sequestered him in the White House, refusing all visitors and access, and the nature of his ailment was never revealed to the public or to most members of the government. Although his mental capacities were obviously impaired, he never relinquished command; thus, the nation was essentially without a president for the final 20 months of his administration. Some historians speculate that he could have persuaded Congress and the public to endorse his proposal for a League of Nations had he not become ill.

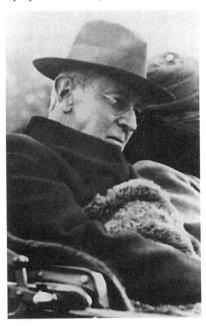

A photographer snapped the above photograph of a haggard, demented President Wilson in one of the rare moments when he was outside the White House, propped against the right side of his automobile, with hat and clothing strategically draped to conceal his left hemiparesis.

54. This man was the smallest U.S. President, standing scarcely over 5 feet tall and weighing little more than 100 pounds, with "a discouraging feebleness of the constitution" much of his life. He was nevertheless a brilliant thinker who reshaped political philosophy and was one of the most intellectual presidents. His wife was renowned for her charm and grace and became one of the most famous First Ladies. He had to overcome the stigma of a lack of military service, which was due to a neurologic condition. **Who was this President, and what was his problem?**

James Madison, the 4th President of the United States, helped frame the Bill of Rights and is known as the "Father of the Constitution." He had many hypochondriacal and hysterical symptoms as a young man, many of which disappeared as he grew older. Among the most prominent was "a constitutional liability to sudden attacks of the nature of epilepsy," which were known by his friends to be bizarre spells that he suffered in response to stress. When he tried to enlist for military service in the Revolutionary War, he was rejected because of his "epileptoid hysteria" and told to go home, study less, and increase his exercise outdoors. These spells disappeared in his 30s, and indeed he enjoyed good health and vigorous leadership as President.

55. The patient is a 35-year-old woman who gradually developed fatigue and dizziness and began complaining of stiffness and pain in her legs, especially in the calves. She developed a fine tremor involving the entire body but most prominent in the limbs—more so in the arms than in the legs. The tremor was present at rest and resembled a trembling or shivering movement. These symptoms progressed over a day or two, at which time she complained of a fairly steady epigastric pain with nausea and then persistent vomiting. By the third day, the fatigue had progressed to lethargy, and she became bedridden. It was noted that her pupils were slightly large and sluggish, and she had developed protracted hiccups. Her general physical examination showed her temperature to be slightly subnormal and her pulse irregular. She had constipation and decreased urine output, and her tongue was large and red. The conjunctivae were also in-fected. Her gastrointestinal distress continued, and she had very diminished bowel sounds. On the fifth day of her illness her lethargy progressed to stupor and she became arousable. She died on the seventh day. The patient lived on a farm, and the middle-aged man and wife on an adjacent farm had died of identical symptoms one week before the onset of the patient's illness. Another neighbor who lived half a mile away died several days later. This patient had directly nursed and cared for both families. **Can you identify this patient and her illness?**

The patient is Nancy Hanks Lincoln, the mother of Abraham Lincoln, who died at age 35 on October 15, 1818, when her son was 9 years old. Apart from the fact that she was born out of wedlock, the illegitimate daughter of Lucy Hanks of Elizabethtown, Kentucky, little is known about Lincoln's mother. There are not even any reliable descriptions of what she looked like.

Nancy Lincoln died of a disease known as the "trembles" or "staggers," named for its pri-macy symptom of tremor. The first references to this disease appeared in colonial days, but the cause was unknown and variously attributed to infections, noxious gases, or poisonings. Outbreaks of the illness occurred frequently as settlers migrated westward, causing "an appalling loss of human life." It was not until 1927 that the cause was finally found to be a toxic substance in the leaves of the white snakeroot plant, a flower that grows native in the Midwest, reaching a height of 2 to 3 feet, with sharp-toothed leaves and white or purple bell-shaped flowers. It grew only in dense woods, and when land was sufficiently cleared for pastures and farming, the plant disappeared. Outbreaks of the disease were caused by settlers moving into an area that had not been cleared sufficiently to provide adequate grazing land for their cattle. The cows would forage in the woods, eat the snakeroot, and the toxin would accumulate and concentrate in their milk. When ingested by humans, this milk would produce the disease. Indeed, the other name for the disease was "milk sickness."

The toxin was named "trematol" because of the tremors which were the primary symptom of the disease. Trematol is an aromatic alcohol with a pleasant odor and a chemical structure of $C_{16}H_{22}O_3$. Ingestion of this compound causes ketosis and elevated acetone levels, but the exact nature of its action in tissues, especially the nervous system, was never determined. Autopsies performed on patients who had died of milk sickness never showed any gross changes in the brain. With the continued westward migration and clearing of land, the natural habitat of the white snakeroot diminished. Although the plant has not become extinct, the last recorded case of milk sickness was in 1938.

INDEX

Page numbers in **boldface type** indicate complete chapters.

Acetazolamide, pseudotumor cerebri management, 281

Acetylcholine
  Alzheimer's disease deficiency, 214
  autonomic nervous system, 184
  central cholinergic synapse function, 5
  peripheral synapse function, 5
  receptor antibodies in myasthenia gravis
    binding sites, 74
    clinical evidence, 73
    experimental evidence, 73
    immunopathology, 73
  receptor classes, 5

Achromatopsia, lesions, 48

Acid-maltase deficiency, features and differential diagnosis, 65

Acoustic neuroma, features, 144–145

Acquired immunodeficiency syndrome (AIDS)
  antiretroviral therapy side effects, 339
  aseptic meningitis, 340
  cryptococcal meningitis, 341
  dementia, 340
  myelopathy with, 119
  peripheral neuropathies, 89, 339–340
  progressive multifocal leukoencephalopathy, 340
  seizures, 340
  syphilis, 341
  toxoplasma encephalitis, 340, 341
  vision effects, 340

Acromegaly, neurologic complications, 318

Acrylamide, peripheral neuropathy induction, 89

Action potential, definition, 2

Acute dystonic reaction (ADR), drug induction, 176

Addison's disease, neurologic complications, 318

ADHD. See Attention deficit hyperactivity disorder

Adhesion molecules, types and mutations in disease, 10

Adrenoleukodystrophy, features, 351

Agnosia
  anosognosia, 227
  Anton's syndrome, 227–228
  definition, 227
  prosopagnosia, 227
  visual agnosia, 227

Agraphia, definition, 226–227

AIDS. See Acquired immunodeficiency syndrome

Alar plate, development, 15

Alexander's disease, features, 352

Alexia, definition, 226

Alpha-bungarotoxin, pharmacologic action, 82

ALS. See Amyotrophic lateral sclerosis

Altitude sickness
  causes, 315
  treatment, 315

Alzheimer's disease (AD)
  amyloid deposits, 214

Alzheimer's disease (AD) (cont.)
  cholinergic hypothesis, 214
  clinical subtypes, 212
  diagnosis
    alcohol dementia differential diagnosis, 211
    blood tests, 211
    classification, 211
    criteria, 211
    imaging studies, 211–212
    lumbar puncture, 212
  Down syndrome association, 213
  electroencephalography, 376
  gene mutations
    apolipoprotein E, 213
    early-onset disease, 212
    late-onset disease, 213
  language disturbances, 212
  motor features, 212
  neuropathology, 213–214
  Parkinson's disease relationship, 159
  progression, 212
  risk factors, 213
  symptoms, 212
  tau protein role, 214
  treatment
    aggressiveness, 215
    anxiety, 215
    depression, 214–215
    donepezil, 215
    nerve growth factor, 214
    respite care, 215
    rivastigmine, 215
    selegiline, 215
    sleep disorders, 214
    tacrine, 215
    vitamin E, 215

Amantadine, Parkinson's disease treatment, 153–154

Amphotericin B
  side effects, 335
  spinal fluid penetration, 335

Amyloid, Alzheimer's disease deposits, 214

Amyotrophic lateral sclerosis (ALS)
  clinical presentation, 96
  diagnosis, 96
  differential diagnosis, 96–97
  electromyography, 392
  etiology, 96
  famous patients, 97
  treatment, 97

Analgesia. See Pain

Anemia, symptoms, 315

Anomic aphasia
  characteristics, 224
  lesions, 224

Anosmia, causes, 43

Anosognosia
  behavioral syndromes with, 227
  definition, 227
Anoxia, electroencephalography, 387
Anterior circulation, arteries, 49
Anterior horn cell, deficits, 97
Anterior spinal artery
  anatomy, 113
  occlusion signs, 114, 126
Antibiotic toxicity, neurologic complications, 332
Anticipation, trinucleotide repeat diseases, 12
Anticonvulsants, pain management, 269–270
Antiphospholipid antibody syndrome
  neurologic complications, 316
  treatment, 316
Anton's syndrome, features, 227–228
Apgar score
  components, 345
  neurologic prognosis, 345–346
Aphasia, **219–228**
  anomic aphasia, 224
  aphemia, 223
  Broca's aphasia, 220
  causes, 219
  children versus adults, 226
  conduction aphasia, 221
  cortical aphasia, 224
  definition, 219
  fluent versus nonfluent, 219, 220
  global aphasia, 223
  jargon aphasia, 220
  multiple languages, 219
  neologism, 220
  paraphasia, 220
  Pitre's law, 219
  progressive aphasia, 225
  Ribot's rule, 219
  subcortical aphasia, 224–225
  thalamic aphasia, 225
  transcortical aphasias
    mixed, 224
    motor, 223–224
    sensory, 223
  Wernicke's aphasia, 221
  word deafness, 221–222
Aphemia
  characteristics, 223
  lesions, 223
Apnea test, brainstem function evaluation, 135
Apneustic breathing
  features, 36, 37
  lesions, 37
Apolipoprotein E, Alzheimer's disease role, 213
Apoptosis, neurons, 10
Apraxia
  constructional apraxia, 227
  definition, 227
  dressing apraxia, 227
  of speech, 227
  types and lesions, 227
Arachnoiditis, following spinal surgery, 109

Argyll Robertson pupil, features, 45
Aristotle, brain function theory, 404
Arnold-Chiari malformation
  complications, 349–350
  types, 350
Arrhythmia
  Guillain-Barré syndrome management, 188
  types with central nervous system disease, 191
Arterial thrombosis, in pregnancy, 326
Artery of Adamkiewicz, anatomy, 113
Aseptic meningitis
  cerebrospinal fluid findings in AIDS, 340
  diagnosis, 337
  ECHO virus, 337
  herpes meningitis, 338
Aspirin
  consumption in United States, 404
  stroke prevention, 244, 245
Asterixis, causes, 179, 312
Astrocyte
  blood-brain barrier, 2
  features, 1
Ataxia, paraneoplastic movement disorder, 18
Ataxia-myokymia syndrome, potassium channel
    defects, 8
Ataxia-telangiectasia, features, 355
Ataxic breathing
  features, 36, 37
  lesions, 37
Attention deficit hyperactivity disorder (ADHD)
  clinical features, 366
  treatment in Tourette's syndrome, 174
Atypical facial pain, causes, 268
Auditory pathway, anatomy, 38
Auricular nerve, stimulation and vagal reflexes, 199
Autism, clinical manifestations, 366
Autonomic dysfunction
  acute pandysautonomia, 189
  failure versus hyperactivity, 183
  genetic causes, 193–195
  history and body systems, 182–183
  in heart transplantation, 192
  mastocytosis differential diagnosis, 200
  norepinephrine assay, 185
  orthostatic hypotension, 197, 198
  paraneoplastic autonomic syndromes, 189–190
  Parkinson's disease, 193
  peripheral neuropathies with, 187–189
  physical examination, 183
  pure autonomic failure versus multiple system
    atrophy, 193
  Sjögren's syndrome, 189
  tetraplegia and autonomic dysreflexia, 199
Autonomic nervous system, **181–200**
Axillary nerve, injury, 24
Axotomy, central nervous system neuron
    regeneration, 13
Azathioprine, chronic immune-related
    demyelinating polyradiculopathy treatment, 92
Azidothymidine (AZT)
  muscle effects, 69–70, 339

Azidothymidine (AZT) *(cont.)*
  seizure effects, 340
AZT. *See* Azidothymidine

Babinski sign, historical perspective, 406
Back pain
  AHCPR diagnostic guidelines, 99
  cervical pain, 104–106
  diagnostics, 106–107
  differential diagnosis, 104
  disabling events, 99
  generators of pain, 100
  mechanical spine pain, 102
  mechanisms, 99
  natural history, 107
  nonoperative treatment, 107–108
  operative treatment, 108–110
  prevalence, 99
  thoracic spine disease, 104
Baclofen, pain management, 270
Bacterial meningitis
  cerebrospinal fluid findings, 329
  cryptococcal meningitis
    with AIDS, 341
    risk factors, 251
  culture studies, 329
  encephalitis differential diagnosis, 329
  hypoglycorrhachia with, 329
  organisms, 329–330
  pediatric disease
    neonatal meningitis, 356
    pathogens, 356
    signs and symptoms, 356
  polymicrobial meningitis, 331
  prophylaxis, 329
  recurrence, 331
Baltic myoclonus, 401
Baroreceptor
  evaluation of function, 196–197
  function, 196
  signaling, 196
Basal ganglia
  aphasia, 224
  blood supply, 50
  components, 147
  corpus striatum, 41
  disorders, **147–180**
  inputs, 41
  lenticular complex, 41
  neurotransmitters, 148
  organization, 147–148
  outputs, 41, 148
  striatal dopamine receptors, 149
  striatal patch and matrix compartments, 148
  subthalamic nucleus function, 148
  transplant surgery in Parkinson's disease
    treatment, 159
Basal plate, development, 15
Behavioral neurology, **219–228**
Behçet's disease, neurologic complications,
  322

Bell's palsy
  herpes simplex virus role, 339
  nerve conduction velocity, 394
  in pregnancy, 326
Black widow spider venom, pharmacologic action, 81
Blood-brain barrier
  accessible regions of brain, 2
  components, 1–2
  compromising conditions, 2
Blood pressure
  aging and hypotension predisposition, 195
  baroreceptors, 196–197
  central nervous system disease effects, 192
  fluctuation management in Guillain-Barré
    syndrome, 188
  maintenance, 195
Botulinum toxin
  dystonia treatment, 170–171
  essential tremor treatment, 165
  indications, 171
  neurologic manifestations, 332
  tension headache treatment, 279
Botulism
  clinical presentation, 81
  infection, 81
Brachial plexus
  cords, 22
  roots, 21, 22
  trunks, 22
Brain abscess
  causes, 330
  clinical presentation, 330
  computed tomography, 330
Brain death
  electroencephalography criteria, 388
  reversible electrocerebral inactivity, 388
Brainstem
  blood supply, 50, 125–126
  cranial nerves, 29–30, 122–123
  functional overview, 121
  medulla anatomy and function, 33–35, 121, 126
  midbrain anatomy and function, 30–32, 122, 126
  parts, 29
  pons anatomy and function, 32–33, 122, 126
Brainstem auditory evoked potentials, multiple
    sclerosis, 203
Brainstem disease, **121–135**
  bulbar palsy, 131
  central pontine myelinolysis, 132
  coma evaluation
    apnea test, 135
    irreversible damage testing, 134–135
    localization of dysfunction, 134
  dorsal midbrain syndrome, 128
  dorsolateral midbrain syndrome, 128
  ependymoma, 131
  glioma, 131
  hemorrhage causes, 129
  history, 56
  internuclear ophthalmoplegia, 130
  lateral medullary syndrome, 126

Brainstem disease *(cont.)*
  lesions
    differential diagnosis, 124
    extra-axial lesions, 124
    intra-axial lesions, 124, 125
    localization approach, 123–124
    magnetic resonance imaging, 124, 125
    signs, 124
    symptoms, 124
  locked-in syndrome, 129
  lower dorsal pontine syndrome, 127
  medial medullary syndrome, 126
  metabolic dysfunction, 131–132
  metastatic lesions, 131
  one-and-a-half syndrome, 130–131
  Parinaud syndrome, 130
  physical examination, 56–57
  pseudobulbar palsy, 131
  reticular formation function, 133–134
  top of the basilar syndrome, 129
  transient ischemic attacks
    causes, 128–129
    symptoms, 128
  upper dorsal pontine syndrome, 127
  ventral midbrain syndrome, 128
  ventral pontine syndrome, 127
  vertigo, 132–133
Brain tumor
  calcification, 253
  chemotherapy, 252
  children, 359–361, 363
  endocrine tumors, 254
  ependymoma
    brainstem, 131
    risk, 253
  glioma
    brainstem, 131
    survival rate, 252
  headache with, 280, 363
  histology, 251
  lymphoma, 253
  markers, 253
  medulloblastoma prognosis, 252–253
  meningioma
    risks, 253
    sites, 253
    treatment, 253
  metastasis
    incidence, 256
    prognosis, 256
    resection, 256
    risks, 253
    sites, 256
  pineal tumors, 253
  primitive neuroectodermal tumors in children,
    252, 253
  radiation therapy, 252, 256, 260
  sites and types, 253, 254, 255
  supratentorial, 251
Breach rhythm, electroencephalography,
  373–374

Broca's aphasia
  clinical features, 220
  lesions, 220
Broca's area
  electrical stimulation effects, 230
  language processing, 48
Brodmann's areas, nomenclature, 404, 405
Bromocriptine
  dopamine receptor specificity, 157, 158
  Parkinson's disease treatment, 157, 158
  side effects, 158
Brown-Sequard syndrome
  features, 114
  historical perspective, 402
Buchanan, James, 413
Bulbar palsy, features, 131

Calcium channel
  diseases, 9
  excitable cell functions, 8
  types, 8–9
Campylobacter jejuni, Guillain-Barré syndrome
  role, 95
Canavan's disease, features, 352
Capsaicin, topical analgesia, 270
Carbon disulfide, peripheral neuropathy induction, 89
Cardiac disease, neurologic complications, 309
Carnitine deficiency
  clinical presentation, 66
  treatment, 66
Carotid endarterectomy, stroke prevention, 245
Carpal tunnel syndrome (CTS)
  definition, 393
  diagnosis, 88, 393
  differential diagnosis, 393
  treatment, 393
Cataplexy, features, 304
Cauda equina, anatomy, 27
Cavernous sinus infection, neurologic
  complications, 331–332
Celiac disease, neurologic complications, 310
Cellular alterations, leading to neurologic disease, 1
Central-core disease, malignant hyperthermia
  relationship, 65
Central neurogenic hyperventilation
  features, 36, 37
  lesions, 37
Central venous thrombosis, in pregnancy, 325–326
Cerebellar disease, **137–146**
  acquired disease etiology, 141–142
  ataxia in childhood, infection role, 357
  cerebellar versus sensory ataxia, 140
  clinical presentation, 139–140
  clinical tests, 140
  hereditary diseases, 142–144
  herniation
    downward, 145
  · treatment, 145
    upward, 145
  history, 57
  infarction and hemorrhage presentation, 144

Cerebellar disease *(cont.)*
  lesion localization principles, 140–141
  neoplasms in degeneration, 250
  paraneoplastic cerebellar degeneration, 145–146
  physical examination, 57
  posterior fossa neoplasm, 144
  speech signs, 232
  syndromes, 141
Cerebellopontine angle, tumors, 255
Cerebellopontine angle syndrome
  causes, 144
  clinical presentation, 144
Cerebellum
  blood supply, 50, 139
  connections, 40, 138
  cortex layers, 39–40
  dentarubrothalamic tract synapse, 40
  essential tremor role, 163–164
  frontopontocerebellar fibers, 40
  functional overview, 137
  hemispheres, 39, 137
  inferior olives afferent, 40
  lobes, 39, 137, 138
  Mollaret's triangle, 40
  nuclei, 40
  peduncles, 138–139
Cerebral arteries, types and anatomy, 49
Cerebral cortex
  Betz cells, 48
  columnar organization, 48
  layers, 46
  line of Gennari, 48
  lobe functions, 48
Cerebral palsy (CP), infection role, 355, 357
Cerebrospinal fluid (CSF). *See also* Lumbar puncture
  adult volumes, 50
  aseptic meningitis findings in AIDS, 340
  bacterial meningitis findings, 329
  cerebral malaria findings, 334
  herpes encephalitis findings, 338
  Listeria infection and management, 331
  multiple sclerosis analysis, 203
  production
    rates, 50
    sites, 50
  route, 51
  syphilis findings, 333
Cervical radiculopathy
  clinical features, 104
  differentiating signs and symptoms by vertebrae, 105
  signs and symptoms, 25–26
  Spurling's maneuver, 105
  surgical management
    anterior cervical diskectomy, 108
    anterior cervical diskectomy and fusion, 108
    anterior cervical diskectomy and fusion with internal fixation, 109
    posterior foraminotomy, 109
Cervical spondylosis
  definition, 116

Cervical spondylosis *(cont.)*
  myelopathy
    clinical presentation, 117
    management, 117
    surgical management, 109
Channelopathies, with epilepsy, 287
Chaperone, functions, 11
Chemotherapy
  brain tumors, 252
  leptomeningeal carcinomatosis, 257
  mental status alterations, 250
  side effects, 259–260
Cherry-red spot, fovea centralis, 352
Cheyne-Stokes breathing
  features, 36, 37
  lesions, 37
Chorea. *See also* Huntington's disease
  autoimmune disease, 175
  speech signs, 230
  Sydenham's chorea, 175
  Wilson's disease, 175
Choroid plexus
  cerebrospinal fluid production, 50
  location, 50
Chronic immune-related demyelinating
      polyradiculopathy (CIDP)
  corticosteroid risks, 92–93
  diagnostic criteria, 92
  differential diagnosis, 94
  immunosuppressive therapy, 92
  interferon therapy, 93
  intravenous immunoglobulin therapy, 93, 94
  plasma exchange, 93
Churg-Strauss syndrome, neurologic complications, 322
Ciguatera, neurologic manifestations, 332
Circle of Willis, vessels, 49
CK. *See* Creatine kinase
Clinical neuroanatomy, **15–51**
Clinical neuroscience, **1–14**
Clonidine, pain management, 270
Clopidogrel, stroke prevention, 245
Cluster breathing
  features, 36, 37
  lesions, 37
Cluster headache
  age of onset, 278
  differential diagnosis, 278
  symptoms, 278
  treatment
    corticosteroids, 278
    lithium, 278
    oxygen, 278
    rhinorrhea and lacrimation, 278
Cluttering, speech, 234
CMAP. *See* Compound motor action potential
CMV. *See* Cytomegalovirus
Cochlea
  fluid pressure wave pathway, 37–38
  perilymph compartments, 37
Cogan's syndrome, neurologic complications, 323

Coma
  brainstem function evaluation
    apnea test, 135
    irreversible damage testing, 134–135
    localization of dysfunction, 134
  electroencephalography
    alpha coma pattern, 387
    brain death criteria, 388
    spindle coma pattern, 387
    theta coma pattern, 387–388
  endocrine diseases with, 317, 319
Complex regional pain syndrome (CRPS)
  clinical stages, 264
  course, 264
  diagnosis, 265
  diagnostic criteria, 263–264
  emotional disturbances, 264
  precipitating events, 264
  sympathetically maintained pain relationship, 265
  sympatholytic procedures, 265
  treatment, 265
  types, 264
Complications, systemic disease, **309–327**
Compound motor action potential (CMAP), normal
    values, 391
Computed tomography (CT)
  brain abscess, 330
  neurocystercosis, 356–357
  spine, 106
  stroke, 239, 246–247
  vascular dementia, 216
Conduction aphasia
  clinical features, 221
  lesions, 221
Conduction block, definition, 392
Cone, arrangement and function, 44
Corpus callosum, agenesis syndromes, 348
Cortical-basal ganglionic degeneration (CBGD),
    features, 162, 218, 234
Corticospinal fibers
  cranial nerve III proximity, 29
  decussation, 29
  origins, 28
  synapse, 29
Corticosteroids
  back pain management, 108
  central nervous system infection management, 332
  chronic immune-related demyelinating
    polyradiculopathy treatment, 92
  cluster headache treatment, 278
  multiple sclerosis management, 205
  myasthenia gravis treatment, 79
  pseudotumor cerebri management, 281
  risk prevention, 92–93
  temporal arteritis treatment, 281
  tuberculosis patients, 335
Cranial nerves
  anatomy and function
    III, 31, 50
    IV, 31, 50
    V, 32

Cranial nerves (cont.)
  anatomy and function (cont.)
    VI, 32
    VII, 32, 33
    VIII, 33
    IX, 33, 34
    X, 33, 34
    XI, 33, 34
    XII, 34–35
  brainstem lesion localization, 123
  dysarthria lesions, 232–233
  external ear canal innervation, 38
  hyperacusis damage, 38
  localization of isolated deficits, 124
  peripheral neuropathies and involvement, 85
  somatic afferents, 30
  somatic efferents, 30
  types and functions, 29–30, 123
  visceral afferents, 30
  visceral efferents, 30
Creatine kinase (CK), elevation
  causes, 60–61
  exercise induction, 61
  in myopathy, 60
  patient work-up, 61
Creutzfeldt-Jakob disease (CJD)
  AIDS dementia differential diagnosis, 340
  diagnosis, 336
  electroencephalography, 336, 376–377
  infection control, 336–337
  lesion features, 336
  mad cow disease, 337
Critical-illness myopathy (CIM), electromyography,
    394–395
Critical-illness polyneuropathy (CIP)
  electromyography, 394–395
  features, 90
Crocodile tear, origins, 406
CRPS. See Complex regional pain syndrome
CSF. See Cerebrospinal fluid
CT. See Computed tomography
CTS. See Carpal tunnel syndrome
Curare, pharmacologic action, 82
Cushing's disease, neurologic complications, 318
Cyclophosphamide, chronic immune-related
    demyelinating polyradiculopathy treatment, 92
Cytomegalovirus (CMV)
  neurologic complications, 251
  retinitis in AIDS, 340

Dale's principle, generalization and exceptions, 4
Decerebrate posturing, 36
Decorticate posturing, 36
Deep brain stimulation (DBS), Parkinson's disease
    treatment, 158
Degenerative spine disease, **99–110**
Dejerine, Jules, 402
Delirium
  definition, 209
  dementia relationship, 209–210
Dementia, **209–218**. See also Alzheimer's disease

Dementia *(cont.)*
  causes, 210
  definitions, 209
  delirium relationship, 209–210
  differential diagnosis, 218
  frontotemporal dementia, 214
  screening instruments, 210
  subcortical dementia, 217–218
  vascular dementia, 216
Demyelinating disease, **201–207**. *See also* Multiple
    sclerosis
  symptom etiology, 201
  types, 201
Denervation supersensitivity, 7
Deprenyl, Parkinson's disease treatment, 153
Dermatome
  definition, 112
  postherpetic neuralgia, 266
  spinal root correlation, 25
Dermatomyositis (DM)
  with cancer, 249
  classification, 62
  clinical presentation, 62
  muscle biopsy, 63
Descartes, Rene
  blink reflex discovery, 404
  view of pineal gland, 404
Development
  milestones, 344–345
  reflexes, 344
Diabetes insipidus, tumor localization in children,
    359
Diabetes mellitus
  coma with, 319
  infection, 332
  nervous system effects, 318–319
  neuropathy
    autonomic neuropathy manifestations, 187
    pain with, 88
    prevalence, 87
    seizures with, 317
  vascular occlusive disease and neurologic
    complications, 319
Diagnostic approach, **53–58**
Dialysis
  dementia, 314
  disequilibrium syndrome, 313
  intracranial hemorrhage, 314
Dickens, Charles, 409
Dimethylaminopropionitrile, peripheral neuropathy
    induction, 89
Diphtheria toxin, neurologic manifestations, 332
Disc
  bulge, 101
  herniation, 101, 102
    lumbar disc, 103
    thoracic disc, 104
  protrusion, 101
DMD. *See* Duchenne muscular dystrophy
Dodgson, Charles Lutwidge, 408
Donepezil, Alzheimer's disease treatment, 215

Dopamine
  functions, 6
  receptors, 6
    striatal D1 and D2 receptors, 149
    types, 148–149
  secretion, 6
  synthesis, 6
  uptake, 6
Doppler ultrasound, stroke, 241
Dorsal column
  decussation, 28
  information types and pathway, 27
Dorsal midbrain syndrome, features, 128
Dorsal nerve root, sensory axons, 24
Dorsal root ganglia, cell types, 25
Dorsal scapular nerve, anatomy, 21, 22
Dorsolateral midbrain syndrome, features,
    128
Dostoyevsky, Fyodor, 410
Down syndrome
  Alzheimer's disease association, 213
  features, 350
Duchenne muscular dystrophy (DMD)
  clinical manifestations, 364
  diagnosis, 364
  dystrophin mutation, 64, 364
  systemic involvement, 64–65
  therapeutic prospects, 364–365
Dysarthria, **229–235**
  brainstem causes, 230
  causes, 229
  cranial nerve lesions, 230–231
  definition, 229
  electrical stimulation studies, 229–230
  muscle disturbances, 231
  nerve damage causes, 230
  prognosis, 229
  spasmodic dysphonia, 231–232
Dysfluency, **229–235**
Dyskinesia
  levodopa induction and management
    diphasic dyskinesia, 156, 157
    off dyskinesia, 156, 157
    peak-dose dyskinesia, 156
    tardive dyskinesia. *See* Tardive dyskinesia
Dyslexia
  definition, 225
  types and lesions, 225
Dysphagia, **229–235**
  causes, 233–234
  definition, 233
  mechanical dysphagia, 233, 234
  neuromotor dysphagia, 233, 234
  swallowing
    reflex, 233
    stages, 233
    vagus nerve role, 233
  symptoms, 233, 234
Dysphonia, definition, 229
Dystonia
  acute dystonic reaction, 176

Dystonia *(cont.)*
  classification, 167
  essential tremor association, 164
  focal dystonia forms, 169–170
  gene mutations, 169
  idiopathic dystonia forms, 168
  secondary dystonia
    causes, 167–168
    clinical presentation, 167
  torsion dystonia, 166–167
  treatment
    botulinum toxin, 170–171
    levodopa, 170
    surgery, 171

Eale's syndrome, neurologic complications, 323
Ear
  external, 37
  inner, 37
  middle, 37
  sensitivity, 407
Echocardiography, stroke evaluation, 240
Eclampsia
  mortality, 324
  neurologic complications, 324
  treatment, 324–325
Edinger-Westphal nucleus
  function, 31
  pupil constriction regulation, 44, 45
Edrophonium test
  myasthenic vs. cholinergic crisis differentiation, 80
  protocol, 77
  rationale, 77
EEG. *See* Electroencephalogram
EKG. *See* Electrocardiogram
Electrocardiogram (EKG)
  beat-to-beat heart rate test, 196–197
  myocardial injury with central nervous system
    disease, 191
  stroke, 240, 248
Electroencephalogram (EEG), **367–388**
  absence seizure, 379
  activating procedures, 380
  Alzheimer's disease, 376
  anoxia, 387
  breach rhythm, 373–374
  coma
    alpha coma pattern, 387
    brain death criteria, 388
    spindle coma pattern, 387
    theta coma pattern, 387–388
  Creutzfeldt-Jakob disease, 336, 376–377
  drugs and beta activity induction, 378
  encephalopathy monitoring, 376
  epilepsy, 289
  epileptiform
    focal spikes, 381
    phantom spike and wave pattern, 385
    positive bursts, 384
    small sharp spike pattern, 386
    theta bursts, 385

Electroencephalogram (EEG) *(cont.)*
  frequencies for recording, 367
  generalized seizure, 284, 384
  hyperventilation response, 380–381
  hypnagogic hypersynchrony, 380
  hypsarrhythmia, 378–379
  K complex, 370
  lambda waves, 382
  Lennox-Gastaut syndrome, 383
  mu rhythm, 373
  normal waking electroencephalogram
    adults, 367
    children, 372–373
    infants, 371
  occipital dominant rhythm, 372
  periodic lateralizing epileptiform discharges, 377
  posterior fossa tumor, 375
  postictal changes, 384
  pseudotumor cerebri, 374
  signal sources, 367
  sleep
    epileptiform discharges during sleep, 384
    nonrapid eye movement sleep, 367–369
    positive occipital sharp transients, 382–383
    rapid eye movement sleep, 369
    spindles, age of onset, 372
  slow triphasic waves, 312
  stroke
    hemispheric infarction, 374–375
    lacunar infarct, 375
    middle cerebral artery infarction, 374
  subacute sclerosing panencephalitis, 376–377
  subdural hematoma, 375
  suppression-burst pattern, 386
  tracé alternant, 372
  tracé discontinu, 371
  triphasic wave significance, 375–376
  vascular dementia, 216
  vertex transients, 372, 382
Electrolyte disorders, neurologic complications,
  319–320
Electromyogram (EMG), **389–395**
  amyotrophic lateral sclerosis, 96, 392
  brachial plexus lesions, 392–393
  C8 root lesion, 394
  critical care patients, 394–395
  denervation effects, 390
  drug myopathy, 395
  endplate activity, 390
  fasciculation potentials, 389
  fibrillation potentials, 389
  F-wave, 391
  Guillain-Barré syndrome, 392
  H-reflex, 391
  inclusion body myositis, 392
  indications, 389
  insertional activity, 389
  myopathy, 390
  myotonic discharges, 68, 390
  nerve conduction velocity. *See* Nerve conduction
    velocity

Electromyogram (EMG) *(cont.)*
nerve transection effects, 390
polymyositis, 392
polyphasic units, 389
positive sharp waves, 390
radiculopathy evaluation, 107
radiculopathy, 393, 394
repetitive nerve stimulation. *See* Repetitive nerve stimulation
single-fiber recording. *See* Single-fiber electromyography
single motor unit potentials, 389
spastic paresis, 392
ulnar nerve entrapment, 393
Emergencies, **399**
EMG. *See* Electromyogram
Encephalitis, viral, 337–338
Endocrine disease, neurologic complications, 316–319
Entacapone, Parkinson's disease treatment, 158
Ependymal cell, features, 1
Ependymoma. *See* Brain tumor
Epilepsy, **283–300**. *See also* Seizure
antiepileptic drug treatment
add-on drug effects, 295–296
blood level monitoring, 297
drug interactions, 295, 296
felbamate, 291, 292
gabapentin, 291, 292
half-lives and dosing, 293
idiosyncratic reactions, 297
indications, 298
initiation, 290
lamotrigine, 291, 292
levetiracetam, 291, 292
mechanisms of action, 293
monotherapy, 294
oxcarbazepine, 291, 292
prophylactic use, 297
rational polytherapy, 294
selection by seizure type, 290–291
side effects, 294
teratogenic risks, 297–298
termination, 290
tiagabine, 291, 292
topiramate, 291, 292
zonisamide, 291, 292
benign childhood epilepsy with centrotemporal spikes, 286
channelopathies, 287
children, 362
definition, 283
diagnosis
electroencephalography, 289
magnetic resonance imaging, 289
positron emission tomography, 290
single-photon emission computed tomography, 290
driving recommendations, 300
head trauma type and risks, 288
historical perspective, 406–407
juvenile myoclonic epilepsy, 286

Epilepsy *(cont.)*
pregnancy management, 326
risk factors, 286
surgery, 300
syndromes, 284–286
Epley maneuver, benign positional vertigo treatment, 133
Equine encephalitis, types, 337–338
Erb's palsy, nerve injury, 22
Ergotamine, migraine treatment, 275, 277
Essential tremor (ET)
brain generators of tremor, 163–164
clinical correlates, 162–163
dystonia association, 164
features, 162
Parkinson's disease association, 164
physiologic tremor differentiation, 163
prevalence, 162
treatment
alcohol, 165
botulinum toxin, 165
primidone, 165
propranolol, 165
variants, 164–165
Ethylene oxide, peripheral neuropathy induction, 89–90
Excitotoxicity hypothesis, 9
Exner's area, lesion effects, 48
Eye movement
saccade, 39
smooth pursuit, 39
vertical, 39

Fabry's disease
clinical presentation, 194
pathogenesis, 194
treatment, 194
Familial amyloidosis, pathogenesis, 194
Familial dysautonomia
diagnostic criteria, 193
prevalence and heredity, 193
Fasciculi proprii, anatomy, 112
Febrile convulsion
benign, 286
complex seizure, 362
consequences, 286, 362
heredity, 286
simple seizure, 362
Felbamate, seizure management, 291, 292
Femoral nerve, anatomy, 19
Fibromyalgia
clinical features, 262, 263
diagnostic criteria, 262
myofascial pain syndrome comparison, 263
treatment, 263
Filum terminale, anatomy, 27
Flare, scratch response mechanism, 198
Flaubert, Gustave, 410
Floppy baby
causes, 348
differential diagnosis, 347

Focal dystonia, forms, 169–170
Folate deficiency, neurologic complications, 311
Fosphenytoin, status epilepticus treatment, 299
Free radical
    neuronal injury, 9
    scavenging, 9–10
Friedreich's ataxia
    clinical features, 143–144
    prevalence, 142
Frontal lobe, functions, 48
Frontooccipital circumference (FOC), growth, 344
Functional cloning, disease genes, 12
Fungal infection
    antifungal agents, 335
    headache with, 334
    meningitis, 335

GABA. See Gamma-aminobutyric acid
Gabapentin
    migraine treatment, 276
    pain management, 270
    seizure management, 291, 292
Gain-of-function mutation, autosomal dominant
        disease, 12–13
Galactosemia, features, 353
Galen malformation, presentations, 358
Gamma-aminobutyric acid (GABA), receptors, 5–6
Gamma efferent nerve fiber, function, 18
Ganser's syndrome, 209
Gastrointestinal disease, neurologic complications,
        309–311
Gaucher's disease, features, 353
GBS. See Guillain-Barré syndrome
Gehrig, Lou, 97
Gene
    allele, 11
    mutation types, 11–12
    polymorphism, 11
Gene therapy, challenges, 14
Genitofemoral nerve, anatomy, 19
Gershwin, George, 411
Gerstmann's syndrome
    clinical features, 227
    lesions, 227
Gilles de la Tourette, George, 404
Glatiramer acetate, multiple sclerosis management,
        206
Glioma. See Brain tumor
Global aphasia
    characteristics, 222
    lesions, 222
Glossopharyngeal neuralgia, clinical features, 267
Glutamate, receptor types, 5
Gower's sign, 60
Granulomatous angiitis, neurologic complications,
        323–324
Guillain-Barré syndrome (GBS)
    autonomic dysfunction
        adynamic ileus, 189
        arrhythmia management, 188
        atonic bladder, 189

Guillain-Barré syndrome (GBS) (cont.)
    autonomic dysfunction (cont.)
        blood pressure fluctuation management, 188
        duration of cardiovascular instability, 188
        incidence, 188
    Campylobacter jejuni infection, 95
    clinical presentation, 94
    electromyography, 392
    forms, 94
    Guillain, George, 401
    immunopathology, 94–95
    laboratory findings, 95
    prognostic indicators, 95
    relapse, 95
    treatment, 95
Gustatory nucleus, anatomy, 34

Hallervorden-Spatz disease, features, 354
Haploinsufficiency, definition, 13
Headache, 273–281. See also Cluster headache;
        Migraine; Tension headache
    analgesia, 273
    brain tumor, 280
    children, 363–364
    cranial structure sensitivity, 273
    incidence, 273
    localization, 273
    postcoital headache, 280
    in pregnancy, 324
    pseudotumor cerebri, 280–281
    serious indications, 273
    sex distribution, 273
    spinal tap headache, 279–280
    temporal arteritis, 291
Heart transplantation, autonomic dysfunction, 192
Hematologic disease, neurologic complications,
        315–316
Hemianopsia, types and lesions, 45
Hemochromatosis, neurologic complications, 312
Hemophilia, neurologic complications, 315
Hepatic encephalopathy
    causes, 311
    treatment, 311
Hepatosplenomegaly, neurodegenerative diseases
        with, 353
Hereditary neuropathy with liability to pressure
        palsy (HNPP), diagnosis, 88
Herpes simplex virus (HSV)
    Bell's palsy role, 339
    encephalitis
        cerebrospinal fluid findings, 338
        clinical features, 338
        histopathologic findings, 338
        neonates, 356
        peripheral viral entry, 339
        treatment, 338
    meningitis, 338
    Ramsey-Hunt syndrome, 338
Hexacarbon solvents, peripheral neuropathy
        induction, 90
Hippocampal sclerosis, with seizures, 300

History, patient
  accuracy in neurologic disease diagnosis, 58
  autonomic dysfunction, 182–183
  brainstem disease, 56
  cerebellar disease, 57
  cortical versus subcortical disease, 57, 58
  lesion localization approaches, 53
  microcephaly, 348
  muscle disease, 53
  neuromuscular junction disease, 54
  pediatric neurology, 343
  peripheral neuropathies, 54
  radiculopathies, 54–55
  spinal cord disease, 55
  stroke, 239
HIV. *See* Human immunodeficiency virus
Horner's syndrome
  clinical presentation, 44
  diagnosis, 44
H-reflex, S1 radiculopathy evaluation, 107
Human immunodeficiency virus (HIV). *See*
    Acquired immunodeficiency syndrome
Huntington's disease (HD)
  clinical presentation, 174–175
  dementia with, 217–218
  genetic testing, 175
  neuropathologic findings, 175
  treatment, 175
  Westphal variant, 175
Hurler's disease, features, 353
Hydrocephalus, communicating versus
    noncommunicating, 50
Hypercalcemia, neurologic complications, 320
Hyperhidrosis
  causes, 199–200
  treatment, 200
Hyperkalemia, neurologic complications, 319
Hypermagnesemia, neurologic complications, 320
Hypernatremia, neurologic complications, 320
Hyperparathyroidism, neurologic complications,
  318
Hypersensitivity angiitis, neurologic complications,
  322–323
Hyperthyroidism, neurologic complications, 317
Hyperventilation, clinical features, 314
Hyperviscosity states, neurologic complications,
  315
Hypnagogic hallucination, features, 304
Hypnagogic hypersynchrony,
  electroencephalography, 380
Hypocalcemia, neurologic complications, 320
Hypoglycorrhachia, causes, 329
Hypokalemia, neurologic complications, 319
Hypomagnesemia, neurologic complications, 320
Hyponatremia, neurologic complications, 320
Hypoparathyroidism, neurologic complications, 318
Hypothermia, neurologic conditions with, 192
Hypothyroidism
  congenital, 354
  neurologic complications, 317
Hypsarrhythmia, electroencephalography, 378–379

Ia nerve fiber, function, 18
Ib nerve fiber
  origination, 18
  synapse, 18
Iliohypogastric nerve
  anatomy, 19
  McBurney's incision risks, 19
Impotence
  differential diagnosis of nonpsychogenic causes,
    191
  neurologic diseases, 327
Inclusion body myositis (IBM)
  clinical presentation, 62–63
  electromyography, 392
  muscle biopsy, 63
Infantile hypotonia. *See* Floppy baby
Infectious disease, **329–341**
Inferior gluteal nerve, anatomy, 20
Insomnia
  causes, 306
  definition, 305
  jet lag management, 306
  treatment, 306
Interferon, chronic immune-related demyelinating
    polyradiculopathy treatment, 93
Intermediolateral cell column, anatomy, 112
Internuclear ophthalmoplegia (INO), features, 130
Intravenous immunoglobulin (IVIG)
  chronic immune-related demyelinating
    polyradiculopathy treatment, 93, 94
  Guillain-Barré syndrome treatment, 95
Intraventricular hemorrhage, neonatal
  complications, 346
  grading, 346
  prognosis, 346
  risk factors, 346
Ion channel. *See also specific channels*
  channelopathy, 7
  conductance, 7
  gating, 7
  permeability, 7
Isaacs syndrome
  clinical presentation, 69
  treatment, 69
Isoniazid, peripheral neuropathy induction, 332
IVIG. *See* Intravenous immunoglobulin

Jet lag, management, 306
Jugular foramen syndrome, clinical presentation,
  34
Junctional scotoma, features, 45

K complex, electroencephalography, 370
Kearns-Sayre syndrome, features, 353
Kennedy, Foster, 402–403
Kidney disease, neurologic complications, 313–314
Kinetic tremor
  causes, 166
  clinical features, 165
  treatment, 166
Klumpke's palsy, nerve injury, 22

Korsakoff's syndrome
  alcohol role, 210
  vitamin deficiency differential diagnosis, 311
Krabbe's disease, features, 351
Kuru, features, 337

Lambda waves, electroencephalography, 382
Lambert-Eaton myasthenic syndrome (LEMS)
  anesthesia precautions, 81
  autoimmune response, 72, 80
  clinical presentation, 80, 249
  neuromuscular junction morphology, 80
  paraneoplastic syndrome, 189–190
  repetitive nerve stimulation, 391
  repetitive nerve stimulation response, 80
  treatment, 81, 190
  tumors with, 80, 189–190
Lamotrigine, seizure management, 291, 292
Language
  compromise, 229
  definition, 219
Larynx, nerve paralysis, 233
Lateral femoral cutaneous nerve
  anatomy, 19
  meralgia paresthetica, 20
Lateral medullary syndrome, features, 126
Lazarus sign, 408
Lead poisoning, neurologic complications, 313
Learning disabilities, children, 366
Left-handedness, prevalence, 219
LELAS syndrome, features, 354
Lennox-Gastaut syndrome
  electroencephalography, 383
  features, 285–286
Leprous neuropathy, prevalence, 87, 88
Leptomeningeal carcinomatosis
  cerebrospinal fluid analysis, 257
  chemotherapy, 257
  clinical presentation, 256
  imaging, 257
  sources, 257
Leptospirosis, clinical presentation, 334
Lesion, localization approaches, 53
Levetiracetam, seizure management, 291, 292
Levodopa
  clinical fluctuations and management, 155, 156
  dyskinesia induction and management
    diphasic dyskinesia, 156, 157
    off dyskinesia, 156, 157
    peak-dose dyskinesia, 156
  dystonia treatment, 170
  initiation of therapy, 154
  Parkinson's disease treatment, 153, 154
  progressive supranuclear palsy treatment, 160
  side effects, 154
  Sinemet CR preparation, 156
Lewy body dementia, features, 218
Lhermitte's sign, 114
Lidoderm, topical analgesia, 270
Limbic lobe, 43
Lincoln, Nancy Hanks, 415–416

Lithium, cluster headache treatment, 278
Liver disease, neurologic complications, 311–313
Locked-in syndrome, features, 129
Logorrhea, definition, 221
Long-term depression (LTD), function, 4
Long-term potentiation (LTP), induction, 4
Long thoracic nerve, anatomy, 21, 22
Loss-of-function mutation, autosomal dominant
  disease, 12–13
Lower dorsal pontine syndrome, features, 127
Lumbar plexus
  branches, 19
  roots, 18
Lumbar puncture
  Alzheimer's disease, 212
  cerebrospinal fluid analysis. See Cerebrospinal fluid
  headache, 279–280, 401
  historical perspective, 401
  site, 51
Lumbar radiculopathy
  differentiating signs and symptoms by vertebrae, 103
  signs and symptoms, 25
  surgical management, 109
Lumbar stenosis
  clinical features, 103
  neurogenic claudication mechanism, 103–104
  straight leg-raising test, 104
  surgical management, 109
Lung disease, neurologic complications, 314–315
Lyme disease
  clinical presentation, 334
  neuropathy types, 89, 334

Macrocephaly, differential diagnosis, 348
Madison, James, 415
Magnetic resonance angiography (MRA), stroke, 239, 241
Magnetic resonance imaging (MRI)
  acoustic neuroma, 145
  brainstem lesions, 124, 125
  epilepsy, 289
  multiple sclerosis, 204
  spine, 106
  stroke, 239
  vascular dementia, 216
  Wilson's disease, 179
Malaria, cerebral, 334
Marcus Gunn pupil
  lesions, 44
  testing, 44–45
Mary Walker phenomenon, myasthenia gravis, 74
Mastocytosis, autonomic dysfunction differential
  diagnosis, 200
Maupassant, Guy de, 409
McArdle's disease
  clinical presentation, 66
  differential diagnosis, 66
  treatment, 66
Medial longitudinal fasciculus (MLF), anatomy, 29
Medial medullary syndrome, features, 126

Medulla
    anatomy and function, 33–35, 121
    blood supply, 126
    lateral medullary syndrome, 126
    medial medullary syndrome, 126
Medulloblastoma, prognosis, 252–253
Megalencephaly, differential diagnosis, 348
Melatonin, synthesis, 6
MEN 2b. *See* Multiple endocrine neoplasia type 2b
Mendelsohn, Felix, 411–412
Ménière's disease, features, 133
Meningioma. *See* Brain tumor
Meningitis. *See* Aseptic meningitis; Bacterial
    meningitis
Meralgia paresthetica, causes, 20
MERRF syndrome, features, 353
Mesencephalon
    adult derivatives, 16
    formation, 15
Metachromatic leukodystrophy (MLD), clinical
    variants, 351
Methyl bromide, peripheral neuropathy induction, 90
Methysergide maleate, migraine treatment, 277
Microcephaly
    history, 348
    laboratory tests, 349
    physical examination, 348
Microglia, features, 1
Midbrain
    anatomy and function, 30–32, 122
    blood supply, 126
    dorsal midbrain syndrome, 128
    dorsolateral midbrain syndrome, 128
    ventral midbrain syndrome, 128
Midrin, migraine treatment, 275
Migraine
    age of onset, 274
    alternating hemiplegia, 363
    aura, 274
    children, 363–364
    classification, 363
    food induction, 275, 363
    fortification spectra, 401
    frequency of attack, 274
    phases, 274
    prophylaxis
        drug selection , 277
        nicardipine, 277
        nifedipine, 277
        propranolol, 276
        tricyclic antidepressants, 276
        valproic acid, 277
        verapamil, 277
    serotonin role, 275
    symptoms, 274
    treatment
        children, 363–364
        ergotamine, 275, 277
        gabapentin, 276
        methysergide maleate, 277
        Midrin, 275

Migraine *(cont.)*
    treatment *(cont.)*
        naratriptan, 276
        pregnant patients, 277
        sumatriptan, 275, 276
        topirimate, 276
        triptans, 275, 276
        vascular theory, 275
Mini-Mental Status Examination (MMSE)
    dementia evaluation, 210
    limitations, 210
Mitoxantrone, multiple sclerosis management, 206
Möbius syndrome, features, 33
Mollaret's triangle, 40
Monoclonal gammopathy of uncertain significance
    (MGUS)
    M-protein types, 92
    neuropathy association, 91–92
Mononeuritis multiplex, causes, 86
Morphine, equianalgesic dose table, 258
Motor unit, components, 17, 59
Movement disorders, **147–180**
MRA. *See* Magnetic resonance angiography
MRI. *See* Magnetic resonance imaging
MS. *See* Multiple sclerosis
Multifocal motor neuropathy (MMN), differential
    diagnosis, 94
Multiple endocrine neoplasia type 2b (MEN 2b)
    clinical features, 195
    gene mutations, 195
Multiple sclerosis (MS)
    brainstem effects, 132
    children, 352
    clinical course, 202
    demyelination mechanism, 201
    diagnosis
        brainstem auditory evoked potentials, 203
        cerebrospinal fluid analysis, 203
        criteria, 203
        magnetic resonance imaging, 204
        somatosensory evoked potentials, 204
        visual evoked potentials, 203
    etiology
        autoimmunity, 205
        epidemiology, 204–205
        infection, 205
    incidence, 201, 204
    optic neuritis relationship, 202
    prognosis, 202
    symptoms, 201–202
    treatment
        cerebellar tremor and ataxia, 207
        corticosteroids, 205
        fatigue, 206
        glatiramer acetate, 206
        immunosuppression, 206
        interferon, 206
        motor deficits, 207
        neurogenic bladder, 207
Multiple sleep latency test (MSLT)
    daytime sleepiness evaluation, 303

Multiple sleep latency test (MSLT) *(cont.)*
    medication effects, 303
    narcolepsy diagnosis, 304
    normal sleep latency, 303
Multiple system atrophy (MSA)
    pure autonomic failure differential diagnosis,
        193
    syndromes, 161
    treatment, 161
Mu rhythm, electroencephalography, 373
Muscarinic acetylcholine receptor, function, 5
Muscle
    A band, 17
    biopsy
        indications, 61
        myositis, 63
        staining, 61
        tubular aggregates, 62
    contraction mechanism, 17
    embryonic origins, 59
    fiber types, 61
    H band, 17
    histologic organization, 16–17
    I band, 17
    innervation, 17–18
    ragged red fibers, 62
    Z line, 17
Myasthenia gravis (MG)
    acetylcholine receptor antibodies
        binding sites, 74
        clinical evidence, 73
        experimental evidence, 73
        immunopathology, 73
    autoimmune response, 72, 73
    children, 365
    congenital syndromes, 76
    corticosteroid therapy, 79
    crises
        cholinergic, 79–80
        myasthenic, 79, 80
    diagnosis, 76–77
    drug avoidance, 78–79
    drug-induced autoimmune disease, 79
    epidemiology, 72–73
    human leukocyte antigen types, 73
    Mary Walker phenomenon, 74
    neonatal disease, 76
    neuromuscular manifestations, 72
    pyridostigmine therapy, 78
    repetitive nerve stimulation, 391
    safety margin of synaptic transmission at motor
        endplate, 74
    speech signs, 233
    thymus
        pathogenesis role, 75
        thymectomy management, 75–76
    tumors with, 75
Myelin
    definition, 401
    function, 201
Myelomeningocele, complications, 349–350

Myelopathy, **111–119**
    causes, 114
    clinical presentation, 114
    radiation myelopathy, 260
Myoblast, structure and function, 59
Myoclonus
    classification, 177–178
    distinguishing from tics and chorea, 177
    treatment, 178–179
Myofascial pain syndrome (MPS)
    clinical features, 262
    fibromyalgia comparison, 263
    treatment, 263
    trigger points, 262
Myofiber, structure and function, 59
Myofibril, structure and function, 59
Myokymia, features, 68
Myopathy, **59–70**
    with cardiac disease, 68
    children, 365
    classification, 62, 65
    clinical presentation, 59
    congenital myopathies, 65
    definition, 59
    drug induction, 69–70
    with dysphagia, 68
    hypertrophy of muscle, 67
    laboratory tests, 60–61
    metabolic myopathies, 65
    mitochondrial myopathies, 66–67
    pain with, 59
    with respiratory failure, 68
    weakness grading, 59–60
Myotome, definition, 112
Myotonic dystrophy
    clinical manifestations, 365
    facial appearance, 63, 365
    gene mutation, 64
    heredity, 365
    neonatal complications, 365
    prevalence, 64
    systemic involvement, 64
Myotube, structure and function, 59

Naratriptan, migraine treatment, 276
Narcolepsy
    diagnosis, 304, 305
    sleep paralysis, 304, 305
    tetrad, 304
    treatment, 304–305
Necrosis, neurons, 10
Neologism, definition, 220
Nernst equation, 2
Nerve conduction velocity
    Bell's palsy, 394
    critical care patients, 394–395
    Guillain-Barré syndrome, 392
    indications, 390
    normal values, 391
Nerve growth factor, Alzheimer's disease treatment,
    214

Neural crest, cell differentiation, 15
Neural tube, formation, 15
Neurapraxia, definition, 392
Neuroanatomy, **15–51**
Neurocystercosis
    clinical presentation, 335
    epidemiology, 334
    pediatric disease, 356–357
Neurofibromatosis
    type I, 354
    type II, 354
Neuroleptic malignant syndrome (NMS)
    clinical presentation, 70, 336
    etiology, 70
    treatment, 70
Neurology, historical perspective, 403
Neuromuscular junction (NMJ)
    active zone, 72
    neurotransmission
        postsynaptic events, 72
        presynaptic events, 71
        synaptic cleft events, 72
    safety margin of synaptic transmission at motor
        endplate, 74
Neuromuscular junction disease, **71–82**. *See also*
    specific diseases
    children, 364–366
    history, 54
    physical examination, 54
Neuromyotonia, features, 68
Neuronal ceroid lipofuscinoses (NCL)
    Finnish snowballs, 407
    types, 353
Neuronal transplantation, barriers, 13–14
Neuro-oncology, **249–260**
    chemotherapy complications, 259–260
    children, 359–361
    leptomeningeal carcinomatosis, 256–257
    metastatic disease, 255–256
    neurologic complications, 249–251
    pain, 257–259
    primary brain tumors, 251–255
Neuropathic tremor, features, 166
Neuroradiology, **397–398**
Neurotransmitter. *See also specific neurotransmitters*
    Dale's principle, 4
    definitive criteria, 4
Neurotrophic factor, types, 10, 11
Nicardipine, migraine prophylaxis, 277
Nicotinic acetylcholine receptor, function, 5
Niemann-Pick disease, features, 353
Nifedipine, migraine prophylaxis, 277
Nocturnal myoclonus, features, 306–307
Nocturnal paroxysmal dystonia, features, 307
Norepinephrine
    age effects on response, 185
    autonomic dysfunction assay, 185
    autonomic nervous system, 184
Nucleus ambiguus, anatomy, 34
Nucleus solitarius, anatomy, 34
Nucleus tractus solitarius (NTS), function, 185

Oat-cell carcinoma, antibodies, 250
Obsessive-compulsive disorder (OCD), treatment in
    Tourette's syndrome, 174
Obstructive sleep apnea
    sleep deprivation, 303
    treatment, 304
Obturator nerve, anatomy, 19
Occipital lobe, functions, 48
Occipital neuralgia, features, 364
OCD. *See* Obsessive-compulsive disorder
Olfaction
    anosmia causes, 43
    pathway anatomy, 43
    receptor cells, 43
    sensitivity in humans, 408
Oligodedroglia, features, 1
Ondine's curse, 407
One-and-a-half syndrome, features, 130–131
Opsoclonus-myoclonus
    features, 180
    neoplasms with, 250
Optic nerve, pathway, 45
Organ of Corti
    audiofrequency analysis, 38
    neuroepithelial cell arrangement, 38
Orthostatic hypotension
    autonomic dysfunction versus hypovolemia, 197
    management, 197
    nonneurogenic causes, 198
    syncope, 197
Orthostatic tremor (OT), features, 164
Ototoxicity, antibiotics, 332
Oxcarbazepine, seizure management, 291, 292

Pain
    acute versus chronic, 261
    analgesics
        adjuvant analgesics, 269–270
        classification, 268
        NSAIDs, 269
        opioids, 268–269
        topical analgesics, 270
    assessment of chronic pain, 262
    cancer patients
        barriers to treatment, 257
        control adequacy, 257
        neuropathic pain treatment, 257–258
    chronic pain management
        behavioral and cognitive therapies, 270
        implantable drug pumps, 271
        neural ablative procedures, 271
        neurostimulation management, 270–271
        overview of strategies, 271–272
    definition, 261
    equianalgesic dose table, 258
    neuropathic pain, 257, 261–262
    nociception comparison, 261
    nociceptive pain, 257, 261
    opioid administration routes, 259
    opioid resistance, 258–259, 268–269
    patient-controlled analgesia, 258

Pain *(cont.)*
polyneuropathy symptoms, 265–266
psychogenic pain, 261
syndromes, **261–272**
Palilalia, features, 234
Pallidotomy, Parkinson's disease treatment, 158–159
PAN. *See* Polyarteritis nodosa
Pandysautonomia, acute, 189
Papez's circuit, 43
Paramedian pontine reticular formation (PPRF),
anatomy, 39
Paraneoplastic autonomic neuropathy, features, 190
Paraneoplastic cerebellar degeneration (PCD)
clinical presentation, 145
etiology, 146
Paraneoplastic intestinal pseudoobstruction,
features, 190
Paraneoplastic movement disorder, types, 180
Paraneoplastic subacute sensory neuropathy,
features and treatment, 190
Parasellar lesions, differential diagnosis, 360
Parasympathetic nervous system
anatomy, 183–184
neurotransmitters, 184–185
stimulation, physiologic responses, 181
Parietal lobe, functions, 48
Parinaud syndrome, features, 130
Parkinson's disease (PD)
autonomic dysfunction, 193
causes, 150–151
clinical diagnosis specificity, 152
clinical fluctuations, 155, 156
dementia with, 159, 217
drug induction, 151, 161, 260
essential tremor association, 164
genetics, 151–152
laboratory tests, 152–153
neurophysiologic changes in basal ganglia, 149
progressive supranuclear palsy differential
diagnosis, 160
signs and symptoms, 149–150, 152
speech signs, 229
treatment
amantadine, 153–154
deprenyl, 153
dopamine agonists, 157–158
levodopa, 153, 154–157
monoamine oxidase inhibitors, 158
surgery, 158–159
vascular parkinsonism, 161
Parsonage-Turner syndrome, symptoms, 22
Pediatric neurology, **343–366**
development
milestones, 344–345
reflexes, 344
history taking, 343
physical examination, 344
Pelizaeus-Merzbacher disease, features, 352
Pergolide
dopamine receptor specificity, 157, 158
Parkinson's disease treatment, 157, 158

Pergolide *(cont.)*
side effects, 158
Perinatal asphyxia, classification, 346–347
Periodic limb movement disorder, features, 306–307
Periodic paralysis
classification, 67
symptoms, 67
treatment, 67
Peripheral neuropathy, **83–97**. *See also specific
neuropathies*
with autonomic dysfunction, 187–189
biopsy
nerve types, 86
sural nerve, 86–87
chemical induction, 89–90
clinical tests for root syndromes, 84–85
conduction block, 84
cranial nerve involvement, 85
critical-illness polyneuropathy, 90
disease classification, 83
hereditary neuropathy and genetic testing, 90, 91
history, 54
hypertrophic nerve conditions, 86
immune-mediated neuropathies, 91–92
infectious disease, 89
mononeuritis multiplex causes, 86
motor neuropathies, 86
patterns of nerve damage, 83
physical examination, 54
proximal versus distal origins, 85
sensory neuropathies, 86
upper extremity origins, 85
Peroneal nerve, anatomy, 21
PET. *See* Positron emission tomography
Phantom limb pain, features, 266
Phenylketonuria, features, 354
Phonation, definition, 219
Phyntanic acid, accumulation in Refsum's disease,
403
Physical examination
accuracy in neurologic disease diagnosis, 58
autonomic dysfunction, 183
brainstem disease, 56–57
cerebellar disease, 57
cortical versus subcortical disease, 57–58
microcephaly, 348
muscle disease, 54
neuromuscular junction disease, 54
pediatric neurology, 344
peripheral neuropathies, 54
radiculopathies, 55
spinal cord disease, 55–56
stroke, 239
Physical therapy, neck and back pain, 107–108
Plasma exchange
chronic immune-related demyelinating
polyradiculopathy treatment, 93
Guillain-Barré syndrome treatment, 95
POEMS syndrome, features, 91
Polio
postpolio syndrome, 339

Polio (cont.)
    Roosevelt, Franklin Delano, 413–414
Polyarteritis nodosa (PAN)
    central nervous system effects, 322
    peripheral nervous system effects, 322
Polymerase chain reaction (PCR), principles, 12
Polymyositis (PM)
    classification, 62
    clinical presentation, 62
    electromyography, 392
    muscle biopsy, 63
Polysomnography
    medication effects, 303
    parameters for measurement, 303
    sleepwalking, 307
Pons
    anatomy and function, 32–33, 122
    blood supply, 126
    central pontine myelinolysis, 132
    locked-in syndrome, 129
    lower dorsal pontine syndrome, 127
    upper dorsal pontine syndrome, 127
    ventral pontine syndrome, 127
Porphyria
    neurologic complications, 312–313
    treatment of acute intermittent porphyria, 313
Porphyria
    autonomic dysfunction, 195
    types, 195
Positional cloning, disease genes, 12
Positron emission tomography (PET)
    epilepsy, 290
    Parkinson's disease, 152–153
    vascular dementia, 216
Postcoital cephalgia
    clinical features, 280
    headache types, 280
    treatment, 280
Posterior circulation, arteries, 49
Posterior femoral cutaneous nerve, anatomy, 20
Posterior fossa
    childhood tumors, 360–361
    electroencephalography of tumors, 375
    neoplasm, 144
Postherpetic neuralgia (PHN)
    atypical facial pain, 268
    clinical features, 266
    dermatomal frequencies, 266
    treatment, 266
Postural tachycardia syndrome (POTS)
    clinical features, 198
    treatment, 198
Potassium channel
    blockers, 7–8
    diseases, 8
    function in neurons, 7
POTS. See Postural tachycardia syndrome
Pramipexole
    dopamine receptor specificity, 157, 158
    Parkinson's disease treatment, 157, 158
    side effects, 158

Pregnancy, neurologic complications, 324–327
Primary lateral sclerosis, features, 97
Primidone, essential tremor treatment, 165
Primitive neuroectodermal tumor (PNET)
    complications, 359
    features, 359
Prion, diseases, 13, 336–337
Progressive multifocal leukoencephalopathy (PML)
    with AIDS, 340
    features, 251
Progressive myoclonus epilepsy, differential
        diagnosis, 288–289
Progressive supranuclear palsy (PSP)
    cause, 160
    clinical features, 159
    dementia with, 218
    Parkinson's disease differential diagnosis, 160
    treatment, 160–161
Prolactinoma, treatment, 254
Propranolol
    essential tremor treatment, 165
    migraine prophylaxis, 276
Prosencephalon
    adult derivatives, 16
    formation, 15
Prosody
    definition, 225
    functional-anatomic correlates, 225
Prosopagnosia
    definition, 226
    lesions, 226
Protein synthesis, molecular biology, 11
Pseudobulbar palsy, features, 131
Pseudodementia
    definition, 209
    with depression, 209, 210
Pseudotumor cerebri
    definition, 280
    diagnosis, 280
    electroencephalography, 374
    etiology, 281
    treatment, 281
    visual complaints, 281
PSP. See Progressive supranuclear palsy
Psychosis, with dementia, 210
Pudendal nerve, anatomy, 21
Pupil
    afferent defects, 44–45
    constriction pathway, 44, 45
    dilatation pathway, 44
    reflex in third-nerve palsy diagnosis, 45
Pyramidal tract, decussation, 112
Pyridostigmine
    adverse effects, 78
    cholinergic crisis, 79–80
    myasthenia gravis treatment, 78
    parenteral versus oral dose, 78
    Timespan formulation for slow release, 78

Q-T syndromes, potassium channel defects, 8
Quadrigeminal plate, anatomy, 30

Rabies
  peripheral viral entry, 339
  postexposure prophylaxis, 339
Radial nerve, crutches injury, 24
Radiation therapy
  brain tumor, 252, 256, 260
  cranial effects in children, 361
  myelopathy onset, 260
  side effects, 260
Radicular pain, versus referred pain, 102
Radiculopathy, **99–110**
  diagnostics, 106–107
  electromyography, 393, 394
  history, 54–55
  physical examination, 55
Ragged red fibers, mitochondrial cytopathies, 353
Ramsey-Hunt syndrome, features, 338
Rapid eye movement (REM) sleep
  cardiovascular autonomic changes, 198
  sleep behavior disorders, 307
Rasagiline, Parkinson's disease treatment, 158
Ravel, Maurice, 410
Red nucleus, function, 31
Referred pain, versus radicular pain, 102
Refsum's disease, phyntanic acid accumulation, 403
REM sleep. *See* Rapid eye movement sleep
Renal transplantation, neurologic complications, 314
Renshaw cell, function, 18
Repetitive nerve stimulation (RNS)
  Lambert-Eaton myasthenic syndrome, 391
  myasthenia gravis, 391
Repolarization, processes affecting, 2
Respiratory insufficiency, neurologic complications, 314
Respite care, Alzheimer's disease, 215
Restless legs syndrome
  clinical features, 308
  treatment, 308
Reticular formation, anatomy, 29
Reticulospinal tract, anatomy, 29
Reye syndrome, neurologic complications, 311–312
Rheumatoid arthritis (RA)
  central nervous system effects, 321
  myelopathy with, 321
  peripheral nervous system effects, 321
Rheumatologic disease, neurologic complications, 320–322
Rhombencephalon
  adult derivatives, 16
  formation, 15
Right-handedness
  dominance theories, 408
  prevalence, 219
Right occipital lobe infarction, vision effects, 46
Riley-Day syndrome. *See* Familial dysautonomia
Riluzole
  amyotrophic lateral sclerosis treatment, 97
  Parkinson's disease treatment, 158
Rinne's test, hearing assessment, 38
Rivastigmine, Alzheimer's disease treatment, 215
Rod, arrangement and function, 44

Roosevelt, Franklin Delano, 413–414
Ropinirole
  dopamine receptor specificity, 157, 158
  Parkinson's disease treatment, 157, 158
  side effects, 158
Rostral basilar artery, occlusion, 129

Saccade, eye movement, 39
Salivatory nucleus, anatomy, 34
Saltatory conduction, definition, 3
Scapular winging, palsies, 88–89
Sciatic nerve, anatomy, 20, 21
Scleroderma, with trigeminal neuropathy, 321–322
Scombroid poisoning
  neurologic manifestations, 333
  toxin features, 333
Seizure, **283–300**. *See also* Epilepsy
  antiepileptic drug treatment
    add-on drug effects, 295–296
    blood level monitoring, 297
    drug interactions, 295, 296
    felbamate, 291, 292
    gabapentin, 291, 292
    half-lives and dosing, 293
    idiosyncratic reactions, 297
    indications, 298
    initiation, 290
    lamotrigine, 291, 292
    levetiracetam, 291, 292
    mechanisms of action, 293
    monotherapy, 294
    oxcarbazepine, 291, 292
    prophylactic use, 297
    rational polytherapy, 294
    selection by seizure type, 290–291
    side effects, 294
    teratogenic risks, 297–298
    termination, 290
    tiagabine, 291, 292
    topiramate, 291, 292
    zonisamide, 291, 292
  causes
    alcohol withdrawal, 288
    by age, 287
    drug induction, 288
    heredity, 288
    metabolic causes, 288
  central nervous system changes, 287
  childbirth, differential diagnosis during, 326
  children, 362–363
  classification, 283
  definition, 283
  with endocrine disease, 316–317
  generalized seizure
    age of onset, 283–284
    causes, 283
    electroencephalography, 284
    types, 284
  neonates, 362
  partial seizure
    complex, 284

Seizure *(cont.)*
  partial seizure *(cont.)*
    simple, 284
    systemic effects, 287
Selective serotonin reuptake inhibitors (SSRIs), pain management, 269
Selegiline, Alzheimer's disease treatment, 215
Senility, definition, 209
Sensory nerve action potential (SNAP), normal values, 391
Serotonin
  melatonin synthesis, 6
  migraine role, 275
  receptors, 6
Sexual dysfunction, neurologic diseases, 327
SFEMG. *See* Single-fiber electromyography
Shaken-baby syndrome, features, 361
Shapiro's syndrome, hypothermia with, 192
Shy-Drager syndrome. *See* Multiple system atrophy
Siamese twins, Chang and Eng, 412
Sickle cell anemia
  cerebrovascular complications in children, 358
  neurologic complications, 315
Single-fiber electromyography (SFEMG)
  indications, 391
  myasthenia gravis diagnosis, 77
Single-photon emission computed tomography (SPECT)
  epilepsy, 290
  Parkinson's disease, 153
  vascular dementia, 216
Sjögren's syndrome
  autonomic dysfunction, 189
  neuromuscular diseases with, 321
Skull
  growing fracture, 361–362
  pressure endurance, 403
SLE. *See* Systemic lupus erythematosus
Sleep. *See also* Rapid eye movement sleep
  brain regulation, 301
  electroencephalogram
    epileptiform discharges during sleep, 384
    nonrapid eye movement sleep, 367–369
    positive occipital sharp transients, 382–383
    rapid eye movement sleep, 369
    spindles, age of onset, 372
  requirements for normal function, 302–303
  stages, 301
  theories for existence, 408
Sleep disorders, **301–308**
  classification, 301
  dyssomnias, 301, 302
  parasomnias, 301, 302
  patient reporting, 302
  sleep paralysis, 304, 305
  sleep terrors, 306
  sleepwalking, 307
Smooth pursuit, eye movement, 39
Sodium, neurologic complications of dysregulation, 319–320

Somatosensory evoked potentials, multiple sclerosis, 204
Spasmodic dysphonia
  causes, 232
  clinical presentation, 232
  definition, 231
  prognosis, 232
Spastic paresis, electromyography, 392
SPECT. *See* Single-photon emission computed tomography
Speech
  compromise, 229
  definition, 219
  motor output of brain, 229
Spina bifida, evaluation and management of neonates, 349
Spinal cord
  ascending tracts, 26
  axial musculature axons, 112
  blood supply, 27, 113, 114
  compression causes, 117
  descending tracts, 26
  divisions, 27
  fasciculi proprii, 112
  gray matter subdivision, 26, 111
  intermediolateral cell column, 112, 186
  intermediomedial cell column, 186
  long tracts and locations, 111, 112
  nerve exits, 27
  nerve relationship to vertebral body, 112
  organization, 26, 111
  pyramidal tract, 112
  subacute combined degeneration, 119
  termination, 27
  tumors, 117
Spinal cord arteritis, neurologic complications, 323
Spinal cord disease
  history, 55
  injury and central dysesthetic syndrome, 267
  physical examination, 55–56
  tumors
    bone metastasis, 255
    compression diagnosis and management, 255
    extramedullary region, 255
    intramedullary region, 255
Spinal epidural abscess
  clinical course, 331
  organisms, 331
Spinal shock, features, 114
Spinal stenosis. *See also* Lumbar stenosis
  causes, 101–102
  pain distribution, 102
  spondytic changes of invertebral disc and posterior joints, 101
Spinocerebellar ataxia (SCA)
  classification, 143
  clinical features, 143
Spinocerebellar tract, proprioception, 28
Spinothalamic tract
  decussation, 28
  information types and pathway, 28

Spinothalamic tract *(cont.)*
  VPL projections, 28
Spondylolisthesis, definition, 101
Spondylolysis, definition, 101
Spondylosis
  cervical spondylosis, 105
  definition, 101
  spinal pathophysiology, 100–101
SSRIs. *See* Selective serotonin reuptake inhibitors
Static encephalopathy
  antenatal risk factors, 347
  perinatal/neonatal risk factors, 347
Status epilepticus
  absence status epilepticus, 298
  brain damage, 299
  causes, 298
  classification, 298
  complex status epilepticus, 298
  epilepsia partialis continua, 299
  treatment, 298–299
Stem cell, origins, 13
Stereotypy, with tardive dyskinesia, 176
Steroid myopathy, forms, 70
Stiff-person syndrome
  clinical presentation, 69, 179
  pathophysiology, 179
  treatment, 69
Strachan's syndrome, features, 310
Stroke, **237–248**. *See also* Subarachnoid
      hemorrhage
  in cancer patients, 250
  cardiac disease association, 309
  causes
    anterior circulation stroke, 239
    posterior circulation stroke, 239
  children, laboratory investigations, 358
  clinical presentation
    anterior circulation stroke, 238
    cardioembolic stroke, 237
    hemiparesis, 237
    hemorrhagic stroke, 237–238
    lacunar stroke, 237
    posterior circulation stroke, 238–239
    thrombotic stroke, 237
  definition, 237
  electroencephalography
    hemispheric infarction, 374–375
    lacunar infarct, 375
    middle cerebral artery infarction, 374
  evaluation
    computed tomography, 239
    Doppler ultrasound, 241
    echocardiography, 240
    electrocardiography, 240
    history, 239
    laboratory tests, 239
    magnetic resonance angiography, 239, 241
    magnetic resonance imaging, 239
    neurologic exam, 239
    physical examination, 239
  historical perspective, 404

Stroke *(cont.)*
  incidence
    overall, 237
    by type, 238
  mortality, 243
  in pregnancy, 325
  prevention
    aspirin, 244, 245
    carotid endarterectomy, 245
    clopidogrel, 245
    primary versus secondary prevention, 245
    ticlopidine, 245
    warfarin prevention in atrial fibrillation patients,
        244
  prognosis by age, 358
  risk factors
    age, 242
    cardiac disease, 242
    cholesterol profile, 242
    clotting system abnormalities, 243
    drug abuse, 242
    hypertension, 242
    oral contraceptives, 243
    overview, 241–242, 243
    smoking, 242
  treatment
    intra-arterial thrombolysis, 244
    surgery, 245
    tissue plasminogen activator, 243
    vascular dementia, 216
Sturge-Weber syndrome, features, 355
Stuttering
  acquisition, 232
  characteristics, 232
  prevalence, 232
Subacute sclerosing panencephalitis,
      electroencephalography, 376–377
Subarachnoid hemorrhage (SAH)
  central nervous system complications, 248
  clinical profile, 246
  computed tomography, 246–247
  focal neurologic signs, 248
  grading, 247–248
  incidence, 245
  lesion locations, 246
  prognosis, 24
  risk factors, 246
  systemic complications, 248
  treatment
    medical management, 247
    ruptured aneurysm, 247
Subdural hematoma
  electroencephalography, 375
  vitamin deficiency risks, 311
Substantia nigra
  anatomy, 31
  Parkinson's disease effects, 31
Sudomotor axon reflex, mechanism, 199
Sumatriptan, migraine treatment, 275, 276
Superior gluteal nerve, anatomy, 20
Superior oblique palsy, head tilt, 32

Superior quadrantanopsia, lesions, 46
Suprascapular nerve, anatomy, 22
Sural nerve, biopsy, 86–87
Swallowing
    reflex, 233
    stages, 233
    vagus nerve role, 233
Sympathetic nervous system
    anatomy, 183–184
    neurotransmitters, 184–185
    stimulation, physiologic responses, 181
Sympathetically maintained pain (SMP)
    complex regional pain syndrome relationship, 265
    sympatholytic procedures, 265
Synapse
    chemical signal transmission, 3
    learning and memory, 4
    modification, 3
    vesicle protein types and functions, 3
Syncope, etiology, 197
Syphilis
    with AIDS, 341
    cerebrospinal fluid findings, 333
    diagnosis, 333
    neurologic manifestations, 334
Syringomyelia
    causes, 116
    clinical presentation, 116
    definition, 115
    primary versus secondary, 116
    treatment, 116
Systemic disease, neurologic complications, 309–327
Systemic lupus erythematosus (SLE)
    central nervous system effects, 320–321
    neurologic sequelae and survival, 321
    peripheral nervous system effects, 321

Tacrine, Alzheimer's disease treatment, 215
Tamoxifen, retinopathy induction, 260
Tapeworm. See Neurocystercosis
Tardive dyskinesia (TD)
    drug induction, 176
    pathogenesis, 176–177
    stereotypy, 176
    treatment, 177
Tau, Alzheimer's disease role, 214
Tay-Sachs disease, clinical features, 352
TCAs. See Tricyclic antidepressants
TD. See Tardive dyskinesia
Temporal arteritis
    clinical features, 281, 323
    complications, 281
    diagnosis, 281, 323, 335
    treatment, 281, 323
Temporal lobe, functions, 48
Tension headache
    causes, 279
    chronic, 279
    episodic, 279
    treatment, 279
Tetanus toxin, neurologic manifestations, 332

Tetraplegia, autonomic dysreflexia, 199
Tetrodotoxin
    neurologic manifestations, 333
    sources, 332
Thalamotomy, Parkinson's disease treatment, 158
Thalamus
    anatomy, 41–42
    aphasia, 224
    blood supply, 50
    Dejerine and Roussy syndrome, 267
    inputs, 42–43
    limbic lobe, 43
    nuclei, 42
    Papez's circuit, 43
    vision role, 45
Thiamine deficiency, brainstem effects, 132
Thoracic outlet syndrome (TOS), features, 24
Thrombocytopenia, neurologic complications, 316
Thrombotic thrombocytopenic purpura (TTP)
    chemotherapy induction, 260
    neurologic complications, 316
Thymoma
    diagnosis, 75
    with myasthenia gravis, 75
TIA. See Transient ischemic attack
Tiagabine, seizure management, 291, 292
Tibial nerve, anatomy, 21
Tic disorders. See also Tourette's syndrome
    classification of tics, 172
    clinical features of tics, 172
    clinical spectrum, 173
    etiologic classification, 172–173
Ticlopidine, stroke prevention, 245
Tissue plasminogen activator (t-PA), stroke
        management, 243
Tizanidine, pain management, 270
Tolcapone, Parkinson's disease treatment, 158
Topiramate
    migraine treatment, 276
    seizure management, 291, 292
TORCH infections, 347
Torsion dystonia, features, 166–167
TOS. See Thoracic outlet syndrome
Tourette's syndrome (TS)
    clinical spectrum, 173
    diagnosis, 173
    heredity, 173–174
    speech signs, 230
    treatment, 174
t-PA. See Tissue plasminogen activator
Tracé alternant, electroencephalography, 372
Tracé discontinu, electroencephalography, 371
Transient ischemic attack (TIA)
    brainstem
        causes, 128–129
        symptoms, 128
    historical perspective, 404
    myocardial infarction association, 309
Transverse myelitis
    causes, 115
    clinical features, 115

Transverse myelitis (cont.)
　management, 115
Trematol, toxicity, 416
Trichloroethylene, peripheral neuropathy induction,
　90
Tricyclic antidepressants (TCAs)
　migraine prophylaxis, 276
　pain management, 269
Trigeminal neuralgia
　clinical features, 267
　treatment, 267
Trigeminal nucleus, subdivisions, 32
Trigeminal sensory neuropathy, connective tissue
　disease relationship, 91
Trinucleotide repeats
　anticipation, 12
　diseases, 12
Trivia, **401–416**
Tropical spastic paraparesis, features, 118
TS. See Tourette's syndrome
TS. See Tuberous sclerosis
TTP. See Thrombotic thrombocytopenic purpura
Tuberculous meningitis, clinical presentation, 335
Tuberous sclerosis (TS), features, 354–355

Ulnar nerve entrapment
　causes, 393
　diagnosis, 393
　differential diagnosis, 394
　treatment, 393–394
Upper dorsal pontine syndrome, features, 127
Uremic encephalopathy, features, 313
Uremic neuropathy, features, 313

Vacor, peripheral neuropathy induction, 90
Valproic acid, migraine prophylaxis, 277
Varicella zoster virus
　lymphoma patient infection, 251
　neurologic complications, 338–339
Vascular disease, **237–248**
Vasculitides, neurologic complications, 322–324
Ventral midbrain syndrome, features, 128
Ventral nerve root, motor axons, 24
Ventral pontine syndrome, features, 127
Ventricles
　adult derivatives, 16
　formation, 15
Verapamil, migraine prophylaxis, 277
Vertigo
　benign positional vertigo, 133
　causes, 132
　central versus peripheral vertigo, 133
　definition, 132
　Ménière's disease, 133
　vestibular neuronitis, 133
Vestibular apparatus
　cold water injection response, 37
　nuclei output, 36, 37

Vestibular apparatus (cont.)
　receptors, 36
　spinal cord tracts, 36
　synapses, 36
Vestibular neuronitis, features, 133
Vestibulospinal tract, anatomy, 29
Vision, sensitivity limits, 401
Visual evoked potentials, multiple sclerosis, 203
Vitamin B6 deficiency, neurologic complications,
　310
Vitamin B12 deficiency
　neurologic complications, 310
　subacute combined degeneration of spinal cord,
　119
Vitamin D deficiency, neurologic complications,
　310–311
Vitamin E, Alzheimer's disease treatment, 215
Vocal cord, paralysis, 231
Vocal folds, musculature, 231
Vogt-Koyanagi-Harada syndrome, features, 336
von Hippel-Lindau syndrome, features, 255, 355
von Münchhausen, Karl, 412–413

Wada test
　handedness effects, 230
　protocol, 230
Wallerian degeneration, features, 83
Warfarin, stroke prevention in atrial fibrillation
　patients, 244
Weber's test, hearing assessment, 38
Wegener's granulomatosis, neurologic
　complications, 323
Wernicke's aphasia
　clinical features, 221
　lesions, 221
Wernicke's area
　electrical stimulation effects, 230
　language processing, 48
Wernicke's encephalopathy
　hypothermia with, 192
　thiamine deficiency, 132, 310
　triad of neurologic complaints, 310
West Nile encephalitis, features, 338
Whipple's disease
　etiology, 336
　neurologic complications, 310, 336
Wilson's disease
　causes, 179
　chorea, 175
　clinical features, 179, 312
　treatment, 180, 312
Wilson's disease, features, 353
Wilson, Woodrow, 414–415
Word deafness
　lesions, 221–222
　types, 221

Zellweger's syndrome, features, 353